# *Theoretical Basis for*
# *NURSING*

Melanie McEwen, PhD, RN
Associate Professor
University of Texas Health Science Center at Houston
School of Nursing
Houston, Texas

Evelyn M. Wills, PhD, RN
Professor
SLEMCO/BoRSF Regents Professor in Nursing
Department of Nursing
College of Nursing and Allied Health Professions
University of Louisiana at Lafayette
Lafayette, Louisiana

## EDITION

## 3

Wolters Kluwer | Lippincott Williams & Wilkins
Health
Philadelphia · Baltimore · New York · London
Buenos Aires · Hong Kong · Sydney · Tokyo

*Senior Acquisitions Editor:* Jean Rodenberger
*Product Manager:* Helen Kogut
*Director of Nursing Production:* Helen Ewan
*Art Director, Design:* Joan Wendt
*Art Director, Illustration:* Brett MacNaughton
*Manufacturing Coordinator:* Karin Duffield
*Vendor Manager:* Beth Martz
*Production Services:* MPS Limited, A Macmillan Company

9 8 7 6 5 4 3 2 1

Printed in China

**Library of Congress Cataloging-in-Publication Data**

McEwen, Melanie.
    Theoretical basis for nursing / Melanie McEwen, Evelyn M. Wills.—3rd ed.
        p. ; cm.
    Includes bibliographical references and indexes.
    ISBN 978-1-60547-323-9
    1. Nursing—Philosophy. 2. Nursing models. I. Wills, Evelyn M. II. Title.
    [DNLM: 1. Nursing Theory. WY 86 M4773t 2011]
    RT84.5.T36 2011
    610.73—dc22
                                                    2009033469

CCS1209

*To Kaitlin and Grant—You have helped me broaden my thoughts and consider all kinds of possibilities; I hope I've done the same for you.*
*Also for Helen and Keith—Our children chose well. Besides, you have given us Madelyn, Logan, Brenna, and Liam; they are gifts beyond words.*

*Melanie McEwen*


*To Tom, Paul, and Vicki, who light up my life, and to Marian, who is my applause. To Teddy, Gwen, Merlyn, and Madelyn who have been so patient and loving during this process.*
*A thousand thank yous to Peggy, who has supported me through this writing process.*

*Evelyn M. Wills*

**Grace M. Bielkiewicz, RN, PMHCNS-BC**
Assistant Professor (Retired)
Department of Nursing
Southern University
Baton Rouge, Louisiana

**Martha Kuhns, PhD, RN, CNS**
Clinical Nurse Specialist
Western Psychiatric Institute & Clinic
Pittsburgh, Pennsylvania

**Melinda Granger Oberleitner, RN, CNS, DNS, APRN**
Associate Dean
College of Nursing and Allied Health Professions
University of Louisiana at Lafayette
Lafayette, Louisiana

**Cynthia Ayres, PhD, RN**
Assistant Professor
Rutgers, The State University of New Jersey
Newark, NJ

**Patricia M. Burbank, DNSc, MS, RN**
Professor
University of Rhode Island
Kingston, RI

**Marcia D. Gragert, PhD, RN**
Associate Professor and Project Director,
    Gerontology NP/CNS Specialty
University of North Dakota
Grand Forks, ND

**Carol S. Humpherys, DNS,
    RN, CNA**
Clinical Assistant Professor and Director
University of Illinois at Chicago
Urbana, IL

**Rae Langford, EdD**
Associate Professor
Texas Woman's University
Houston, TX

**Joanne K. Olson, PhD, RN**
Professor and Associate Dean
University of Alberta
Edmonton, Alberta

**Hélène Sylvain, PhD**
Director, Nursing Department
Université du Québec è Rimouski
Rimouski, Québec

Many graduate nursing students respond with a cringing expression or a resounding "ugh!" when faced with the requirement of taking a course on theory. Indeed, many fail to see theory's relevance to the "real world" of nursing practice and often have difficulty applying the information in later courses and in their research. This book resulted from the frustration felt by a group of nursing instructors who met to adopt a textbook for a theory course. Indeed, because of student complaints and faculty dissatisfaction, we were changing textbooks yet again. A fairly lengthy discussion arose in which we concluded that the available books did not meet the needs of our students or course faculty. At the end of the discussion, it was determined that we would require three different books and recommend two others. Once again, students complained, and we concurred. To gather more data on theory courses and related information from a wider group of theory instructors, a nationwide survey was conducted. This survey corroborated the frustration felt by our small group of theory instructors, and gave us additional information to use in creating a new, and hopefully better, mousetrap.

As in past editions, an ongoing review of trends in nursing theory and nursing science has shown an increasing emphasis on middle range theory, evidence-based practice, and situation-specific theories. To remain current and timely, in this third edition, we have enhanced the discussion of those topics.

## ORGANIZATION OF THE TEXT

*Theoretical Basis for Nursing* is designed to be a basic nursing theory textbook that includes the essential information students need to understand and apply theory.

The book is divided into four units. **Unit I, Introduction to Theory,** provides the background needed to understand what theory is and how it is used in nursing. It outlines tools and techniques used to develop, analyze, and evaluate theory so that it can be used in nursing practice, research, administration and management, and education. In this unit, we have provided a balanced view of "hot" topics (e.g., philosophical world views and utilization of borrowed theory). Also, rather than espousing one strategy for activities such as concept development and theory evaluation, we have included a variety of strategies.

**Unit II, Nursing Theories,** focuses largely on the grand nursing theories, and begins with a chapter describing their historical development. This unit divides the grand nursing theories into three groups based on their focus (human needs, interactive process, and unitary process). The works of many of the grand theorists are briefly summarized in Chapters 7, 8, and 9. We acknowledge that these analyses are not comprehensive; rather, they are intended to provide the reader with enough information to understand the basis of the work and to whet the reader's appetite to select one or more for further study.

Chapters 10 and 11 cover the significant topic of middle range nursing theory. Chapter 10 presents a detailed overview of the origins and growth of middle range theory in nursing and gives numerous examples of how middle range theories have been developed by nurses. Chapter 11 provides an overview of some of the growing number of middle range nursing theories. The theories presented include some of the most commonly used middle range nursing theories (e.g., Pender's Health Promotion Model and Leininger's Culture Care Diversity Model) as well as some that are less well known but have a growing body of research support (e.g., the Theory of Unpleasant Symptoms, the Uncertainty in Illness Theory). The intent is to provide a broad range of middle range theories to familiarize the reader with examples and to encourage them to search for others appropriate to their practice or research. Ultimately, it is hoped that readers will be challenged to develop new theories that can be used by nurses.

**Unit III, Borrowed Theories Used by Nurses,** is rather unique in nursing literature. Our book acknowledges that "borrowed" or "shared" theories are essential to nursing and negates the idea that the use of borrowed theory in practice or research is detrimental. In this unit, we have identified some of the most significant theories that have been developed outside of the discipline of nursing but are continually used in nursing. We have organized these theories based on broad disciplines: theories from the sociologic sciences, behavioral sciences, and biomedical sciences, as well as from administration and management and learning. Each of these chapters was written by a nurse with both educational and practical experience in his or her respective area. These theories are presented with sufficient information to allow the reader to understand the theories and to recognize those that might be appropriate for her or his own work. These chapters also provide original references and give examples of how the concepts, theories, and models described have been used by other nurses.

Finally, **Unit IV, Application of Theory in Nursing Practice,** explains how theories are applied in nursing. Separate chapters cover nursing practice, nursing research, nursing administration and management, and nursing education. These chapters include many specific examples for the application of theory and are intended to be a practical guide for theory use. The heightened development of practice theories and evidence-based practice (EVP) guidelines are critical to theory application in nursing today so these areas have been expanded. The unit concludes with a chapter that discusses some of the future issues in theory within the discipline.

## KEY FEATURES

In addition to numerous tables and boxes that highlight and summarize important information, *Theoretical Basis for Nursing* contains case studies, learning activities, exemplars, Internet resources, and illustrations.

- **Case Studies:** At the end of Chapter 1 and the beginning of Chapters 2 to 21, case studies help the reader understand how the content in the chapter relates to the everyday experience of the nurse, whether in practice, research, or other aspects of nursing.
- **Learning Activities:** At the end of each chapter, learning activities pose critical thinking questions, propose individual and group projects related to topics covered in the chapter, and stimulate classroom discussion.
- **Exemplars:** In five chapters, an exemplar discusses a scholarly study from the perspectives of concept analysis (Chapter 3); theory development (Chapter 4); theory analysis and evaluation (Chapter 5); middle range theory development (Chapter 10); and theory generation via research, theory testing via research, and use of a theory as the conceptual framework for a research study (Chapter 18).
- **Internet Resources:** Because of the importance of the Internet as a resource, whenever appropriate we have included web addresses that will direct the reader to sites that contain additional information about the topic at hand.
- **Illustrations:** Diagrams and models are included throughout the book to help the reader better understand the many different theories presented.

## NEW TO THIS EDITION

- Expanded discussions of situation-specific theories
- More detailed explanation of EVP and its relationship to theory in nursing
- Numerous recent examples of application of theories in nursing practice, nursing research, leadership/administration, and education
- NEW instructional support

Visit thePoint at **http://thePoint.lww.com** to learn about a variety of resources that are available for students and instructors.

In summary, the focus of this book is on the application of theory rather than on the study, analysis, and critique of grand theorists or a presentation of a specific aspect of theory (e.g., construction or evaluation). It is hoped that practicing nurses, nurse researchers, and nursing scholars, as well as graduate students and theory instructors, will use this book to gain a better understanding and appreciation of theory.

*Melanie McEwen, PhD, RN*
*Evelyn Wills, PhD, RN*

# Acknowledgments

**Our heartfelt** thanks to Product Manager Helen Kogut for her assistance, patience, and persistence in helping us complete this project. She has made a difficult task seem easy! We also want to thank Senior Acquisitions Editor Jean Rodenberger for her continued support and assistance with this edition. Finally, a huge word of thanks to our contributors who have diligently worked to present the notion of "theory" in a manner that will engage graduate nursing students, and to look for new examples and applications to help make theory fresh and relevant.

# Contents

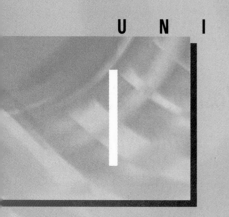

*Introduction to Theory*

# 1

# Philosophy, Science, and Nursing

## Melanie McEwen

*L*argely due to the work of nursing scientists, nursing theorists, and nursing scholars over
*the past five decades, nursing has been recognized as both an emerging profession and
an academic discipline. Crucial to the attainment of this distinction have been
numerous discussions regarding the phenomena of concern to nurses and countless efforts to
enhance involvement in theory utilization, theory generation, and theory testing to direct
research and improve practice.*

*A review of the nursing literature from the late 1970s until the present shows sporadic
discussion of whether nursing is a profession, a science, or an academic discipline. These
discussions are sometimes pleading, frequently esoteric, and occasionally confusing. Questions
that have been raised include: What defines a profession? What constitutes an academic
discipline? What is nursing science? Why is it important for nursing to be seen as a profession
or an academic discipline?*

## Nursing as a Profession

In the past, there has been considerable discussion about whether nursing is a profession or an occupation. This is important for nurses to consider for several reasons. An occupation is a job or a career, whereas a profession is a learned vocation or occupation that has a status of superiority and precedence within a division of work. In general terms, occupations require widely varying levels of training or education, varying levels of skill, and widely variable defined knowledge bases. Indeed, all professions are occupations, but not all occupations are professions (Logan, Franzen, Pauling, & Butcher, 2004; Schwirian, 1998).

Professions are valued by society because the services professionals provide are beneficial for members of the society. Characteristics of a profession include (1) a defined knowledge base, (2) power and authority over training and education, (3) registration, (4) altruistic service, (5) a code of ethics, (6) lengthy socialization, and (7) autonomy (Rutty, 1998). A profession must also have an institutionalized goal or social mission as well as a group of scholars, investigators, or researchers who work to continually advance the knowledge of the profession with the goal of improving practice (Schlotfeldt, 1989). In addition, professionals are responsible and accountable to the public for their work (Northrup et al., 2004). Traditionally, professions have included the clergy, law, and medicine.

Until recently, nursing was viewed as an occupation rather than a profession. Nursing has had difficulty being deemed a profession because the services provided by nurses have been perceived as an extension of those offered by wives and mothers. Additionally, historically nursing has been seen as subservient to medicine, and nurses have delayed in identifying and organizing professional knowledge. Furthermore, the education for nurses is not yet standardized, and the three-tier entry-level system into practice that persists (diploma, associate degree, and bachelor's degree) may have hindered professionalization. Finally, autonomy in practice is incomplete because nursing is still dependent on medicine to direct much of its practice.

On the other hand, many of the characteristics of a profession can be observed in nursing. Indeed, nursing has a social mandate to provide health care for clients at different points in the health–illness continuum. There is a growing knowledge base, authority over education, altruistic service, a code of ethics, and registration requirements for practice. Although the debate is ongoing, it can be successfully argued that nursing is an aspiring, evolving profession (Logan et al., 2004; Rutty, 1998; Smith, 2000; Wolf, 2006).

## Nursing as an Academic Discipline

Disciplines are distinctions between bodies of knowledge found in academic settings. A *discipline* is "a branch of knowledge ordered through the theories and methods evolving from more than one worldview of the phenomenon of concern" (Parse, 1997, p. 74). It has also been termed a field of inquiry characterized by a unique perspective and a distinct way of viewing phenomena (Holzemer, 2007; Parse, 1999).

Viewed another way, a discipline is a branch of educational instruction or a department of learning or knowledge. Institutions of higher education are organized around disciplines into colleges, schools, and departments (e.g., business administration, chemistry, history, and engineering).

Disciplines are organized by structure and tradition. The structure of the discipline provides organization and determines the amount, relationship, and ratio of each type of knowledge that comprises the discipline. The tradition of the discipline provides the content, which includes ethical, personal, esthetic, and scientific knowledge (Northrup et al., 2004; Riegel et al., 1992). Characteristics of disciplines include (1) a distinct perspective and syntax, (2) determination of what phenomena are of interest, (3) determination of the context in which the phenomena are viewed, (4) determination of what questions to ask, (5) determination of what methods of study are used, and (6) determination of what evidence is proof (Donaldson & Crowley, 1978).

Knowledge development within a discipline proceeds from several philosophical and scientific perspectives or worldviews (Newman, Sime, & Corcoran-Perry, 1991; Parse, 1997, 1999). These worldviews may serve to divide or segregate members of a discipline. For example, in psychology practitioners might consider themselves behaviorists, Freudians, or any one of a number of other divisions.

Several ways of classifying academic disciplines have been proposed. For instance, they may be divided into the basic sciences (physics, biology, chemistry, sociology, anthropology) and the humanities (philosophy, ethics, history, fine arts). In this classification scheme, it is arguable that nursing has characteristics of both.

Distinctions may also be made between academic disciplines (e.g., physics, physiology, sociology, mathematics, history, philosophy) and professional disciplines (e.g., medicine, law, nursing, social work). In this classification scheme, the academic disciplines aim to "know," and their theories are descriptive in nature. Research in academic disciplines is both basic and applied. Conversely, the professional disciplines are practical in nature, and their research tends to be more prescriptive and descriptive (Donaldson & Crowley, 1978).

Nursing's knowledge base draws from many disciplines. In the past, nursing has depended heavily on physiology, sociology, psychology, and medicine to provide academic standing and to inform practice. In recent years, however, nursing has been seeking what is unique to nursing and developing those aspects into an academic discipline. Areas that identify nursing as a distinct discipline are as follows:

- An identifiable philosophy.
- At least one conceptual framework (perspective) for delineation of what can be defined as nursing.
- Acceptable methodologic approaches for the pursuit and development of knowledge (Oldnall, 1995).

To begin the quest to validate nursing as both a profession and an academic discipline, this chapter provides an overview of the concepts of science and philosophy. It examines the schools of philosophical thought that have influenced nursing and explores the epistemology of nursing to explain why recognizing the multiple "ways of knowing" is an important concept in the quest for development and application of theory in nursing. Finally, the chapter presents issues related to how philosophical worldviews affect knowledge development through research. The chapter concludes with a case study that depicts how "the ways of knowing" in nursing are used on a day-to-day, even moment-by-moment, basis by all practicing nurses.

## Introduction to Science and Philosophy

*Science* is concerned with causality (cause and effect). The scientific approach to understanding reality is characterized by observation, verifiability, and experience; hypothesis testing and experimentation are considered scientific methods. In contrast, *philosophy* is concerned with the purpose of human life, the nature of being and reality, and the theory and limits of knowledge. Intuition, introspection, and reasoning are examples of philosophical methodologies. Science and philosophy share the common goal of increasing knowledge (Fawcett, 1999; Silva, 1977). The science of any discipline is tied to its philosophy, which provides the basis for understanding and developing theories for science (Gustafsson, 2002; Silva & Rothbert, 1984).

### OVERVIEW OF SCIENCE

Science is both a process and a product. Parse (1997) defines science as the "theoretical explanation of the subject of inquiry and the methodological process of sustaining knowledge in a discipline" (p. 74). Science has also been described as a way of explaining observed phenomena as well as a system of gathering, verifying, and systematizing information about reality (Streubert-Speziale & Carpenter, 2006). As a process, science is characterized by systematic inquiry that relies heavily on empirical

---

**BOX 1-1**  *Characteristics of Science*

1. Science must show a certain coherence.
2. Science is concerned with definite fields of knowledge.
3. Science is preferably expressed in universal statements.
4. The statements of science must be true or probably true.
5. The statements of science must be logically ordered.
6. Science must explain its investigations and arguments.

Source: Silva (1977).

---

observations of the natural world. As a product, it has been defined as empirical knowledge that is grounded and tested in experience and is the result of investigative efforts (Johnson, 1991). Furthermore, science is conceived as being the consensual, informed opinion about the natural world, including human behavior and social action (Gortner & Schultz, 1988).

Science has come to represent knowledge, and it is generated by the application of a variety of procedures or methods to acquire that knowledge. Citing Van Laer, Silva (1977) lists six characteristics of science (Box 1-1).

Science has been classified in several ways. These include pure or basic science, natural science, human or social science, and applied or practice science. The classifications are not mutually exclusive and are open to interpretation based on philosophical orientation. Table 1-1 lists examples of a number of sciences by this manner of classification.

Some sciences defy classification. For example, computer science is arguably applied or perhaps pure. Law is certainly a practice science, but it is also a social science. Psychology might be a basic science, a human science, or an applied science, depending on what aspect of psychology one is referring to.

There are significant differences between the human and natural sciences. Human sciences refer to the fields of psychology, anthropology, and sociology and may even extend to economics and political science. These disciplines deal with various aspects of humans and human interactions. Natural sciences, on the other hand, are concentrated on elements found in nature that do not relate to the totality of the individual. There are inherent differences between the human and natural sciences that make the research techniques of the natural sciences (i.e., laboratory experimentation) improper or potentially problematic for human sciences (Gortner & Schultz, 1988).

It has been posited that although nursing draws on the basic and pure sciences (e.g., physiology and chemistry) and has many characteristics of social sciences, it is an applied or practice science. However, it is important to note that it is also synthesized,

TABLE 1-1 *Classifications of Science*

| Natural sciences | Chemistry, physics, biology, physiology, geology, meteorology |
|---|---|
| Basic or pure sciences | Mathematics, logic, chemistry, physics, English (language) |
| Human or social sciences | Psychology, anthropology, sociology, economics, political science, history, religion |
| Practice or applied sciences | Architecture, engineering, medicine, pharmacology, law |

in that it draws on the knowledge of other established disciplines—including other practice disciplines (Holzemer, 2007; Oldnall, 1995).

## OVERVIEW OF PHILOSOPHY

Within any discipline, both scholars and students should be aware of the philosophical orientations that are the basis for developing theory and advancing knowledge (DiBartolo, 1998; Northrup et al., 2004). Rather than a focus on solving problems or answering questions related to that discipline (which are tasks of the discipline's science), the philosophy of a discipline studies the concepts that structure the thought processes of that discipline with the intent of recognizing and revealing foundations and presuppositions (Blackburn, 2005; Cronin & Rawlings-Anderson, 2004).

Philosophy has been defined as "a study of problems that are ultimate, abstract, and general. These problems are concerned with the nature of existence, knowledge, morality, reason, and human purpose" (Teichman & Evans, 1999, p. 1). Philosophy tries to discover knowledge and truth, and attempts to identify what is valuable and important.

Modern philosophy is usually traced to Rene Descartes, Francis Bacon, Baruch Spinoza, and Immanuel Kant (circa 1600–1800). Descartes (1596–1650) and Spinoza (1632–1677) were early rationalists. Rationalists believe that reason is superior to experience as a source of knowledge. Rationalists attempt to determine the nature of the world and reality by deduction and stress the importance of mathematical procedures.

Bacon (1561–1626) was an early empiricist. Like rationalists, he supported experimentation and scientific methods for solving problems.

The work of Kant (1724–1804) set the foundation for many later developments in philosophy. Kant believed that knowledge is relative and that the mind plays an active role in knowing. Other philosophers have also influenced nursing and the advance of nursing science. Several are discussed later in the chapter.

Although there is some variation, traditionally the branches of philosophy include metaphysics (ontology and cosmology), epistemology, logic, esthetics, and ethics or axiology. Political philosophy and philosophy of science are added by some authors (Rutty, 1998; Teichman & Evans, 1999). Table 1-2 summarizes the major branches of philosophy.

TABLE 1-2 *Branches of Philosophy*

| Metaphysics | Study of the fundamental nature of reality and existence—general theory of reality |
|---|---|
| Ontology | Study of theory of being (what is or what exists) |
| Cosmology | Study of the physical universe |
| Epistemology | Study of knowledge (ways of knowing, nature of truth, and relationship between knowledge and belief) |
| Logic | Study of principles and methods of reasoning (inference and argument) |
| Ethics (axiology) | Study of nature of values; right and wrong (moral philosophy) |
| Esthetics | Study of appreciation of the arts or things beautiful |
| Philosophy of science | Study of science and scientific practice |
| Political philosophy | Study of citizen and state |

Sources: Blackburn (2005); Teichman and Evans (1999).

## Science and Philosophical Schools of Thought

The concept of science as understood in the 21st century is relatively new. In the period of modern science, three philosophies of science dominate: rationalism, empiricism, and human science/phenomenology. Rationalism and empiricism are often termed *received view* and human science/phenomenology and related worldviews (i.e., historicism) are considered *perceived view* (Hickman, 2002; Meleis, 2005; Moody, 1990).

### RECEIVED VIEW (EMPIRICISM, POSITIVISM, LOGICAL POSITIVISM)

*Empiricism* has its roots in the writings of Francis Bacon, John Locke, and David Hume, who valued observation, perception by senses, and experience as sources of knowledge (Gortner & Schultz, 1988). Empiricism is founded on the belief that what is experienced is what exists, and its knowledge base requires that these experiences be verified through scientific methodology (Gustafsson, 2002; Wainwright, 1997). This knowledge is then passed on to others in the discipline and subsequently built on. The term *received view* or *received knowledge* denotes that individuals learn by being told or receiving knowledge.

Empiricism holds that truth corresponds to observable, reduction, verification, control, and bias-free science. It emphasizes mathematic formulas to explain phenomena and prefers simple dichotomies and classification of concepts. Additionally, everything can be reduced to a scientific formula with little room for interpretation (DiBartolo, 1998; Gortner & Schultz, 1988).

Empiricism focuses on understanding the parts of the whole in an attempt to understand the whole. It strives to explain nature through testing of hypotheses and development of theories. Theories are made to describe, explain, and predict phenomena in nature and to provide understanding of relationships between phenomena. Concepts must be operationalized in the form of propositional statements, thereby making measurement possible. Instrumentation, reliability, and validity are stressed in empirical research methodologies. Once measurement is determined, it is possible to test theories through experimentation or observation, which results in verification or falsification (Cull-Wilby & Pepin, 1987; Suppe & Jacox, 1985).

*Positivism* is often equated with empiricism. Like empiricism, positivism supports mechanistic, reductionist principles, where the complex can be best understood in terms of its basic components (Gortner, 1993). *Logical positivism* was the dominant empirical philosophy of science between the 1880s and 1950s. Logical positivists recognized only the logical and empirical bases of science and stressed that there is no room for metaphysics, understanding, or meaning within the realm of science (Polifroni & Welch, 1999). Logical positivism maintained that science is value free, independent of the scientist, and obtained using objective methods. The goal of science is to explain, predict, and control. Theories are either true or false, subject to empirical observation, and capable of being reduced to existing scientific theories (Riegel et al., 1992; Rutty, 1998).

#### Contemporary Empiricism/Postpositivism

Positivism came under criticism in the 1960s when positivistic logic was deemed faulty (Rutty, 1998). An overreliance on strictly controlled experimentation in artificial settings produced results that indicated that much significant knowledge or information was missed. In recent years, scholars have determined that the positivist view of science is outdated and misleading in that it contributes to overfragmentation in knowledge and theory development (DiBartolo, 1998). It has been observed that positivistic analysis of theories is fundamentally defective due to insistence on analyzing the logically ideal, which results in findings that have little to do with actual science and reality. It was maintained that the context of discovery was artificial and that theories and explanations can be understood only within their discovery contexts (Suppe & Jacox, 1985). Also, scientific inquiry is inherently value-laden, as even choosing what to investigate and/or what techniques to employ will reflect the values of the researcher.

The current generation of postpositivists accept the subjective nature of inquiry, but still support rigor and objective study through quantitative research methods. Indeed, it has been observed that modern empiricists or postpositivists are concerned with explanation and prediction of complex phenomena, recognizing contextual variables (Powers & Knapp, 2006; Reed, 2008).

### Nursing and Empiricism

As a new and emerging discipline, nursing followed established disciplines (i.e., physiology) and the medical model in stressing logical positivism. Early nurse scientists embraced the importance of objectivity, control, fact, and measurement of smaller and smaller parts. Based on this influence, acceptable methods for knowledge generation in nursing have stressed traditional, orthodox, and preferably experimental methods.

Positivism continues to heavily influence nursing science (Riegel et al., 1992). This viewpoint has been challenged in recent years, however. As DiBartolo (1998) stated, "the majority of nursing scholars now concur that the received view is fundamentally incompatible with the discipline's complex philosophical commitment to holism and the humanistic approach, therefore it has been essentially discarded as a basis for the science of nursing" (p. 353). Consequently, postpositivism has become a more contemporary worldview in nursing.

## PERCEIVED VIEW (HUMAN SCIENCE, PHENOMENOLOGY, CONSTRUCTIVISM, HISTORICISM)

In the late 1960s and early 1970s, several philosophers including Kuhn, Feyerbend, and Toulmin challenged the positivist view by arguing that the influence of history on science should be emphasized. The perceived view of science, which may also be referred to as the interpretive view, includes phenomenology, constructivism, and historicism. The interpretive view focuses on the perceptions of both the subject being studied and the researcher and tends to de-emphasize reliance on strict control and experimentation in laboratory settings (Monti & Tingen, 1999).

The perceived view of science centers on descriptions that are derived from collectively lived experiences, interrelatedness, human interpretation, and learned reality, as opposed to artificially invented reality (Rutty, 1998). It is argued that the pursuit of knowledge and truth is naturally historical, contextual, and value-laden. Thus, there is no single truth. Rather, knowledge is deemed true if it withstands practical tests of utility and reason (DiBartolo, 1998).

*Phenomenology* is the study of phenomena and emphasizes the appearance of things as opposed to the things themselves. In phenomenology, understanding is the goal of science, with the objective of recognizing the connection between one's experience, values, and perspective. It maintains that each individual's experience is unique, and there are many interpretations of reality (Gortner & Schultz, 1988; Monti & Tingen, 1999; Polifroni & Welch, 1999). Inquiry begins with individuals and their experiences with phenomena. Perceptions, feelings, values, and the meanings that have come to be attached to things and events are the focus.

For social scientists, the *constructivist* approaches of the perceived view focus on understanding the actions and meaning of individuals. What exists depends on what

TABLE 1-3 *Comparison of the Received and Perceived Views of Science*

| Received View of Science—Hard Sciences | Perceived View of Science—Soft Sciences |
|---|---|
| Empiricism/positivism/logical positivism | Historicism/phenomenology |
| Reality/truth/facts considered acontextual | Reality/truth/facts considered in context |
| Reality/truth/facts considered ahistorical | Reality/truth/facts considered with regard to history |
| Objective | Subjective |
| Deductive | Inductive |
| Prediction and control | Description and understanding |
| One truth | Multiple truths |
| Validation and replication | Trends and patterns |
| Reductionism | Constructivism |
| Quantitative research methods | Qualitative research methods |

Sources: Meleis (2005); Moody (1990).

individuals perceive to exist. Knowledge is subjective and created by individuals. Thus, research methodology entails the investigation of the individual's world (Wainwright, 1997). There is an emphasis on subjectivity, multiple truths, trends and patterns, discovery, description, and understanding.

Feminism and critical social theory are also considered to be perceived view. These philosophical schools of thought recognize the influence of gender, culture, society, and shared history as being essential components of science (Riegel et al., 1992). Critical social theorists contend that reality is dynamic and shaped by social, political, cultural, economic, ethnic, and gender values (Streubert-Speziale & Carpenter, 2006). This was graphically illustrated by the dramatic differences in perspective or world-views which led to the September 11, 2001 terrorist attacks. Critical social theory and feminist theories will be described in more detail in Chapter 12.

### Nursing and Phenomenology

Because they examine phenomena within context, phenomenology as well as other perceived view of philosophies are conducive to discovery and knowledge development inherent to nursing. Phenomenology is open, variable, and relativistic and based on human experience and personal interpretations. As such, it is a guiding paradigm for nursing practice theory and education (DiBartolo, 1998).

In nursing science, the dichotomy of philosophic thought between the received, empirical view of science and the perceived, interpretative view of science has persisted. This may have resulted, in part, because nursing draws heavily from both natural sciences (physiology, biology) and social sciences (psychology, sociology). Table 1-3 compares the two dominant philosophical views of science in nursing.

## Nursing Philosophy, Nursing Science, and Philosophy of Science in Nursing

The terms *nursing philosophy*, *nursing science*, and *philosophy of science* in nursing are sometimes used interchangeably. The differences, however, in the general meaning of these concepts are important to recognize.

## NURSING PHILOSOPHY

Nursing philosophy has been described as "a statement of foundational and universal assumptions, beliefs and principles about the nature of knowledge and thought (epistemology) and about the nature of the entities represented in the metaparadigm (i.e., nursing practice and human health processes [ontology])" (Reed, 1995, p. 76). Nursing philosophy, then, refers to the belief system of the profession and provides perspectives for practice, scholarship, and research (Gortner, 1990).

No single dominant philosophy has prevailed in the discipline of nursing. Many nursing scholars and nursing theorists have written extensively in an attempt to identify the overriding belief system, but to date, none have been universally successful.

## NURSING SCIENCE

Barrett (2002) defined nursing science as "the substantive, discipline-specific knowledge that focuses on the human-universe-health process articulated in the nursing frameworks and theories" (p. 57). In general, nursing science refers to the system of relationships of human responses in health and illness addressing biologic, behavioral, social, and cultural domains (Gortner & Schultz, 1988). The goal of nursing science is to represent the nature of nursing—to understand it, to explain it, and to use it for the benefit of humankind. It is nursing science that gives direction to the future generation of substantive nursing knowledge, and it is nursing science that provides the knowledge for all aspects of nursing (Barrett, 2002; Holzemer, 2007).

## PHILOSOPHY OF SCIENCE IN NURSING

Philosophy of science in nursing helps to establish the meaning of science through an understanding and examination of nursing concepts, theories, laws, and aims as they relate to nursing practice. It seeks to understand truth; to describe nursing; to examine prediction and causality; to critically relate theories, models, and scientific systems; and to explore determinism and free will (Nyatanga, 2005; Polifroni & Welch, 1999).

## Knowledge Development and Nursing Science

Development of nursing knowledge reflects the interface between nursing science and research. The ultimate purpose of knowledge development is to improve nursing practice. Approaches to knowledge development have three facets: ontology, epistemology, and methodology. Ontology refers to the study of being: what is or what exists. Epistemology refers to the study of knowledge or ways of knowing. Methodology is the means of acquiring knowledge (Powers & Knapp, 2006). The following sections discuss nursing epistemology and issues related to methods of acquiring knowledge.

## EPISTEMOLOGY

*Epistemology* is the study of the theory of knowledge. Epistemologic questions include: What do we know? What is the extent of our knowledge? How do we decide whether we know? and What are the criteria of knowledge? (Schultz & Meleis, 1988).

According to Streubert-Speziale and Carpenter (2006), it is important to understand the way in which nursing knowledge develops to provide a context in which to judge the appropriateness of nursing knowledge and methods that nurses use to develop that knowledge. This in turn will refocus methods for gaining knowledge as well as establishing the legitimacy or quality of the knowledge gained.

## Ways of Knowing

In epistemology, there are several basic types of knowledge. These include the following:

- Empirics—the scientific form of knowing. Empirical knowledge comes from observation, testing, and replication.
- Personal knowledge—a priori knowledge. Personal knowledge pertains to knowledge gained from thought alone.
- Intuitive knowledge—includes feelings and hunches. Intuitive knowledge is not guessing, but relies on nonconscious pattern recognition and experience.
- Somatic knowledge—knowing of the body in relation to physical movement. Somatic knowledge includes experiential use of muscles and balance to perform a physical task.
- Metaphysical (spiritual) knowledge—seeking the presence of a higher power. Aspects of spiritual knowing include magic, miracles, psychokinesis, extrasensory perception, and near-death experiences.
- Esthetics—knowledge related to beauty, harmony, and expression. Esthetic knowledge incorporates art, creativity, and values.
- Moral or ethical knowledge—knowledge of what is right and wrong. Values and social and cultural norms of behavior are components of ethical knowledge.

## Nursing Epistemology

Nursing epistemology has been defined as "the study of the origins of nursing knowledge, its structure and methods, the patterns of knowing of its members, and the criteria for validating its knowledge claims" (Schultz & Meleis, 1988, p. 21). Like most disciplines, nursing has both scientific knowledge and knowledge that can be termed conventional wisdom (knowledge that has not been empirically tested).

Traditionally, only what stands the test of repeated measures constitutes truth or knowledge. Classical scientific processes (i.e., experimentation), however, are not suitable for creating and describing all types of knowledge. Social sciences, behavioral sciences, and the arts rely on other methods to establish knowledge. Because it has characteristics of social and behavioral sciences, as well as biologic sciences, nursing must rely on multiple ways of knowing.

In a classic work, Carper (1978) identified four fundamental patterns for nursing knowledge: (1) empirics—the science of nursing, (2) esthetics—the art of nursing, (3) personal knowledge in nursing, and (4) ethics—moral knowledge in nursing.

*Empirical knowledge* is objective, abstract, generally quantifiable, exemplary, discursively formulated, and verifiable. When verified through repeated testing over time, it is formulated into scientific generalizations, laws, theories, and principles that explain and predict (Carper, 1978, 1992). It draws on traditional ideas that can be verified through observation and proved by hypothesis testing.

Empirical knowledge tends to be the most emphasized way of knowing in nursing, because there is a need to know how knowledge can be organized into laws and theories for the purpose of describing, explaining, and predicting phenomena of concern to nurses. Most theory development and research efforts are engaged in seeking and generating explanations that are systematic and controllable by factual evidence (Carper, 1978, 1992).

*Esthetic knowledge* is expressive, subjective, unique, and experiential rather than formal or descriptive. Esthetics includes sensing the meaning of a moment. It is evident through actions, conduct, attitudes, and interactions of the nurse in response to another. It is not expressed in language (Carper, 1978).

Esthetic knowledge relies on perception. It is creative and incorporates empathy and understanding. It is interpretive, contextual, intuitive, and subjective and requires synthesis rather than analysis. Furthermore, esthetics goes beyond what is explained by principles and creates values and meaning to account for variables that cannot be quantitatively formulated (Carper, 1978, 1992).

*Personal knowledge* refers to the way in which nurses view themselves and the client. Personal knowledge is subjective and promotes wholeness and integrity in personal encounters. Engagement, rather than detachment, is a component of personal knowledge.

Personal knowledge incorporates experience, knowing, encountering, and actualizing the self within the practice. Personal maturity and freedom are components of personal knowledge, which may include spiritual and metaphysical forms of knowing. Because personal knowledge is difficult to express linguistically, it is largely expressed in personality (Carper, 1978, 1992).

*Ethics* refers to the moral code for nursing and is based on obligation to service and respect for human life. Ethical knowledge occurs as moral dilemmas arise in situations of ambiguity and uncertainty, and when consequences are difficult to predict. Ethical knowledge requires rational and deliberate examination and evaluation of what is good, valuable, and desirable as goals, motives, or characteristics (Carper, 1978, 1992). Ethics must address conflicting norms, interests, and principles and provide insight into areas that cannot be tested.

Fawcett, Watson, Neuman, Walkers, and Fitzpatrick (2001) stress that integration of all patterns of knowing are essential for professional nursing practice and that no one pattern should be used in isolation from others. Indeed, they are interrelated and interdependent because there are multiple points of contact between and among them (Carper, 1992). Thus, nurses should view nursing practice from a broadened perspective that places value on ways of knowing beyond the empirical (Silva, Sorrell, & Sorrell, 1995). Table 1-4 summarizes selected characteristics of Carper's patterns of knowing in nursing.

### Other Views of Patterns of Knowledge in Nursing

Although Carper's work is considered classic, it is not without critics. Schultz and Meleis (1988) observed that Carper's work did not incorporate practical knowledge into the ways of knowing in nursing. Because of this and other concerns, they described three patterns of knowledge in nursing: clinical, conceptual, and empirical.

*Clinical knowledge* refers to the individual nurse's personal knowledge. It results from using multiple ways of knowing while solving problems during client care provision. Clinical knowledge is manifested in the acts of practicing nurses and results from combining personal knowledge and empirical knowledge. It may also involve intuitive and subjective knowing. Clinical knowledge is communicated retrospectively through publication in journals (Schultz & Meleis, 1988).

*Conceptual knowledge* is abstracted and generalized beyond personal experience. It explicates patterns revealed in multiple client experiences, which occur in multiple situations, and articulates them as models or theories. In conceptual knowledge, concepts are drafted and relational statements are formulated. Propositional statements are supported by empirical or anecdotal evidence or defended by logical reasoning.

Conceptual knowledge uses knowledge from nursing and other disciplines. It incorporates curiosity, imagination, persistence, and commitment in the accumulation of

TABLE 1-4 *Characteristics of Carper's Patterns of Knowing in Nursing*

| Pattern of Knowing | Relationship to Nursing | Source or Creation | Source of Validation | Method of Expression | Purpose or Outcome |
|---|---|---|---|---|---|
| Empirics | Science of nursing | Direct or indirect observation and measurement | Replication | Facts, models, scientific principles, laws, statements, theories, descriptions | Description, explanation, and prediction |
| Esthetics | Art of nursing | Creation of value and meaning, synthesis of abstract and concrete | Appreciation; experience; inspiration; perception of balance, rhythm, proportion, and unity | Appreciation; empathy; esthetic criticism; engaging, intuiting, and envisioning | Move beyond what can be explained, quantitatively formulated, understanding, balance |
| Personal knowledge | Therapeutic use of self | Engagement, opening, centering, actualizing self | Response, reflection, experience | Empathy, active participation | Therapeutic use of self |
| Ethics | Moral component of nursing | Values clarification, rational and deliberate reasoning, obligation, advocating | Dialogue, justification, universal generalizability | Principles, codes, ethical theories | Evaluation of what is good, valuable, and desirable |

Sources: Carper (1978); Carper (1992); Chinn and Kramer (2008).

facts and reliable generalizations that pertain to the discipline of nursing. Conceptual knowledge is communicated in propositional statements (Schultz & Meleis, 1988).

*Empirical knowledge* results from experimental, historical, or phenomenological research and is used to justify actions and procedures in practice. The credibility of empirical knowledge rests on the degree to which the researcher has followed procedures accepted by the community of researchers, and on the logical, unbiased derivation of conclusions from the evidence. Empirical knowledge is evaluated through systematic review and critique of published research and conference presentations (Schultz & Meleis, 1988).

Chinn and Kramer (2008) also expanded on Carper's patterns of knowing to include "emancipatory knowing"—what they designate as the "praxis of nursing." In their view, emancipatory knowing refers to human's ability to critically examine the current status quo and to determine why it currently exists. This, in turn, supports identification of inequities in social and political institutions and clarification of cultural values and beliefs to improve conditions for all. In this view, emancipatory knowledge is expressed in actions that are directed toward changing existing social structures and establishing practices that are more equitable and favorable to human health and well-being.

In another work, Moch (1990) identified these patterns: experiential knowing (becoming aware of participation or being in the world), interpersonal knowing (an increased awareness that occurs through intense interaction with others), and intuitive knowing (the immediate knowing of something that does not appear to involve conscious reasoning).

Finally, following an in-depth examination of Carper's work, White (1995) added the element of "context" or the sociopolitical environment of the persons (both the nurse and the patient) and their interaction. She focused her observations of the need to recognize the situation in which the interaction takes place.

### Summary of Ways of Knowing in Nursing

For decades, the importance of the multiple ways of knowing has been recognized in the discipline of nursing. If nursing is to achieve a true integration between theory, research, and practice, theory development and research must integrate different sources of knowledge. Kidd and Morrison (1988) state that in nursing, synthesis of theories derived from different sources of knowledge will

1. Encourage the use of different types of knowledge in practice, education, theory development and research
2. Encourage the use of different methodologies in practice and research
3. Make nursing education more relevant for nurses with different educational backgrounds
4. Accommodate nurses at different levels of clinical competence
5. Ultimately promote high-quality client care and client satisfaction

## Research Methodology and Nursing Science

Being heavily influenced by logical empiricism, as nursing began developing as a scientific discipline in the mid-1900s, quantitative methods were used almost exclusively in research. In the 1960s and 1970s, schools of nursing aligned nursing inquiry with scientific inquiry in a desire to bring respect to the academic environment, and nurse researchers and nurse educators valued quantitative research methods over other forms.

A debate over methodology began in the 1980s, however, when some nurse scholars asserted that nursing's ontology (what nursing is) was not being adequately and sufficiently explored using quantitative methods in isolation. Subsequently, qualitative research methods began to be put into use. The assumptions were that qualitative methods showed the phenomena of nursing in ways that were naturalistic and unstructured and not misrepresented (Holzemer, 2007; Rutty, 1998).

The manner in which nursing science is conceptualized determines the priorities for nursing research and provides measures for determining the relevance of various scientific research questions. Therefore, the way in which nursing science is conceptualized also has implications for nursing practice. The philosophical issues regarding methods of research relate back to the debate over the worldviews of received versus perceived views of science, and whether nursing is a practice or applied science, a human science, or some combination as described previously. The notion of evidence-based practice has emerged in over the last few years, largely in response to these and related concerns. Evidence-based practice will be described in Chapter 17.

### NURSING AS A PRACTICE SCIENCE

In early years, the debate focused on whether nursing was a basic science or an applied science. The goal of basic science is the attainment of knowledge. In basic research, the investigator is interested in understanding the problem and produces knowledge for knowledge's sake. It is analytical and the ultimate function is to analyze a conclusion backward to its proper principles (Johnson, 1991).

Conversely, an applied science is one that uses the knowledge of basic sciences for some practical end. Engineering, architecture, and pharmacology are examples. In applied research, the investigator works toward solving problems and producing solutions for the problem. In practice sciences, research is largely clinical and action oriented (Moody, 1990). Thus, as an applied or practical science, nursing requires research that is applied and clinical (Fawcett, 1999).

## NURSING AS A HUMAN SCIENCE

The term *human science* is traced to philosopher Wilhelm Dilthey (1833–1911). Dilthey proposed that the human sciences require concepts, methods, and theories that are fundamentally different from those of the natural sciences. Human sciences study human life by valuing the lived experience of persons and seek to understand life in its matrix of patterns of meaning and values. Some scholars believe that there is a need to approach human sciences differently from conventional empiricism and contend that human experience must be understood in context (Cody & Mitchell, 2002; Mitchell & Cody, 1992).

In human sciences, scientists hope to create new knowledge to provide understanding and interpretation of phenomena. In human sciences, knowledge takes the form of descriptive theories regarding the structures, processes, relationships, and traditions that underlie psychological, social, and cultural aspects of reality. Data are interpreted within context to derive meaning and understanding (Wolfer, 1993). Humanistic scientists value the subjective component of knowledge. They recognize that humans are not capable of total objectivity and embrace the idea of subjectivity (Streubert-Speziale & Carpenter, 2006). The purpose of research in human science is to produce descriptions and interpretations to help understand the nature of human experience.

Increasingly, nursing is being referred to as a human science (Cody & Mitchell, 2002; Mitchell & Cody, 1992). Indeed, the discipline has examined issues related to behavior and culture, as well as biology and physiology, and sought to recognize associations among factors that suggest explanatory variables for human health and illness (Gortner, 1993). Thus, it fits the pattern of other humanistic sciences (i.e., anthropology, sociology).

## QUANTITATIVE VERSUS QUALITATIVE METHODOLOGY DEBATE

Nursing scholars accept the premise that scientific knowledge is generated from systematic study. The research methodologies and criteria used to justify the acceptance of statements or conclusions as true within the discipline result in conclusions and statements that are appropriate, valid, and reliable for the purpose of the discipline.

Two dominant forms of scientific inquiry have been identified in nursing: (1) empiricism, which objectifies experience and may test propositions or hypotheses in controlled experimentation; and (2) phenomenology and other forms of qualitative research (i.e., grounded theory, hermeneutics, historical research, ethnography), which study lived experiences and meanings of events (Gortner & Schultz, 1988; Monti & Tingen, 1999). Reviews of the scientific status of nursing knowledge usually contrast the positivist–deductive–quantitative approach with the interpretive–inductive–qualitative alternative.

Although nursing theorists and nursing scientists emphasize the importance of sociohistorical contexts and person–environment interactions, they tend to focus on "hard science" and the research process. It has been argued that there is an overvaluation of the empirical/quantitative view because it is seen as "true science" (Tinkle & Beaton, 1983). Indeed, the experimental method is held in the highest regard. A viewpoint has persisted into the 21st century in which scholars assume that descriptive or qualitative research should be performed only where there is little information available or when the science is young. Correlational research may follow, and then experimental methods can be used when the two lower ("less rigid" or "less scientific") levels have been explored.

### Quantitative Methods

Traditionally, science has been uniquely quantitative. The quantitative approach has been justified by its success in measuring, analyzing, replicating, and applying the knowledge gained (Streubert-Speziale & Carpenter, 2006). According to Wolfer (1993), science should incorporate methodologic principles of objective observation/description, accurate measurement, quantification of variables, mathematical and statistical analysis, experimental methods, and verification through replication whenever possible.

Kidd and Morrison (1988) state that in their haste to prove the credibility of nursing as a profession, nursing scholars have emphasized reductionism and empirical validation through quantitative methodologies, emphasizing hypothesis testing. In this framework, the scientist develops a hypothesis about a phenomenon and seeks to prove or disprove it.

### Qualitative Methods

The tradition of using qualitative methods to study human phenomena is grounded in the social sciences. Phenomenology and other methods of qualitative research arose because aspects of human values, culture, and relationships were unable to be described fully using quantitative research methods. It is generally accepted that qualitative research findings answer questions centered on social experience and give meaning to human life. Beginning in the 1970s, nursing scientists were challenged to explain phenomena that defy quantitative measurement, and qualitative approaches, which emphasize the importance of the client's perspective, began to be used in nursing research (Kidd & Morrison, 1988).

Repeatedly, scholars have stated that nursing research should incorporate means for determining interpretation of the phenomena of concern from the perspective of the client or care recipient. Contrary to the assertions of early scientists, many later nurse scientists believe that qualitative inquiry contains features of good science including theory and observation, logic, precision, clarity, and reproducibility (Gortner, 1990; Monti & Tingen, 1999).

### Methodologic Pluralism

In many respects nursing is still undecided about which methodologic approach (qualitative or quantitative) best demonstrates the essence and uniqueness of nursing, because both methods have strengths and limitations. Munhall (2007), Oldnall (1995), and Sandelowski (2000), among others, believe that the two approaches may be considered complementary and appropriate for nursing as a research-based discipline. Indeed it has repeatedly been argued that both approaches are equally important and even essential for nursing science development (Foss & Ellefsen, 2002; Shih, 1998; Thurmond, 2001; Young, Taylor, & Renpenning, 2001).

Basic philosophical viewpoints have guided and directed research strategies in the past. More recently scholars have called for theoretical and methodologic pluralism in nursing philosophy and nursing science. Pluralism of research designs is essential for reflecting the uniqueness of nursing, and multiple approaches to theory development and testing should be encouraged. Because there is not one best method of developing knowledge, it is important to recognize that valuing one standard as exclusive or superior restricts the ability to progress (Cull-Wilby & Pepin, 1987).

## Summary

Nursing is an evolving profession, an academic discipline, and a science. There has not yet been a concerted effort to identify and obtain agreement about the currently available knowledge that is fundamental to nursing. The knowledge that constitutes the discipline has not yet been identified and structured, and agreement has not been reached concerning appropriate and needed inclusions (Schlotfeldt, 1992).

Entering the 21st century, nurses are split on whether to emphasize a humanistic, holistic focus or an objective, scientifically derived means of comprehending reality. What is needed is an open philosophy that ties empirical concepts that are capable of being validated through the senses with theoretical concepts of meaning and value.

It is important that future nursing leaders and novice nurse scientists possess an understanding of nursing's philosophical foundations. The legacy of philosophical positivism continues to drive beliefs in the scientific method and research strategies, but it is time to move forward to face the challenges of the increasingly complex and volatile health care environment.

## Case Study

The following is adapted from a paper written by a graduate student describing an encounter in nursing practice that highlights Carper's (1978) ways of knowing in nursing.

In her work, Carper (1978) identified four patterns of knowing in nursing: empirical knowledge (science of nursing), esthetic knowledge (art of nursing), personal knowledge, and ethical knowledge. Each is essential and depends on the others to make the whole of nursing practice, and it is impossible to state which of the patterns of knowing is most important. If nurses focus exclusively on empirical knowledge, for example, nursing care would become more like medical care. But without an empirical base, the art of nursing is just tradition. Personal knowledge is gained from experience and requires a scientific basis, understanding, and empathy. Finally, the moral component is necessary to determine what is valuable, ethical, and compulsory. Each of these ways of knowing is illustrated in the following scenario.

*Mrs. Smith was a 24-year-old primigravida who presented to our unit in early labor. Her husband, and father of her unborn child, had abandoned her two months prior to delivery, and she lacked close family support. I cared for Mrs. Smith throughout her labor and assisted during her delivery.*

*During this process, I taught breathing techniques to ease pain and improve coping. Position changes were encouraged periodically, and assistance was provided as needed. Mrs. Smith's care included continuous fetal monitoring, intravenous hydration, analgesic administration, back rubs, coaching and encouragement, assistance while getting an epidural, straight catheterization as needed, vital sign monitoring per policy, oxytocin administration after delivery, newborn care, and breastfeeding assistance, among many others. All care was explained in detail prior to rendering.*

*Empirical knowledge was clearly utilized in Mrs. Smith's care. Examples would be those practices based on the Association of Women's Health, Obstetric and Neonatal Nurses (AWHONN) evidence-based standards. These include guidelines for fetal heart rate monitoring and interpretation, assessment and management of Mrs. Smith while receiving her epidural analgesia, the assessment and management of side effects secondary to her regional analgesia, and even frequency for monitoring vital signs. Other examples would be assisting Mrs. Smith to an upright position during her second stage of labor to facilitate delivery and delaying nondirected pushing once she was completely dilated.*

*Esthetic knowledge, or the art of nursing, is displayed in obstetrical nursing daily. Rather than just responding to biologic developments or spoken requests, the whole person was valued and cues were perceived and responded to for the good of the patient. The care I gave Mrs. Smith was holistic; her social, spiritual, and psychological and physical needs were all addressed in a comprehensive and seamless fashion. The empathy conveyed to the patient took into account her unique self and situation, and the care provided was reflexively tailored to her needs. I recognized the profound experience of which I was a part, and adapted my actions and attitude to honor the patient and value the larger experience.*

*Many aspects of personal knowledge seem intertwined with esthetics, though more emphasis seems to be on the meaningful interaction between the patient and nurse. As above, the patient was cared for as a unique individual. Though secondary to the awesome nature of birth, much of the experience revolved around the powerful interpersonal relationship established. Mrs. Smith was accepted as herself. Though efforts were made by me to manage certain aspects of the experience, Mrs. Smith was allowed control and freedom of expression and reaction. She and I were both committed to the mutual though brief relationship. This knowledge stems from my own personality and ability to accept others, willingness to connect to others, and desire to collaborate with the patient regarding her care and ultimate experience.*

*The ethical knowledge of nursing is continuously utilized in nursing care to promote the health and well-being of the patient; and in this circumstance, the unborn child as well. Every decision made must be weighed against desired goals and values, and nurses must strive to act as advocates for each patient. When caring for a patient and an unborn child, there is a constant attempt to do no harm to either, while balancing the care of both. A very common example is the administration of medications for the mother's comfort that can cause sedation and respiratory depression in the neonate. This case involved fewer ethical considerations than many others in obstetrics. These include instances in which physicians do not respond when the nurse feels there is imminent danger and the chain of command must be utilized, or when assistance is required for the care of abortion patients or in other situations that may be in conflict with the nurses moral or religious convictions.*

*A close bond was formed while I cared for Mrs. Smith and her baby. Soon after admission, she was holding my hand during contractions and had shared very intimate details of her life, separation, and fears. Though she had shared her financial concerns and had a new baby to provide for, a few weeks after her delivery I received a beautiful gift basket and card. In her note she shared that I had touched her in a way she had never expected and she vowed never to forget me; I've not forgotten her either.*

Contributed by Shelli Carter, RN, MSN

## LEARNING ACTIVITIES

1. Reflect on the above case study. Think of a situation from personal practice in which multiple ways of knowing were used. Write down the anecdote and share it with classmates.

2. With classmates, discuss whether nursing is a profession or an occupation. What can current and future nurses do to enhance nursing's standing as a profession?

3. Debate with classmates the two predominant philosophical schools of thought in nursing (received view and perceived view). Which worldview best encompasses the profession of nursing? Why?

4. With classmates, discuss instances in which you have observed conflicts between/among health care providers (e.g., nurses and physicians) or between health care providers and patients. Analyze the situation to determine if the root source of the conflict might be related to differing "worldview" perspectives of the parties involved. For example, why does an elderly diabetic patient not follow the advice of health care providers regarding how to manage diabetes?

## REFERENCES

Barrett, E. A. M. (2002). What is nursing science? *Nursing Science Quarterly, 15*(1), 51–60.

Blackburn, S. (2005). *Oxford dictionary of philosophy* (2nd ed.). New York: Oxford University Press.

Carper, B. A. (1978). Fundamental patterns of knowing in nursing. *Advances in Nursing Science, 1*(1), 13–24.

Carper, B. A. (1992). Philosophical inquiry in nursing: An application. In J. F. Kikuchi & H. Simmons (Eds.), *Philosophic inquiry in nursing* (pp. 71–80). Newbury Park, CA: Sage.

Chinn, P. L., & Kramer, M. K. (2008). *Theory and nursing: Integrated knowledge development* (7th ed.). St. Louis: Mosby.

Cody, W. K., & Mitchell, G. J. (2002). Nursing knowledge and human science revisited: Practical and political considerations. *Nursing Science Quarterly, 15*(1), 4–13.

Cronin, P., & Rawlings-Anderson, K. (2004). *Knowledge for contemporary nursing practice.* London: Mosby.

Cull-Wilby, B. L., & Pepin, J. I. (1987). Towards a coexistence of paradigms in nursing knowledge development. *Journal of Advanced Nursing, 12*(4), 515–522.

DiBartolo, M. C. (1998). Philosophy of science in doctoral nursing education revisited. *Journal of Professional Nursing, 14*(6), 350–360.

Donaldson, S. K., & Crowley, D. M. (1978). The discipline of nursing. *Nursing Outlook, 26*(2), 113–120.

Fawcett, J. (1999). The state of nursing science: Hallmarks of the 20th and 21st centuries. *Nursing Science Quarterly, 12*(4), 311–318.

Fawcett, J., Watson, J., Neuman, B., Walkers, P. H., & Fitzpatrick, J. (2001). On nursing theories and evidence. *Journal of Nursing Scholarship, 3*(2), 115–119.

Foss, C., & Ellefsen, B. (2002). The value of combining qualitative and quantitative approaches in nursing research by means of method triangulation. *Journal of Advanced Nursing, 40*(2), 242–248.

Gortner, S. R. (1990). Nursing values and science: Toward a science philosophy. *Image: Journal of Nursing Scholarship, 22*(2), 101–105.

Gortner, S. R. (1993). Nursing's syntax revisited: A critique of philosophies said to influence nursing theories. *International Journal of Nursing Studies, 30*(6), 477–488.

Gortner, S. R., & Schultz, P. R. (1988). Approaches to nursing science methods. *Image: Journal of Nursing Scholarship, 20*(1), 22–24.

Gustafsson, B. (2002). The philosophy of science from a nursing-scientific perspective. *Theoria: Journal of Nursing Theory, 11*(2), 3–13.

Hickman, J. S. (2002). An introduction to nursing theory. In J. George (Ed.). *Nursing theories: The base for professional nursing practice* (5th ed., pp. 1–20). Upper Saddle River, NJ: Prentice-Hall.

Holzemer, W. L. (2007). Towards understanding nursing science. *Japan Journal of Nursing Science, 4*(1), 57–59.

Johnson, J. L. (1991). Nursing science: Basic, applied, or practical? Implications for the art of nursing. *Advances in Nursing Science, 14*(1), 7–16.

Kidd, P., & Morrison, E. F. (1988). The progression of knowledge in nursing research: A search for meaning. *Image: Journal of Nursing Scholarship, 20*(4), 222–224.

Logan, J., Franzen, D., Pauling, C., & Butcher, H. K. (2004). Achieving professionhood through participation in professional organizations. In L. Haynes, T. Boese, & H. Butcher (Eds.), *Nursing in contemporary society: Issues, trends, and transition to practice* (pp. 52–70). Upper Saddle River, NJ: Prentice-Hall.

Meleis, A. I. (2005). *Theoretical nursing: Development and progress* (3rd ed.). Philadelphia: Lippincott Williams & Wilkins.

Mitchell, G. J., & Cody, W. K. (1992). Nursing knowledge and human science: Ontological and epistemological considerations. *Nursing Science Quarterly, 5*(2), 54–61.

Moch, S. D. (1990). Personal knowing: Evolving research in nursing. *Scholarly Inquiry for Nursing Practice, 4*(2), 155–163.

Monti, E. J., & Tingen, M. S. (1999). Multiple paradigms of nursing science. *Advances in Nursing Science, 21*(4), 64–80.

Moody, L. E. (1990). *Advancing nursing science through research.* Newbury Park, CA: Sage.

Munhall, P. L. (2007). *Nursing research: A qualitative perspective* (4th ed.). Boston: Jones & Bartlett Publishers.

Newman, M. A., Sime, A. M., & Corcoran-Perry, S. A. (1991). The focus of the discipline of nursing. *Advances in Nursing Science, 14*(1), 1–6.

Northrup, D. T., Tschanz, C. L., Olynyk, V. G., Makaroff, K. L. S., Szabo, J., & Biasio, H. A. (2004). Nursing: Whose discipline is it anyway? *Nursing Science Quarterly, 17*(1), 55–62.

Nyatanga, L. (2005). Nursing and the philosophy of science. *Nurse Education Today, 25,* 670–674.

Oldnall, A. S. (1995). Nursing as an emerging academic discipline. *Journal of Advanced Nursing, 21,* 605–612.

Parse, R. R. (1997). The language of nursing knowledge: Saying what we mean. In I. M. King & J. Fawcett (Eds.), *The language of nursing theory and metatheory* (pp. 73–77). Indianapolis, IN: Center Nursing Press.

Parse, R. R. (1999). Nursing: The discipline and the profession. *Nursing Science Quarterly, 12*(4), 275–276.

Polifroni, E. C., & Welch, M. (1999). *Perspectives on philosophy of science in nursing.* Philadelphia: Lippincott Williams & Wilkins.

Powers, B. A., & Knapp, T. R. (2006). *Dictionary of nursing theory and research* (3rd ed.). New York: Springer Publishing.

Reed, P. G. (1995). A treatise on nursing knowledge development in the 21st century: Beyond postmodernism. *Advances in Nursing Science, 17*(3), 70–84.

Reed, P. G. (2008). Adversity and advancing nursing knowledge. *Nursing Science Quarterly, 21*(2), 133–139.

Riegel, B., Omery, A., Calvillo, E., Elsayed, N. G., et al. (1992). Moving beyond: A generative philosophy of science. *Image: Journal of Nursing Scholarship, 24*(2), 115–119.

Rutty, J. E. (1998). The nature of philosophy of science, theory and knowledge relating to nursing and professionalism. *Journal of Advanced Nursing, 28*(2), 243–250.

Sandelowski, M. (2000). Combining qualitative and quantitative sampling, data collection, and analysis techniques in mixed-method studies. *Research in Nursing & Health, 23*(3), 246–255.

Schlotfeldt, R. M. (1989). Structuring nursing knowledge: A priority for creating nursing's future. *Nursing Science Quarterly, 1*(1), 35–38.

Schlotfeldt, R. M. (1992). Answering nursing's philosophical questions: Whose responsibility is it? In J. F. Kikuchi & H. Simmons (Eds.), *Philosophic inquiry in nursing* (pp. 97–104). Newbury Park, CA: Sage.

Schultz, P. R., & Meleis, A. I. (1988). Nursing epistemology: Traditions, insights, questions. *Image: Journal of Nursing Scholarship, 20*(4), 217–221.

Schwirian, P. M. (1998). *Professionalization of nursing: Current issues and trends* (3rd ed.). Philadelphia: Lippincott Williams & Wilkins.

Shih, F. J. (1998). Triangulation in nursing research: Issues of conceptual clarity and purpose. *Journal of Advanced Nursing, 28*(3), 631–641.

Silva, M. C. (1977). Philosophy, science, theory: Interrelationships and implications for nursing research. *Image: Journal of Nursing Scholarship, 9*(3), 59–63.

Silva, M. C., & Rothbert, D. (1984). An analysis of changing trends of philosophies of science on nursing theory development and testing. *Advances in Nursing Science, 6*(2), 1–13.

Silva, M. C., Sorrell, J. M., & Sorrell, C. D. (1995). From Carper's patterns of knowing to ways of being: An ontological philosophical shift in nursing. *Advances in Nursing Science, 18*(1), 1–13.

Smith, L. S. (2000). Is nursing an academic discipline? *Nursing Forum, 35*(1), 25–28.

Streubert-Speziale, H. J., & Carpenter, D. R. (2006). *Qualitative research in nursing: Advancing the humanistic imperative* (4th ed.). Philadelphia: Lippincott Williams & Wilkins.

Suppe, F., & Jacox, A. (1985). Philosophy of science and development of nursing theory. In H. H. Werley & J. J. Fitzpatrick (Eds.), *Annual review of nursing research.* New York: Springer.

Teichman, J., & Evans, K. C. (1999). *Philosophy: A beginner's guide* (3rd ed.). Cambridge, MA: Blackwell.

Thurmond, V. A. (2001). The point of triangulation. *Journal of Nursing Scholarship, 33*(3), 253–258.

Tinkle, M. B., & Beaton, J. L. (1983). Toward a new view of science: Implications for nursing research. *Advances in Nursing Science, 5*(2), 27–36.

Wainwright, S. P. (1997). A new paradigm for nursing: The potential of realism. *Journal of Advanced Nursing, 26*(6), 1262–1271.

White, J. (1995). Patterns of knowing: Review, critique, and update. *Advances in Nursing Science, 17*(4), 73–86.

Wolf, K. A. (2006). The slow march to professional practice. In L. C. Andrist, P. K. Nicholas, & K. A. Wolf (Eds.), *A history of nursing ideas* (pp. 305–318). Boston: Jones and Bartlett Publishers.

Wolfer, J. (1993). Aspects of reality and ways of knowing in nursing: In search of an integrating paradigm. *Image: Journal of Nursing Scholarship, 25*(2), 141–146.

Young, A., Taylor, S. G., & Renpenning, K. M. (2001). *Connections: Nursing research, theory and practice.* St. Louis: Mosby.

# 2

# Overview of Theory in Nursing

## Melanie McEwen

*M*att Ng has been an emergency room nurse for almost 6 years and recently decided to enroll in a master's degree program to become an acute care nurse practitioner. As he read over the degree requirements, Matt was somewhat bewildered. One of the first courses required by his program was titled Theory Application in Nursing. He was interested in the courses in advanced pharmacology, advanced physical assessment, and pathophysiology and was excited about the advanced practice clinical courses, but a course that focused on nursing theory did not appear applicable to his goals.

Looking over the syllabus for the theory application course did little to reassure him, but he was determined to make the best of the situation and went to the first class with an open mind. The first few class periods were mildly interesting as the students and instructor discussed the historical evolution of the discipline of nursing and the stages of nursing theory development. But as the course progressed, topics became more interesting. The students learned ways to analyze and evaluate theories and examined a number of different types of theories used by nurses. There were several assignments including a concept analysis, an analysis of a middle range nursing theory, and a synthesis paper that examined the use of non-nursing theories in nursing research.

By the end of the semester, Matt was able to recognize the importance of the study of theory. He understood how theoretical principles and concepts affected his current practice and how they would be essential to consider as he continued his studies to become an advanced practice nurse.

When asked about theory, many nurses and nursing students, and often even nursing faculty will respond with a furrowed brow, a pained expression, and a resounding "ugh"! When questioned about their negative response, most will admit that the idea of studying theory is confusing, that they see no practical value, and that theory is, in essence, too theoretical.

Likewise, some nursing scholars believe that nursing theory is practically nonexistent, whereas others recognize that many practitioners have not heard of nursing theory. Some nurses lament that nurse researchers use theories and frameworks from other disciplines, whereas others ask why they bother with theory. Questions and debates about theory in nursing abound in the literature.

Myra Levine, one of the pioneer nursing theorists, recently wrote that "the introduction of the idea of theory in nursing was sadly inept" (Levine, 1995, p. 11). She stated,

> *In traditional nursing fashion, early efforts were directed at creating a procedure—a recipe book for prospective theorists—which then could be used to decide what was and was not a theory. And there was always the thread of expectation that the great, grand, global theory would appear and end all speculation. Most of the early theorists really believed they were achieving that. (p. 11)*

Levine went on to explain that every new theory posited new central concepts, definitions, relational statements, and goals for nursing, then attracted a chorus of critics. This resulted in nurses finding themselves confused about the substance and intention of the theories. Indeed, "in early days, theory was expected to be obscure. If it was clearly understandable, it wasn't considered a very good theory" (Levine, 1995, p. 11).

The drive to develop nursing theory has been marked by nursing theory conferences, the proliferation of theoretical and conceptual frameworks for nursing, and the formal teaching of theory development in graduate nursing education. It has resulted in the development of many systems for theory analysis and evaluation, a fascination with the philosophy of science, and confusion about theory development strategies and division of choice of research methodologies.

There is debate and confusion over the types of theories that should be used by nurses. Should they be only nursing theories or can nurses use theories borrowed from other disciplines? There is debate over terminology such as *conceptual framework, conceptual model,* and *theory.* There have been heated discussions concerning the appropriate level of theory for nurses to develop, as well as how, why, where, and when to test, measure, analyze, and evaluate these theories/models/conceptual frameworks. The question has been repeatedly asked: Should nurses adopt a single theory, or do multiple theories serve them best? It is no wonder, then, that graduate nursing students display consternation, bewilderment, and even anxiety when presented with the prospect of studying theory.

To be useful, theory must be meaningful and relevant, but above all, it must be understandable. This chapter discusses many of the issues described above. It presents the rationale for studying and using theory in practice, research, management/administration, and education; gives definitions of key terms; provides an overview of the history of development of theory utilization in nursing; describes the scope of theory and levels of theory; and, finally, introduces the widely accepted nursing metaparadigm.

## Overview of Theory

Most scholars agree that it is the unique theories and perspectives used by a discipline that distinguish it from other disciplines. The theories used by members of a profession clarify basic assumptions and values shared by its members and define the nature, outcome, and purpose of practice (Alligood, 2006; Rutty, 1998).

Definitions of the term *theory* abound in the nursing literature. At a basic level, theory has been described as a systematic explanation of an event in which constructs and concepts are identified and relationships are proposed and predictions made

(Streubert-Speziale & Carpenter, 2006). Theory has also been defined as a "creative and rigorous structuring of ideas that project a tentative, purposeful and systematic view of phenomena" (Chinn & Kramer, 2008, p. 305). Finally, theory has been called a set of interpretative assumptions, principles, or propositions that help explain or guide action (Young, Taylor, & Renpenning, 2001).

In their classic work, Dickoff and James (1968) state that theory is invented, rather than found in or discovered from reality. Furthermore, theories vary according to the number of elements, the characteristics and complexity of the elements, and the kind of relationships between or among the elements.

## The Importance of Theory in Nursing

Before the advent of development of nursing theories, nursing was subsumed under medicine. Nursing practice was prescribed by others and highlighted by traditional, ritualistic tasks with little regard to rationale. The initial work of theorists was aimed at clarifying the complex intellectual and interactional domains that distinguish expert nursing from the mere doing of tasks (Omrey, Kasper, & Page, 1995). It was believed that conceptual models and theories could create mechanisms by which nurses would communicate their professional convictions, provide a moral/ethical structure to guide actions, and foster a means of systematic thinking about nursing and its practice (Chinn & Kramer, 2008; DeKeyser & Medoff-Cooper, 2001; Peterson, 2008; Thorne, Canam, Dahinten, Hall, Henderson, & Kirkham, 1998; Ziegler, 2005). The idea that a single, unified model of nursing—a worldview of the discipline—might emerge was encouraged by some (Tierney, 1998).

It is widely believed that use of theory offers structure and organization to nursing knowledge and provides a systematic means of collecting data to describe, explain, and predict nursing practice. Use of theory also promotes rational and systematic practice by challenging and validating intuition. Theories make nursing practice more overtly purposeful by stating not only the focus of practice, but specific goals and outcomes. Theories define and clarify nursing and the purpose of nursing practice to distinguish it from other caring professions by setting professional boundaries. Finally, use of a theory of nursing leads to coordinated and less fragmented care (Alligood, 2006; Chinn & Kramer, 2008; McKenna, 1993; Ziegler, 2005).

Ways in which theories and conceptual models developed by nurses have influenced nursing practice are described by Fawcett (1992), who stated that in nursing they:

- Identify certain standards for nursing practice
- Identify settings in which nursing practice should occur and the characteristics of what the model's author considers recipients of nursing care
- Identify distinctive nursing processes and technologies to be used, including parameters for client assessment, labels for client problems, a strategy for planning, a typology of intervention, and criteria for evaluation of intervention outcomes
- Direct the delivery of nursing services
- Serve as the basis for clinical information systems including the admission database, nursing orders, care plan, progress notes, and discharge summary
- Guide the development of client classification systems
- Direct quality assurance programs

## Terminology of Theory

Young, Taylor, and Renpenning (2001) write that in nursing, conceptual models or frameworks detail a network of concepts and describe their relationships, thereby explaining broad nursing phenomena. Theories, they believe, are the narrative that accompanies the conceptual model. These theories typically provide a detailed description of all of the components of the model and outline relationships in the form of propositions. Critical components of the theory or narrative include definitions of the central concepts or constructs, propositions or relational statements, the assumptions on which the framework is based, and the purpose, indications for use or application. Many conceptual frameworks and theories will also include a schematic drawing or model depicting the overall structure of or interactivity of the components (Chinn & Kramer, 2008).

Some terms may be new to students of theory and others need clarification. Table 2-1 lists definitions for a number of terms that are encountered in writings on theory. Many of these terms will be described in more detail later in the chapter and in subsequent chapters.

## Historical Overview: Theory Development in Nursing

### FLORENCE NIGHTINGALE

Most nursing scholars credit Florence Nightingale with being the first modern nursing theorist. Nightingale was the first to delineate what she considered nursing's goal and practice domain, and she postulated that "to nurse" meant having charge of the personal health of someone. She believed the role of the nurse was seen as placing the client "in the best condition for nature to act upon him" (Hilton, 1997, p. 1211).

Nightingale received her formal training in nursing in Kaiserswerth, Germany in 1851. Following her renowned service for the British army during the Crimean War, she returned to London and established a school for nurses. According to Nightingale, formal training for nurses was necessary to "teach not only what is to be done, but how to do it." She was the first to advocate the teaching of symptoms and what they indicate. Further, she taught the importance of rationale for actions and stressed the significance of "trained powers of observation and reflection" (Kalisch & Kalisch, 2004, p. 36).

In *Notes on Nursing*, published in 1859, Nightingale proposed basic premises for nursing practice. In her view, nurses were to make astute observations of the sick and their environment, record observations, and develop knowledge about factors that promoted healing. Her framework for nursing emphasized the utility of empirical knowledge, and she believed that knowledge developed and used by nurses should be distinct from medical knowledge. She insisted that trained nurses control and staff nursing schools and manage nursing practice in homes and hospitals (Chinn & Kramer, 2008; Kalisch & Kalisch, 2004).

### STAGES OF THEORY DEVELOPMENT IN NURSING

Subsequent to Nightingale, almost a century passed before other nursing scholars attempted the development of philosophical and theoretical works to describe and define nursing and to guide nursing practice. Kidd and Morrison (1988) described five stages in the development of nursing theory and philosophy: (1) silent knowledge, (2) received knowledge, (3) subjective knowledge, (4) procedural knowledge, and (5) constructed knowledge. Table 2-2 gives an overview of characteristics of each of

TABLE 2-1 *Definitions and Characteristics of Theory Terms and Concepts*

| Term | Definition and Characteristics |
| --- | --- |
| Assumptions | Assumptions are beliefs about phenomena one must accept as true to accept a theory about the phenomena as true. Assumptions may be based on accepted knowledge or personal beliefs and values. Although assumptions may not be susceptible to testing, they can be argued philosophically. |
| Borrowed or shared theory | A borrowed theory is a theory developed in another discipline that is not adapted to the worldview and practice of nursing. |
| Concept | Concepts are the elements or components of a phenomenon necessary to understand the phenomenon. They are abstract and derived from impressions the human mind receives about phenomena through sensing the environment. |
| Conceptual model/conceptual framework | A conceptual model is a set of interrelated concepts that symbolically represents and conveys a mental image of a phenomenon. Conceptual models of nursing identify concepts and describe their relationships to the phenomena of central concern to the discipline. |
| Construct | Constructs are the most complex type of concept. They are comprised of more than one concept and typically built or constructed by the theorist or philosopher to fit a purpose. The terms *concept* and *construct* are often used interchangeably, but some authors use concept as the more general term—all constructs are concepts, but not all concepts are constructs. |
| Empirical indicator | Empirical indicators are very specific and concrete identifiers of concepts. They are actual instructions, experimental conditions, and procedures used to observe or measure the concept(s) of a theory. |
| Epistemology | Epistemology refers to theories of knowledge or how people come to have knowledge; in nursing it is the study of the origins of nursing knowledge. |
| Hypotheses | Hypotheses are tentative suggestions that a specific relationship exists between two concepts or propositions. As the hypothesis is repeatedly confirmed, it progresses to an empirical generalization and ultimately to a law. |
| Knowledge | Knowledge refers to the awareness or perception of reality acquired through insight, learning, or investigation. In a discipline, knowledge is what is collectively seen to be a reasonably accurate understanding of the world as seen by members of the discipline. |
| Laws | A law is a proposition about the relationship between concepts in a theory that has been repeatedly validated. Laws are highly generalizable. Laws are found primarily in disciplines that deal with observable and measurable phenomena, such as chemistry and physics. Conversely, social and human sciences have few laws. |
| Metaparadigm | A metaparadigm represents the worldview of a discipline—the global perspective that subsumes more specific views and approaches to the central concepts with which the discipline is concerned. The metaparadigm is the ideology within which the theories, knowledge, and processes for knowing find meaning and coherence. Nursing's metaparadigm is generally thought to consist of the concepts of person, environment, health, and nursing. |
| Middle range theory | Middle range theory refers to a part of a discipline's concerns related to particular topics. The scope is narrower than that of broad-range or grand theories. |

*(Continued)*

TABLE 2-1 *Definitions and Characteristics of Theory Terms and Concepts (Continued)*

| Term | Definition and Characteristics |
| --- | --- |
| Model | Models are graphic or symbolic representations of phenomena that objectify and present certain perspectives or points of view about nature or function or both. Models may be theoretical (something not directly observable—expressed in language or mathematics symbols) or empirical (replicas of observable reality—model of an eye, for example). |
| Ontology | Ontology is concerned with the study of existence and the nature of reality. |
| Paradigm | A paradigm is an organizing framework that contains concepts, theories, assumptions, beliefs, values, and principles that form the way a discipline interprets the subject matter with which it is concerned. It describes work to be done and frames an orientation within which the work will be accomplished. A discipline may have a number of paradigms. The term paradigm is associated with Kuhn's *Structure of Scientific Revolutions.* |
| Phenomena | Phenomena are the designation of an aspect of reality; the phenomena of interest become the subject matter that are the primary concerns of a discipline. |
| Philosophy | A philosophy is a statement of beliefs and values about human beings and their world. |
| Practice or microtheory | A practice or microtheory deals with a limited range of discrete phenomena that are specifically defined and are not expanded to include their link with the broad concerns of a discipline. |
| Praxis | Praxis is the application of a theory to cases encountered in experience. |
| Relationship statements | Relationship statements indicate specific relationships between two or more concepts. They may be classified as propositions, hypotheses, laws, axioms, or theorems. |
| Taxonomy | A taxonomy is a classification scheme for defining or gathering together various phenomena. Taxonomies range in complexity from simple dichotomies to complicated hierarchical structures. |
| Theory | Theory refers to a set of logically interrelated concepts, statements, propositions, and definitions, which have been derived from philosophical beliefs of scientific data and from which questions or hypotheses can be deduced, tested, and verified. A theory purports to account for or characterize some phenomenon. |
| Worldview | Worldview is the philosophical frame of reference used by a social or cultural group to describe that group's outlook on and beliefs about reality. |

Sources: Blackburn (2005); Chinn and Kramer (2008); Powers and Knapp (2006); Tomey and Alligood (2006).

these stages in the development of nursing theory, and each stage is described in the following sections.

### Silent Knowledge Stage

Recognizing the impact of the poorly trained nurses on the health of soldiers during the Civil War, in 1868 the American Medical Association advocated the formal training of nurses and suggested that schools of nursing be attached to hospitals with

TABLE 2-2 *Stages in the Development of Nursing Theory*

| Stage | Source of Knowledge | Impact on Theory and Research |
|---|---|---|
| Silent knowledge | Blind obedience to medical authority | Little attempt to develop theory. Research was limited to collection of epidemiologic data. |
| Received knowledge | Learning through listening to others | Theories were borrowed from other disciplines. As nurses acquired non-nursing doctoral degrees, they relied on the authority of educators, sociologists, psychologists, physiologists, and anthropologists to provide answers to nursing problems. |
| | | Research was primarily educational research or sociologic research. |
| Subjective knowledge | Authority was internalized and a new sense of self emerged | A negative attitude toward borrowed theories and science emerged. |
| | | Nurse scholars focused on defining nursing and on developing theories about and for nursing. |
| | | Nursing research focused on the nurse rather than on clients and clinical situations. |
| Procedural knowledge | Includes both separate and connected knowledge | Proliferation of approaches to theory development. Application of theory in practice was frequently underemphasized. Emphasis was placed on the procedures used to acquire knowledge, with overattention to the appropriateness of methodology, the criteria for evolution, and statistical procedures for data analysis. |
| Constructed knowledge | Integration of different types of knowledge (intuition, reason, and self-knowledge) | Nursing theory should be based on prior empirical studies, theoretical literature, client reports of clinical experiences and feelings, and the nurse scholar's intuition or related knowledge about the phenomenon of concern. |

Source: Kidd and Morrison (1988).

instruction being provided by medical staff and resident physicians. The first training school for nurses in the United States was opened in 1872 at the New England Hospital. Three more schools, located in New York, New Haven, and Boston, opened shortly thereafter (Kalisch & Kalisch, 2004). Most schools were under the control of hospitals and superintended by hospital administrators and physicians. Education and practice were based on rules, principles, and traditions that were passed along through an apprenticeship form of education.

There followed rapid growth in the number of hospital-based training programs for nurses, and by 1909 there were 1006 such programs (Kalisch & Kalisch, 2004). In these early schools, a meager amount of theory was taught by physicians and practice was taught by experienced nurses. The curricula contained some anatomy and physiology and occasional lectures on special diseases. Few nursing books were available and the emphasis was on carrying out physicians' orders. Nursing education and practice focused on the performance of technical skills and application of a few basic principles, such as aseptic technique and principles of mobility. Nurses depended on physicians' diagnosis and orders, and as a result, largely adhered to the medical model, which views body and mind separately and focuses on cure and treatment of pathologic problems (Kenney, 1995). Hospital administrators saw nurses as inexpensive labor. Nurses were exploited both as students and as experienced workers. They were taught to be submissive and obedient, and they learned to fulfill their responsibilities to physicians without question (Chinn & Kramer, 2008).

Unfortunately, with a few exceptions, this model of nursing education persisted for more than 80 years. One exception was Yale University, which started the first autonomous school of nursing in 1924. At Yale, and in other later collegiate programs, professional training was strengthened by in-depth exposure to the underlying theory of disease as well as the social, psychological, and physical aspects of client welfare. The growth of collegiate programs lagged, however, due to opposition from many physicians who argued that university-educated nurses were overtrained. Hospital schools continued to insist that nursing education meant acquisition of technical skills, and knowledge of theory was unnecessary and might actually handicap the nurse (Andrist, 2006; Chinn & Kramer, 2008; Kalisch & Kalisch, 2004).

### Received Knowledge Stage

It was not until after World War II that substantive changes were made in nursing education. During the late 1940s and into the 1950s, serious nursing shortages were fueled by a decline in nursing school enrollments. A 1948 report, *Nursing for the Future*, by Esther Brown, PhD, compared nursing with teaching. She noted that the current model of nursing education was central to the problems of the profession and recommended that efforts be made to focus nursing education in universities, with formal education, as opposed to the apprenticeship system that existed in most hospital programs (Kalisch & Kalisch, 2004).

Other factors during this time challenged the tradition of hospital-based training for nurses. One of these factors was a dramatic increase in the number of hospitals resulting from the Hill-Burton Act, which worsened the ongoing and sometimes critical nursing shortage. In addition, professional organizations for nurses were restructured and began to grow. It was also during this time that state licensure testing for registration took effect, and by 1949, 41 states required testing. The registration requirement necessitated that education programs review the content matter they were teaching to determine minimum criteria and some degree of uniformity. In addition, the processes used in instruction were also reviewed and evaluated (Kalisch & Kalisch, 2004).

Over the next decade a number of other events occurred that altered nursing education and nursing practice. In 1950, the journal *Nursing Research* was first published. The American Nurses Association began a program to encourage nurses to pursue graduate education to study nursing functions and practice. Books on research methods and explicit theories of nursing began to appear. In 1956, the Health Amendments Act authorized funds for financial aid to promote graduate education for full-time study to prepare nurses for administration, supervision, and teaching. These events resulted in a slow but steady increase in graduate nursing education programs.

The first doctoral programs in nursing originated within schools of education at Teachers College, Columbia University (1933) and New York University (1934). But it would be 20 more years before the first doctoral program in nursing began at the University of Pittsburgh (1954). Doctoral programs grew fairly slowly over the next two decades, but by 1970 there were 20 such programs. Beginning in the late 1980s and throughout the 1990s, the number of doctoral programs grew fairly steadily. Beginning in the early 21st century, however, their number has dramatically increased, and by

2007, there were 107 doctoral programs granting a PhD or DNS/DSN/DNSc. In addition, there were 73 doctorate of nursing practice (DNP) programs with many more being planned (American Association of Colleges of Nursing, 2008).

This growth in graduate nursing education allowed nurse scholars to debate ideas, viewpoints, and research methods in the nursing literature. As a result, nurses began to question the ideas that were taken for granted in nursing and the traditional basis in which nursing was practiced.

### Subjective Knowledge Stage

Until the 1950s, nursing was principally derived from social, biologic, and medical theories. With the exceptions of Nightingale's work in the 1850s, nursing theory had its beginnings with the publication of Hildegard Peplau's book in 1952. Peplau described the interpersonal process between the nurse and the client. This started a revolution in nursing, and in the late 1950s and 1960s a number of nurse theorists emerged seeking to provide an independent conceptual framework for nursing education and practice (Hilton, 1997). The nurse's role came under scrutiny during this decade as nurse leaders debated the nature of nursing practice and theory development.

During the 1960s, the development of nursing theory was heavily influenced by three philosophers, James Dickoff, Patricia James, and Ernestine Weidenbach, who, in a series of articles, described theory development and the nature of theory for a practice discipline. Other approaches to theory development combined direct observations of practice, insights derived from existing theories and other literature sources, and insights derived from explicit philosophical perspectives about nursing and the nature of health and human experience. Early theories were characterized by a functional view of nursing and health. They attempted to define what nursing is, describe the social purposes nursing serves, explain how nurses function to realize these purposes, and identify parameters and variables that influence illness and health (Chinn & Kramer, 2008).

In the 1960s, a number of nurse leaders (Abdellah, Orlando, Widenbach, Hall, Henderson, Levine, & Rogers) developed and published their views of nursing. Their descriptions of nursing and nursing models evolved from their personal, professional, and educational experiences, and reflected their perception of ideal nursing practice.

### Procedural Knowledge Stage

By the 1970s, the nursing profession viewed itself as a scientific discipline evolving toward a theoretically based practice focusing on the client. In the late 1960s and early 1970s, several nursing theory conferences were held. Also, significantly, in 1972, the National League for Nursing implemented a requirement that nursing curricula be based on conceptual frameworks. During these years, many nursing theorists published their beliefs and ideas about nursing and some developed conceptual models. The views of nursing of theorists such as Orem, King, Neuman, and Roy often were more idealistic than practical and realistic, and nurses had difficulty applying them to practice (Kenney, 1995).

During the 1970s, a consensus developed among nursing leaders regarding common elements of nursing. These were the nature of nursing (roles/actions), the individual recipient of care (client), the context of nurse–client interactions (environment), and health. Nurses debated whether there should be one conceptual model for nursing or several models to describe the relationships among the nurse, client, environment, and health (Fawcett, 1993; Kenney, 1995). Books were written for nurses on how to critique, develop, and apply nursing theories. Graduate schools developed courses on analysis and application of theory, and researchers identified nursing theories as conceptual frameworks for their studies. Through the late 1970s and early 1980s, theories moved to characterizing nursing's role from what they do to what nursing is. This moved nursing from a context-dependent, reactive position to a context-independent, proactive arena (Chinn & Kramer, 2008).

### Constructed Knowledge Stage

During the late 1980s, scholars began to concentrate on the need to develop substantive theory that provides meaningful foundation for nursing practice. There was a call to develop substance in theory and to focus on nursing concepts grounded in practice and linked to research. The 1990s and into the early 21st century saw an increasing emphasis on philosophy and philosophy of science in nursing. Attention shifted from grand theories to middle range and practice or situation-specific theories, as well as application of theory in research and practice.

This is the current stage of theory development in nursing. It is anticipated that the importance of application of middle range and practice theories in research and practice will continue to be stressed. Correspondingly, less attention will be given to grand theories and conceptual frameworks.

## SUMMARY OF STAGES OF NURSING THEORY DEVELOPMENT

A number of events and individuals have had an impact on the development and utilization of theory in nursing practice, research, and education. Table 2-3 provides a summary of significant events.

Beginning in the early 1950s, efforts to represent nursing theoretically produced broad conceptualizations of nursing practice. These conceptual models or frameworks proliferated during the 1960s and 1970s. Although the conceptual models were not developed using traditional scientific research processes, they did provide direction for nursing by focusing on a general ideal of practice that served as a guide for research and education. Table 2-4 lists the works of many of the nursing theorists and the titles and year of key theoretical publications. The works of a number of the major theorists are discussed in Chapters 7, 8, and 9. Reference lists and bibliographies outlining application of their work to research, education, and practice are described in those chapters.

## Classification of Theories in Nursing

Over the last 40 years, a number of methods for classifying theory in nursing have been described. These include classification based on range/scope or abstractness (grand or macrotheory to practice or situation-specific theory) and type or purpose of the theory (descriptive, predictive, or situation-producing theory). Both of these classification schemes are discussed in the following sections.

## SCOPE OF THEORY

One method for classification of theories in nursing that has become common is to differentiate theories based on scope, which refers to complexity and degree of abstraction. The scope of a theory includes its level of specificity and the concreteness of its concepts and propositions. This classification scheme typically uses the terms *metatheory, philosophy,* or *worldview* to describe the philosophical basis of the discipline, *grand theory* or *macrotheory* to describe the comprehensive conceptual

TABLE 2-3 *Significant Events in Theory Development in Nursing*

| Event | Year |
|---|---|
| Nightingale published *Notes on Nursing* | 1859 |
| American Medical Association advocated formal training for nurses | 1868 |
| Teacher's College—Columbia University—Doctorate in Education degree for nursing | 1920 |
| Yale University began the first collegiate school of nursing | 1924 |
| Report by Dr. Esther Brown—"Nursing for the Future" | 1948 |
| State licensure for registration became standard | 1949 |
| *Nursing Research* first published | 1950 |
| H. Peplau published *Interpersonal Relations in Nursing* | 1952 |
| University of Pittsburgh began the first PhD program in nursing | 1954 |
| Health Amendments Act passed—funded graduate nursing education | 1956 |
| Process of theory development discussed among nursing scholars (works published by Abdellah, Henderson, Orlando, Wiedenbach, and others) | 1960–1966 |
| First symposium on Theory Development in Nursing (published in *Nursing Research* in 1968) | 1967 |
| Symposium Theory Development in Nursing | 1968 |
| Dickoff, James, and Weidenbach—"Theory in a Practice Discipline" | |
| First Nursing Theory Conference | 1969 |
| Second Nursing Theory Conference | 1970 |
| Third Nursing Theory Conference | 1971 |
| National League for Nursing adopts Requirement for Conceptual Framework for Nursing Curricula | 1972 |
| Key articles published in *Nursing Research* (Hardy—Theories: Components, Development and Evaluation; Jacox—Theory Construction in Nursing; and Johnson—Development of Theory) | 1974 |
| Nurse educator conferences on nursing theory | 1975, 1978 |
| *Advances in Nursing Science* first published | 1979 |
| Books written for nurses on how to critique theory, develop theory, and apply nursing theory | 1980s |
| Graduate schools of nursing develop courses on how to analyze and apply theory in nursing | 1980s |
| Research studies in nursing identify nursing theories as frameworks for study | 1980s |
| Publication of numerous books on analysis, application, evaluation, and development of nursing theories | 1980s |
| Philosophy and philosophy of science courses offered in doctoral programs | 1990s |
| Increasing emphasis on middle range and practice theories for nursing | 1990s |
| Nursing literature described the need to establish interconnections among central nursing concepts | 1990s |
| *Philosophy of Nursing* first published | 1999 |
| Books published describing, analyzing, and discussing application of middle range theory and evidence-based practice | 2000s |

Sources: Bishop and Hardin (2006); Kalisch and Kalisch (2004); Kenney (1995); Meleis (2005); Moody (1990).

TABLE 2-4 *Chronology of Publications of Selected Nursing Theorists*

| Theorist | Year | Title of Theoretical Writings |
|---|---|---|
| Florence Nightingale | 1859 | *Notes on Nursing* |
| Hildegard Peplau | 1952 | *Interpersonal Relations in Nursing* |
| Virginia Henderson | 1955 | *Principles and Practice of Nursing,* 5th edition |
| | 1966 | *The Nature of Nursing: A Definition and Its Implications for Practice, Research and Education* |
| | 1991 | *The Nature of Nursing: Reflections After 25 Years* |
| Dorothy Johnson | 1959 | *A Philosophy of Nursing* |
| | 1980 | *The Behavioral System Model for Nursing* |
| Faye Abdellah | 1960 | *Patient-Centered Approaches to Nursing* |
| | 1968 | 2nd edition |
| Ida Jean Orlando | 1961 | *The Dynamic Nurse–Patient Relationship* |
| Ernestine Wiedenbach | 1964 | *Clinical Nursing: A Helping Art* |
| Lydia E. Hall | 1964 | *Nursing: What is it?* |
| Joyce Travelbee | 1966 | *Interpersonal Aspects of Nursing* |
| | 1971 | 2nd edition |
| Myra E. Levine | 1967 | *The Four Conservation Principles of Nursing* |
| | 1973 | *Introduction to Clinical Nursing* |
| | 1989 | *The Conservation Principles: Twenty Years Later* |
| Martha Rogers | 1970 | *An Introduction to the Theoretical Basis of Nursing* |
| | 1980 | *Nursing: A Science of Unitary Man* |
| | 1983 | *Science of Unitary Human Being: A Paradigm for Nursing* |
| | 1989 | *Nursing: A Science of Unitary Human Beings* |
| Dorthea E. Orem | 1971 | *Nursing: Concepts of Practice* |
| | 1980 | 2nd edition |
| | 1985 | 3rd edition |
| | 1991 | 4th edition |
| | 1995 | 5th edition |
| | 2001 | 6th edition |
| Imogene M. King | 1971 | *Toward a Theory for Nursing: General Concepts of Human Behavior* |
| | 1981 | *A Theory for Nursing: Systems, Concepts, Process* |
| | 1989 | *King's General Systems Framework and Theory* |
| Betty Neuman | 1974 | *The Betty Neuman Health-Care Systems Model: A Total Person Approach to Patient Problems* |
| | 1982 | *The Neuman Systems Model* |
| | 1989 | 2nd edition |
| | 1995 | 3rd edition |
| | 2002 | 4th edition |

TABLE 2-4 *Chronology of Publications of Selected Nursing Theorists (Continued)*

| Theorist | Year | Title of Theoretical Writings |
|---|---|---|
| Evelyn Adam | 1975 | *A Conceptual Model for Nursing* |
| | 1980 | *To Be a Nurse* |
| | 1991 | 2nd edition |
| Callista Roy | 1976 | *Introduction to Nursing: An Adaptation Model* |
| | 1980 | *The Roy Adaptation Model* |
| | 1984 | *Introduction to Nursing: An Adaptation Model,* 2nd edition |
| | 1991 | *The Roy Adaptation Model* |
| | 1999 | 2nd edition |
| Josephine Paterson and Loretta Zderad | 1976 | *Humanistic Nursing* |
| Jean Watson | 1979 | *Nursing: The Philosophy and Science of Caring* |
| | 1985 | *Nursing: Human Science and Human Care* |
| | 1989 | *Watson's Philosophy and Theory of Human Caring in Nursing* |
| | 1999 | *Human Science and Human Care* |
| Margaret A. Newman | 1979 | *Theory Development in Nursing* |
| | 1983 | *Newman's Health Theory* |
| | 1986 | *Health as Expanding Consciousness* |
| | 2000 | 2nd edition |
| Madeleine Leininger | 1980 | *Caring: A Central Focus of Nursing and Health Care Services* |
| | 1988 | *Leininger's Theory of Nursing: Cultural Care Diversity and Universality* |
| | 2001 | *Culture Care Diversity and Universality* |
| | 2006 | 2nd edition |
| Joan Riehl Sisca | 1980 | *The Riehl Interaction Model* |
| | 1989 | 2nd edition |
| Rosemary Parse | 1981 | *Man-Living-Health: A Theory for Nursing* |
| | 1985 | *Man-Living-Health: A Man-Environment Simultaneity Paradigm* |
| | 1987 | *Nursing Science: Major Paradigms, Theories, Critiques* |
| | 1989 | *Man-Living-Health: A Theory of Nursing* |
| | 1999 | *Illuminations: The Human Becoming Theory in Practice and Research* |
| Joyce Fitzpatrick | 1983 | *A Life Perspective Rhythm Model* |
| | 1989 | 2nd edition |
| Helen Erickson et al. | 1983 | *Modeling and Role Modeling* |
| Nancy Roper, Winifred Logan, and Alison Tierney | 1983 | *A Model for Nursing* |
| | 1983 | *The Roper/Logan/Tierney Model for Nursing* |
| | 1996 | *The Elements of Nursing: A Model for Nursing Based on a Model of Living* |
| | 2000 | *The Roper/Logan/Tierney Model for Nursing* |

*(Continued)*

TABLE 2-4 *Chronology of Publications of Selected Nursing Theorists (Continued)*

| Theorist | Year | Title of Theoretical Writings |
|---|---|---|
| Patricia Benner and Judith Wrubel | 1984 | *From Novice to Expert: Excellence and Power in Clinical Nursing Practice* |
| | 1989 | *The Primacy of Caring: Stress and Coping in Health and Illness* |
| Anne Boykin and Savina Schoenhofer | 1993 | *Nursing as Caring* |
| | 2001 | 2nd edition |
| Barbara Artinian | 1997 | *The Intersystem Model: Integrating Theory and Practice* |

Sources: Chinn and Kramer (2008); Hickman (2002); Hilton (1997).

frameworks, *middle range* or *midrange* theory to describe frameworks that are relatively more focused than the grand theories, and *microtheory, situation-specific theory,* or *practice theory* to describe those smallest in scope (Higgins & Moore, 2000; Peterson, 2008). Theories differ in complexity and scope along a continuum from microtheories to grand theories. Figure 2-1 compares the scope of nursing theory by level of abstractness.

### Metatheory

Metatheory refers to a theory about theory. In nursing, metatheory focuses on broad issues such as the processes of generating knowledge and theory development, and it is a forum for debate within the discipline (Chinn & Kramer, 2008; Powers & Knapp, 2006). Philosophical and methodologic issues at the metatheory or worldview level include identifying the purposes and kinds of theory needed for nursing, developing and analyzing methods for creating nursing theory, and proposing criteria for evaluating theory (Brix, 1993; Hickman, 2002; Walker & Avant, 2005).

Walker and Avant (2005) presented an overview of historical trends in nursing metatheory. Beginning in the 1960s, metatheory discussions involved nursing as an academic discipline and the relationship of nursing to basic sciences. Later discussions addressed the predominant philosophical worldviews (received view versus perceived view) and methodologic issues related to research (see Chapter 1). Recent metatheoretical issues relate to the philosophy of nursing and address what levels of theory development are needed for nursing practice, research, and education (i.e., grand theory versus middle range and practice theory) and the increasing focus on the philosophical perspectives of critical theory and feminism.

| Theory | Level of Abstraction |
|---|---|
| Metatheory | Most abstract |
| Grand theories | |
| Middle range theories | |
| Practice theories | Least abstract |

FIGURE 2-1 Comparison of the scope of nursing theories.

## Grand Theories

Grand theories are the most complex and broadest in scope. They attempt to explain broad areas within a discipline and may incorporate numerous other theories. The term *macrotheory* is used by some authors to describe a theory that is broadly conceptualized and is usually applied to a general area of a specific discipline (Higgins & Moore, 2000; Peterson, 2008).

Grand theories are nonspecific and comprised of relatively abstract concepts that lack operational definitions. Their propositions are also abstract and are not generally amenable to testing. Grand theories are developed through thoughtful and insightful appraisal of existing ideas as opposed to empirical research (Fawcett, 2000). The majority of the nursing conceptual frameworks (i.e., Orem, Roy, Rogers) are considered to be grand theories. Chapters 6 through 9 discuss many of the grand nursing theories.

## Middle Range Theories

Middle range theory lies between the nursing models and more circumscribed, concrete ideas (practice theories). Middle range theories are substantively specific and encompass a limited number of concepts and a limited aspect of the real world. They are comprised of relatively concrete concepts that are operationally defined and relatively concrete propositions that may be empirically tested (Higgins & Moore, 2000; Peterson, 2008; Whall, 2005).

Fawcett (2000) states that a middle range theory may be (1) a description of a particular phenomenon, (2) an explanation of the relationship between phenomena, or (3) a prediction of the effects of one phenomenon or another. Many investigators favor working with propositions and theories characterized as middle range rather than with conceptual frameworks because they provide the basis for generating testable hypotheses related to particular nursing phenomena and to particular client populations (Chinn & Kramer, 2008; Ketefian & Redman, 1997). Examples of middle range theories used in nursing include social support, quality of life, and health promotion. Chapters 10 and 11 describe middle range theory in detail.

## Practice Theories

Practice theories are also called microtheories, prescriptive theories, or situation-specific theories and are the least complex. Practice theories are more specific than middle range theories and produce specific directions for practice (Higgins & Moore, 2000; Peterson, 2008; Whall, 2005). They contain the fewest concepts and refer to specific, easily defined phenomena. They are narrow in scope, explain a small aspect of reality, and tend to be prescriptive. They are usually limited to specific populations or fields of practice and often use knowledge from other disciplines (McKenna, 1993). Examples of practice theories developed and used by nurses are theories of infant bonding and oncology pain management. Chapter 17 provides more information on practice theories.

## Partial Theories

Some writers also describe partial theories. *Partial theories* are those in the development stage. In a partial theory some concepts have been identified and some relationships between them have been identified, but the theory is not complete. Keck (1998) states, "theories derived from the social sciences, including nursing, are probably exclusively partial theories because there are few, if any, phenomena that have been totally and completely explained" (p. 23).

## TYPE OR PURPOSE OF THEORY

In their seminal work, Dickoff and James (1968) defined theories as intellectual inventions designed to describe, explain, predict, or prescribe phenomena. They described four kinds of theory, each of which builds on the other. These are:

- Factor-isolating theories (descriptive theories)
- Factor-relating theories (explanatory theories)
- Situation-relating theories (predictive theories or promoting or inhibiting theories)
- Situation-producing theories (prescriptive theories)

Dickoff and James (1968) stated that nursing as a profession should go beyond the level of descriptive or explanatory theories and attempt to attain the highest levels—that of situation-producing and situation-relating theories.

### Factor-Isolating Theories

Factor-isolating theories are those that describe, observe, and name concepts, properties, and dimensions. Descriptive theory identifies and describes the major concepts of phenomena but does not explain how or why the concepts are related. The purpose of factor-isolating theory is to provide observation and meaning regarding the phenomena. It is generated and tested by descriptive research techniques including concept analysis, case studies, literature review phenomenology, ethnography, and grounded theory (Fawcett, 1999; Young, Taylor, & Renpenning, 2001).

Examples of descriptive theories are readily found in the nursing literature. Bu and Jezewski (2006), for example, used the process of concept analysis to develop a middle range theory of patient advocacy. Using a grounded theory methodology, Sun and colleagues (2006) developed a theory-based guide to enable nurses to initiate and maintain therapeutic relationships and direct care for patients at risk for suicide. Weiss and others (2008) also used grounded theory to construct a theory explaining sexual decision-making behaviors and beliefs among adolescent females. Robles-Silva (2008) used ethnography to construct a conceptual model explaining the multiple phases that caregivers experience while working with poor, chronically ill adults in Mexico. Finally, comprehensive literature review was used by Register and Herman (2006) to develop a middle range theory for generative quality of life for elders and by Hess and Insel (2007) to develop a conceptual model for chemotherapy-related change in cognitive function.

### Factor-Relating Theories

Factor-relating theories, or explanatory theories, are those that relate concepts to one another, describe the interrelationships among concepts or propositions, and specify the associations or relationships among some concepts. Further explication of the logical and empirical adequacy of the relationships is necessary. They attempt to tell how or why the concepts are related and may deal with cause and effect and correlations or rules that regulate interactions. They are developed by correlational research (Fawcett, 1999).

An example of an explanatory theory is a proposed Theory of Diversity of Human Field Pattern (Hastings-Tolsma, 2006). This theory was developed from a descriptive, correlational study that examined the relationships between risk-taking behavior (e.g., change) and time movement, within the context of energy flow and field patterns. It was determined that risk-taking and time experience were specific patterns deemed indicative of the individual's participation in field patterning. Another example of an explanatory theory is the Thriving Model (Haight, Barba, Tesh, & Courts, 2002), which builds on previous work related to failure to thrive in elders by defining the constructs thriving and failure to thrive, and describing how thriving results from engagement, and supportive and harmonious concordance between the person and their human and nonhuman environments.

### Situation-Relating Theories

Situation-relating theories are achieved when the conditions under which concepts are related are stated and the relational statements are able to describe future outcomes consistently. Situation-relating theories move to prediction of precise relationships between concepts. Experimental research is used to generate and test them (Fawcett, 1999).

Predictive theories are relatively difficult to find in the nursing literature. In one example, Chang, Wung, and Crogan (2008) used a quasi-experimental research design to create a theoretical model supporting an intervention designed to improve elderly nursing home resident's ability to provide self-care. Their research validated the premise that the theory-based intervention improved performance of activities of daily living among residents in the study group compared with a control group.

Another example of a situation-relating or predictive theory in nursing can be found in the Caregiving Effectiveness Model. The process outlining development of this theory was described by Smith, Pace, Kochinda, Kleinbeck, Loehler, and Popkess-Vawter (2002) and combined numerous steps in theory construction and empirical testing and validation. In the model, caregiving effectiveness is dependent on the interface of a number of factors including the characteristics of the caregiver, interpersonal interactions between the patient and caregiver, and the educational preparedness of the caregiver, combined with adaptive factors such as economic stability, and the caregiver's own health status and family adaptation and coping mechanisms. The model itself graphically details the interaction of these factors and depicts how they collectively work to impact caregiving effectiveness.

### Situation-Producing Theories

Situation-producing theories are those that prescribe activities necessary to reach defined goals. Prescriptive theories address nursing therapeutics and consequences of interventions. They include propositions that call for change and predict consequences of nursing interventions. They should describe the prescription, the consequence(s), the type of client, and conditions (Meleis, 2005).

Prescriptive theories are among the most difficult to identify in the nursing literature. One example is a work by Auvil-Novak (1997) that presented the development of a middle range theory of chronotherapeutic intervention for postsurgical pain based on three experimental studies of pain relief among postsurgical clients. The theory uses a time-dependent approach to pain assessment and provides directed nursing interventions to address postoperative pain.

## Issues in Theory Development in Nursing

A number of issues related to use of theory in nursing have received significant attention in the literature. The first is the issue of borrowed versus unique theory in nursing. A second issue is nursing's metaparadigm, and a third is the importance of the concept of caring in nursing.

## BORROWED VERSUS UNIQUE THEORY IN NURSING

Since the 1960s, the question of borrowing theory from other disciplines has been raised in the discussion of nursing theory. The debate over borrowed theory centers in the perceived need for theory unique to nursing discussed by many nursing theorists.

The main premise held by those opposed to borrowed theory is that only theories that are grounded in nursing should guide the actions of the discipline. A second premise that supports the need for unique theory is that any theory that evolves out of the practice arena of nursing is substantially nursing. Although one might borrow theory and apply it to the realm of nursing actions, it is transformed into nursing theory because it addresses phenomena within the arena of nursing practice.

Opponents of using borrowed theory believe that nursing knowledge should not be tainted by using theory from physiology, psychology, sociology, and education. Furthermore, they believe borrowing requires returning, and that the theory is not in essence nursing if concepts are borrowed (Levine, 1995).

Proponents of using borrowed theory in nursing believe that knowledge belongs to the scientific community and to society at large, and it is not the property of individuals or disciplines (Powers & Knapp, 2006). Indeed, these individuals feel that knowledge is not the private domain of one discipline, and the use of knowledge generated by any discipline is not borrowed, but shared. Further, shared theory does not lessen nursing scholarship, but enhances it (Levine, 1995).

Furthermore, advocates of borrowed or shared theory believe that, like other applied sciences, nursing depends on the theories from other disciplines for its theoretical foundations. For example, general systems theory is used in nursing, biology, sociology, and engineering. Different theories of stress and adaptation are valuable to nurses, psychologists, and physicians.

In reality, all nursing theories incorporate concepts and theories shared with other disciplines to guide theory development, research, and practice. However, simply adopting concepts or theories from another discipline does not convert them into nursing concepts or theories. It is important, therefore, for theorists, researchers, and practitioners to use concepts from other disciplines appropriately. Emphasis should be placed on redefining and synthesizing the concepts and theories according to a nursing perspective (Bowie, 2003; Levine, 1995).

## NURSING'S METAPARADIGM

The most abstract and general component of the structural hierarchy of nursing knowledge is what Kuhn (1977) called the *metaparadigm*. A metaparadigm is the global perspective of a discipline that identifies the primary phenomena of interest to that discipline and explains how the discipline deals with those phenomena in a unique manner (Fawcett, 2000). The metaparadigm includes major philosophical orientations or worldviews of a discipline, the conceptual models and theories that guide research and other scholarly activities, and the empirical indicators that operationalize theoretical concepts (Fawcett & Malinski, 1996). The purpose or function of the metaparadigm is to summarize the intellectual and social missions of the discipline and place boundaries on the subject matter of that discipline (Kim, 1989). Fawcett and Malinski (1996) identified four requirements for a metaparadigm. These are listed in Box 2-1.

According to Fawcett and Malinski (1996), in the 1970s and early 1980s, a number of nursing scholars identified a growing consensus that the dominant phenomena within the science of nursing revolved around the concepts of man (person), health, environment, and nursing. Fawcett first wrote on the central concepts of nursing in 1978

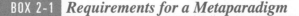

| BOX 2-1 | *Requirements for a Metaparadigm* |

1. A metaparadigm must identify a domain that is distinctive from the domains of other disciplines—the concepts and propositions represent a unique perspective for inquiry and practice.
2. A metaparadigm must encompass all phenomena of interest to the discipline in a parsimonious manner—the concepts and propositions are global and there are no redundancies in concepts or propositions.
3. A metaparadigm must be perspective-neutral—the concepts and propositions do not represent a specific perspective (i.e., a specific paradigm or conceptual model or combination)
4. A metaparadigm must be international in scope and substance—the concepts and propositions do not reflect particular national, cultural, or ethnic beliefs and values.

and formalized them as the metaparadigm of nursing in 1984. This articulation of four metaparadigm concepts (person, health, environment, and nursing) served as an organizing framework around which conceptual development proceeded (Thorne et al., 1998).

Wagner (1986) examined the nursing metaparadigm in depth. Her sample of 160 doctorate-prepared chairpersons, deans, or directors of programs for bachelor's of science in nursing revealed that between 94% and 98% of the respondents agreed that the concepts that comprise the nursing metaparadigm are person, health, nursing, and environment. She concluded that these findings indicated a consensus within the discipline of nursing that these are the dominant phenomena within the science. A summary of definitions for each term is presented here.

*Person* refers to a being composed of physical, intellectual, biochemical, and psychosocial needs; a human energy field; a holistic being in the world; an open system; an integrated whole; an adaptive system; and a being who is greater than the sum of his parts (Wagner, 1986). Nursing theories are often most distinguishable from each other by the various ways in which they conceptualize the person or recipient of nursing care. Although some nursing writers have expanded to include family or community as the focus, most nursing models organize data about the individual person as a focus of the nurse's attention (Thorne et al., 1998).

*Health* is the ability to function independently; successful adaptation to life's stressors; achievement of one's full life potential; and unity of mind, body, and soul (Wagner, 1986). Health has been a phenomenon of central interest to nursing since its inception. Nursing literature indicates great diversity in the explication of health and quality of life (Thorne et al., 1998).

*Environment* typically refers to the external elements that affect the person; internal and external conditions that influence the organism; significant others with whom the person interacts; and an open system with boundaries that permit the exchange of matter, energy, and information with human beings (Wagner, 1986). Many nursing theories have a narrow conceptualization of the environment as the immediate surroundings or circumstances of the individual. This view limits understanding by making the environment rigid, static, and natural. A multilayered view of the environment encourages understanding of an individual's perspective and immediate context and incorporates the sociopolitical and economic structures and underlying ideologies that influence reality (Thorne et al., 1998).

*Nursing* is a science, an art, and a practice discipline, and involves caring. Goals of nursing include care of the well, care of the sick, assisting with self-care activities, helping individuals attain their human potential, and discovering and using nature's laws of health. The purposes of nursing care include placing the client in the best condition for nature to restore health, promoting the adaptation of the individual, facilitating the development of an interaction between the nurse and the client in which jointly set goals are met, and promoting harmony between the individual and the environment (Wagner, 1986). Furthermore, nursing practice facilitates, supports, and assists individuals, families, communities, and societies to enhance, maintain, and recover health and to reduce and ameliorate the effects of illness (Thorne et al., 1998).

In addition to these definitions, many grand nursing theorists, and virtually all of the theoretical commentators, incorporate these four terms into their conceptual or theoretical frameworks. Table 2-5 presents theoretical definitions of the metaparadigm concepts from selected nursing conceptual frameworks and other writings.

### Relationships Among the Metaparadigm Concepts

The concepts of nursing's metaparadigm have been linked in four propositions identified in the writings of Donaldson and Crowley (1978) and Gortner (1980). These are as follows:

1. Person and health: Nursing is concerned with the principles and laws that govern the life-process, well-being, and optimal functioning of human beings, sick or well.
2. Person and environment: Nursing is concerned with the patterning of human behavior in interaction with the environment in normal life events and critical life situations.
3. Health and nursing: Nursing is concerned with the nursing action or processes by which positive changes in health status are effected.
4. Person, environment, and health: Nursing is concerned with the wholeness or health of human beings, recognizing that they are in continuous interaction with their environments (Fawcett & Malinski, 1996).

In addressing how the four concepts meet the requirements for a metaparadigm, Fawcett and Malinski (1996) state that the first three propositions represent recurrent themes identified in the writings of Nightingale and other nursing scholars. Furthermore, the four concepts and propositions identify the unique focus of the discipline of nursing and encompass all relevant phenomena in a parsimonious manner. Finally, the concepts and propositions are perspective-neutral because they do not reflect a specific paradigm or conceptual model and they do not reflect the beliefs and values of any one country or culture.

### Other Viewpoints on Nursing's Metaparadigm

There is some dissension in the acceptance of person/health/environment/nursing as nursing's metaparadigm. Kim (1987, 1989) identified four domains (client, client–nurse, practice, and environment) as an organizing framework or typology of nursing. In this framework, the most significant difference appears to be in placing health issues (i.e., health care experiences and health care environment) within the client domain and differentiating the nursing practice domain from the client–nurse domain. The latter focuses specifically on interactions between the nurse and the client.

Meleis (2005) maintained that nursing encompasses seven central concepts: interaction, nursing client, transitions, nursing process, environment, nursing therapeutics, and health. Addition of the concepts of interaction, transitions, and nursing

TABLE 2-5 *Selected Theoretical Definitions of the Concepts of Nursing's Metaparadigm*

| Metaparadigm Concept | Author/Source of Definition | Definition |
|---|---|---|
| Person/human being/client | D. Johnson | A behavioral system with patterned, repetitive, and purposeful ways of behaving that link person to the environment. |
| | B. Neuman | A dynamic composite of the interrelationships between physiological, psychological, sociocultural, developmental, spiritual, and basic structure variables. May be an individual, group, community, or social system. |
| | D. Orem | Are distinguished from other living things by their capacity (1) to reflect upon themselves and their environment, (2) to symbolize what they experience, and (3) to use symbolic creations (ideas, words) in thinking, in communicating, and in guiding efforts to do and to make things that are beneficial for themselves or others. |
| | M. Rogers | An irreducible, indivisible, pandimensional energy field identified by pattern and manifesting characteristics that are specific to the whole and that cannot be predicted from knowledge of the parts. |
| Nursing | M. Leininger | A learned humanistic and scientific profession and discipline that is focused on human care phenomena and activities to assist, support, facilitate, or enable individuals or groups to maintain or regain their well-being (or health) in culturally meaningful and beneficial ways, or to help people face handicaps or death. |
| | M. Newman | Caring in the human health experience. |
| | D. Orem | A specific type of human service required whenever the maintenance of continuous self-care requires the use of special techniques and the application of scientific knowledge in providing care or in designing it. |
| | J. Watson | A human science of persons and human health–illness experiences that are mediated by professional, personal, scientific, esthetic, and ethical human care transactions. |
| Health | M. Leininger | A state of well-being that is culturally defined, valued, and practiced, and that reflects the ability of individuals (or groups) to perform their daily role activities in culturally expressed, beneficial, and patterned lifeways. |
| | M. Newman | A pattern of evolving, expanding consciousness regardless of the form or direction it takes. |
| | C. Roy | A state and process of being and becoming an integrated and whole person. It is a reflection of adaptation, that is, the interaction of the person and the environment. |
| | J. Watson | Unity and harmony within the mind, body, and soul. Health is also associated with the degree of congruence between the self as perceived and the self as experienced. |
| Environment | M. Leininger | The totality of an event, situation, or particular experience that gives meaning to human expressions, interpretations, and social interactions in particular physical, ecologic, sociopolitical, and cultural settings. |

*(Continued)*

TABLE 2-5 *Selected Theoretical Definitions of the Concepts of Nursing's Metaparadigm (Continued)*

| Metaparadigm Concept | Author/Source of Definition | Definition |
|---|---|---|
| | B. Neuman | All internal and external factors of influences that surround the client or client system. |
| | M. Rogers | An irreducible, pandimensional energy field identified by pattern and integral with the human field. |
| | C. Roy | All conditions, circumstances, and influences that surround and affect the development and behavior of human adaptive systems with particular consideration of person and earth resources. |

Sources: Johnson (1980); Leininger (1991); Neuman (1995); Newman (1990); Orem (2001); Rogers (1990); Roy and Andrews (1999); Watson (1985).

process denotes the greatest difference between this framework and the more commonly described person/health/environment/nursing framework.

## CARING AS A CENTRAL CONSTRUCT IN THE DISCIPLINE OF NURSING

A final debate that will be discussed in this chapter centers on the place of the concept of caring within the discipline and science of nursing. This debate has been escalating over the last decade and has been motivated by the perceived urgency of identifying nursing's unique contribution to the health care disciplines and revolves around the defining attributes and roles within the practice of nursing (Thorne et al., 1998).

The concept of caring has occupied a prominent position in nursing literature and has been touted as the essence of nursing by renowned nursing scholars including Leininger, Watson, and Erikkson. Indeed, it has been proposed that nursing be defined as the study of caring in the human health experience (Newman, Sime, & Corcoran-Perry, 1991).

Although some theorists (i.e., Watson, Leininger, and Boykin) have gone so far as to identify caring as the essence of nursing, there is little if any rejection of caring as *a* central concept for nursing, although not necessarily *the* most significant concept. Thorne and colleagues (1998) cited three major areas of contention in the debate about caring in nursing. The first is the diverse views on the nature of caring. These range from caring as a human trait to caring as a therapeutic intervention and differ according to whether the act of caring is conceptualized as being client-centered, nurse-centered, or both.

A second major issue in the caring debate concerns the use of caring terminology to conceptualize a specialized role. It has been asked whether there is a compelling reason to lay claim to caring as nursing's unique domain when so many professions describe their function as involving caring, and the concept of caring is prominent in the work of many other disciplines (e.g., medicine, social work, psychology) (Thorne et al., 1998).

A third issue centers around the implications for the future development of the profession should nursing espouse caring as its unique mandate. It has been observed that nurses should ask themselves if it is politically astute to be the primary interpreters of a construct that is both gendered and devalued (Meadows, 2007; Thorne et al., 1998).

Thus, it is argued by Fawcett and Maliniski (1996) that although caring is included in several conceptualizations of the discipline of nursing, it is not a dominant term in every conceptualization and therefore does not represent a discipline-wide viewpoint. Furthermore caring is not uniquely a nursing phenomenon, and caring behaviors may not be generalizable across national and cultural boundaries.

## Summary

Like Matt Ng, the graduate nursing student described in the opening case study, nurses who are in a position to learn more about theory, and to recognize how and when to apply it, must often be convinced of the relevance of such study and to understand the benefits. The study of theory requires exposure to many new concepts, principles, thoughts, and ideas, as well as a student who is willing to see how theory plays an important role in nursing practice, research, education, and administration.

Although study and use of theoretical concepts in nursing dates back to Nightingale, little progress in theory development was made until the 1960s. Indeed, the past five decades have produced significant advancement in theory development for nursing. This chapter has presented an overview of this evolutionary process. In addition, the basic types of theory and purposes of theory were described. Subsequent chapters will explain many of the concepts introduced here to assist advanced practice nurses to understand the relationship among theory, practice, and research and to further develop the discipline, the science, and the profession of nursing.

## LEARNING ACTIVITIES

1. Examine early issues of *Nursing Research* (1950s and 1960s) and determine whether theories or theoretical frameworks were used as a basis for research. What types of theories were used? Review current issues to analyze how this has changed.

2. Examine early issues of *American Journal of Nursing* (1900–1950). Determine if and how theories were used in nursing practice. What types of theories were used? Review current issues to analyze how this has changed.

3. Find reports that present middle range or practice theories in the nursing literature. Identify if these theories are descriptive, explanatory, predictive, or prescriptive in nature.

4. With classmates, debate whether caring should or should not be part of the nursing metaparadigm.

## INTERNET RESOURCES

The Hahn School of Nursing Theory Page—contains links to sites for information on many grand and middle range nursing theories.
http://www.sandiego.edu/academics/nursing/theory/

Nurse Scribe's Nursing Theory Page—contains links to many grand nursing theorists' home pages as well as links to other reference materials related to nursing theory.
http://www.enursescribe.com/nurse_theorists.htm

Clayton College Department of Nursing's Nursing Theory Link Page—contains comprehensive links to sites containing information for grand and middle range nursing theories.
http://healthsci.clayton.edu/eichelberger/nursing.htm

## REFERENCES

Alligood, M. R. (2006). Introduction to nursing theory: Its history, significance and analysis. In A. M. Tomey & M. R. Alligood (Eds.), *Nursing theorists and their work* (6th ed., pp. 3–15). St. Louis: Mosby.

American Association of Colleges of Nursing (AACN). (2008). Institutions offering doctoral programs in nursing and degrees conferred, Fall, 2007. Available at: http://www.aacn.nche.edu/IDS/pdf/DOC.pdf. Accessed July 30, 2008.

Andrist, L. C. (2006). The history of the relationship between feminism and nursing. In L. C. Andrist, P. K. Nicholas, & K. A. Wolfe (Eds.), *A history of nursing ideas.* Boston: Jones & Bartlett Publishers.

Auvil-Novak, S. E. (1997). A middle range theory of chronotherapeutic intervention for postsurgical pain. *Nursing Research, 46*(2), 66–71.

Bishop, S. M., & Hardin, S. R. (2006). History and philosophy of science. In A. M. Tomey & M. R. Alligood (Eds.), *Nursing theorists and their work* (6th ed., pp. 16–24). St. Louis: Mosby.

Blackburn, S. (2005). *Oxford dictionary of philosophy.* New York: Oxford University Press.

Bowie, B. H. (2003). Letter to the editor. *Nursing Science Quarterly, 16*(3), 279.

Brix, E. C. (1993). Critical thinking and theory-based practice. *Holistic Nursing Practice, 7*(3), 21–27.

Bu, X., & Jezewski, M. A. (2006). Developing a mid-range theory of patient advocacy through concept analysis. *Journal of Advanced Nursing, 57*(110), 101–112.

Chang, S. H., Wung, S. F., & Crogan, N. L. (2008). Improving activities of daily living for nursing home elder persons in Taiwan. *Nursing Research, 57*(3), 191–198.

Chinn, P. L., & Kramer, M. K. (2008). *Integrated theory and knowledge development in nursing* (7th ed.). St. Louis: Mosby.

DeKeyser, F. G., & Medoff-Cooper, B. (2001). A nontheorist's perspective on nursing theory: Issues of the 1990s. *Scholarly Inquiry for Nursing Practice: An International Journal, 15*(4), 329–341.

Dickoff, J., & James, P. (1968). A theory of theories: A position paper. *Nursing Research, 17*(3), 197–203.

Donaldson, S. K., & Crowley, D. M. (1978). The discipline of nursing. *Nursing Outlook, 26*(2), 113–120.

Fawcett, J. (1992). Contemporary conceptualizations of nursing: Philosophy or science? In J. F. Kikuchi & H. Simmons (Eds.), *Philosophic inquiry in nursing* (pp. 64–70). Newbury Park, CA: Sage.

Fawcett, J. (1993). *Analysis and evaluation of nursing theories.* Philadelphia: Davis.

Fawcett, J. (1999). *The relationship of theory and research* (3rd ed.). Philadelphia: Davis.

Fawcett, J. (2000). *Analysis and evaluation of contemporary nursing knowledge: Nursing models and theories.* Philadelphia: Davis.

Fawcett, J., & Malinski, V. M. (1996). On the requirements for a metaparadigm: An invitation to dialogue. *Nursing Science Quarterly, 9*(3), 94–97, 100–101.

Gortner, S. R. (1980). Nursing science in transition. *Nursing Research, 29*(3), 180–183.

Haight, B. K., Barba, B. E., Tesh, A. S., & Courts, N. F. (2002). Thriving: A life span theory. *Journal of Gerontological Nursing, 28*(3), 14–22.

Hastings-Tolsma, M. (2006). Toward a theory of diversity of human field pattern. *Visions, 14*(2), 34–46.

Hess, L. M., & Insel, K. C. (2007). Chemotherapy-related change in cognitive function: A conceptual model. *Oncology Nursing Forum, 34*(5), 981–990.

Hickman, J. S. (2002). An introduction to nursing theory. In J. George (Ed.), *Nursing theories: The base for professional nursing practice* (5th ed., pp. 1–20). Upper Saddle River, NJ: Prentice-Hall.

Higgins, P. A., & Moore, S. M. (2000). Levels of theoretical thinking in nursing. *Nursing Outlook, 48*(4), 179–183.

Hilton, P. A. (1997). Theoretical perspective of nursing: A review of the literature. *Journal of Advanced Nursing, 26*(6), 1211–1220.

Johnson, D. E. (1980). The behavioral system model for nursing. In J. P. Riehl & C. Roy (Eds.), *Conceptual models for nursing practice* (2nd ed., pp. 209–216). New York: Appleton-Century-Crofts.

Kalisch, P. A., & Kalisch, B. J. (2004). *The advance of American nursing* (4th ed.). Philadelphia: Lippincott Williams & Wilkins.

Keck, J. F. (1998). Terminology of theory development. In A. M. Tomey & M. R. Alligood (Eds.), *Nursing theorists and their work* (4th ed., pp. 16–24). St. Louis: Mosby.

Kenney, J. W. (1995). Relevance of theory-based nursing practice. In P. J. Christensen & J. W. Kenney (Eds.), *Nursing process: Application of conceptual models* (4th ed., pp. 3–17). St. Louis: Mosby.

Ketefian, S., & Redman, R. W. (1997). Nursing science in the global community. *Image: Journal of Nursing Scholarship, 29*(1), 11–16.

Kidd, P., & Morrison, E. F. (1988). The progression of knowledge in nursing research: A search for meaning. *Image: Journal of Nursing Scholarship, 20*(4), 222–224.

Kim, H. S. (1987). Structuring the nursing knowledge system: A typology of four domains. *Scholarly Inquiry for Nursing Practice, 1*(2), 99–110.

Kim, H. S. (1989). Theoretical thinking in nursing: Problems and prospects. *Recent Advances in Nursing, 24,* 106–122.

Kuhn, T. S. (1977). Second thought on paradigms. In F. Suppe (Ed.), *The structure of scientific theory* (pp. 459–482). Urbana, IL: University of Illinois Press.

Leininger, M. (1991). *Culture care diversity and universality: A theory of nursing.* New York: National League for Nursing.

Levine, M. E. (1995). The rhetoric of nursing theory. *Image: Journal of Nursing Scholarship, 27*(1), 11–14.

McKenna, G. (1993). Unique theory—Is it essential in the development of a science of nursing? *Nurse Education Today, 15,* 121–127.

Meadows, R. (2007). Beyond caring. *Nursing Administration Quarterly, 31*(2), 158–161.

Meleis, A. I. (2005). *Theoretical nursing: Development and progress* (3rd ed.). Philadelphia: Lippincott Williams & Wilkins.

Moody, L. E. (1990). *Advancing nursing science through research*. Newbury Park, CA: Sage.

Neuman, B. (1995). *The Neuman systems model* (3rd ed.). Norwalk, CT: Appleton & Lange.

Newman, M. A. (1990). Newman's theory of health as praxis. *Nursing Science Quarterly, 3*(1), 37–41.

Newman, M. A., Sime, A. M., & Corcoran-Perry, S. A. (1991). The focus of the discipline of nursing. *Advances in Nursing Science, 14*(1), 1–6.

Omrey, A., Kasper, C. E., & Page, G. G. (1995). *In search of nursing science*. Thousand Oaks, CA: Sage.

Orem, D. E. (2001). *Nursing: Concepts of practice* (6th ed.). St. Louis: Mosby.

Peplau, H. (1952). *Interpersonal relations in nursing*. New York: Putnam's Sons.

Peterson, S. J. (2008). Introduction to the nature of nursing knowledge. In S. J. Peterson & T. S. Bredow (Eds.), *Middle range theories: Application to nursing research* (2nd ed., pp. 3–41). Philadelphia: Lippincott Williams & Wilkins.

Powers, B. A., & Knapp, T. R. (2006). *A dictionary of nursing theory and research* (3rd ed.). New York: Springer Publishing.

Register, M. E., & Herman, J. (2006). A middle range theory of generative quality of life for the elderly. *Advances in Nursing Science, 29*(4), 340–350.

Robles-Silva, L. (2008). The caregiving trajectory among poor and chronically ill people. *Qualitative Health Research, 18*(3), 358–368.

Rogers, M. E. (1990). Nursing: Science of unitary, irreducible, human beings: Update 1990. In E. A. M. Barrett (Ed.), *Visions of Rogers' science-based nursing* (pp. 5–11). New York: National League for Nursing.

Roy, C., & Andrews, H. A. (1999). *The Roy adaptation model* (2nd ed.). Norwalk, CT: Appleton & Lange.

Rutty, J. E. (1998). The nature of philosophy of science, theory and knowledge relating to nursing and professionalism. *Journal of Advanced Nursing, 28*(2), 243–250.

Smith, C. E., Pace, K., Kochinda, C., Kleinbeck, S. V. M., Loehler, J., & Popkess-Vawter, S. (2002). Caregiving effectiveness model evolution to a midrange theory of home care: A process for critique and replication. *Advances in Nursing Science, 25*(1), 50–64.

Streubert-Speziale, H. J., & Carpenter, D. R. (2006). *Qualitative research in nursing: Advancing the humanistic imperative* (4th ed.). Philadelphia: Lippincott Williams & Wilkins.

Sun, F. K., Long, A., Boore, J., & Tsao, L. I. (2006). A theory for the nursing care of patients at risk of suicide. *Journal of Advanced Nursing, 53*(6), 680–690.

Thorne, S., Canam, C., Dahinten, S., Hall, W., Henderson, A., & Kirkham, S. R. (1998). Nursing's metaparadigm concepts: Disimpacting the debates. *Journal of Advanced Nursing, 27*(6), 1257–1268.

Tierney, A. F. (1998). Nursing models: Extant or extinct? *Journal of Advanced Nursing, 28*(1), 77–85.

Tomey, A. M., & Alligood, M. R. (2006). *Nursing theorists and their work* (6th ed.). St. Louis: Mosby.

Wagner, J. (1986). *Nurse scholar's perceptions of nursing's metaparadigm*. Dissertation, Ohio State University.

Walker, L. O., & Avant, K. C. (2005). *Strategies for theory construction in nursing* (4th ed.). Upper Saddle River, NJ: Prentice-Hall.

Watson, J. (1985). *Nursing: Human science and human care*. Norwalk, CT: Appleton-Century-Crofts.

Weiss, J. A., Jampol, M. L., Lievano, J. A., Smith, S. M., & Wurster, J. L. (2008). Normalizing risky sexual behaviours: A grounded theory study. *Pediatric Nursing, 34*(2), 163–167.

Whall, A. L. (2005). The structure of nursing knowledge: Analysis and evaluation of practice, middle range and grand theory. In J. J. Fitzpatrick & A. L. Whall (Eds.), *Conceptual models of nursing: Analysis and application* (4th ed., pp. 5–20). Upper Saddle River, NJ: Prentice-Hall.

Young, A., Taylor, S. G., & Renpenning, K. M. (2001). *Connections: Nursing research, theory and practice*. St. Louis: Mosby.

Ziegler, S. M. (2005). *Theory-directed nursing practice* (2nd ed.). New York: Springer Publishing.

# 3

# Concept Development: Clarifying Meaning of Terms

## Evelyn Wills and Melanie McEwen

*M*ary Talbot is a home health nurse with several years of experience. Recently Mary was assigned to care for Mrs. Janet Benson, who had had a mastectomy. The pathology report revealed a slow-growing, noninvasive carcinoma in situ; there were no involved nodes, and further tests showed no metastasis. Mrs. Benson was thankful that she was most likely free of the disease.

In the hospital, Mrs. Benson progressed well. But after she was discharged and began chemotherapy, she would frequently weep over things that seemed trivial. Her husband called Mary because he was concerned as this was not Mrs. Benson's usual behavior. Typically, she was self-contained, stoic, and accepting of life's circumstances, seldom demonstrating excessive emotion. To try to better understand Mrs. Benson's response, and to plan care accordingly, Mary consulted Rebecca Wallis, a certified oncology nurse specialist (ONS). After discussing the case with Mary, Rebecca set up an appointment with the Bensons. To gather data from both Mr. and Mrs. Benson's viewpoints, Rebecca asked each of them to explain how they felt about Mrs. Benson's cancer. Mr. Benson replied that the loss of his wife's breast was a small matter to him; he loved her for herself, and he was grateful that she was getting well.

Mrs. Benson seemed relieved by his pronouncement. In response to Rebecca's questioning, she focused on her sadness and inquired if this was common in women who had had a mastectomy. Rebecca explained that the reaction was quite common and that oncology nurses in the region used the term postmastectomy grief (PMG) reaction to describe it. The ONSs had worked out a protocol of nursing therapy for PMG, but it had not been formally tested. In the protocol they requested that the physician oncologist refer the patient to a psychiatric home health nurse for an assessment. The psychiatric home health nurse would confer with the oncologist and the nurse practitioner and, if needed, would request a referral to a licensed therapist. Additionally, a group called "Breast Cancer Support" had been organized in the area by women who had undergone a mastectomy. In this group, problems such as sadness were discussed by women who had experienced them, and support given to those who were going through recovery from breast cancer surgery. Rebecca recommended that the Bensons attend a meeting.

*Mrs. Benson's case, and the problem of PMG reaction in general, prompted Rebecca to seek more information about this reaction of breast cancer patients. Her review of the literature suggested that the phenomena needed further study to develop the knowledge base for practice. Because of her education, she realized that she first needed to define and name the problem. To this end, she chose to use concept development strategies she had learned in her graduate nursing program to initiate preparation for a formal research study.*

---

Experienced nurses, although focused on the practical application of nursing knowledge, demonstrate an inclination toward generalizing what they have learned from a group of clients to other clients with similar problems. This is obvious in the professional discussions of clinical nurses, particularly those educated for advanced practice, who might state, "we see certain phenomenon frequently enough in practice that we have developed clinical protocols or interventions."

These observed phenomena are considered by nurses to be reliable, enduring, and stable features of practical experience, whether or not they have acquired a name and whether or not they have been studied in research (Kim, 2000, 2006). Expert practice and enhanced education lead advanced practice nurses to recognize commonalities in phenomena that suggest the need for inquiry. This, in turn, may guide development of clinical hypotheses and testing of interventions (Cutcliffe & Mckenna, 2005; Wilson & Raines, 1999). With the current focus on evidence-based practice, clear delineation of the concepts under study in research requires that the linkages among phenomena, concepts, and practice be clarified (Hupcey & Penrod, 2008).

For the nurse who desires to discriminately, formally, and concretely examine a phenomenon in depth, such as described above, the most logical place to start is by defining the phenomenon or concept for further study. This is not an easy task, however, and significant time, research, and effort must be made to adequately define nursing concepts (Duncan, Cloutier, & Baily, 2007; Kim, 2006). To simplify the process, a number of strategies and methods for concept analysis, concept development, and concept clarification have been proposed and used by nursing scholars for many years.

The rationale for concept development and several methods commonly used by nurses are discussed in this chapter. This will allow advanced practice nurses to develop or clarify meanings for the phenomena encountered in practice. The outcome can then serve as the basis for further development of theory for research and practice.

## The Concept of "Concept"

Concepts are terms that refer to phenomena that occur in nature or in thought. *Concept* has been defined as an abstract term derived from particular attributes (Kerlinger, 1986) and "a symbolic statement describing a phenomenon or a class of phenomena" (Kim, 2000, p. 15). Concepts may be abstract (e.g., hope, love, desire) or relatively concrete (e.g., airplane, body temperature, pain). Concepts are formulated in words that enable people to communicate their meanings about realities in the world (Cutcliff & McKenna, 2005; Kim, 2000; Parse, 1999; Penrod & Hupcey, 2005) and give meaning to phenomena that can directly or indirectly be seen, heard, tasted, smelled, or touched (Fawcett, 1999). A concept may be a word (e.g., grief, empathy, power, pain), two words (e.g., job satisfaction, need fulfilment, role strain), or a phrase (e.g., maternal role attachment, biomarkers of preterm labor, health-promoting behaviors). Finally, when they are operationalized, concepts become variables used in hypotheses to be tested in research.

Concepts have been compared to bricks in a wall that lend structure to science (Hardy, 1973). Chinn and Kramer (2008) believe that concepts are more than terms, and constructing conceptual meaning is a vital approach to theory building in which mental constructions or ideas are used to represent experiences. Similarly, Parse (2006) agrees that formal study of concepts enhances knowledge development for nursing through naming, creating, and confirming the phenomena of interest.

Although it was once thought that concepts could be defined once and for all, that idea has been disputed (Penrod & Hupcey, 2005; Rodgers & Knafl, 2000). Theorists now understand that conceptual meaning is created by scholars to assist in imparting the meaning to their readers and, ultimately, to benefit the discipline. Conceptual fluidity and dependence on the context is common in writings on concept analysis in current literature (Duncan, Cloutier, & Bailey, 2007; Penrod & Hupcey, 2005). This makes it imperative that scholars and researchers define concepts clearly and distinctly so that their readers may thoroughly and accurately comprehend their work. Because conceptual meanings are dynamic, they should be defined for each specific use the writer or researcher makes of the term. Indeed, concepts are defined and their meanings are understood only within the framework of the theory of which they are a part (Hardy, 1973).

## TYPES OF CONCEPTS

Concepts explicate the subject matter of the theories of a discipline. For example, concepts from psychology include personality, intelligence, and cognition; concepts from biology include cell, species, and protoplasm (Jacox, 1974). Dubin (1978) explained the differences between various types of concepts, characterizing them as enumerative, associative, relational, statistical, and summative. Table 3-1 shows characteristics and examples of each of these types of concepts.

In nursing, concepts have been borrowed or derived from other disciplines (i.e., adaptation, culture, homeostasis) as well as developed directly from nursing practice and research (i.e., maternal–infant bonding, health-promoting behaviors, breastfeeding

TABLE 3-1 *Types of Concepts*

| Concept | Characteristics | Examples |
|---|---|---|
| Enumerative concepts | Are always present and universal | Age, height, weight |
| Associative concepts | Exist only in some conditions within a phenomenon; may have a zero value | Income, presence of disease, anxiety |
| Relational concepts | Can be understood only through the combination or interaction of two or more enumerative or associative concepts | Elderly (must combine concepts of age and longevity) Mother (must combine man, woman, and birth) |
| Statistical concepts | Relate the property of one thing in terms of its distribution in the population rate | Average blood pressure HIV/AIDS prevalence rate |
| Summative concepts | Represent an entire complex entity of a phenomenon; are complex and not measurable | Nursing, health, and environment |

Source: Dubin (1978).

attrition). In nursing literature, concepts have been categorized in several ways. For example, they have been described as concrete or abstract, variable or nonvariable (Hardy, 1973), and as operationally or theoretically defined.

### Abstract Versus Concrete Concepts

Concepts may be viewed on a continuum from concrete (specific) to abstract (general). At one end of the continuum are concrete concepts, which have simple, directly observable empirical referents, that can be seen, felt, or heard (e.g., a chair, the color red, jazz music). Concrete concepts are limited by time and space and are observable in reality.

At the other end of the continuum are abstract concepts (i.e., art, social support, personality, role). These are not clearly observable directly or indirectly and must be defined in terms of observable concepts (Jacox, 1974). Abstract concepts are independent of time and space. The more abstract a concept is, the more it transcends time and geography (Meleis, 2007).

Some concepts are formed from direct experiences with reality, whereas others are formed from indirect experiences. Relatively concrete or "empirical" concepts are formed from direct observations of objects, properties, or events. Concepts describing objects (i.e., desk or dog) or properties (i.e., cold, hard) are more empirical because the object or property that represents the idea (the empirical indicator) can be directly observed. Slightly more abstract properties such as height, weight, and gender can also be observed or measured.

As concepts become more abstract, their empirical indicators become less concrete and less directly measurable, and assessment of abstract concepts increasingly depends on indirect measures. For example, cardiovascular fitness, social support, and self-esteem are not directly observable properties or objects. To study these and similar concepts, their empirical referents must be defined and means must be identified or developed to measure them.

### Variable (Continuous) Versus Nonvariable (Discrete) Concepts

Concepts may be categorized as variable or nonvariable (Hardy, 1973). Concepts that describe phenomena according to some dimensions of the phenomena are termed *variables*. A discrete (noninterval level) concept identifies categories or classes of characteristics. Discrete concepts include gender, ethnic background, religion, and marital status. Discrete variables can be single variable categories that may be answered as "yes" or "no" (i.e., either one is pregnant or not pregnant; one is a nurse or is not a nurse), or fits into a predefined category (e.g., religion, marital status, educational attainment).

Continuous (variable) concepts permit classification of dimension or graduation of phenomena on a continuum (i.e., blood pressure, pain) (Bishop, 2002). Variable concepts include sex-role orientation, level of well-being, and degree of cultural identity (Meleis, 2007). An examination of recent nursing research led to numerous examples of continuous or variable concepts that were being studied. These included the concepts of hope, quality of life, resilience, and grief. In each case, the concept was defined operationally and measured by tools, scales, or some other indicator to show where the respondent's level of the variable fell relative to others or relative to a predefined norm.

### Theoretically Versus Operationally Defined Concepts

Concepts may be theoretically or operationally defined. A theoretical definition gives meaning to a term in context of a theory and permits any reader to assess the validity of the definition. The operational definition tells how the concept is linked to concrete situations and describes a set of procedures that will be performed to assign a value for the concept. Operational definitions permit the concept to be measured and allow hypotheses to be tested. Thus, operational definitions form the bridge

TABLE 3-2 *Examples of Theoretically and Operationally Defined Concepts*

| Concept | Theoretical Definition | Operational Definition | Source |
|---|---|---|---|
| Spirituality | An awareness of one's inner self and a sense of connection to a higher being, nature, others, or to some purpose greater than oneself | Score on the Spiritual Perspectives Scale | Humphreys, J. (2000). Spirituality and distress in sheltered battered women. *Image: The Journal of Nursing Scholarship, 32*(3), 273–278. |
| Quality of life | A complex, multidimensional concept in which a person's sense of well-being stems from satisfaction or dissatisfaction with the areas of life that are most important to him/her | Score on the Quality of Life Index | Schreier, A. M., & Williams, S. A. (2004). Anxiety and quality of life in women who receive radiation or chemotherapy for breast cancer. *Oncology Nursing Forum, 31*(1), 127–130. |
| Abuse | Any intentional physical attack by a perpetrator that resulted in injury or pain | Score on the Abuse Assessment Screen | Dunn, L. L., & Oths, K. S. (2004). Prenatal predictors of intimate partner abuse. *Journal of Obstetric Gynecology, and Neonatal Nursing, 33*(1), 54–63. |
| Coping | Cognitive and behavioral efforts to manage specific external and/or internal demands that are appraised as taxing and exceeding the resources of the person | Score on the Coping Health Inventory for Children | Vinson, J. A. (2002). Children with asthma: Initial developing of the child resilience model. *Pediatric Nursing, 28*(2), 149–157. |
| Self-esteem | A persons' sense of self-worth or value | Score on the Rosenberg Self-Esteem Scale | Wesley, Y. (2003). Desire for children among black women with and without HIV infection. *Journal of Nursing scholarship, 35*(1), 37–43. |

between the theory and the empirical world (Hardy, 1973). Examples of theoretically and operationally defined concepts are shown in Table 3-2.

## SOURCES OF CONCEPTS

When beginning a review of concepts found in nursing practice, research, education, and administration, one may look to several places or sources for relevant concepts. Indeed, the source of nursing concepts may be from the natural world, from research, or derived from other disciplines.

Naturalistic concepts are concepts seen in nature or in nursing practice such as body weight, thermoregulation, hematologic complications, depression, pain, and spirituality. These may be on a continuum from concrete to abstract and some may be measurable in fact (i.e., body weight, temperature) and others (i.e., pain or spirituality) measurable only indirectly and only in principle.

TABLE 3-3 *Sources of Concepts*

| Concept | Source | Characteristics | Examples from Nursing Literature |
|---------|--------|-----------------|----------------------------------|
| Naturalistic concepts | Present in nursing practice | May be defined and developed for use in research and theory development. Often have medical implications as well as nursing use | Body weight, pain, thermoregulation, depression, hematologic complications, circadian dysregulation |
| Research-based concepts | Developed through a qualitative research processes (i.e., grounded theory or existential phenomenology) | Often relate to a nursing specialty | Hope, grief, cultural competence, chronic pain |
| Existing concepts | Borrowed from other disciplines | Developed for nursing practice, but are useful in research and theory | Job satisfaction, quality of life, abuse, adaptation, stress |

Sources: Cowles and Rogers (1993); Parse (1999); Verhulst and Swartz-Barcott (1993); Wang (2000).

Research-based concepts are the result of conceptual development that is grounded in research processes. The theorist/researcher studies the realm of interest and identifies themes. Through qualitative, phenomenological, or grounded theory approaches, the researcher may uncover meanings of the phenomena of interest and their theoretical relationships (Parse, 1999; Rodgers, 2000). Examples include health-related quality of life (Ferrans, Zerwic, Wilbur, & Larson, 2005), grief (Reed, 2003), cultural competence (Shu, 2004), and adaptation to chronic pain (Dunn, 2005).

Existing concepts are the final type of concept. The nursing literature is filled with adapted concepts, more or less well synthesized through derivation from other disciplines. Such concepts include human needs from Maslow's (1954) hierarchy of needs, and stress from Selye's (1956) physiologic theory of the stress of life. Theories of bodily function come from the study of physiology (Guyton & Hall, 1996). Borrowed concepts from medicine are clearly seen in clinical practice, especially in critical care areas of institutions. Other existing concepts commonly used in nursing research, administration, and practice are empathy, suffering, abuse, hope, and burnout. Table 3-3 summarizes the three sources of concepts for nursing.

## Concept Analysis/Concept Development

Concept analysis, concept development, concept synthesis, and other terms refer to the rigorous process of bringing clarity to the definition of the concepts used in science. Concept analysis and concept development are the terms used most commonly in nursing and are generally applied to the process of inquiry that examines concepts for their level of development as revealed by their internal structure, use, representativeness, and relationship to other concepts. Thus, concept analysis/concept development explores the meaning of concepts to promote understanding.

## PURPOSES OF CONCEPT DEVELOPMENT

Clarifying, recognizing, and defining concepts that describe phenomena is the purpose of concept development or concept analysis. These processes serve as the basis for development of conceptual frameworks and research studies.

Because a considerable portion of the conceptual basis of nursing theory, research, and practice has been constructed using concepts adopted from other disciplines, reexamination of these concepts for relevance and fit is important. The process of applying borrowed concepts may have altered their meaning, and it is important to review them for appropriateness of application (Hupcey, Morse, Lenz, & Tason, 1996). Also, as knowledge is continually developing, new concepts are being introduced and accepted, and concepts are continually being investigated and refined. Furthermore, some concepts are poorly defined with characteristics that have not been described, whereas other concepts that have been defined will present with inconsistency between the definition and its use in research (Morse, Hupcey, Mitcham, & Lenz, 1996).

In summary, concept analysis can be used to evaluate the level of maturity or development of nursing concepts by

- Identifying gaps in nursing knowledge
- Determining the need to refine or clarify a concept when it appears to have multiple meanings
- Evaluating the adequacy of competing concepts in their relation to other phenomena
- Examining the congruence between the definition of the concept and the way it has been operationalized
- Determining the fit between the definition of the concept and its clinical application (Morse et al., 1996)

## CONTEXT FOR CONCEPT DEVELOPMENT

In the course of nursing practice, and specifically in advanced nursing practice, multiple instances of a problem will be seen as shown in the opening case study. When talking among peers, nurses may clarify a problem so that colleagues can understand the situation. Eventually the nurse will develop a term, a word, or a phrase as a name for the problem. Thus begins the most elemental method for identifying a theoretical phenomena—concept naming.

In refining the phenomenon so that the phenomenon can be studied, the steps of the concept development process are instituted. In this process, instances of the phenomenon are collected, the similarities and differences between the concept being studied and other concepts are reviewed, and those that are material to the use of the concept are extracted and the concept is defined from its existence in nature (Lincoln & Guba, 1985). Isolating specific information from all the surrounding information (the context) is important, but nurses must see the concept emerging and take note of the context in which the concept occurs.

In the case study at the beginning of the chapter, the nurses recognized the problem of women with breast cancer and their periodic sadness and noted the context in which the phenomenon occurred. It was important to include only those situations that were relevant. Questions that might be asked to assess the context include: Did the women have nonsupportive husbands? Were their lives threatened by nodal involvement and metastasis? What were the previous experiences of the women with disease or injury? What is the history of cancer in the women's families?

## CONCEPT DEVELOPMENT AND CONCEPTUAL FRAMEWORKS

Once concepts have been identified, named, and developed, the practitioner can test them in descriptive studies, particularly qualitative studies to further develop the concept and make explicit its use in real situations. The concept can be analyzed for its relation to many facets of the nursing discipline and the meaning made explicit for the nurse's use in daily work or scholarly endeavors.

Conceptual frameworks are structures that relate concepts together in a meaningful way. Although relationships are posited in conceptual frameworks, frequently neither the direction nor the strength of the relationships is made explicit for use in practice or for testing in a research project (Meleis, 2007). Chapter 4 provides a detailed discussion of the processes used in the development of theories and conceptual frameworks.

## CONCEPT DEVELOPMENT AND RESEARCH

A common language is necessary for communicating the meanings of concepts that comprise theories. Theory, research, and practice are linked, and most scholars recognize that they cannot be separated. Researchers relate concepts together into structures that are called models and theories and derive from them testable relationships called hypotheses (Kerlinger, 1986).

Hickman (2002) points out that nursing research, theory, and practice form a cycle and that entry into this cycle may be at any point. Research both precedes theory and is guided by theory. Both theory and research direct practice and conversely research and theory are derived from practice situations. Thus, theory, while guiding research, is simultaneously being tested in the research process. The conceptual elements of the theory that guide the research or are being tested by the research are named and defined during concept analysis.

Difficulties with studying a problem in nursing may be related to the exactness with which the terms in use are developed and defined. Poorly defined concepts may lead to faulty construction of research instruments and methods (Morse, 1995). Frequently, a nursing problem does not lend itself exactly to existing terminology. In this situation, the nurse should engage in the effort of concept development. Furthermore, if one cannot successfully define the problem so that other professionals can understand it, concept development is necessary.

## Strategies for Concept Analysis and Concept Development

There are multiple methods of constructing meaning for concepts. This can be accomplished through review of research literature, scholarly critique, and thoughtful definition. When a formal or detailed meaning is warranted, however, a more structured method for concept development will need to be used.

In the early 1960s, Wilson (1963) developed a process for defining concepts to improve communication and comprehension of the meanings of terms in scientific use. Wilson used 11 steps, or techniques, to guide the concept analysis process. Two recent examples, which used Wilson's method of concept development, were discovered in the nursing literature. Sachse (2007) used Wilson's method to study the concept of hope, and Maijala, Munnukka, and Nikkonen (2000) used Wilson's method to study the concept of envy.

---

**BOX 3-1** *Steps in Concept Analysis*

1. Select a concept.
2. Determine the aims or purposes of analysis.
3. Identify all the uses of the concept possible.
4. Determine the defining attributes.
5. Identify model case.
6. Identify borderline, related, contrary, invented, and illegitimate cases.
7. Identify antecedents and consequences.
8. Define empirical referents.

Source: Walker and Avant (2005, p. 65).

---

Building on the process presented by Wilson, nurses have published several techniques, methods, and strategies for concept development. Strategies devised by several nurse scholars will be presented briefly in the following sections, and examples of published works using these methods will be provided where available.

## WALKER AND AVANT

Walker and Avant first explicated the process of concept analysis for nurses in 1983. Their procedures were based on Wilson's method and clarified his methods so that graduate students could apply them to examine phenomena of interest to nurses. Three different processes were described by Walker and Avant (2005): concept analysis, concept synthesis, and concept derivation.

### Concept Analysis

*Concept analysis* is an approach espoused by Walker and Avant (2005) to clarify the meanings of terms and to define terms (concepts) so that writers and readers share a common language. Concept analysis should be conducted when concepts require clarification or further development to define them for a nurse scholar's purposes, whether that is research, theory development, or practice. This method for concept analysis requires an eight-step approach, as listed in Box 3-1.

### Concept Synthesis

*Concept synthesis* is used when concepts require development based on observation or other forms of evidence. The individual must develop a way to group or order the information about the phenomenon from his or her own viewpoint or theoretical requirement. Three methods of synthesizing concepts are as follows:

1. Qualitative synthesis—relies on sensory data and looking for similarities, differences, and patterns among the data to identify the new concept
2. Quantitative synthesis—requires numerical data to delineate those attributes that belong to the concept and those that do not
3. Literary synthesis—involves reviewing a wide range of the literature to acquire new insights about the concept or to find new concepts (Walker & Avant, 2005)

### Concept Derivation

*Concept derivation* from Walker and Avant's (2005) perspective is often necessary when there are few concepts currently available to a nurse that explain a problem area. It is applicable when a comparison or analogy can be made between one field or area

**BOX 3-2** *Steps in Concept Derivation*

1. Become thoroughly familiar with the existing literature.
2. Search other fields of interest for new ways of viewing the topic.
3. Select a parent concept that gives an insightful view of the topic.
4. Redefine the concept(s) in terms of the topic of interest.

Source: Walker and Avant (2005, p. 55).

that is conceptually defined and another that is not. Concept derivation can be helpful in generating new ways of thinking about a phenomenon of interest. A four-step plan for the work of moving likely concepts from disciplines outside nursing into the nursing lexicon has been developed (Box 3-2).

### Examples of Concept Analysis Using Walker and Avant's Techniques

Walker and Avant's techniques have been taught for more than two decades in graduate nursing programs, and it is the most common technique used for concept analysis in nursing. Table 3-4 lists several examples from recent nursing literature. In their most recent edition, Walker and Avant (2005) outlined the processes for each of the methods described in depth and provide a number of examples for clarification. The reader is referred to their work, as well as to the examples listed, for more information.

## RODGERS

Rodgers first published her evolutionary method for concept analysis in 1989 (Rodgers, 1989). According to Rodgers (2000), concept analysis is necessary because

TABLE 3-4 *Examples of Concept Analyses Using Walker and Avant's Methods*

| Concept | Reference |
|---|---|
| Art of nursing | Finfgeld-Connet, D. (2008). Concept synthesis of the art of nursing. *Journal of Advanced Nursing, 62*(3), 381–388. |
| Care dependency | Bogatz, T., Dijkstra, A., Lohrman, C., & Dassen, T. (2007). The meaning of care dependency as shared by care givers and care recipients: A concept analysis. *Journal of Advanced Nursing, 60*(5), 561–569. |
| Grief | Sullivan, K. (2005). Grief: An analysis of the concept as it relates to bereavement. In J. R. Cutcliffe & H. P. Mckenna (Eds.), *The essential concepts of nursing* (pp. 161–178). New York: Elsevier. |
| Loneliness | Brown, R. (2005). An analysis of loneliness as a concept if importance for dying persons. In J. R. Cutcliffe & H. P. Mckenna (Eds.), *The essential concepts of nursing* (pp. 229–242). New York: Elsevier. |
| Patient advocacy | Bu, X., & Jezewski, M. A. (2007). Developing a midrange theory of patient advocacy through concept analysis. *Journal of Advanced Nursing, 57*(1), 101–110. |
| Preserving dignity | Anderberg, P., Lepp, M., Berglund, A., & Segsten, K. (2007). Preserving dignity in caring for older adults: A concept analysis. *Journal of Advanced Nursing, 59*(6), 635–643. |
| Teamwork | Xyrichis, A., & Ream, E. (2008). Teamwork: A concept analysis. *Journal of Advanced Nursing, 61*(2), 232–241. |
| Therapeutic relationships | Chambers, M. (2005). A concept analysis of therapeutic relationships. In J. R. Cutcliffe & H. P. Mckenna (Eds.), *The essential concepts of nursing* (pp. 301–316). New York: Elsevier. |

BOX 3-3 *Steps in Rodgers' Process of Concept Analysis*

1. Identify the concept and associated terms.
2. Select an appropriate realm (a setting or a sample) for data collection.
3. Collect data to identify the attributes of the concept and the contextual basis of the concept (i.e., interdisciplinary, sociocultural, and temporal variations).
4. Analyze the data regarding the characteristics of the concept.
5. Identify an exemplar of the concept, if appropriate.
6. Identify hypotheses and implications for further development.

Source: Rodgers (2000, p. 85).

concepts are dynamic, "fuzzy," and context dependent and possess some pragmatic utility or purpose. Furthermore, because phenomena, needs, and goals change, concepts must be continually refined and variations introduced to achieve a clearer and more useful meaning.

Rodgers (2000) examined two viewpoints or schools of thought regarding concept development and showed that the methods of each differ significantly. She termed these methods "essentialism" and "evolutionary" viewpoints. In her work, she contrasted the essentialist method of concept development as exemplified by Wilson (1963) and Walker and Avant (1995) with concept development using the evolutionary method.

The evolutionary method of concept development is a concurrent task approach. In it, the tasks may be going on all at the same time, rather than a sequence of specific steps that are completed before going to the next step. The activities involved in the evolutionary method are listed in Box 3-3.

Rodgers (2000) defined many terms and explained the process of concept analysis using the evolutionary view. The goal of the concept analysis will, to an extent, determine how the researcher *identifies the concept of interest* and terms and expressions selected. The incorporation of a new term into a nurse's way of viewing a client situation is often a circumstance warranting analysis of a new concept.

The goal of the analysis will also influence *selection of the setting and sample* for data collection. For instance, the setting may be a library and the sample might be literature. The sampling might be time-oriented, say literature from the previous 5 years. In any case, the researcher's goal is to develop a rigorous design consistent with the purpose of the analysis. The selection of literature from related disciplines might include those that typically use the concept. An exhaustive review includes all the indexed literature using the concept and may be limited by a time frame such as several years.

A randomization process is then used to select the sample across each discipline over time. In *collecting and managing the data* a discovery approach is preferred. The focus of the data analysis is on identifying the attributes, antecedents, and consequences and related concepts or surrogate terms. The attributes located by this means constitute a "real definition as opposed to a nominal or dictionary definition" (Rodgers, 2000, p. 91).

Rodgers defines *surrogate terms* as ways of expressing the concept other than by the term of interest. She distinguishes between surrogate terms and *related concepts* by showing that surrogate terms are different words that express the concept, whereas "related concepts are part of a network that provide a background" and "lend significance to the concept of interest" (Rodgers, 2000, p. 92).

*Analyzing the data* can go on simultaneously with its collection according to Rodgers (2000), or it can be delayed until all the data are collected. The latter is allowed in concept analysis using the evolutionary process because data are currently available, rather than being constantly created by the subjects as in qualitative research study. The researcher must beware of considering the data "saturated," that is, redundant, too early.

*Identifying an exemplar* from the literature, field observation, or interview is important and will provide a clear example of the concept. Examples of real cases are preferred over constructed cases (in contrast to Wilson's [1963] method). The goal is to illustrate the characteristics of the concept in relevant contexts to enhance the clarity and effective application of the concept.

*Interpreting the results* involves gaining insight on the current status of the concept and generating implications for inquiry based on this status and identified gaps. Interpreting the results may involve interdisciplinary comparison, temporal comparison, and assessment of the social context within which the concept analysis was conducted.

*Identifying implications* for further development and formal inquiry may be the result. The results of the analysis may direct further inquiry rather than giving the final answer on the meaning of the concept. The implications of this form of research-based concept analysis may yield questions for further research, or hypotheses may be extracted from the findings. The major outcome of the evolutionary method of concept analysis is the generation of further questions for research rather than the static definition of the concept. Table 3-5 lists a number of references for concept analyses using this method. For more information, the reader is referred to Rodgers (2000).

TABLE 3-5 *Examples of Concept Analyses Using Rodgers' Methods*

| Concept | Reference |
| --- | --- |
| Cancer survivorship | Doyle, N. (2008). Cancer survivorship: Evolutionary concept analysis. *Journal of Advanced Nursing, 62*(4), 499–509. |
| Chronic fatigue | Jorgenson, R. (2008). Chronic fatigue: An evolutionary concept analysis. *Journal of Advanced Nursing, 63*(2), 199–207. |
| Empathetic response | Campbell-Yeo, M., Latimer, M., & Johnston, C. (2008). The empathetic response in nurses who treat pain: Concept analysis. *Journal of Advanced Nursing, 61*(6), 711–719. |
| Forgiveness | Recine, A. G., Werner, J. S., & Recine, L. (2007). Concept analysis of forgiveness with a multicultural emphasis. *Journal of Advanced Nursing, 59*(3), 308–316. |
| Hope | Johnson, S. (2007). Hope in terminal illness: An evolutionary concept analysis. *International Journal of Palliative Nursing, 13*(9), 451–459. |
| Information need | Timmins, F. (2006). Exploring the concept of information need. *International Journal of Nursing Practice, 12*(6), 375–381. |
| Renal supportive care | Noble, H., Kelly, D., Rawlings-Anderson, K., & Meyer, J. (2007). A concept analysis of renal supportive care: The changing world of nephrology. *Journal of Advanced Nursing, 59*(6), 644–653. |
| Routine | Zisberg, A., Young, H., Schepp, K., & Zysberg, L. (2007). A concept of routine: Relevance to nursing. *Journal of Advanced Nursing, 57*(4), 442–453. |
| Self-monitoring | Wilde, M. H., & Garvin, S. (2007). A concept analysis of self-monitoring. *Journal of Advanced Nursing. 57*(3), 339–350. |
| Stigma | Butt, G. (2008). Stigma in the context of hepatitis C: Concept analysis. *Journal of Advanced Nursing, 62*(6), 712–724. |

TABLE 3-6 *Phases of Swartz-Barcott and Kim's Hybrid Model of Concept Development*

| Phase | Activities |
|---|---|
| Theoretical phase | Select a concept |
| | Review the literature |
| | Determine meaning and measurement |
| | Choose a working definition |
| Fieldwork phase | Set the stage |
| | Negotiate entry into a setting |
| | Select cases |
| | Collect and analyze data |
| Final analytical phase | Weigh findings |
| | Write report |

Source: Swartz-Barcott and Kim (2000).

## SWARTZ-BARCOTT AND KIM

A hybrid model of concept development was initially presented by Swartz-Barcott and Kim in 1986 and expanded and revised in 1993 and 2000. This method for concept development involves a three-phase process, which is summarized in Table 3-6.

### Theoretical Phase

In the theoretical phase, a borrowed concept, an underdeveloped nursing concept, or a concept from clinical practice may be selected. The main consideration is that the concept has relevance for nursing. A clinical encounter may be described in detail to arrive at the concept through analysis. *The literature is searched* broadly and systematically across disciplines that may use the concept. A set of questions that provides inquiry into the essential nature of the concept, the means of clear definition, and ways to enhance its measurability focuses on questions of measurement and definition. *Meaning and measurement* are dealt with. This requires thought for comparing and contrasting the data. *A working definition* is chosen to be used in the final phase. The definition should maintain a nursing perspective.

### Fieldwork Phase

In the *fieldwork* phase, the concept is corroborated and refined. The fieldwork phase integrates with the literature phase and expands into a modified qualitative research approach (i.e., participant observation). The steps of this phase are setting the stage, negotiating entry, selecting cases, and collecting and analyzing the data.

### Analytical Phase

The final analytical phase includes examination of the details in the light of the literature review. The researcher reviews the findings with the original purpose in view. Three questions guide the final analysis:

1. How much is the concept applicable and important to nursing?
2. Does the initial selection of the concept seem justified?

**3.** To what extent do the review of literature, theoretical analysis, and empirical findings support the presence and frequency of the concept within the population selected for empirical study? (Swartz-Barcott & Kim, 2000, p. 147)

The final step of the process is to *write up the findings*. The work may be reported as either fieldwork or as a concept analysis. Elements the researcher must consider when writing the findings are length of the study, the intended audience, timing, pacing of the authorship process, anticipated length of the manuscript, how much detail of the process to include, and ethics of the interpretation of the analysis (Swartz-Barcott & Kim, 2000).

Several results can be realized by this type of analysis:

**1.** The current meaning of the concept can be supported or refined.
**2.** A different definition than previously used may stand out.
**3.** The concept may be completely redefined.
**4.** A new or refined way of measuring the concept may be the result (Swartz-Barcott & Kim, 1993).

Examples of published reports using this model are listed in Table 3-7.

## MELEIS

Meleis (2007) described three strategies to develop conceptual meaning for use in nursing theory, research, and practice. These are concept exploration, concept clarification, and concept analysis.

### Concept Exploration

*Concept exploration* is used when concepts are new and ambiguous in a discipline, when concepts are camouflaged by being embedded in the daily nursing discussion, or when a concept from another discipline is being redesigned for use in nursing. Concept exploration may awaken nurses to a new concept or revitalize the meanings

TABLE 3-7 *Examples of Concept Analyses Using Swartz-Barcott and Kim's Hybrid Method*

| Concept | Reference |
|---|---|
| Being sensitive | Sayers, K. L., & de Vries, K. (2008). A concept development of "being sensitive" in nursing. *Nursing Ethics, 15*(3), 289–303. |
| Coping with arthritic pain | Seomun, G. A., Chang, S. O., Lee, P. S., Lee, S. J., & Sin, H. J. (2006). Concept analysis of coping with arthritic pain by South Korean older adults: Development of a hybrid model. *Nursing and Health Sciences, 8*(1), 10–19. |
| Family resilience | Lee, I., Lee., E. O., Kim, H. S., Park, Y. S., Song, M., & Park, Y. H. (2004). Concept development of family resilience: A study of Korean families with a chronically ill child. *Journal of Clinical Nursing, 13*(5), 636–645. |
| Nursing information | Erdley, W. S. (2005). Concept development of nursing information. *CIN: Computers, Informatics, Nursing, 23*(2), 93–99. |
| Service awareness | Crist, J. D., Michaels, C., Gelfand, D. E., & Phillips, L. R. (2007). Defining and measuring service awareness among elders and caregivers of Mexican descent. *Research and Theory for Nursing Practice, An International Journal, 21*(2), 119–129. |

BOX 3-4  *Process of Concept Clarification*

1. Clarify the boundaries of the concept including what attributes should be included and what excluded.
2. Critically review the properties of the concept.
3. Bring to light new dimensions that had not been considered.
4. Compare, contrast, delineate, and differentiate these properties and provide exemplars of the concept.
5. Identify assumptions and philosophical bases and "what events trigger the phenomenon and propose questions from a nursing perspective" (p. 167).

Source: Meleis (2007, p. 167).

of an overused concept to make it explicit for practice, research, and theory building. The steps Meleis (2007) suggests for this endeavor are as follows:

1. Identifying the major components and dimensions of the concept
2. Raising appropriate questions about the concept
3. Proposing triggers for continuing the exploration
4. Identifying and defining the advantages to the discipline of continuing the exploration of this concept (p. 165)

### Concept Clarification

*Concept clarification* is used to "refine concepts that have been used in nursing without a clear, shared, and conscious agreement on the properties of meanings attributed to the concept" (Meleis, 2007, p. 167). Concept clarification is a way to refine existing concepts when they lack clarity for a specific nursing endeavor. The processes involved in concept clarification allow for reduction of ambiguities while critically reviewing the properties. The processes are presented in Box 3-4.

### Concept Analysis

*Concept analysis,* according to Meleis (2007), assumes that the concept has been introduced into nursing literature but is ready to move to the level of development for research. This process implies that the concept will be broken down to its essentials and then reconstructed for its contribution to the nursing lexicon. The goal of the analysis is to bring the concept close to use in research or clinical practice and to ultimately contribute to instrument development and theory testing.

Meleis (2007) focused on an integrated approach to concept development, which includes defining, differentiating, delineating antecedents and consequences, modeling, analogizing, and synthesizing. Table 3-8 lists each of these components and presents related activities or tasks to be accomplished for each phase. Clark and Robinson (2000) used Meleis's earlier work to describe the concept of multiculturalism, and Felten and Hall (2001) used Meleis's strategies to describe the concept of resilience in elderly women.

## MORSE

In response to concerns that some concepts in the nursing lexicon had been derived and not developed adequately for nursing, or had become overused by those who did not clarify them, Morse (1995) developed a method of concept development to enhance clarity and distinctiveness of nursing concepts. In this method, she used the term "advanced techniques of concept analysis" and described the processes of concept delineation, concept comparison, and concept clarification.

TABLE 3-8 *Meleis' Processes for Concept Development*

| Process | Task or Activity |
|---|---|
| Defining | Creating theoretical and operational definitions that clarify ambiguities, enhance precision, and relate concepts to empirical referents |
| Differentiating | Sorting in and out similarities and differences between the concept being developed and other like concepts |
| Delineating antecedents | Defining the contextual conditions under which the concept is perceived and expected to occur |
| Delineating consequences | Defining events, situations, or conditions that may result from the concept |
| Modeling | Defining and identifying exemplars (i.e., clinical referents or research referents) to illustrate some aspect of the concept. Models may be same or like models, or contrary models |
| Analogizing | Describing the concept through another concept or phenomenon that is similar and has been studied more extensively |
| Synthesizing | Bringing together findings, meanings, and properties that have been discovered and describing future steps in theorizing |

Source: Meleis (2007, pp. 179–180).

### Concept Delineation

*Concept delineation* is a strategy that requires an extensive literature search and assists in separating two terms that seem closely linked. The concepts are then compared and contrasted to identify commonalities, similarities, and differences such that distinctions may be drawn between the terms (Morse, 1995).

### Concept Comparison

*Concept comparison* clarifies competing concepts, again using an extensive literature review and keeping the literature for each concept separate. Three phases are used in the comparison:

1. Preconditions—the status of the concept in nursing and its use in teaching or clinical practice
2. Process—the type of nursing response to the concept, at what level of consciousness it occurs, and, if it is identified with the client, at what level
3. Outcomes—whether the concept was used to identify process or product, its accuracy in prediction, the client's condition, and the client's experience with the concept (Morse, 1995, pp. 39–41)

### Concept Clarification

For Morse (1995), *concept clarification* is used with concepts that are "mature" and have a large body of literature identifying and using them. The concept clarification process requires a "literature review to identify the underlying values and to identify, describe and compare and contrast the attributes of each" (p. 41).

Published reports using Morse's methods for concept development are becoming increasingly common. Olson and Morse (2005) delineated the concept of fatigue using a system of analytic questions pertinent to the concept to reach a new conceptualization of fatigue; Whitehead (2004) used Morse's method to analyze health promotion and health education; Fasnacht (2003) used Morse's methods to "refine"

| BOX 3-5 | *Four Principles of Concept Analysis* |
|---------|----------------------------------------|

**Epistemological principle** is based on the question: "Is the concept clearly defined and well differentiated from other concepts?" (p. 405).

**Pragmatic principle** in which the question to be answered is: "Is the concept applicable and useful within the scientific realm or inquiry? Has it been operationalized?" In this principle, they believe that an operationalized concept has achieved a level of maturity (p. 405).

**Linguistic principle** asks "Is the concept used consistently and appropriately within

context?" (p. 406). Similarly to Morse and to Rogers, they find that context or lack of context is a factor important in this type of analysis (p. 406).

**Logical principle** applies the question: "Does the concept hold its boundaries through theoretical integration with other concepts?" (p. 406). The authors require that the concept not be blurred with respect to other concepts, but that it remains logically clear and distinct.

Source: From Penrod and Hupcey (2005, pp. 405–406).

the concept of creativity; and Kunyk and Olson (2001) used concept clarification to examine empathy. In other published reports using Morse's methods, trust was studied by Hupcey and colleagues (2001) and uncertainty in illnesses was analyzed by McCormick (2002).

## PENROD AND HUPCEY

Penrod and Hupcey (2005) built on Morse's method and termed their method "principle-based concept analysis." Explaining their intent to "determine and evaluate the state of the science surrounding the concept" (p. 405) and "produce evidence that reveals scholars' best estimate of 'probable truth' in the scientific literature" (p. 406), they outlined four principles for their method: epistemological, pragmatic, linguistic, and logical (Box 3-5).

Penrod and Hupcey (2005) explain that in their method of concept analysis, the findings "are summarized as a theoretical definition that integrates an evaluative summary of each of the criteria posed by the four over-arching principles." To do this, the researcher must consider three issues: (1) selection of appropriate disciplinary literature for review, (2) assurance of the adequacy and appropriateness of the sample derived from the literature, and (3) employment of "within- and across-discipline analytic techniques." They have elucidated that this advanced level of concept development seems to be more relevant to the research endeavor, as it is a research-based concept analysis.

Despite being developed very recently, examples of published works using Penrod and Hupcey's (2005) method for concept analysis can readily be found. For example, Bell, Lucas, and White-Traut (2008) used the Principle-Based Method to clarify the term "neonatal neurobehavioral organization" and Larkin, de Casterlé, and Schotsmans (2007) evaluated "Transience in Relation to Palliative Care" using this method. Lastly, Penrod (2007) advanced the concept of "living with uncertainty" using the Penrod and Hupcey method.

## COMPARISON OF MODELS FOR CONCEPT DEVELOPMENT

The nursing literature contains several comparisons and critiques of the various models and methods for concept development/concept analysis. Indeed, Hupcey and colleagues (1996) and Morse and coworkers (1996) provided a detailed and well-researched

TABLE 3-9 *Comparison of Selected Methods of Concept Development*

| Author(s) | Method | Purpose | Number of Steps | Constructed Cases | Other Factors/Steps |
|---|---|---|---|---|---|
| Walker and Avant | Concept analysis | Clarify meaning of terms | 8 | Model, borderline, related, contrary | Identify empirical referents and defining attributes; delineate antecedents and consequences |
| Rodgers | Evolutionary concept analysis | Refine and clarify concepts for use in research and practice | 5 | Model only (Identified— not constructed) | Identify appropriate realm (setting and sample); analyze data about characteristics, conduct interdisciplinary or temporal comparisons; identify hypotheses and implications for further study |
| Swartz-Barcott and Kim | Hybrid model of concept development | Support or refine the meaning of a concept and/or develop a new or refined way to measure a concept | 3 phases | Model case, contrary case | Develop working definitions, search literature, participant observation, collect and analyze data, write findings |
| Meleis | Concept development | Define concepts theoretically and operationally, clarify ambiguities, relate concepts to empirical referents | 7 | Same or like models; contrary models | Define concept, use an analogy to describe a similar concept, synthesize findings; differentiate similarities and differences between like concepts; delineate antecedents and consequences |
| Morse | Concept comparison | Clarifies the meaning of competing concepts | 3 phases | Not specified | Uses extensive literature review to examine and describe preconditions (status of use of the concepts in teaching or practice), process, and outcomes of use of the concept |
| Penrod and Hupcey | Principle-based concept analysis | Concept analysis | 4 phases based on principles | Not specified | Sampling within bodies of large multidisciplinary literature yields a theoretically based scientific definition |

comparison of the techniques presented by Walker and Avant (1986), Swartz-Barcott and Kim (1993), and Rodgers (1989). Strengths and weaknesses of each method were described in their papers. More recently Duncan, Cloutier, and Bailey (2007) reviewed the history of concept analysis comparing the major methods in common use.

A number of works comparing two different methods of concept analysis were found in the literature. For example, Fu, LeMone, and McDaniel (2004) used an integrative approach combining the methods of Walker and Avant and Rodgers to analyze symptom management. Penrod (2007) advanced the concept of living with uncertainty using the methods espoused by Morse and Penrod and Hupcey, and Shin and White-Traut (2007) analyzed the concept of transition to motherhood in the neonatal intensive care unit combining elements from Rogers' evolutionary method and Swartz-Barcott and Kim's Hybrid Model. Table 3-9 on page 63 compares the various formats for concept development/concept analysis described earlier.

## Summary

Rebecca Wallis, one of the nurses from the opening case study, identified what she thought was a new phenomenon that was pertinent to her practice of oncology nursing and decided to develop the concept more fully. By applying techniques of concept analysis to the PMG reaction, she began the process of formulating information on this concept that could ultimately be used by other nurses in practice or research.

The process of developing concepts includes reviewing the nurse's area of interest, examining the phenomena closely, pondering the terms that are relevant and that fit together with reality, and operationalizing the concept for practice, research, or educational use. Whether advanced practice nurses or nursing scholars elect to use the methods proposed by Wilson (1963), Walker and Avant (1986, 1995, 2005), Morse (1995), Rodgers (2000), Swartz-Barcott and Kim (2000), Meleis (2007), or Penrod and Hupcey (2005), or a combination, it is clear that the process of developing, clarifying, comparing and contrasting, and integrating well-derived and defined concepts is necessary for theory development and to guide research studies. This will, in turn, ultimately benefit practice. Chapter 4 builds on the process of concept development by describing the processes used to link concepts to form relationship statements and to construct conceptual models, frameworks, and theories.

## CONCEPT ANALYSIS EXEMPLAR

The following is an outline delineating the steps of a concept analysis using Rodgers' evolutionary method.

Breen, J. (2002). Transitions in the concept of chronic pain. *Advances in Nursing Science, 24*(4), 48–59.

1. *Identify the concept and associated terms*

*Concept:* Chronic pain (noncancerous pain in adults)
*Associated terms:* Chronic pain, persistent pain, intractable pain, and continuous pain

2. *Select an appropriate realm (setting) for data collection*

The realm for the study was nursing, psychology, and neurophysiology professional journal publications between the years 1969 and 1999. Included were case studies, qualitative and quantitative studies, review articles, and meta-analyses.

3. *Identify the attributes of the concept and the contextual basis of the concept*

*Attributes of chronic pain:* Their primary dimensions (physical, behavioral, and psychological)
Physical dimension is characterized by quantity, intensity (level or severity), neurological transmission, and anatomic patterns of chronic pain.

Behavioral dimension is characterized by expressive, movement, and functional behaviors.

Psychological dimension is characterized by affective and evaluative components.

4. *Specify the characteristics of the concept*

Characteristics of chronic pain include:

Relative language (e.g., "ache") and modifiers (e.g., "annoying" or "dull").

*Behaviors:* Expressive behaviors (moaning and use of pain words); movement behaviors (grimacing, massaging, protective movements, rhythmic movements); functional behaviors (use of socially defined sick-role behaviors such as decreased mobility, inactivity, and bed rest).

*Time dimension:* Include onset and frequency or rhythm of pain episodes.

*Antecedents:* No specific physical or psychological characteristics were noted that were antecedents of chronic pain. Although trauma sometimes precedes chronic pain, trauma is not necessary or sufficient to cause chronic pain. Chronic pain may be related to alterations in the production and regulation of cortisol, serotonin, and endogenous opioids and in the synthesis and release of sensory neuropeptides.

*Consequences:* Two themes: living with chronic pain results in alterations of psychological life patterns including depression, anger, anxiety, grief, hopelessness, and helplessness; social pattern alterations may result in isolation and loneliness; there may be loss of work, and consequently, loss of insurance and money to pay for medical expenses; and *coping with chronic pain*—effective coping—decreases the adverse effects of chronic pain by reducing stress and thereby reducing pain intensity. Strategies include distraction, meditation, positive thinking, counseling, and use of alternative treatments (e.g., acupuncture, massage, herbal medications, meditation, and imagery).

5. *Identify an exemplar of the concept*

Chronic pain is a subjective, multidimensional, bio/psycho/social syndrome that can be recognized by physical, psychological, and behavioral patterns. Chronic pain results in physical, psychological, and social alterations of function to varying degrees. There is no known purpose and there is no single explanation of the symptoms.

6. *Identify hypotheses and implications for development*

Research is needed to understand the relationship between intensity, quality and duration of pain, and central nervous system function.

Research is needed to explore body–brain–mind interactions in the development, persistence, and consequences of chronic pain.

Research is needed to identify the subjective symptoms that may differentiate chronic pain from acute pain. If early symptoms can be identified, studies can be conducted to determine interventions that may stop the development of chronic pain.

## LEARNING ACTIVITIES

1. From a literature search or clinical practice, choose a term or concept of interest. Review the literature for discussion of the concept. Discriminate between the concept of interest and associated terms and write a scholarly paper that defines and develops the concept.

2. Obtain a copy of Walker and Avant's (2005), or Rodgers' (2000) work that presents methods for analyzing, synthesizing, or deriving a concept. Work through each step and summarize a new definition of a concept. Formulate the work into a scholarly paper suitable for publication using the selected system.

3. For a scholarly or clinical research project, clarify a concept of interest using one of the above methods of concept development, clarification, or analysis. As an empirical part of the paper, locate an instrument with which the concept may be measured or operationalized.

4. As a thesis or research project use one of the above methods of advanced concept development to derive a concept for the discipline of nursing. Exhaustively review the literature and collect data from either clients or other professionals to use to develop the concept and determine empirical referents. Determine a method to measure the concept and analyze the data using quantitative and qualitative methods. Write a paper summarizing the process suitable for publication to inform the nursing profession of the newly derived concept.

# REFERENCES

Bell, A. F., Lucas, R., & White-Traut, R. C. (2008). Concept clarification of neonatal neurobehavioral organization. *Journal of Advanced Nursing, 61*(5), 570–581.

Bishop, S. M. (2002). Theory development process. In A. M. Tomey & M. R. Alligood (Eds.), *Nursing theorists and their work* (5th ed., pp. 50–61). St. Louis: Mosby.

Chinn, P. L., & Kramer, M. K. (2008). *Theory and nursing: Integrated knowledge development* (7th ed.). St. Louis: Mosby.

Clark, C., & Robinson, T. (2000). Multiculturalism as a concept in nursing. *Journal of National Black Nurses' Association, 11*(2), 39–43.

Cowles, K. V. & Rogers, B. L. (1993). The concept of grief: An evolutionary perspective. In B. L. Rogers & K. A. Knafl (Eds.). *Concept development in nursing: Foundations techniques, and applications.* Philadelphia: Saunders.

Cutcliffe, J. R., & McKenna, H. P. (2005). *The essential concepts of nursing: Building blocks for practice.* New York: Elsevier.

Dubin, R. (1978). *Theory building.* New York: Free Press.

Duncan, C., Cloutier, J. D., & Bailey, P. H. (2007). Concept analysis: The importance of differentiating the ontological focus. *Journal of Advanced Nursing, 58*(3), 293–300.

Dunn, K. S. (2005). Testing a middle-range theoretical model of adaptation to chronic pain. *Nursing Science Quarterly, 18*(2), 146–156.

Fasnacht, P. H. (2003). Creativity: A refinement of the concept for nursing practice. *Journal of Advanced Nursing, 41*(2), 195–202.

Fawcett, J. (1999). *The relationship of theory and research* (3rd ed.). Philadelphia: Davis.

Felten, B. S., & Hall, J. M. (2001). Conceptualizing resilience in women older than 85: Overcoming adversity from illness or loss. *Journal of Gerontological Nursing, 27*(11), 46–53.

Ferrans, C. E., Zerwic, J. J., Wilbur, J. E., & Larson, J. L. (2005). Conceptual model of health-related quality of life. *Journal of Nursing Scholarship, 37*(4), 336–342.

Fu, M. R., LeMone, P., & McDaniel, R. W. (2004). An integrated approach to an analysis of symptom management in patients with cancer. *Oncology Nursing Forum, 31*(1), 65–70.

Guyton, A. C., & Hall, J. E. (1996). *Textbook of medical physiology* (9th ed.). Philadelphia: Saunders.

Hardy, M. (1973). Theories: Components, development, evaluation. *Theoretical foundations for nursing.* New York: MSS Information Systems.

Hickman, J. S. (2002). An introduction to nursing theory. In J. George (Ed.), *Nursing theories: The base for professional nursing practice* (5th ed., pp. 1–20). Upper Saddle River, NJ: Prentice-Hall.

Hupcey, J. E., Morse, J. M., Lenz, E. R., & Tason, M. C. (1996). Wilsonian methods of concept analysis: A critique. *Scholarly Inquiry for Nursing Practice, 10*(3), 185–210.

Hupcey, J. E., & Penrod, J. (2008). Enhancing methodological clarity: Principle-based concept analysis. *Journal of Advanced Nursing, 50*(4), 403–409.

Hupcey, J. E., Penrod, J., Morse, J. M., & Mitcham, C. (2001). An exploration and advancement of the concept of trust. *Journal of Advanced Nursing, 36*(2), 282–293.

Jacox, A. K. (1974). Theory construction in nursing: An overview. *Nursing Research, 23*(1), 4–13.

Kerlinger, F. N. (1986). *Foundations of behavioral research* (3rd ed.). New York: Holt, Rinehart & Winston.

Kim, H. S. (2000). *The nature of theoretical thinking in nursing* (2nd ed.). New York: Springer.

Kim, H. S. (2006). The concept of holism. In H. S. Kim & I. Kollak (Eds.), *Nursing theories: Conceptual and philosophical foundations* (2nd ed.) (chap. 7, pp. 89–108). New York: Springer.

Kunyk, D., & Olson, J. K. (2001). Clarification of conceptualizations of empathy. *Journal of Advanced Nursing, 35*(3), 317–325.

Larkin, P. J., de Casterlé, B. D., & Schotsmans, P. (2007). Towards a conceptual evaluation of transience in relation to palliative care. *Journal of Advanced Nursing, 59*(1), 86–96.

Lincoln, Y. S., & Guba, E. G. (1985). *Naturalistic inquiry.* Beverly Hills, CA: Sage.

Maijala, H., Munnukka, T., & Nikkonen, M. (2000). Feeling of "lacking" as the core of envy: A conceptual analysis of envy. *Journal of Advanced Nursing, 31*(6), 1342–1350.

Maslow, A. H. (1954). *Motivation and personality.* New York: Harper.

McCormick, K. M. (2002). A concept analysis of uncertainty in illness. *Journal of Nursing Scholarship, 34*(2), 127–131.

Meleis, A. I. (2007). *Theoretical nursing: Development and progress* (4th ed.). Philadelphia: Lippincott Williams & Wilkins.

Morse, J. M. (1995). Exploring the theoretical basis of nursing using advanced techniques of concept analysis. *Advances in Nursing Science, 17*(3), 31–46.

Morse, J. M., Hupcey, J. E., Mitcham, C., & Lenz, E. R. (1996). Concept analysis in nursing research: A critical appraisal. *Scholarly Inquiry for Nursing Practice, 10*(3), 253–277.

Olson, K., & Morse, J. M. (2005). *Delineating the concept of fatigue using a pragmatic utility approach.* In J. R. Cutcliffe & H. P. McKenna (Eds.), *The essential concepts of nursing.* New York: Elsevier.

Parse, R. R. (1999). *Hope: An international human becoming perspective.* Sudbury, MA: Jones & Bartlett and National League for Nursing.

Parse, R. R. (2006). Concept inventing: Continuing clarification. *Nursing Science Quarterly, 19*(4), 289.

Penrod, J. (2007). Living with uncertainty: Concept advancement. *Journal of Advanced Nursing, 57*(6), 658–557.

Penrod, J., & Hupcey, J. E. (2005). Enhancing methodological clarity: Principle-based concept analysis. *Journal of Advanced Nursing, 50*(4), 403–409.

Reed, K. S. (2003). Grief is more than tears. *Nursing Science Quarterly, 16*(1), 77–81.

Rodgers, B. L. (1989). Concept analysis and the development of nursing knowledge: The evolutionary cycle. *Journal of Advanced Nursing, 14*(4), 330–335.

Rodgers, B. L. (2000). Concept analysis: An evolutionary view. In B. L. Rodgers & K. A. Knafl (Eds.), *Concept development in nursing: Foundations, techniques, and applications* (2nd ed., pp. 77–102). Philadelphia: Saunders.

Rodgers, B. L., & Knafl, K. A. (2000). *Concept development in nursing: Foundations, techniques, and applications* (2nd ed.). Philadelphia: Saunders.

Sachse, D. (2007). Hope: More than a refuge in a storm. *International Journal of Psychiatric Nursing Research, 13*(11), 1546–1553.

Selye, H. (1956). *The stress of life.* New York: McGraw-Hill.

Shin, H., & White-Traut, R. (2007). The conceptual structure of transition to motherhood in the neonatal intensive care unit. *Journal of Advanced Nursing, 58*(1), 90–98.

Shu, E. E. (2004). The model of cultural competence through an evolutionary concept analysis. *Journal of Transcultural Nursing, 15*(2), 93–102.

Swartz-Barcott, D., & Kim, H. S. (1986). A hybrid model for concept development. In P. L. Chinn (Ed.), *Nursing research methodology: Issues and implementation.* Rockville, MD: Aspen.

Swartz-Barcott, D., & Kim, H. S. (1993). An expansion and elaboration of the hybrid model of concept development. In B. L. Rodgers & K. A. Knafl (Eds.), *Concept development in nursing* (pp. 107–133). Philadelphia: Saunders.

Swartz-Barcott, D., & Kim, H. S. (2000). An expansion and elaboration of the hybrid model of concept development. In B. L. Rodgers & K A. Knafl (Eds.), *Concept development in nursing* (2nd ed., pp. 129–160). Philadelphia: Saunders.

Verhulst, G., Swartz-Barcott, D. (1993). A Concept analysis of withdrawal: Application of the hybrid model of concept development. In B. L. Rogers & K. A. Knafl (Eds.) *Concept development in nursing: Foundations techniques, and applications,* (pp. 135–158). Philadelphia: Saunders.

Walker, L. O., & Avant, K. (1986). *Strategies for theory construction in nursing* (1st ed.). Norwalk, CT: Appleton & Lange.

Walker, L. O., & Avant, K. (1995). *Strategies for theory construction in nursing* (3rd ed.). Norwalk, CT: Appleton & Lange.

Walker, L. O., & Avant, K. (2005). *Strategies for theory construction in nursing* (4th ed.). Upper Saddle River, NJ: Prentice-Hall.

Wang, C. H. (2000). Developing a concept of hope from a human science perspective. *Nursing Science Quarterly, 13*(3), 248–251.

Whitehead, D. (2004). Health promotion and health education: Advancing the concepts. *Journal of Advanced Nursing, 47*(3), 311–320.

Wilson, J. (1963). *Thinking with concepts.* Cambridge, UK: Cambridge University Press.

Wilson, A. H., & Raines, K. H. (1999). Contributions of graduate students to nursing knowledge in women's health. *Image: Journal of Nursing Scholarship, 31*(4), 403.

# 4

# Theory Development: Structuring Conceptual Relationships in Nursing

## Melanie McEwen

*J*ill Watson is enrolled in a master's nursing program and beginning work on her thesis. As an occupational health nurse at a large telecommunication manufacturing company for the past 7 years, Jill has concentrated much of her practice in the area of health promotion. She has organized numerous health fairs, led countless health help sessions, regularly posted health information on central bulletin boards, and provided screening programs for many illnesses. Despite her efforts to improve the health of the workers, many still smoke, are overweight, do not exercise, and have other negative lifestyle habits. Realizing that lack of information about health-related issues is not a problem, Jill has focused on trying to understand why people choose not to engage in positive health practices. As a result, she became interested in the concept of motivation.

In one of her early courses in her master's program, Jill completed an analysis of the concept of health motivation. During this exercise she defined the concept; identified antecedents, consequences, and empirical referents; and developed a number of case studies including a model case, a related case, and a contrary case.

As her studies progressed, Jill reviewed the literature from nursing, psychology, and sociology on health beliefs and health motivation and discovered several related theories. The Health Belief Model appeared to best describe her impressions of the issues at hand, but the model had not been developed for nursing and did not completely fit her conceptualization of the variables and issues in health motivation. For her thesis she decided to modify the Health Belief Model to focus on the concept of health motivation and to develop an instrument to measure the variables she had generated in her earlier work.

---

In nursing, theories are systematic explanations of events in which constructs and concepts are identified; relationships are proposed; and predictions are made to describe, explain, predict, or prescribe practice and research (Dickoff, James, & Wiedenbach,

1968; Streubert-Speziale & Carpenter, 2008). Without nursing theory, nursing activities and interventions are guided by rote, tradition, some outside authority, hunches, or they may simply be random.

Theories are not discovered; instead, they are invented to describe, explain, or understand phenomena or solve nagging problems (e.g., Why don't people apply knowledge of positive health practices?). In the past, nursing leaders saw theory development as a means of clearly establishing nursing as a profession, and throughout the last 50 years, many nursing scholars developed models and theories to guide nursing practice, nursing research, nursing administration and management, and nursing education. As discussed in Chapter 2, these models and theories have been created at different levels (grand, middle range, practice) and for different purposes (description, explanation, prediction, etc.).

Theory development seeks to help the nurse understand practice in a more complete and insightful way and provides a method of identifying and expressing key ideas about the essence of practice. Theories help organize existing knowledge and aid in making new and important discoveries to advance practice (Walker & Avant, 2005). As illustrated in the above case study, development and application of nursing theory are essential to revise, update, and refine the practice of nursing and to further advance the profession.

## Overview of Theory Development

Several terms related to the creation of theory are found in the nursing literature. Theory construction, theory development, theory building, and theory generation are sometimes used synonymously or interchangeably. In other cases (Cesario, 1997; Walker & Avant, 2005), authors have differentiated the concepts or subsumed one term as a component or process within another. In this chapter, the term *theory development* is used as the global term to refer to the processes and methods used to create, modify, or refine a theory. *Theory construction* is used to describe one of the final steps of theory development in which the components of the theory are organized and linkages specified.

Theory development is a complex, time-consuming process that covers a number of stages or phases from inception of concepts to testing of theoretical propositions through research (Powers & Knapp, 2006). In general, the process of theory development begins with one or more concepts that are derived from within a discipline's metatheory or philosophy. These concepts are further refined and related to one another in propositions or statements that can be submitted to empirical testing (Chinn & Kramer, 2008; Peterson, 2008; Reynolds, 1971).

## Categorizations of Theory

As described in Chapter 2, theories are often categorized using different criteria. Theories may be grouped based on scope or level of abstraction (grand theory, middle range theory, practice theory), the purpose of the theory, or the source or discipline in which the theory was developed.

### CATEGORIZATION BASED ON SCOPE OR LEVEL OF ABSTRACTION

An overview of "levels of theory" was presented in Chapter 2. In nursing, theories are often viewed based on scope or level of abstraction, where the most global or abstract level is the philosophical, or metatheory, level, followed by grand theory, middle range theory, and practice theory. In the early years of nursing theory (1950–1980), theory development was largely at the metatheory and grand theory levels. Recently, however, there has been a significant shift with recognition of the need to focus more on middle range and practice (situation-specific) theories that are more relevant to nursing practice and more amenable to testing through research. The following sections will review and expand on each level of theory.

### Philosophy, Worldview, or Metatheory

*Metatheory* refers to the philosophical and methodologic questions related to developing a theoretical base for nursing. It has also been termed "worldview" by some (Hickman, 2002). According to Walker and Avant (2005), metatheory deals with the processes of generating knowledge and debating broad issues related to the nature of theory, types of theory needed, and suitable criteria for theory evaluation. Chapter 1 discussed a number of philosophical issues related to a worldview or metatheory in nursing including epistemology, research methods, and related questions.

### Grand Theories

In nursing, grand theories are composed of relatively abstract concepts that are not operationally defined and attempt to explain or describe very comprehensive aspects of human experience and response. Grand theories consist of conceptual frameworks defining broad perspectives for practice and ways of looking at nursing phenomena based on these perspectives. They provide global viewpoints for nursing practice, education, and research, but they are limited because of their generality and abstractness. Because of their level of abstraction, these theories are generally difficult to apply to the daily practice of nurses and are difficult to test (Hickman, 2002; Higgins & Moore, 2000; Peterson, 2008; Walker & Avant, 2005).

Early grand nursing theories focused on the nurse–client relationship and the role of the nurse. Later grand theories expanded to more encompassing concepts (holistic perspective, interpersonal relations, social systems, and health). Recent grand theories have attempted to address phenomenological aspects of nursing (caring, transcultural issues) (Moody, 1990). Chapters 6 through 9 provide an examination of grand nursing theories.

### Middle Range Theories

The need for practice disciplines to develop middle range theories was first proposed in the field of sociology in the 1960s. In nursing, development of middle range theory is growing to fill the gaps between grand nursing theories and nursing practice.

Compared to grand theories, middle range theories contain limited numbers of concepts and are limited in scope. Within the scope of middle range theories, however, some degree of generalization is possible across specialty areas and settings. Propositions are clear, and testable hypotheses can be derived. Middle range theories cover such concepts as pain, symptom management, cultural issues, and health promotion (Higgins & Moore, 2000; Peterson, 2008; Walker & Avant, 2005). Chapters 10 and 11 provide a detailed discussion of middle range theories and their application in nursing.

### Practice Theories

Practice theories (microtheories, situation-specific, or prescriptive theories) explain prescriptions or modalities for practice. The essence of practice theory is a defined or identified goal and prescriptions for interventions or activities to achieve this goal

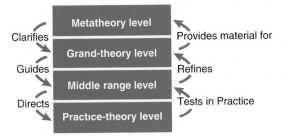

| Clarifies | Metatheory level | Provides material for |
| Guides | Grand-theory level | Refines |
| Directs | Middle range level | Tests in Practice |
| | Practice-theory level | |

FIGURE 4-1 Relationship among levels of theory. (From Walker, L. O., & Avant, K. C. (2005). *Strategies for theory construction in nursing* (4th ed.). Upper Saddle River, NJ: Prentice-Hall. Reprinted by permission of Pearson Education, Inc., Upper Saddle River, NJ.)

(Walker & Avant, 2005). Practice theories can cover particular elements of a specialty, such as oncology nursing, obstetric nursing, or operating room nursing, or they may relate to another aspect of nursing such as nursing administration or nursing education. Such theories typically describe specific elements of nursing care, such as cancer pain relief, or a specific experience, such as dying and end-of-life care.

Practice theories contain few concepts, are narrow in scope, and explain a relatively small aspect of reality. They are derived from middle range theories, practice experiences and empirical testing (Peterson, 2008). Furthermore, when the concepts and statements are operationally defined, they may be tested by appropriate research strategies (Higgins & Moore, 2000).

### Relationship Among Levels of Theory in Nursing

Walker and Avant (2005) state that the four levels of theory may be linked to direct and focus the discipline of nursing. As they describe, metatheory (worldview or philosophy) clarifies the methodologies and roles for each subsequent level of theory development (grand, middle range, practice). Each level of theory provides material for further analysis and clarification at the level of metatheory. Grand nursing theories guide the phenomena of concern at the middle range level. Middle range theories assist in refinement of grand theories and direct prescriptions of practice theories. Practice theories are constructed from scientifically based propositions about reality and test the empirical validity of those propositions as they are incorporated into client care (Higgins & Moore, 2000). Figure 4-1 illustrates the relationships among the levels of theory in nursing.

## CATEGORIZATION BASED ON PURPOSE

As discussed in Chapter 2, Dickoff and James (1968) described four kinds of theory: factor-isolating theories (descriptive theories), factor-relating theories (explanatory theories), situation-relating theories (predictive theories), and situation-producing theories (prescriptive theories). Each higher level of theory builds on the lower levels (Dickoff et al., 1968), and each is reviewed in the following sections.

### Descriptive Theories

Descriptive theories describe, observe, and name concepts, properties, and dimensions, but they do not explain the interrelationships among the concepts or propositions, and they do not indicate how changes in one concept affect other concepts. According to Barnum (1998), descriptive theory is the first and most important level of theory development because it determines what will be perceived as the essence of the phenomenon under study. Subsequent theory development expands or refines those elements and specifies relationships that are determined to be important in the descriptive phase. Thus, it is critical that the most significant constituents of the phenomenon be recognized and named in this earliest phase of theory development.

The two types of descriptive theory are naming and classification. *Naming theories* describe the dimension or characteristics of a phenomenon. *Classification theories* describe dimensions or characteristics of a phenomenon that are structurally interrelated and are sometimes referred to as typologies or taxonomies (Barnum, 1998; Fawcett, 1999).

Descriptive theories are generated and tested by descriptive or explanatory research. Techniques for generating and testing descriptive theory include concept analysis, case studies, comprehensive literature review, surveys, phenomenology, ethnography, grounded theory, and historical inquiry (Fawcett, 1999). Examples of descriptive theory found in recent nursing literature include the development of a model for the HELLP syndrome (hemolysis, elevated liver enzymes, and low platelets) in pregnant women (phenomenology) (Kidner & Flanders-Stepans, 2004); development of a model for understanding caregiving changes among poor, chronically ill Mexicans (ethnography) (Robles-Silva, 2008); and the proposed middle range Theory for Generative Quality of Life for the Elderly (comprehensive literature review) (Register & Herman, 2006). In other examples, Zauderer (2008) used a case study approach to examine the phenomenon of altered maternal–newborn attachment and Rew (2003) used grounded theory to explore self-care behaviors of homeless youth.

### Explanatory Theories

Explanatory theory is the second level in theory development. Once phenomena have been identified and named, they can be viewed in relation to other phenomena. Explanatory theories relate concepts to one another and describe and specify some of the associations or interrelations between and among the concepts. Further, explanatory theories attempt to tell how or why the concepts are related and may deal with causality, correlations, and rules that regulate interactions (Barnum, 1998; Dickoff et al., 1968).

Explanatory theories can be developed only after the parts of the phenomena have been identified and tested, and they are generated and tested by correlational research. Correlational research requires collection or measurement of data gathered by observation or self-report instruments that will yield either qualitative or quantitative data (Fawcett, 1999). Examples of explanatory theories from recent nursing literature include development of a theory of diversity of human field pattern (Hastings-Tolsma, 2006); an examination of resilience among operating room nurses (Gillespie, Chaboyer, Wallis, & Grimbeek, 2007); and a practice theory identifying the cues that trigger participation in prostate screening (Nivens, Herman, Weinrich, & Weinrich, 2001). In a qualitative study, Olshansky (2003) developed a theoretical model through combining previously described constructs of "identity as infertile" and "vulnerability to depression." Similarly, Moore and Coty (2006) developed a model of breastfeeding behavior involving such constructs as breastfeeding attitude, support for breastfeeding, breastfeeding behavioral control, and barriers and problems encountered with breastfeeding.

### Predictive Theories

Predictive theories describe precise relationships between concepts and are the third level of theory development. Predictive theories presuppose the prior existence of the more elementary types of theory. They result after concepts are defined and relational statements are generated and are able to describe future outcomes consistently. Predictive theories include statements of causal or consequential relatedness (Dickoff et al., 1968).

Predictive theories are generated and tested by experimental research involving manipulation of a phenomenon to determine how it affects or changes some dimension or characteristic of another phenomenon (Fawcett, 1999). Different research designs may be used in this process. These include pretest–posttest designs, quasi-experiments, and true experiments. These research studies produce quantifiable data that are statistically analyzed. Examples of predictive theories include a model examining patient satisfaction with nurse practitioner care (Green & Davis, 2005), a model identifying social cognitive factors that predict elders' health (Zauszniewski, Chung, & Krafcik, 2001), and a model predicting physical activity in older adults with hypertension (Lee & Laffrey, 2006). In an interesting work, Tourangeau (2005) synthesized research literature from multiple sources to propose a theoretical model predicting patient mortality. She identified the following contributing or determining factors to mortality: nurses' staffing, burnout, satisfaction, skill mix, experience and role support, as well as such factors as physician expertise, hospital location, and patient characteristics (e.g., age, gender, comorbidity, socioeconomic status, and chronicity).

### Prescriptive Theories

Prescriptive theories are perceived to be the highest level of theory development (Dickoff et al., 1968). Prescriptive theories prescribe activities necessary to reach defined goals. In nursing, prescriptive theories address nursing therapeutics and predict the consequence of interventions (Meleis, 2007). Prescriptive theories have three basic components: (1) specified goals or outcomes, (2) explicit activities to be taken to meet the goal, and (3) a survey list that articulates the conceptual basis of the theory (Dickoff et al., 1968).

According to Dickoff et al. (1968), the outcome or goal of a prescriptive theory serves as the norm or standard by which to evaluate activities. The goal must articulate the context of the situation, and this provides the basis for testing to determine whether the goal has been achieved. The specified actions or activities are those nursing interventions that should be taken to realize the goal. The goal will not be realized without the activity, and prescriptions for activities directly affect the goals.

The survey list augments and supplements the prescribed activities. In addition, it serves to prepare for future prescriptive activities. The survey list asks six questions about the prescribed activity that relate to the delineated goal (Box 4-1).

Examples of prescriptive theory are becoming more common in the literature, enhanced by the expanding volume of nursing research and increasing calls for evidence-based practice. The descriptions of feeding, pelvic floor exercise, therapeutic touch, and latex precautions are only a few of many excellent examples of nursing interventions

---

**BOX 4-1** | *Survey List of Questions for Prescriptive Theories*

1. Who performs the activity? (agency)
2. Who or what is the recipient of the activity? (patiency)
3. In what context is the activity performed? (framework)
4. What is the end point of the activity? (terminus)
5. What is the guiding procedure, technique, or protocol of the activity? (procedure)
6. What is the energy source for the activity? (dynamics)

Source: Dickoff et al. (1968).

presented by Bulechek, Butcher, & Dochterman (2008). Lefort's (2000) model to assist self-help in adults with chronic pain is another example.

## CATEGORIZATION BASED ON SOURCE OR DISCIPLINE

Theories may be classified based on the discipline or source of origin. As briefly discussed in Chapter 1, many of the theories used in nursing are borrowed, shared, or derived from theories developed in other disciplines. Because nursing is a human science and a practice discipline, incorporation of shared theories into practice and modification of them for use and testing are common.

Nurses use theories and concepts from the behavioral sciences, biologic sciences, and sociologic sciences, as well as learning theories and organizational and management theories, among others. In many cases these concepts and theories will overlap. For example, adaptation and stress are concepts found in both the behavioral and biologic sciences, and multiple theories have been developed using these concepts. Additionally, some theories defy placement in one discipline, but relate to many. These include such basic concepts as systems theory, change theory, and chaos.

This book discusses a number of theories and concepts organized in terms of sociologic sciences, behavioral sciences, biomedical sciences, administration and management sciences, and learning theories. Table 4-1 presents examples of theories from each of these areas. Although by no means exhaustive, Chapters 12 through 16 provide information on many of the shared theories commonly used in nursing practice, research, education, and administration.

### TABLE 4-1 *Shared Theory Used in Nursing Practice and Research*

| Disciplines | Examples of Theories Used by Nurses |
| --- | --- |
| Theories from sociologic sciences | Family systems theory |
| | Feminist theory |
| | Role theory |
| | Critical social theory |
| Theories from behavioral sciences | Attachment theory |
| | Theories of self-determination |
| | Lazrus and Folkman's theory of stress, coping, and adaptation |
| | Theory of planned behavior |
| Theories from biomedical sciences | Pain |
| | Self-regulation theory |
| | Immune function |
| | Symptomology |
| | Germ theory |
| Theories from administration and management sciences | Donabedian's quality framework |
| | Theories of organizational behavior |
| | Models of conflict and conflict resolution |
| | Job satisfaction |
| Learning theories | Bandura's social cognitive learning theory |
| | Developmental learning theory |
| | Prospect theory |

## Components of a Theory

A theory has several components, including purpose, concepts and definitions, theoretical statements, structure/linkages and ordering, and assumptions (Bishop & Hardin, 2006; Chinn & Kramer, 2008; Powers & Knapp, 2006). Creation of conceptual models is also a component of theory development that is promoted to further explain and define relationships, structure, and linkages.

### PURPOSE

The purpose of a theory explains why the theory was formulated and specifies the context and situations in which it should be applied. The purpose might also provide information about the sociopolitical context in which the theory was developed, circumstances that influenced its creation, the theorist's past experiences, settings in which the theory was formulated, and societal trends. The purpose of the theory is usually explicitly described and should be found within the discussion of the theory (Chinn & Kramer, 2008).

### CONCEPTS AND CONCEPTUAL DEFINITIONS

Concepts and concept development are described in detail in Chapter 3. Concepts are linguistic labels that are assigned to objects or events and are considered to be the building blocks of theories. The theoretical definition defines the concept in relation to other concepts and permits the description and classification of phenomena. Operationally defined concepts link the concept to the real world and identify empirical referents (indicators) of the concept that will permit observation and measurement (Bishop & Hardin, 2006; Chinn & Kramer, 2008; Walker & Avant, 2005). Theories should include explicit conceptual definitions to describe and clarify the phenomenon and explain how the concept is expressed in empirical reality.

### THEORETICAL STATEMENTS

Once a concept is fully developed and presented, it can be combined with other concepts to create statements to describe the real world. Theoretical statements, or propositions, are statements about the relationship between two or more concepts and are used to connect concepts to devise the theory. Statements must be formulated before explanations or predictions can be made, and development of statements asserting a connection between two or more concepts introduces the possibility of analysis (Bishop & Hardin, 2006). The several types of theoretical statements include propositions, laws, axioms, empirical generalizations, and hypotheses (Table 4-2).

Theoretical statements can be classified into two groups. The first group consists of statements that claim the *existence* of phenomena referred to by concepts (existence statements). The second group describes *relationships* between concepts (relational statements) (Reynolds, 1971).

#### Existence Statements

Existence statements and definitions relate to specific concepts and make existence claims about that concept (e.g., that chair is brown or that man is a nurse). Each statement has a concept and is identified by a term that is applied to another object or

TABLE 4-2 *Types of Relationship Statements*

| Type of Statement | Characteristics |
| --- | --- |
| Axioms | Consist of a basic set of statements or propositions that state the general relationship between concepts. Axioms are relatively abstract; therefore, they are not directly observed or measured. |
| Empirical generalizations | Summarize empirical evidence. Empirical generalizations provide some confidence that the same pattern will be repeated in concrete situations in the future under the same conditions. |
| Hypotheses | Statements that lack support from empirical research but are selected for study. The source of hypotheses may be a variation of a law or a derivation from an axiomatic theory, or they may be generated by a scientist's intuition (a hunch). All concepts in a hypothesis must be measurable, with operational definitions in concrete situations. |
| Laws | Well-grounded with strong empirical support and evidence of empirical regulatory. Laws contain concepts that can be measured or identified in concrete settings. |
| Propositions | Statements of a constant relationship between two or more concepts or facts. |

Sources: Hardy (1973); Jacox (1974); Reynolds (1971).

phenomena. Existence statements serve as adjuncts to relational statements and clarify meanings in the theory. Existence statements are also termed nonrelational statements and may be right or wrong depending on the circumstances (Reynolds, 1971).

### Relational Statements

Existence statements can only name and classify objects. Knowing the existence of one concept may be used to convey information about the existence of other concepts. Relational statements assert that a relationship exists between the properties of two or more concepts. This relationship is basic to development of theory and is expressed in terms of relational statements that explain, predict, understand, or control.

Like concepts, statements may have different levels of abstraction (theoretical and operational). The more general statements contain theoretically defined concepts. If the theoretical concepts are replaced with operational definitions, then the statement is "operationalized." The two broad groups of relational statements are those that describe an *association* between two concepts and those that describe a *causal relationship* between two concepts (Reynolds, 1971).

*Associational or Correlational Relationships.* Associational statements describe concepts that occur or exist together (Reynolds, 1971; Walker & Avant, 2005). The nature of the association/correlation may be positive (when one concept occurs or is high, the other concept occurs or is high). For example, as the external temperature rises during the summer, consumption of ice cream increases. An example in human beings is a positive correlation between height and weight—as people get taller, in general their weight will increase.

The association may be neutral when the occurrence of one concept provides no information about the occurrence of another concept. For example, there is no correlation between gender and scores on a pharmacology examination. Finally, the association may be negative. In this case, when one concept occurs or is high, the other concept is low and vice versa. For example, failure to use condoms regularly is associated with an increase in the occurrence of sexually transmitted diseases.

*Causal Relationships.* In causal relationships, one concept is considered to cause the occurrence of a second concept. For example, as caloric intake increases, weight increases. In scientific research, the concept or variable that is the cause is typically referred to as the independent variable and the variable that is affected is referred to as the dependent variable.

In science, there is often disagreement about whether a relationship is causal or simply highly correlated. A classic example is the relationship between cigarette smoking and lung cancer. As early as the 1940s, an association between smoking and lung cancer was recognized, but not until the 1980s was it determined that smoking actually *caused* lung cancer. Likewise, genetic predisposition is *associated* with development of heart disease; it has not been shown to *cause* heart disease.

## STRUCTURE AND LINKAGES

Structuring the theory by logical arrangement and specifying linkages of the theoretical concepts and statements is critical to the development of theory. The structure of a theory provides overall form to the theory. Theory structuring includes determination of the order of appearance of relationships, identification of central relationships, and delineation of direction, strength, and quality of relationships (Chinn & Kramer, 2008).

Although theoretical statements assert connections between concepts, the rationale for the stated connections needs to be developed. Theoretical linkages offer a reasoned explanation of why the variables in the theory may be connected in some manner, which brings plausibility to the theory. When developed operationally, linkages contribute to the testability of the theory by specifying how variables are connected. Thus, conceptual arrangement of statements and linkages can lead to hypotheses (Bishop & Hardin, 2006).

## ASSUMPTIONS

Assumptions are notations that are taken to be true without proof. They are beliefs about a phenomenon that one must accept as true to accept a theory, and although they may not be empirically testable, they can be argued philosophically. The assumptions of a theory are based on what the theorist considers to be adequate empirical evidence to support propositions, on accepted knowledge, or on personal beliefs or values (Jacox, 1974; McKenna & Slevin, 2008; Powers & Knapp, 2006). Assumptions may be in the form of factual assertions or they may reflect value positions. Factual assumptions are those that are known through experience. Value assumptions assert or imply what is right, or good, or ought to be (Chinn & Kramer, 2008).

In a given theory, assumptions may be implicit or explicit. In many nursing theories, they must be "teased out." Furthermore, it is often difficult to separate assumptions that are implicit or integrated into the narrative of the theory from relationship statements (Powers & Knapp, 2006).

## MODELS

Models are schematic representations of some aspect of reality. Various media are used in construction of models; they may be three-dimensional objects, diagrams, geometric formulas, or words. Empirical models are replicas of observable reality (e.g., a plastic model of a uterus or an eye). Theoretical models represent the real world through language or symbols and directional arrows.

Artinian (1982) described the rationale for creating a theoretical or conceptual model. She determined that models help illustrate the processes through which outcomes occur by specifying the relationships among the variables in graphic form where they can be examined for inconsistency, incompleteness, or errors. By creating a model of the concepts and relationships, it is possible to trace the effect of certain variables on the outcome variable rather than making assertions that each variable under study is related to every other variable. Furthermore, the model depicts a process that starts somewhere and ends at a logical point. Using the model, a person should be able to explain what happened, predict what will happen, and interpret what is happening. Finally, Artinian stated that once a model has been conceptually illustrated, the phenomenon represented can be examined in different settings testing the usefulness and generalizability of the underlying theory. The figure in the exemplar at the end of the chapter shows a model illustrating the relationships between the variables of the Caregiving Effectiveness Model.

## Theory Development

Several factors are vital for nurses to examine the process of theory development. First, an understanding of the relationship among theory, research, and practice should be recognized. Second, the nurse should be aware that there are various approaches to theory development, based on the source of initiation (i.e., practice, theory, or research). Finally, the process of theory development should be understood. Each of these factors is discussed in the following sections.

### RELATIONSHIP AMONG THEORY, RESEARCH, AND PRACTICE

Many nurses lack a true understanding of the interrelationship among theory, research, and practice and its importance to the continuing development of nursing as a profession (Pryjmachuk, 1996). As early as the 1970s, nursing scholars commented on the relationships among theory, research, and practice. Indeed, at that time nursing leaders urged that nursing research be combined with theory development to provide a rational basis for practice (Flaskerud, 1984; Moody, 1990).

In applied disciplines such as nursing, practice is based on the theories that are validated through research. Thus, theory, research, and practice affect each other in a reciprocal, cyclical, and interactive way (Hickman, 2002; Marrs & Lowry, 2006) (Figure 4-2).

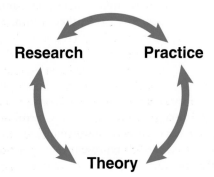

FIGURE 4-2 Research-theory-practice cycle.

### Relationship Between Theory and Research

Research validates and modifies theory. In nursing, theories stimulate nurse scientists to explore significant problems in the field of nursing. In doing so, the potential for the development of nursing knowledge increases (Meleis, 2007). Theories can be used to formulate a set of generalizations to explain relationships among variables. When empirically tested, the results of research can be used to verify, modify, disprove, or support a theoretical proposition.

### Relationship Between Theory and Practice

Theory guides practice. One of the primary uses of theory is to contribute insights about nursing practice situations through provision of goals for assessment, diagnosis, and intervention. Likewise, through practice, nursing theory is shaped and guidelines for practice evolve. Theory renders practice more efficient and more effective, and the ultimate benefit of theory application in nursing is the improvement in client care (Meleis, 2007).

### Relationship Between Research and Practice

Research is the key to the development of a discipline. Middle range and practice theories may be tested in practice through clinical research (Hickman, 2002). If individual practitioners are to develop expertise, they must participate in research. In summary, there is a need to encourage nurses to test and refine theories and models to develop their own personal models of practice (Marrs & Lowry, 2006; Pryjmachuk, 1996).

## APPROACHES TO THEORY DEVELOPMENT

Several different approaches may be used to initiate the process of theory development. Meleis (2007) cites four major strategies differentiated by their origin (theory, practice, or research) and by whether sources from outside of nursing were used to develop the theory. These approaches are theory–practice–theory, practice–theory, research–theory, and theory–research–theory. She then proposes employment of an integrated approach to theory development. Table 4-3 summarizes these different approaches.

### Theory–Practice–Theory

The theory–practice–theory approach to theory development begins with a theory (typically nonnursing) that describes a phenomenon of interest. This approach assumes that the theory can help describe or explain the phenomenon, but it is not completely congruent with nursing and is not directly defined for nursing practice; the focus of the theory is different from the focus needed for nursing.

Using the theory–practice–theory strategy, the nurse would select a theory that may be used to explain or describe a clinical situation (e.g., adaptation, stress, health beliefs). The nurse could modify concepts and consider relationships between concepts that were not proposed in the original theory. To accomplish this, the nurse would need to (1) have a basic knowledge of the theory; (2) analyze the theory by reducing it into components where each component is defined and evaluated; (3) use assumptions, concepts, and propositions to describe the clinical area; (4) redefine assumptions, concepts, and propositions to reflect nursing; and (5) reconstruct a theory using exemplars representing the redefined assumptions, concepts, and propositions (Meleis, 2007). Examples of a theory–practice–theory strategy include Benner's use of Dreyfus's Model of Skill Acquisition to describe novice to expert practice (Benner, 2001) and Roy's use of Helson's Adaptation Theory to describe human responses

TABLE 4-3 *Strategies for Theory Development*

| Origin of Theory | Basis for Development | Type of Theory | Methods for Development |
|---|---|---|---|
| Theory–practice–theory | An existing theory (nonnursing) that can help describe and explain a phenomenon, but the theory is not complete or not completely developed for nursing | Borrowed or shared theory | Theorist selects a nonnursing theory; analyzes the theory; defines and evaluates each component; redefines assumptions, concepts, and propositions to reflect nursing |
| Practice–theory | Existing theories are not useful in describing the phenomenon of interest; theory is derived from clinical situations | Grounded theory | Researcher observes phenomenon of interest, analyzes similarities and differences, compares and contrasts responses, and develops concepts and linkages |
| Research–theory | Development of theory is based on research; theories evolve from replicated and confirmed research findings | Scientific theory | Researcher selects a common phenomenon, lists and measures characteristics of the phenomenon in a variety of situations, analyzes the data to determine if there are patterns that need further study, and formalizes patterns as theoretical statements |
| Theory–research–theory | Theory drives the research questions; the result of the research informs and modifies the theory | Theory testing | Theorist defines a theory and determines propositions for testing; the theory is modified, refined, or further developed based on research findings; in some cases a new theory will be formed |

Source: Meleis (2007).

(Roy & Roberts, 1981). Other examples of theory–practice–theory in recent nursing literature include a work that applied the Theory of Planned Behavior to develop a situation-specific theory of breastfeeding (Nelson, 2006) and Peters' (2006) theory of chronic stress emotions, which was derived from Lazarus's theory of stress using a descriptive, correlational design.

### Practice–Theory

If no appropriate theory appears to exist to describe or explain a phenomenon, theories may be inductively developed from clinical practice situations. The practice–theory approach is based on the premise that in a given situation existing theories are not useful in describing the phenomenon of interest. It assumes that the phenomenon is important enough to pursue and that there is a clinical understanding about it that has not been articulated. Furthermore, insight gained from describing the phenomenon has potential for enhancing the understanding of other similar situations through development of a set of propositions (Meleis, 2007).

This strategy is a grounded theory approach, which begins with a question evolving from a practice situation. It relies on observation of new phenomena in a practice situation, development of concepts, and then labeling, describing, and articulating properties of these concepts. To accomplish this, the researcher observes the phenomenon, analyzes similarities and differences, and then compares and contrasts responses. Following this, the researcher may develop concepts and propositional statements and propose linkages (Meleis, 2007). Examples of the practice–theory strategy of theory development include a situation-specific theory of Caucasian cancer patients' pain experience (Im, 2006), and a proposed theory of "keeping the spirit alive" among children with cancer and their families (Woodgate & Degner, 2003).

### Research–Theory

The research–theory strategy is the most accepted strategy for theory development in nursing, largely due to the early emphasis on empiricism described in Chapter 1. For empiricists, theory development is considered a product of research because theories evolve from replicated and confirmed research findings. The research–theory strategy assumes that there is truth in real life, that the truth can be captured through the senses, and that the truth can be verified (Meleis, 2007). Furthermore, the purpose of scientific theories is to describe, explain, predict, or control a part of the empirical world.

In the research–theory strategy for theory development, the researcher selects a phenomenon that occurs in the discipline and lists characteristics of the phenomenon. A method to measure the characteristics of the phenomenon is developed and implemented in a controlled study. The results of the measurement are analyzed to determine if there are any systematic patterns, and once patterns have been discovered, they are formalized into theoretical statements (Meleis, 2007). Examples of the research–theory strategy from nursing include the development of a taxonomy of passive behaviors in people with Alzheimer's disease (Colling, 2000), a report outlining a conceptual framework for caring in nursing practice (McCance, 2003), and a theoretical look at the involvement of relatives in palliative care (Andershed & Ternestedt, 2001).

### Theory–Research–Theory

In the theory–research–theory approach, theory drives the research questions and the results of the research are used to modify the theory. In this approach, the theorist will begin by defining a theory and determining propositions for testing. If carried through, the research findings may be used to further modify and develop the original theory (Meleis, 2007).

In this process, a theory is selected to explain the phenomenon of interest. The theory is a framework for operational definitions, variables, and statements. Concepts are redefined and operationalized for research. Findings are synthesized and used to modify, refine, or develop the original theory, or in some cases, to create a new theory. The goal is to test, refine, and develop theory and to use theory as a framework for research and theory modification. The researcher/theorist concludes the investigation with a refined, modified, or further developed explanation of the theory (Meleis, 2007). Examples of the theory–research–theory approach from recent nursing literature include a theory of genetic vulnerability developed from Roy's Adaptation Model using grounded theory methodology (Hamilton & Bowers, 2007), and Dunn's (2004, 2005) middle range theory of adaptation to chronic pain, which was also derived from Roy's Adaptation Model. Another example includes the theory of diversity of human field pattern, which was developed from Martha Rogers' Science of Unitary Human Beings using a quantitative research design (Hastings-Tolsma, 2006).

### Integrated Approach

An integrated approach to theory development describes an evolutionary process that is particularly useful in addressing complex clinical situations. It requires gathering of data from the clinical setting, identification of exemplars, discovery of solutions, and recognition of supportive information from other sources (Meleis, 2007).

Integrated theory development is rooted in clinical practice. Practice drives the basic questions and provides opportunities for clinical involvement in research that is designed to answer the questions. In this process for theory development, hunches and conceptual ideas are communicated with other clinicians or participants to allow for critique and further development. Among other strategies, the integrated approach uses skills and tools from clinical practice, various research methods, clinical diaries, descriptive journals, and collegial dialogues in developing a framework or conceptualization (Meleis, 2007).

## PROCESS OF THEORY DEVELOPMENT

The process of theory development has been described in some detail by several nursing scholars (Chinn & Jacobs, 1978; Chinn & Kramer, 1995; Jacox, 1974; Walker & Avant, 2005). Despite slight variations related to terminology and sequencing, the sources are similar in explaining the processes used to develop theory. The three basic steps are concept development, statement/proposition development, and theory construction. Chinn and Kramer (2008) add two additional steps that involve validating, confirming, or testing of the theory and application of theory in practice. Each of the steps are described in the following sections and Table 4-4 summarizes the theory development process.

### Concept Development: Creation of Conceptual Meaning

This first step or process of theory development involves creating conceptual meaning. This provides the foundation for theory development and includes specifying, defining, and clarifying the concepts used to describe the phenomenon of interest (Jacox, 1974).

Creating conceptual meaning uses mental processes to create mental structures or ideas to be used to represent experience. This produces a tentative definition of the concept(s) and a set of criteria for determining if the concept(s) exists in a particular

TABLE 4-4 *Process of Theory Development*

| Step | Description |
|---|---|
| Concept development | Specifying, defining, and clarifying the concepts used to describe a phenomenon of interest |
| Statement development | Formulating and analyzing statements explaining relationships between concepts; also involves determining empirical referents that can validate them |
| Theory construction | Structuring and contextualizing the components of the theory; includes identifying assumptions and organizing linkages between and among the concepts and statements to form a theoretical structure |
| Testing theoretical relationships | Validating theoretical relationships through empirical testing |
| Application of theory in practice | Using research methods to assess how the theory can be applied in practice; research should provide evidence to evaluate the theory's usefulness |

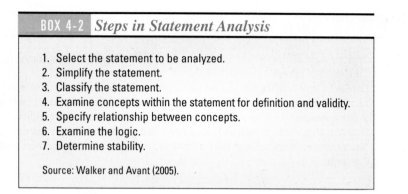

BOX 4-2 *Steps in Statement Analysis*

1. Select the statement to be analyzed.
2. Simplify the statement.
3. Classify the statement.
4. Examine concepts within the statement for definition and validity.
5. Specify relationship between concepts.
6. Examine the logic.
7. Determine stability.

Source: Walker and Avant (2005).

situation (Chinn & Kramer, 2008). Methods of concept development are described in detail in Chapter 3.

### Statement Development: Formulation and Validation of Relational Statements

Relational statements are the skeletons of theory; they are the means by which the theory comes together. The process of formulation and validation of relational statements involves developing the relational statements and determining empirical referents that can validate them.

After a statement has been delineated initially, it should be scrutinized or analyzed. Statement analysis is a process described by Walker and Avant (2005) to thoroughly examine relational statements. Statement analysis classifies statements and examines the relationships between the concepts and helps direct theoretical construction. There are seven steps in the process of statement analysis (Box 4-2). Following the process of statement analysis, the statements are refined and may be operationalized.

### Theory Construction: Systematic Organization of the Linkages

The third stage in theory development involves structuring and contextualizing the components of the theory. This includes formulating systematic linkages between and among concepts, which results in a formal, coherent theoretical structure. The format used depends on what is known or assumed to be true about the phenomena in question (Chinn & Kramer, 2008). Aspects of theory construction include identifying and defining the concepts, identifying assumptions, clarifying the context within which the theory is placed, designing relationship statements, and delineating the organization, structure, or relationship among the components.

Theory synthesis is a theory construction strategy developed by Walker and Avant (2005). In theory synthesis, concepts and statements are organized into a network or whole. The purposes of theory synthesis are to represent a phenomenon through an interrelated set of concepts and statements, to describe the factors that precede or influence a particular phenomenon or event, to predict effects that occur after some event, or to put discrete scientific information into a more theoretically organized form.

Theory synthesis can be used to produce a compact, informative graphic representation of research findings on a topic of interest, and synthesized theories may be expressed in several ways such as graphic or model form. The three steps in theory synthesis are summarized in Box 4-3.

### Validating and Confirming Theoretical Relationships in Research

Chinn and Kramer (2008) include the process of validating and confirming theoretical relationships as a component of theory development. Validating theoretical relationships involves empirically refining concepts and theoretical relationships, identifying

---

**BOX 4-3**  *Steps in Theory Synthesis*

1. Select a topic of interest and specify focal concepts (may be one concept/variable or a framework of several concepts).
2. Conduct a review of the literature to identify related factors and note their relationships. Identify and record relationships indicating whether they are bidirectional, unidirectional, positive, neutral or negative, weak or ambiguous, or strong in support evidence.
3. Organize concepts and relational statements into an integrated representation of the phenomena of interest. Diagrams may be used to express the relationships among the concepts.

Source: Walker and Avant (2005).

---

empirical indicators, and testing relationships through empirical methods. In this step, the focus is on correlating the theory with demonstrable experiences and designing research to validate the relationships. Additionally, alternative explanations are considered, based on the empirical evidence.

### Validation and Application of Theory in Practice

An important final step in theory development identified by Chinn and Kramer (2008) is applying the theory in practice. In this step, research methods are used to assess how the theory can be applied in practice. The theoretical relationships are examined in the practice setting and results are recorded to determine how well the theory achieves the desired outcomes. The research design should provide evidence of the effect of the interventions on the well-being of recipients of care. Questions to be considered in this step include: Are the theory's goals congruent with practice goals? Is the intended context of the theory congruent with the practice situation? Are explanations of the theory sufficient for use in the nursing situation? Is there research evidence supporting use of the theory?

## Summary

Jill Watson, the nurse/graduate student introduced in the case study at the beginning of this chapter, was unable to identify a theory or conceptual model that completely met the needs for her study on health motivation. Because of this, she determined that it would be appropriate and feasible to use theory development techniques to revise an existing theory to use in her research project.

Theory development is an important but complex and time-consuming process. This chapter has presented a number of issues related to the process of theory development. These issues included the purpose of developing theory and the components of a theory. Discussion focused on concepts, theoretical statements, assumptions, and model development and explained the relationships among theory, research, and practice. Finally, the process of theory development was presented.

To further illustrate the process of theory development, a summary report of a theory recently published in the nursing literature is presented. In the following exemplar, each of the components of the theory is clearly identified. In addition, Chapter 5 expands on the process of theory development by examining the processes of theory analysis and evaluation.

## THEORY DEVELOPMENT EXEMPLAR

Smith, C. E., Pace, K., Kochinda, C., Kleinbeck, S. V. M., Koehler, J., & Popkess-Vawter, S. (2002). Caregiving effectiveness model evolution to a midrange theory of home care: A process for critique and replication. *Advances in Nursing Science, 25* (1), 50–64.

Smith and colleagues developed the "Caregiving Effectiveness Model" to be applied to home care situations in which the patient requires "technologically based treatment." Provided here is a summary of the components of this theory outlined by the criteria described in this chapter.

*Scope of theory:* Middle range

*Purpose:* "To explain and predict outcomes of technology-based home caregiving provided by family members" (p. 50). Outcomes of the model are "to help nurses develop relevant nursing interventions to support positive patient and caregiver outcomes" (p. 51).

Concepts and definitions are listed in the following table.

| Concept | Definition | Empirical Indicator |
|---|---|---|
| Caregiving effectiveness | The provision of technical, physical, and emotional care by family members that results in outcomes of optimal patient condition, yet maintains the well-being of caregivers | Caregiving Context Concepts Measures + Adaptive Context Concepts Measures = Caregiving Effectiveness Outcomes |
| ***Caregiving Context Concepts*** | | |
| Caregiving characteristics | Personal characteristics potentially affecting caregiving | Age, gender, education level |
| Caregiving/care-receiving interactions | Quality of relationships between caregivers and patients (mutuality) and motivation to provide home care | Mutuality Scale Motivation to Help |
| Home care management strategies | Educational preparation; health professional teaching and resource management | Preparedness Scale Efficient use of resources (DEA coefficient) |
| ***Adaptive Context Concepts*** | | |
| Family economic stability | Income adequacy; degree of health care services use | Health care services use/cost |
| Caregiver health status | Mental health status (presence or absence of depression); physical health status | Quality of Life Index Depression Score (CES-D Scale) |
| Family adaptation | Family coping and problem-solving skills | Family Coping Scale |
| Reactions to caregiving | Caregiving esteem | Caregiver Reactions Scale |

### *Theoretical Statement and Linkages*

1. Caregiving Effectiveness Outcomes are the result of the variables in the Caregiving Context being mediated by Adaptive Context Variables.
2. Caregiving characteristics mediated by the caregiver mental health status (depression) affect Caregiving Effectiveness Outcomes.

3. Home care management strategies (preparedness) mediated by reactions to caregiving influence patient condition.
4. Caregiving Effectiveness Outcome of Efficient Use of Resources is influenced by caregiving and adaptive context variables.

*Model:* Smith et al.'s schematic diagram combines the statements to illustrate linkages and gives the theory structure as follows.

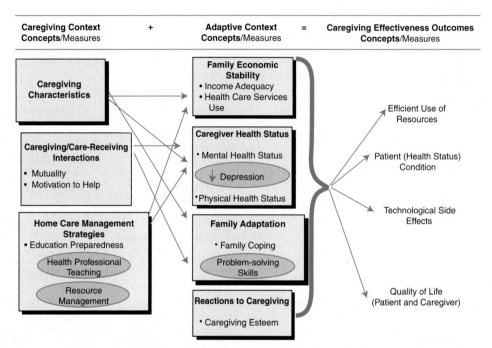

Concepts in the respecified Caregiving Effectiveness Model. Rectangles enclose concepts in the model; ellipses enclose recommended interventions derived from the model and found efficacious in clinical trial; and efficient use of resources is added as an outcome.

### Assumptions

1. Caregiving with complex technological home care is stressful and disruptive to usual family activities.
2. Families prefer home technological care as opposed to institutional care.
3. Model concepts are clinically relevant for nursing practice with patients and their caregivers.
4. Models about caregiving of terminally ill and frail or cognitively impaired older persons are not directly applicable to technology-dependent patients.

## LEARNING ACTIVITIES

1. Find an example of a nursing theory in a current book or periodical. Review the theory and classify it based on scope or level of abstraction (grand theory, middle range theory, practice theory), the purpose of the theory (describe, explain, predict, control), and the source or discipline in which the theory was developed.

2. Find an example of a middle range nursing theory (see Chapter 10 or 11 for ideas). Following the above exemplar, identify the components of the theory (i.e., scope of the theory, purpose, concepts and definitions, etc.).

3. Find an example of a middle range theory that does not contain a model. With classmates, try to create a model that depicts the relationships between and among the concepts. Discuss the challenges posed by this exercise.

## REFERENCES

Andershed, B., & Ternestedt, B. M. (2001). Development of a theoretical framework describing relatives' involvement in palliative care. *Journal of Advanced Nursing, 34*(4), 554–562.

Artinian, B. (1982). Conceptual mapping: Development of the strategy. *Western Journal of Nursing Research, 4*(4), 379–393.

Barnum, B. S. (1998). *Nursing theory: Analysis, application, evaluation* (5th ed.). Philadelphia: Lippincott Williams & Wilkins.

Benner, P. (2001). *From novice to expert: Excellence and power in clinical nursing practice* (commemorative edition). Upper Saddle River, NJ: Prentice-Hall.

Bishop, S. M., & Hardin, S. R. (2006). Theory development process. In A. M. Tomey & M. R. Alligood (Eds.), *Nursing theorists and their work* (6th ed., pp. 35–49). St. Louis: Mosby.

Bulechek, G. M., Butcher, H. K., & Dochterman, G. M. (2008). *Nursing interventions classification* (5th ed.). St. Louis: Mosby.

Cesario, S. (1997). The impact of the electronic domain on theory construction. *Journal of Theory Construction and Testing, 1*(2), 60–63.

Chinn, P. L., & Jacobs, M. K. (1978). A model for theory development in nursing. *Advances in Nursing Science, 1*(1), 1–11.

Chinn, P. L., & Kramer, M. K. (1995). *Theory and nursing integrated knowledge development* (4th ed.). St. Louis: Mosby.

Chinn, P. L., & Kramer, M. K. (2008). *Integrated knowledge developing in nursing* (6th ed.). St. Louis: Mosby.

Colling, K. B. (2000). A taxonomy of passive behaviors in people with Alzheimer's disease. *Image: Journal of Nursing Scholarship, 32*(3), 239–244.

Dickoff, J., & James, P. (1968). A theory of theories: A position paper. *Nursing Research, 17*(3), 197–203.

Dickoff, J., James, P., & Wiedenbach, E. (1968). Theory in a practice discipline part II: Practice oriented research. *Nursing Research, 17*(6), 545–554.

Dunn, K. S. (2004). Toward a middle range theory of adaptation to chronic pain. *Nursing Science Quarterly, 17*(1), 78–84.

Dunn, K. S. (2005). Testing a middle-range theoretical model of adaptation to chronic pain. *Nursing Science Quarterly, 18*(2), 146–156.

Fawcett, J. (1999). *The relationship of theory and research* (3rd ed.). Philadelphia: Davis.

Flaskerud, J. H. (1984). Nursing models as conceptual frameworks for research. *Western Journal of Nursing Research, 6*(2), 153–155.

Gillespie, B. M., Chaboyer, W., Wallis, M., & Grimbeek, P. (2007). Resilience in the operating room: Developing and testing of a resilience model. *Journal of Advanced Nursing, 59*(4), 427–438.

Green, A., & Davis, S. (2005). Toward a predictive model of patient satisfaction with nurse practitioner care. *Journal of the American Academy of Nurse Practitioners, 17*(4), 139–148.

Hamilton, R. J., & Bowers, B. J. (2007). The theory of genetic vulnerability: A Roy model exemplar. *Nursing Science Quarterly, 20*(3), 254–264.

Hardy, M. E. (1973). The nature of theories. *Theoretical foundations for nursing.* New York: MSS Information Systems.

Hastings-Tolsma, M. (2006). Toward a theory of diversity of human field pattern. *Visions, 14*(2), 34–46.

Hickman, J. S. (2002). An introduction to nursing theory. In J. B. George (Ed.), *Nursing theories: The base for professional nursing practice* (5th ed., pp. 1–20). Upper Saddle River, NJ: Prentice-Hall.

Higgins, P. A., & Moore, S. M. (2000). Levels of theoretical thinking in nursing. *Nursing Outlook, 48*(4), 179–183.

Im, E. O. (2006). A situation-specific theory of Caucasian cancer patients' pain experience. *Advances in Nursing Science, 29*(3), 232–244.

Jacox, A. K. (1974). Theory construction in nursing: An overview. *Nursing Research, 23*(1), 4–13.

Kidner, M. C., & Flanders-Stepans, M. B. (2004). A model for the HELLP syndrome: The maternal experience. *Journal of Obstetric, Gynecologic, and Neonatal Nursing, 33*(1), 44–53.

Lee, Y. S., & Laffrey, S. C. (2006). Predictors of physical activity in older adults with borderline hypertension. *Nursing Research, 55*(2), 110–120.

LeFort, S. M. (2000). A test of Braden's self-help model in adults with chronic pain. *Journal of Nursing Scholarship, 32*(2), 153–160.

Marrs, J., & Lowry, L. W. (2006). Nursing theory and practice: Connecting the dots. *Nursing Science Quarterly, 19*(1), 44–50.

McCance, T. V. (2003). Caring in nursing practice: The development of a conceptual framework. *Research and Theory for Nursing Practice, 17*(2), 101–116.

McKenna, H. P., & Slevin, O. D. (2008). *Nursing models, theories and practice.* United Kingdom: Blackwell Publishing.

Meleis, A. I. (2007). *Theoretical nursing: Development and progress* (4th ed.). Philadelphia: Lippincott Williams & Wilkins.

Moody, L. E. (1990). *Advancing nursing science through research.* Newbury Park, CA: Sage Publications.

Moore, E. R., & Coty, M. B. (2006). Prenatal and postpartum focus groups with primiparas: Breastfeeding attitudes, support, barriers, self-efficacy and intention. *Journal of Pediatric Health Care, 20*(1), 35–46.

Nelson, A. M. (2006). Toward a situation-specific theory of breastfeeding. *Research and Theory for Nursing Practice: An International Journal, 20*(1), 9–19.

Nivens, A. S., Herman, J., Weinrich, S., & Weinrich, M. C. (2001). Cues to participation in prostate cancer screening: A theory for practice. *Oncology Nursing Forum, 28*(9), 1449–1456.

Olshansky, E. (2003). A theoretical explanation for previously infertile mothers' vulnerability to depression. *Journal of Nursing Scholarship, 35*(3), 263–268.

Peters, R. M. (2006). The relationship of racism, chronic stress emotions and blood pressure. *Journal of Nursing Scholarship, 38*(3), 234–240.

Peterson, S. J. (2008). Introduction to the nature of nursing knowledge. In S. J. Peterson and T. S. Bredow (Eds.), *Middle range theories: Application to nursing research* (2nd ed., pp. 3–41). Philadelphia: Lippincott Williams & Wilkins.

Powers, B. A., & Knapp, T. R. (2006). *Dictionary of nursing theory and research* (3rd ed.). New York, NY: Springer Publishing.

Pryjmachuk, S. (1996). A nursing perspective on the interrelationships between theory, research and practice. *Journal of Advanced Nursing, 23*, 679–684.

Register, M. E., & Herman, J. (2006). A middle range theory for generative quality of life for the elderly. *Advances in Nursing Science, 29*(4), 340–350.

Rew, L. (2003). A theory of taking care of oneself grounded in experiences of homeless youth. *Nursing Research, 52*(4), 234–241.

Reynolds, P. D. (1971). *A primer in theory construction.* New York: Macmillan.

Robles-Silva, L. (2008). The caregiving trajectory among poor and chronically ill people. *Qualitative Health Research, 18*(3), 358–368.

Roy, C., & Roberts, S. (1981). *Theory construction in nursing: An adaptation model.* Englewood Cliffs, NJ: Prentice-Hall.

Streubert-Speziale, H. J., & Carpenter, D. R. (2008). *Qualitative research in nursing: Advancing the humanistic imperative* (4th ed.). Philadelphia: Lippincott Williams & Wilkins.

Tourangeau, A. E. (2005). A theoretical model of the determinants of mortality. *Advances in Nursing Science, 28*(1), 58–69.

Walker, L. O., & Avant, K. C. (2005). *Strategies for theory construction in nursing* (4th ed.). Norwalk, CT: Appleton & Lange.

Woodgate, R. L., & Degner, L. F. (2003). A spirit within children with cancer and their families. *Journal of Pediatric Oncology Nursing, 20*(3), 103–119.

Zauderer, C. R. (2008). A case study of postpartum depression & altered maternal-newborn attachment. *The American Journal of Maternal Child Nursing, 33*(3), 172–177.

Zauszniewski, J. A., Chung, C., & Krafcik, K. (2001). Social cognitive factors predicting the health of elders. *Western Journal of Nursing Research, 23*(5), 490–503.

# 5

# Theory Analysis and Evaluation

## Melanie McEwen

*Jerry Thompson is nearing completion of his master's degree in nursing. He is currently a case manager for a home health agency and his goal is to become an agency director after he completes his degree. For his research application project, Jerry wants to compare the effectiveness of health teaching in the hospital setting with the effectiveness of health teaching in the home setting. He has identified several areas to examine. These include the quality and type of health information provided, professional competencies of the nurses providing the information, the client's support system, and environmental resources. Outcome variables he will measure focus on utilization of health care (e.g., length of time on home health service, hospital readmissions, development of complications).*

*As his research project began to take shape, Jerry realized he needed a conceptual framework for the project. His advisor suggested Pender's Health Promotion Model. To determine if the model would be appropriate for his study, Jerry obtained the latest edition of Pender's book (Pender, Murdaugh, & Parsons, 2006), which described the model in depth. He then read commentaries in nursing theory books that analyzed her work and completed a literature search to find examples of research studies using the Health Promotion Model as a conceptual framework. After he had compiled these data, Jerry summarized his findings by using Whall's (2005) criteria for analysis and evaluation of middle range theories.*

*This exercise helped Jerry gain insight into the major concepts of the model and let him examine its important assumptions and linkages. From the evaluation, he determined that the model would be appropriate for use as the conceptual framework for his research study.*

---

As nurses began to participate in the processes of theory development in the 1960s, they realized that there was a corresponding need to identify criteria or develop mechanisms to determine if those theories served their intended purpose. As a result, the first method to describe, analyze, and critique theory was published in 1968. Over the following decades, a number of methods or techniques for theory evaluation were proposed. A general understanding of these methods will help the advanced practice nurse select an evaluation method for theory, which is appropriate to the stage of theory development and for the application of the theory (research, practice, administration, or education). This will, in turn, help ensure that the theory is valid and is being used correctly. It will also provide information for developing and testing new theories by identifying gaps and inconsistencies.

## Definition and Purpose of Theory Evaluation

Theory evaluation has been defined as the process of systematically examining a theory. Criteria for this process are variable, but they generally include examination of the theory's origins, meaning, logical adequacy, usefulness, generalizability, and testability. Theory evaluation does not generate new information outside the confines of the theory, but it often leads to new insights about the theory being examined.

Theory evaluation identifies a theory's degree of usefulness to guide practice, research, education, and administration. Such evaluation gives insight into relationships among concepts and their linkages to each other and allows the reviewer to determine the strengths and weaknesses of a theory. It also assists in identifying the need for additional theory development or refinement. Finally, theory evaluation provides a systematic, objective way of examining a theory that may lead to new insights and new formulations that will add to the body of practice or research (Walker & Avant, 2005). The ultimate goal of theory evaluation is to determine the potential contribution of the theory to scientific knowledge.

In nursing practice, theory evaluation may provide a clinician with additional knowledge about the soundness of the theory. It also helps identify which theoretical relationships are supported by research, provides guidelines for the choice of appropriate interventions, and gives some indication of their efficacy. In research, theory evaluation helps clarify the form and structure of a theory being tested or will allow the researcher to determine the relevance of the content of a theory for use as a conceptual framework, as described in the case study. Evaluation will also identify inconsistencies and gaps in the theory used in practice or research (Walker & Avant, 2005).

Various methods have been outlined to assist with this process. The methods are described by several overlapping terms or terms that are used in different ways by different authors. For example, theory analysis, theory description, theory evaluation, and theory critique all describe the process of critically reviewing a theory to assess its relevance and applicability to nursing practice, research, education, and administration. In this chapter, theory evaluation is used as a global term to discuss the process of reviewing theory.

Theory evaluation has been described as a single-phase process (theory analysis) by Alligood (2006) as well as Hardy (1974) (theory evaluation); a two-phase process (theory analysis and theory critique/evaluation) by Fawcett (2005) and Duffey and Muhlenkamp (1974); or a three-phase process (theory description, theory analysis, and theory critique/evaluation) by scholars including Meleis (2007) and Moody (1990). It should be noted that the methods are similar whether they describe one, two, or three phases. A three-phase process is outlined briefly in the following section. Later sections provide more detailed discussions of each phase.

### THEORY DESCRIPTION

Theory description is the initial step in the evaluation process. In theory description, the works of a theorist are reviewed with a focus on the historical context of the theory

(Hickman, 2002). In addition, related works by others are examined to gain a clear understanding of the structural and functional components of the theory. The structural components include assumptions, concepts, and propositions. The functional components consist of the concepts of the theory and how they are used to describe, explain, predict, or control (Meleis, 2007; Moody, 1990).

## THEORY ANALYSIS

Theory analysis is the second phase of the evaluation process. It refers to a systematic process of objectively examining the content, structure, and function of a theory. Theory analysis is conducted if the theory or framework has potential for being useful in practice, research, administration, or education. Theory analysis is a nonjudgmental, detailed examination of a theory, the main aim of which is to understand the theory (Fawcett, 1993; Meleis, 2007).

## THEORY EVALUATION

Theory evaluation, or theory critique, is the final step of the process. Evaluation follows analysis and assesses the theory's potential contribution to the discipline's knowledge base (Fawcett, 1993, 2005; Walker & Avant, 2005). In theory evaluation, critical reflection involves ascertaining how well a theory serves its purpose, with the process of evaluation resulting in a decision or action about use of the theory (Chinn & Kramer, 2008). This involves evaluation of how the theory is used to direct nursing practice and interventions and whether or not it contributes to favorable outcomes (Hickman, 2002).

## Historical Overview of Theory Analysis and Evaluation

Since the late 1960s, a number of nursing scholars have published systems or methods for theory analysis/evaluation. Table 5-1 provides a list of these works. Basic components of the processes described by each are presented in the following sections.

It should be noted that most of the processes/methods for theory analysis and theory evaluation were implicitly or explicitly developed to review grand nursing theories and conceptual frameworks. Only in recent years have the processes and methods been applied to middle range theories and, rarely, practice theories. This observation, however, does not negate the need for analysis and evaluation (whether formal or informal) of middle range and practice theories. Furthermore, the processes should be applicable to all levels of theory.

### CHARACTERISTICS OF SIGNIFICANT THEORIES: ELLIS

Probably the first nursing scholar to document criteria for analyzing theories for use by nurses was Rosemary Ellis. Although not specifically describing a process or method of theory analysis or evaluation, Ellis (1968) identified characteristics of significant theories. The characteristics she specified were scope, complexity, testability, usefulness, implicit values of the theorist, information generation, and meaningful terminology. Her discussion of these characteristics produced the foundation on which later writers developed their criteria.

TABLE 5-1 *Publications of Methods for Nursing Theory Analysis and Evaluation*

| Nursing Scholar | Dates of Publications | Techniques Described (Most Recent Publication) |
| --- | --- | --- |
| Rosemary Ellis | 1968 | Characteristics of significant theories |
| Margaret Hardy | 1974, 1978 | Theory evaluation |
| Mary Duffey and Ann Muhlenkamp | 1974 | Theory analysis and theory evaluation |
| Barbara Barnum (Stevens) | 1979, 1984, 1990, 1994, 1998 | Theory evaluation—internal criticism, external criticism |
| Lorraine Walker and Kay Avant | 1983, 1988, 1995, 2005 | Theory analysis |
| Jacqueline Fawcett | 1980, 1993, 1995, 2000, 2005 | Theory (conceptual framework) analysis and theory (conceptual framework) evaluation |
| Peggy Chinn and Maenoa Kramer (Jacobs) | 1983, 1987, 1991, 1995, 1999, 2004, 2008 | Theory description and critical reflection |
| Afaf Meleis | 1985, 1991, 1997, 2007 | Theory description, theory analysis, theory critique |
| Joyce Fitzpatrick and Ann Whall | 1989, 1996, 2005 | Analysis and evaluation of practice theory, middle range theory and nursing models |
| Sharon Dudley-Brown | 1997 | Theory evaluation |

## THEORY EVALUATION: HARDY

A few years after Ellis, Margaret Hardy (1974) wrote that theory should be evaluated according to certain universal standards. In her writings, Hardy provided a more detailed description of criteria for theory evaluation and presented personal insight on the processes needed. Criteria or standards she suggested for theory evaluation were as follows:

- Meaning and logical adequacy
- Operational and empirical adequacy
- Testability
- Generality
- Contribution to understanding
- Predictability
- Pragmatic adequacy

In a later work (1978), Hardy discussed logical adequacy (diagramming) and stated that because a theory is a set of interrelated concepts and statements, its structure can be analyzed for internal consistency by examining the syntax of the theory as well as its content. Diagramming involves identifying all major theoretical terms (concepts, constructs, operational definitions, referents). Once identified, each component can be represented by a symbol, and a model may be drawn illustrating relationships or linkages between or among the terms. These linkages should specify the direction, the type of relationship (whether positive or negative), and the form of the relationship.

According to Hardy (1974), empirical adequacy is the single most important criterion for evaluating a theory applied in practice. Assessing empirical adequacy requires reviewing literature and critically reading relevant research; it is necessary to

---

**BOX 5-1** | *Questions for Theory Analysis and Theory Evaluation: Duffey and Muhlenkamp*

**THEORY ANALYSIS**
1. What is the origin of the problem(s) with which the theory is concerned?
2. What methods were used in theory development (induction, deduction, synthesis)?
3. What is the character of the subject matter dealt with by the theory?
4. What kind of outcomes of testing propositions are generated by the theory?

**THEORY EVALUATION**
1. Does the theory generate testable hypotheses?
2. Does the theory guide practice or can it be used as a body of knowledge?
3. Is the theory complete in terms of subject matter and perspective?
4. Are the biases or values underlying the theory made explicit?
5. Are the relationships among the propositions made explicit?
6. Is the theory parsimonious?

---

determine if hypotheses testing the theory are clearly deduced from the theory. The entire body of relevant studies should be evaluated in terms of the extent to which it supports the theory or a part of the theory. Finally, the criteria of usefulness and significance refer to the theory's use in controlling, altering, or manipulating major variables and conditions specified by the theory to realize a desired outcome.

## THEORY ANALYSIS AND THEORY EVALUATION: DUFFEY AND MUHLENKAMP

Writing at approximately the same time as Hardy, Duffey and Muhlenkamp (1974) published a two-phase approach to critically examining nursing theory. Theory analysis was the first phase for which they posited four questions for examination. For theory evaluation they suggested six additional questions (Box 5-1).

## THEORY EVALUATION: BARNUM

Barbara Barnum (Stevens) first published her ideas for theory evaluation in 1979. Subsequent editions were published in 1984, 1990, 1994, and 1998. Barnum suggested a method of theory evaluation that differentiates internal and external criticisms. Internal criticism examines how the components of the theory fit with each other; external criticism examines how a theory relates to the extant world. Box 5-2 lists points to be examined for both.

---

**BOX 5-2** | *Theory Evaluation Criteria: Barnum*

**INTERNAL CRITICISM**

Clarity
Consistency
Adequacy
Logical development
Level of theory development

**EXTERNAL CRITICISM**

Reality convergence (how the theory
   relates to the real world)

Utility
Significance
Discrimination (differentiation between
   nursing and other health professions)
Scope
Complexity

TABLE 5-2 *Theory Analysis: Walker and Avant*

| Step | Questions or Tasks |
| --- | --- |
| Determine the origins of the theory | Identify the basis of the original development of the theory. Why was it developed? Was the process of development inductive or deductive? Is there evidence to support or refute the theory? |
| Examine the meaning of the theory | Identify concepts. Examine definitions and their use (theoretical and operational definitions). Identify statements. Examine relationships. |
| Analyze the logical adequacy of the theory | Determine if scientists agree on predictive ability of the theory. Determine if the content makes sense. Identify any logical fallacies. |
| Determine the usefulness of the theory | Is the theory practical and helpful to nursing? Does it contribute to understanding and predicting outcomes? |
| Define the degree of generalizability | Is the theory highly generalizable or specific? |
| Determine if the theory is parsimonious | Can the theory be stated briefly and simply or is it complex? |
| Determine the testability of the theory | Can the theory be supported with empirical data? Can testable hypotheses be generated from the theory? |

Source: Walker and Avant (2005).

## THEORY ANALYSIS: WALKER AND AVANT

Lorraine Walker and Kay Avant first presented their detailed methods for theory analysis in 1983. Their work was subsequently revised in 1988, 1995, and 2005. Building on a multiphase background of concept and statement development, which involves concept and statement analysis, synthesis, and derivation, they expanded the processes to include theory analysis. Table 5-2 gives a brief synopsis of the process of theory analysis they propose.

## THEORY ANALYSIS AND EVALUATION: FAWCETT

Jacqueline Fawcett (1980, 1993, 1995, 2000, 2005) used a two-phase process for analysis and evaluation of theories and conceptual frameworks. In her writings she noted that analysis is a nonjudgmental, detailed examination of a theory. In Fawcett's (2005) most recent work, components of the analysis process include the theory's origins, unique focus, and content. The theory's "origins" refers to the historical evolution of the model/theory, the author's motivation, philosophical assumptions about nursing, the author's inclusion of works of nursing and non-nursing scholars, and the worldview reflected by the model.

The unique focus refers to distinctive views of the metaparadigm concepts, different problems in nurse–patient situations or interactions, and differences in modes of nursing interventions. She notes that theories can be categorized as developmental, systems, interaction, needs, client-focused, person–environment interaction focused, or nursing therapeutics focused. The content of the model is examined to analyze the abstract and general concepts and propositions. Fawcett's method of theory analysis specifically identifies whether and how the concepts and propositions of the metaparadigm (nursing, environment, health, person) are included in the theory. Representative questions to be addressed relative to the content include: "How are human beings defined and described? How is environment defined and described? How is health defined? … What is the goal of nursing? … and What statements are made about the relations among the four metaparadigm concepts?" (Fawcett, 2005, p. 53).

Theory evaluation requires judgments to be made about a theory's significance (Fawcett, 1993) based on how it satisfies certain criteria (Fawcett, 2005). Evaluation is based on review of previously published critiques, research reports, and reports of practical application of the theory. During the process of theory evaluation, the criteria to be examined are the explication of the origins of the theory, the comprehensiveness of the content, its logical congruence, how well it can lead to generation of new theory, its credibility, and how it has contributed to nursing (Fawcett, 2005).

## THEORY DESCRIPTION AND CRITIQUE: CHINN AND KRAMER

Peggy Chinn and Maenoa Kramer (Jacobs) initially wrote on the processes used to analyze theory in 1983. They used the terms theory description and critical reflection to describe a two-phase process. Theory description has six elements: purpose, concepts, definitions, relationships, structure, and assumptions. Table 5-3 presents these elements and their defining characteristics.

"Critical reflection" of a theory involves determining how well a theory serves its purpose. Critical reflection analyzes clarity and consistency of the theory as well as its complexity, generality, accessibility, and importance. In assessing clarity and consistency, Chinn and Kramer's (2008) critical reflection would examine:

- Semantic clarity—Are the concepts defined? Do the concepts establish empirical meaning?
- Semantic consistency—Are the concepts used consistently? Are the concepts congruent with their definitions?
- Structural clarity—Are the connections and reasoning within the theory understandable?
- Structural consistency—Is the structure of the theory consistent in its form?
- Simplicity or complexity—Is the theory simple? Is the theory complex?
- Generality—Does the theory cover a wide scope of experiences and phenomena?
- Accessibility—How accessible is the theory? How well are concepts grounded in empirically identifiable phenomena?
- Importance—How can the theory contribute to nursing practice, research, and education?

TABLE 5-3 *Components of Theory Description: Chinn and Kramer*

| Component | Characteristics |
| --- | --- |
| Purpose | The purpose of the theory should be stated explicitly or at least be identifiable in the text of the theory. |
| Concepts | The concepts of the theory should be linguistically expressed. |
| Definitions | Meanings of concepts are conveyed in theoretical definitions; these definitions give character to the theory. |
| Relationships | Concepts are structured into a systematic form that links each concept with others. |
| Structure | The relationships are linked to form a whole when the ideas of the theory interconnect; structure makes it possible to follow the reasoning of the theory. |
| Assumptions | Assumptions refer to underlying truths that determine the nature of concepts, definitions, purpose, relationship, and structure; may not be explicitly stated. |

Source: Chinn and Kramer (2008).

## THEORY DESCRIPTION, ANALYSIS, AND CRITIQUE: MELEIS

According to Meleis (1985, 2007), there are three stages involved in theory evaluation: theory description, theory analysis, and theory critique. During the process of theory description, the reviewer closely examines the structural and functional components of the theory. The structural components include assumptions (implicit and explicit), concepts, and propositions. The functional assessment considers the anticipated consequence of the theory and its purpose. Components that should be examined are the focus of the theory, and how it addresses the client, nursing, health, the nurse–client interactions, environment, nursing problems, and nursing therapeutics.

Theory analysis involves considering important variables that may have influenced the development of the theory. These include the theorist, paradigmatic origins of the theory, and internal dimensions of the theory. During the analysis procedure, Meleis (2007) recommends reviewing external and internal factors that influenced the theorist, as well as the theorist's experiential background, educational background, and employment history. Likewise, a reconstruction of the professional and academic networks that surrounded the theorist while the theory was evolving should be examined.

Second, Meleis argues that careful consideration of use of theories from other fields or paradigms is to be encouraged. To identify the paradigms from which the theory may have evolved, or to recognize other theorists who may have influenced the development of the theory, the reviewer would consider references, educational and experiential background of the theorist, and the sociocultural context of the theory as it was developed.

Finally, internal dimensions of the theory should be analyzed. This will provide information about the rationale on which the theory is built, systems of relationships, content of the theory, goal of the theory, scope of the theory, context of the theory, abstractness of the theory, and method of development.

Critique of a theory may follow analysis, and Meleis (2007) identified five elements to consider in this phase: the relationship between structure and function, diagram of the theory, circle of contagiousness, usefulness, and external components. The relationship between structure and function involves evaluating the theory's clarity and consistency, level of simplicity or complexity, and tautology/teleology. In assessing the tautology of the theory, the reviewer would observe for needless repetition of an idea in different parts of the theory, which Meleis claims will decrease the clarity of the theory. Teleology occurs when definitions of concepts, conditions, and events are described by consequences rather than properties and dimensions; this should be avoided.

Although not all theories contain models graphically or pictorially depicting the structure of the theory, Meleis (2007) states that theories and models are enhanced by visual representation. The reviewer should determine if the model does indeed help clarify linkages among the concepts and propositions and, thereby, enhance clarity of the theory.

The circle of contagiousness refers to if, and to what extent, the model or theory has been adopted by other experts in the field. In evaluating usefulness, Meleis suggests analysis of the theory's usefulness in practice, research, education, and administration.

The final component of this method is the review of external components of the theory. These include implicit and explicit personal values of both the theorist and the critic. It also refers to congruence with other professional values as well as with social values. Finally, the critic would determine if the theory has social significance.

## ANALYSIS AND EVALUATION OF PRACTICE THEORY, MIDDLE RANGE THEORY, AND NURSING MODELS: WHALL

Whall (2005) is the only nurse scholar to explicitly outline three separate criteria for analysis and evaluation for the three levels of nursing theory. In her most recent edition, she noted that middle range and practice theories have achieved status equal to that of nursing conceptual models, but it has only been nursing models that have been systematically examined. Following this observation, she outlined distinct, although similar, criteria for evaluation of all three levels of nursing theory using a three-phase approach that reviews basic considerations, internal analysis and evaluation, and external analysis and evaluation.

According to Whall (2005), practice theory is produced from practice and deduced from middle range theory as well as from research. Because practice theory is designed for immediate application to practice, questions regarding the fit with empirical data are important in the evaluation process. Operational definitions and descriptions of how to apply practice theory are also important. Internal analysis of practice theory may be accomplished by diagramming the interrelationships of all concepts to detect lapses and inconsistencies in the theory's structure. The assumptions of the theory should be considered in light of historical and current perspectives of nursing. This should include ethical and cultural implications of the theory. External analysis should compare standards of care with the theory and examine nursing research to determine if it supports the theory, is neutral, or is in opposition.

Analysis and evaluation of middle range theory modifies the guidelines used for nursing conceptual models. It examines if the theory fits with the existing nursing perspective and domains. Propositional statements should be examined to determine if they are causal or associative in nature, to assess their relative importance, and to find missing linkages between concepts. It is suggested that diagramming of the relationships may help identify missing relationships. Concepts should be operationally defined to support empirical adequacy. External analysis refers to congruence with more global theories and other related middle range theories. Examination of ethical, cultural, and social policy implications is crucial.

Whall (2005) believes nursing conceptual models should be assessed from a postmodern view. In addition, conceptual models should consider the major paradigm concepts (person, environment, health, and nursing) as well as additional concepts specific to the model. Analysis should examine whether the definitions of the concepts and statements are consistently used throughout the model and whether the interrelationships among the concepts are consistent. Internal analysis considers the assumptions and philosophical basis of the model and looks at the uniformity of discussion throughout the model. External consistency examines the model in relation to views external to the model (i.e., whether the model is being evaluated consistent with other nursing conceptual models and with nursing intervention classification systems). Table 5-4 lists some of the questions for consideration by Whall in analysis and evaluation of all three levels of nursing theory.

## THEORY EVALUATION: DUDLEY-BROWN

One of the most contemporary methods for theory evaluation was presented by Dudley-Brown (1997), who strongly relied on Kuhn's (1977) criteria for theory evaluation. In this method, evaluation should consider accuracy, consistency, fruitfulness, simplicity/complexity, scope, acceptability, and sociocultural utility.

To Dudley-Brown (1997), *accuracy* is essential because the theory should describe nursing as it exists today—not the nursing of the future or of the past. The theory should contain a worldview of nursing consistent with the present reality. *Consistency* relates to the importance of the nursing theory being internally consistent. There should be logical order; terms, concepts, and statements should be used consistently and defined operationally; they should be coherent, and presented logically.

TABLE 5-4 *Criteria for Analysis and Evaluation of Theory: Whall*

| Level of Theory | Basic Considerations | Internal Analysis and Evaluation | External Analysis and Evaluation |
|---|---|---|---|
| Practice theory | Can the concepts be operationalized? Are operationalized concepts congruent with empirical data? Do statements lead to directives for nursing care? Are statements sufficient to practice and not contradictory? | Are there gaps or inconsistencies within the theory that may lead to conflicts and difficulties? Are assumptions congruent with nursing's historical perspective? Are assumptions congruent with ethical standards and social policy? Are assumptions in conflict with given cultural groups? | Is the theory produced with existing nursing standards? Is the theory consistent with existing standards of education within nursing? Is the theory related to nursing diagnoses and nursing intervention practices? Is the theory supported by existing research internal and external to nursing? |
| Middle range theory | What are the definitions and relative importance of major concepts? What is the type and relative importance of major theoretical statements? | What are the assumptions of the theory? What is the relationship of the theory to philosophy of science positions? Are concepts related/not related via statements? Is there internal consistency and congruency of all component parts of the theory? What is the empirical adequacy of the theory? Has the theory been examined in practice and research and has it held up to this scrutiny? | What is the congruency with related theory and research internal and external to nursing? What is the congruence with the perspective of nursing, the domains, and the persistent questions? What ethical, cultural, and social policy issues are related to the theory? |
| Nursing models | What are the definitions of person, nursing, health, and environment? What are additional understandings of the metaparadigm concepts? What are the interrelationships among the metaparadigm concepts? What are the descriptions of other concepts found in the model? | What are the underlying assumptions of the model? What are the definitions of other components of the model? What is the relative importance of basic concepts or other components of the model? What are the analyses of internal and external consistency? What are the analyses of adequacy? | Is nursing research based on the model or related to the model? Is nursing education based on the model or related to the model? Is nursing practice based on the model? What is the relationship to existing nursing diagnoses and interventions systems? |

Another criterion Dudley-Brown (1997) identifies for evaluation is *fruitfulness*. For this criterion, the theory should be useful in generating information and significant in contributing to the development of nursing knowledge.

*Simplicity/complexity* is a fourth criterion for evaluation. Both simple and complex theories are needed. In general, a theory should be balanced and logical. The theory should describe the phenomenon consistently in terms of simplicity or complexity.

*Scope* is a fifth criterion because theories of both broad and limited scope are needed. Scope should be dependent on the phenomenon and its context. Acceptance refers to the adoption of the theory by others. Theories should be useful in practice, education, research, or administration.

*Sociocultural utility* is the final criterion for evaluation. Social congruence encompasses the beliefs, values, and expectations of different cultures. The theory should be measured against the criterion of social utility according to the culture for which it was proposed. Theories proposed for Western societies need to be evaluated for their philosophical and theoretical relevance in other societies and cultures.

## Comparisons of Methods

Several authors (Dudley-Brown, 1997; Moody, 1990; Alligood, 2006) have compared many of the theory analysis and evaluation methods described here. A number of similarities can be found between and among all the methods. Table 5-5 provides a list of the methods reviewed and criteria specified by each author. It is important to note that different authors use different terms for similar concepts; thus, some interpretation of meaning of terms was necessary for the comparison.

As Table 5-5 shows, the most common criteria identified among the theory evaluation methods were an examination of complexity/simplicity (7 of 9) and scope/generality (7 of 9 methods). Other common criteria were inclusion of meaningful terminology, definitions of concepts (6 of 9), consistency (6 of 9), contribution to understanding (5 of 9), usefulness (6 of 9), testability (4 of 9), logical adequacy (4 of 9), and validity/accuracy/empirical adequacy (4 of 9). Criteria mentioned in only one or two methods were implicit values of the theorist, information generation, reality convergence, discrimination between nursing and other health professions, consequences, method of development, correspondence to existing standards, origins of the theory, context, pragmatic adequacy, and application of or to nursing therapeutics.

There appears to be an evolution of the processes over the past three decades. Similarities of criteria were evident based on time of initial writing. Ellis, Duffey and Muhlenkamp, and Hardy were the first nurses to describe the processes of theory evaluation and their criteria are similar. The methods proposed by Walker and Avant are also consistent with those of Hardy and Ellis. Fawcett's model is similar to Chinn and Kramer's approach and to Barnum's internal criticism criteria. Meleis and Whall present the most detailed methods. Meleis' system has three components (description, analysis, and critical reflection) and Whall's examines three levels of theory. Barnum and Whall are similar in that they describe separate internal and external dimensions. The later works of Whall, Meleis, and Dudley-Brown are similar because they include characteristics of circle of contagion and consideration of social and cultural significance as evaluation criteria.

Most methods for analysis and evaluation were developed and used to review grand nursing theories. Indeed, a literature review resulted in no published report of theory evaluation in nursing beyond those in nursing theory textbooks. Books that focus on analysis and evaluation of grand nursing theories include those by Fawcett (1993, 1995, 2000, 2005), Fitzpatrick and Whall (1996), Whall (2005), George (2002), McQuiston and Webb (1995), and Tomey and Alligood (2006). Peterson and Bredow (2008) and Tomey and Alligood (2006) also analyze/evaluate selected middle range nursing theories in their works.

## Synthesized Method of Theory Evaluation

Following the detailed review and comparison of the many methods for theory analysis and evaluation, a method specifically designed to evaluate middle range and practice theories was developed (Box 5-3). These criteria were synthesized from the works of noted nursing scholars described above and are intended to be contemporary and responsive to both recent and anticipated changes in use of theory in nursing practice, research, education, and administration.

TABLE 5-5 *Comparison of Theory Evaluation Criteria*

| Evaluation Criteria | Ellis | Hardy | Barnum | Walker and Avant | Fawcett | Chinn and Kramer | Meleis | Whall | Dudley-Brown |
|---|---|---|---|---|---|---|---|---|---|
| Complexity/simplicity | X | | X | X | X | X | X | | X |
| Testability | X | X | | X | X | | | | |
| Generality/scope | X | X | X | X | X | X | | | X |
| Usefulness | X | X | X | X | | X | X | | |
| Contribution to understanding | | X | X | | X | X | | | X |
| Implicit values | X | | | | | | X | | |
| Information generation | X | | | | | | | | |
| Meaningful terminology (definitions) | X | | | X | X | X | X | X | |
| Logical adequacy | | X | X | X | | | | X | |
| Validity/accuracy/empirical adequacy | | X | | | X | | | X | X |
| Predictability/tested | | X | | | | X | | X | |
| Origins | | | | X | | | X | | |
| Clarity | | X | | | X | X | | | |
| Consistency | | X | | X | X | X | X | X | |
| Context | | | | X | | X | | | |
| Pragmatic adequacy | | | | X | | | X | | |
| Reality convergence | | X | | | | | | | |
| Discrimination | | X | | | | | | | |
| Metaparadigm concepts | | | | X | | X | X | | |
| Assumptions | | | | | X | X | X | | |
| Purpose | | | | | X | X | | | |
| Consequences | | | | | | X | | | |
| Nursing therapeutics interventions | | | | | | X | X | | |
| Method of development | | | | | | X | | | |
| Circle of contagion | | | | | | X | X | X | |
| Social/cultural significance | | | | | | X | X | X | |
| Correspondence to standards/professional values | | | | | | X | X | | |

## Summary

Nurses in clinical practice, as well as graduate students like Jerry Thompson from the case study, should know how to analyze or evaluate a theory to determine if it is reliable and valid and to determine when and how to apply it in practice, research, administration, or education. This chapter has presented and analyzed a number of different

## BOX 5-3  *Synthesized Method for Theory Evaluation*

### THEORY DESCRIPTION

What is the purpose of the theory? (describe, explain, predict, prescribe)

What is the scope or level of the theory? (grand, middle range, practice)

What are the origins of the theory?

What are the major concepts?

What are the major theoretical propositions?

What are the major assumptions?

Is the context for use described?

### THEORY ANALYSIS

Are concepts theoretically and operationally defined?

Are statements theoretically and operationally defined?

Are linkages explicit?

Is the theory logically organized?

Is there a model/diagram? Does the model contribute to clarifying the theory?

Are the concepts, statements, and assumptions used consistently?

Are outcomes or consequences stated or predicted?

### THEORY EVALUATION

Is the theory congruent with current nursing standards?

Is the theory congruent with current nursing interventions or therapeutics?

Has the theory been tested empirically? Is it supported by research? Does it appear to be accurate/valid?

Is there evidence that the theory has been used by nursing educators, nursing researchers, or nursing administrators?

Is the theory socially relevant?

Is the theory relevant cross-culturally?

Does the theory contribute to the discipline of nursing?

What are implications for nursing related to implementation of the theory?

---

methods for evaluation of theory. Like many issues in the study of use of theory in nursing, the process of theory evaluation, although important, is often confusing. In addition, with very few exceptions, the methods or techniques were developed and used almost exclusively to analyze and evaluate grand nursing theories. It is hoped that with the current emphasis on development and use of both practice and middle range theories, there will be a concurrent emphasis on the analysis and evaluation of those theories.

The most commonly used methods were described in some detail and compared. Following this comparison, a synthesized and simplified method for examination of theory was presented. To further help the reader understand this process, this chapter presents an exemplar of the proposed theory evaluation method.

## THEORY EVALUATION EXEMPLAR: THEORY OF CHRONIC SORROW

Burke, M. L., Eakes, G. G., & Hainsworth, M. A. (1999). Milestones of chronic sorrow: Perspectives of chronically ill and bereaved persons and family caregivers. *Journal of Family Nursing, 5* (4), 374–387.

Eakes, G. G. (1993). Chronic sorrow: A response to living with cancer. *Oncology Nursing Forum, 20* (9), 1327–1334.

Eakes, G. G. (1995). Chronic sorrow: The lived experience of parents of chronically mentally ill individuals. *Archives of Psychiatric Nursing, 9* (2), 77–84.

Eakes, G. G. (2009). Chronic sorrow. In S. J. Peterson and T. S. Bredow (Eds.), *Middle range theories: Application to nursing research* (2nd ed., pp 149–160). Philadelphia: Lippincott Williams & Wilkins.

Eakes, G. G, Burke, M. L., & Hainsworth, M. A. (1998). Middle-range theory of chronic sorrow. *Image: Journal of Nursing Scholarship, 30* (2), 179–185.

Hainsworth, M. A. (1995). Chronic sorrow in women with chronically mentally disabled husbands. *Journal of the American Psychiatric Nurses Association, 1*(4), 120–124.

Hobdell, E. (2004). Chronic sorrow and depression in parents of children with neural tube defects. *Journal of Neuroscience Nursing, 36* (2), 82–84.

Hobdell, E. F., Grant, M. L., Valencia, I., Mare, J., Kothare, S. V., Legido, A., & Khurana, D. S. (2007). Chronic sorrow and coping in families of children with epilepsy. *Journal of Neuroscience Nursing, 39* (2), 76–83.

Isaksson, A. K., & Ahlstrom, G. (2008). Managing chronic sorrow: Experiences of patients with multiple sclerosis. *Journal of Neuroscience Nursing, 40* (3), 180–192.

Kendall, L. C. (2005). The experience of living with ongoing loss: Testing the Kendall chronic sorrow instrument (Doctoral dissertation, Virginia Commonwealth University).

Langridge, P. (2002). Reduction of chronic sorrow: A health promotion role for children's community nurses? *Journal of Child Health Care, 6* (3), 157–170.

Lowes, L., & Lyne, P. (2000). Chronic sorrow in parents of children with newly diagnosed diabetes: A review of the literature and discussion of the implications for nursing practice. *Journal of Advanced Nursing, 32* (1), 41–48.

Melvin, C. S., & Heater, B. S. (2004). Suffering and chronic sorrow: Characteristics and a paradigm for nursing interventions. *International Journal for Human Caring, 8* (2), 41–47.

Northington, L. (2000). Chronic sorrow in caregivers of school aged children with sickle cell disease: A grounded theory approach. *Issues in Comprehensive Pediatric Nursing, 23* (2), 141–154.

Schreier, A. M., & Droes, N. S. (2006). Georgene Gaskill Eakes, Mary Lermann Burke, and Margaret A. Hainsworth: Theory of Chronic Sorrow. In A. M. Tomey & M. R. Alligood (Eds.), *Nursing theorists and their work* (6th ed., pp. 679–695). St. Louis: Mosby.

## Theory Description

*Scope of theory*: Middle range

*Purpose of theory*: Explanatory theory—"to explain the experiences of people across the lifespan who encounter ongoing disparity because of significant loss" (p. 179).

*Origins of theory*: "Chronic sorrow" appeared in the literature in 1962 to describe recurrent grief experienced by parents of children with disabilities. A number of research projects were conducted in the 1980s and 1990s describing chronic sorrow among various groups with loss situations. The resulting Theory of Chronic Sorrow, therefore, was inductively developed using concept analysis, extensive review of the literature, critical review of research, and validation in 10 qualitative studies of various loss situations.

*Major concepts*: Chronic sorrow, loss experience, disparity, trigger events (milestones), external management methods, internal management methods. All are defined and explained.

*Major theoretical propositions are as follows*:

1. Disparity between a desired relationship and an actual relationship or a disparity between current reality and desired reality is created by loss experiences.
2. Trigger events bring the negative disparity into focus or exacerbate the experience of disparity.
3. For individuals with chronic or life-threatening illnesses, chronic sorrow is most often triggered when the individual experiences disparity with accepted norms (social, developmental, or personal).
4. For family caregivers, disparity between the idealized and actual is associated with developmental milestones.
5. For bereaved individuals, disparity from the ideal is created by the absence of a person who was central in the life of the bereaved.

*Major assumptions*: Not stated

*Context for use*: "Experienced by individuals across the lifespan"; implied that it may be used in multiple settings and nursing situations.

### Theory Analysis

*Theoretical definitions for major concepts*:

Chronic sorrow—the periodic recurrence of permanent, pervasive sadness or other grief-related feelings associated with ongoing disparity resulting from a loss experience

Loss experience—a significant loss, either actual or symbolic, that may be ongoing, with no predictable end, or a more circumscribed single-loss event

Disparity—a gap between the current reality and the desired as a result of a loss experience

Trigger events or milestones—a situation, circumstance, or condition that brings the negative disparity resulting from the loss into focus or exacerbates the disparity

External management methods—interventions provided by professionals to assist individuals to cope with chronic sorrow

Internal management methods—positive personal coping strategies used to deal with the periodic episodes of chronic sorrow

*Operational definitions for major concepts*: No operational definitions are provided.

*Statements theoretically defined*: Theoretical propositions are implicitly stated in the body of the text.

*Statements operationally defined*: Theoretical propositions are not operationally defined.

*Linkages explicit*: Linkages are described in the text and explicated in the model.

*Logical organization*: Theory is logically organized and described in detail.

*Model/diagram*: A model is provided and assists in explaining linkages of the concepts (see p. xx).

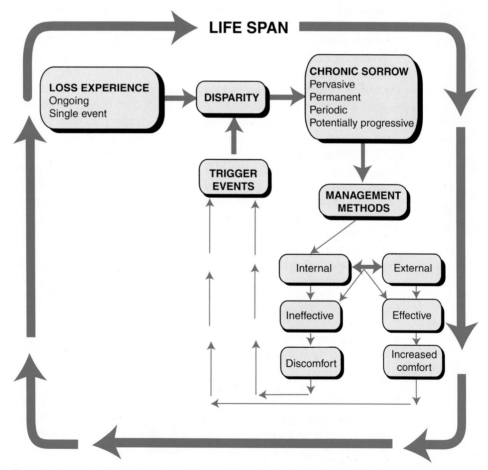

Theoretical model of chronic sorrow. (Source: Eakes, G. G., Burke, M. L., & Haninsworth, M. A. (1998). Middle range theory of chronic sorrow. *Image: Journal of Nursing Scholarship, 30*(2), 179–184.)

*Consistent use of concepts, statements, and assumptions:* Concepts and propositions are used consistently. Assumptions are not explicitly addressed.

*Predicted or stated outcomes or consequences:* Outcomes are stated.

### Theory Evaluation

*Congruence with nursing standards:* The theory appears congruent with nursing standards. A number of articles were identified in recent nursing literature describing how the construct of chronic sorrow has been identified among various aggregates (Eakes, 2009).

*Congruence with current nursing interventions or therapeutics:* Literature-based descriptions of application of components of the theory in nursing practice include caring for bereaved persons and family caregivers (Burke, Eakes, & Hainsworth, 1999), a discussion of caring for children with newly diagnosed diabetes (Lowes & Lyne, 2000), interventions for community nurses to help assist families resolving chronic sorrow (Langridge, 2002), and interventions for suffering related to chronic sorrow (Melvin & Heater, 2004).

*Evidence of empirical testing/research support/validity:* The theory was derived from multiple research studies and a review of the literature.

The Burke/CCRCS Chronic Sorrow Questionnaire is an interview guide comprising 10 open-ended questions that explore the theory's concepts.

Research using the questionnaire includes investigation of chronic sorrow among cancer patients (Eakes, 1993), chronic sorrow in chronically mentally ill individuals (Eakes, 1995), chronic sorrow in women with mentally disabled husbands (Hainsworth, 1995), chronic sorrow in parents of children with neural tube defects (Hobdell, 2004), chronic sorrow and cooping in families of children with epilepsy (Hobdell et al., 2007), and chronic sorrow among patients with multiple sclerosis (Isaksson & Ahlstrom, 2008). Further, a second instrument designed to measure chronic sorrow (Kendall, 2005) has been developed.

*Use by nursing educators, nursing researchers, or nursing administrators:* The above references indicate that the theory has been used in practice and research. Other studies have cited the work of Eakes, Burke, and Hainsworth related to chronic sorrow (e.g., Northington, 2000).

*Social relevance:* Theory is relevant to individuals, families, and groups, irrespective of age or socioeconomic status.

*Transcultural relevance:* Theory is potentially relevant across cultures; theorist notes that "relevance for various cultural groups should be explored" (Eakes, Burke, & Hainsworth, 1998, p. 184).

*Contribution to nursing:* Authors note that the theory is applicable to different groups, but more study is needed to test the theory and to identify strategies to reduce disparity created by loss (prescriptive interventions). Despite the relative newness of the theory, there is a growing body of nursing literature reporting on use both related to interventions and research (Eakes, 2009).

*Conclusions and implications:* The theory is useful and appropriate for nurses practicing in a variety of settings. Implications for research were described and implications for education can be inferred. Further development of the theory is warranted to better explicate relationships and operationalize the concepts and propositions to allow testing.

## LEARNING ACTIVITIES

1. Obtain the original works of two of the nursing scholars whose theory analysis/ evaluation strategies are discussed. Use the strategies to evaluate a recently published middle range nursing theory (see Chapter 11 for examples). How are the conclusions similar? How are they different?

2. For one of the nursing scholars who has published several versions or editions of her work (e.g., Fawcett, Chinn & Kramer, Meleis), obtain a copy of the oldest

version and a copy of the most recent version and compare the strategies suggested. Have they changed?

3. Use the synthesized method for theory evaluation to evaluate a grand nursing theory. Compare findings with published evaluations of the same theory. How are conclusions similar? How are they different?

4. Search the literature for examples of published accounts of nursing theory evaluation or theory analysis. Share your findings with classmates.

## REFERENCES

Alligood, M. R. (2006). Introduction to nursing theory: Its history, significance and analysis. In A. M. Tomey & M. R. Alligood (Eds.), *Nursing theorists and their work* (6th ed., pp. 3–15). St. Louis: Mosby.

Barnum, B. S. (1984). *Nursing theory: Analysis, application, evaluation* (2nd ed.). Boston: Little Brown.

Barnum, B. S. (1990). *Nursing theory: Analysis, application, evaluation* (3rd ed.). Glenview, IL: Scott, Foresman/ Little, Brown Higher Education.

Barnum, B. S. (1994). *Nursing theory: Analysis, application, evaluation* (4th ed.). Philadelphia: Lippincott.

Barnum, B. S. (1998). *Nursing theory: Analysis, application, evaluation* (5th ed.). Philadelphia: Lippincott Williams & Wilkins.

Chinn, P. L., & Kramer, M. K. (1987). *Theory and nursing: A systematic approach* (2nd ed.). St. Louis: Mosby.

Chinn, P. L., & Kramer, M. K. (1991). *Theory and nursing: A systematic approach* (3rd ed.). St. Louis: Mosby.

Chinn, P. L., & Kramer, M. K. (1995). *Theory and nursing: A systmetic approach* (4th ed.). St. Louis: Mosby.

Chinn, P. L., & Kramer, M. K. (1999). *Theory and nursing: Integrated knowledge development* (5th ed.). St. Louis: Mosby.

Chinn, P. L., & Kramer, M. K. (2004). *Integrated theory and knowledge development in nursing* (6th ed.). St. Louis: Mosby.

Chinn, P. L., & Kramer, M. K. (2008). *Integrated theory and knowledge development in nursing* (7th ed.). St. Louis: Mosby.

Dudley-Brown, S. L. (1997). The evaluation of nursing theory: A method for our madness. *International Journal of Nursing Studies, 34*(1), 76–83.

Duffey, M., & Muhlenkamp, A. F. (1974). A framework for theory analysis. *Nursing Outlook, 22*(9), 570–574.

Ellis, R. (1968). Characteristics of significant theories. *Nursing Research, 17*(3), 217–222.

Fawcett, J. (1980). A framework of analysis and evaluation of conceptual models of nursing. *Nurse Educator, 5*(6), 10–14.

Fawcett, J. (1993). *Analysis and evaluation of nursing theories*. Philadelphia: Davis.

Fawcett, J. (1995). *Analysis and evaluation of conceptual models of nursing* (3rd ed.). Philadelphia: Davis.

Fawcett, J. (2000). *Analysis and evaluation of contemporary nursing knowledge: Nursing models and theories.* Philadelphia: Davis.

Fawcett, J. (2005). *Contemporary nursing knowledge: Analysis and evaluation of nursing models and theories* (2nd ed.). Philadelphia: F. A. Davis.

Fitzpatrick, J. J., & Whall, A. (1989). *Conceptual models of nursing: Analysis and application* (2nd ed.). Norwalk, CT: Appleton & Lange.

Fitzpatrick, J. J., & Whall, A. L. (1996). *Conceptual models of nursing: Analysis and application* (3rd ed.). Norwalk, CT: Appleton & Lange.

Fitzpatrick, J. J., & Whall, A. (2005). *Conceptual models of nursing: Analysis and application* (4th ed.). Upper Saddle River, NJ: Prentice Hall.

George, J. B. (2002). *Nursing theories: The base for professional nursing practice* (5th ed.). Upper Saddle River, NJ: Prentice-Hall.

Hardy, M. E. (1974). Theories: Components, development, evaluation. *Nursing Research, 23,* 100–107.

Hardy, M. E. (1978). Perspectives on nursing theory. *Advances in Nursing Science, 1*(1), 27–48.

Hickman, J. S. (2002). An introduction to nursing theory. In J. B. George (Ed.), *Nursing theories: The base for professional nursing practice* (5th ed.). Upper Saddle River, NJ: Prentice-Hall.

Kuhn, T. S. (1977). Second thoughts on paradigms. In F. Suppe (Ed.), *The structure of scientific theory* (pp. 459–482). Urbana, IL: University of Illinois Press.

McQuiston, C. M., & Webb, A. A. (1995). *Foundations of nursing theory: Contributions of 12 key theorists.* Thousand Oaks, CA: Sage.

Meleis, A. I. (1985). *Theoretical nursing: Development and progress*. Philadelphia: J. B. Lippincott.

Meleis, A.I. (1991). *Theoretical nursing: Development and progress* (2nd ed.). Philadelphia: Lippincott Williams & Wilkins.

Melies, A. I. (1997). *Theoretical nursing: Development and progress* (3rd ed.). Philadelphia: Lippincott Williams & Wilkins.

Meleis, A. I. (2007). *Theoretical nursing: Development and progress* (5th ed.). Philadelphia: Lippincott Williams & Wilkins.

Moody, L. E. (1990). *Advancing nursing science through research*. Newbury Park, CA: Sage.

Pender, N. J., Murdaugh, C. L., & Parsons, M. H. (2006). *Health promotion in nursing practice* (5th ed.). Upper Saddle River, NJ: Prentice-Hall.

Peterson, S. J., & Bredow, T. S. (2008). *Middle range theories: Application to nursing research* (2nd ed.). Philadelphia: Lippincott Williams & Wilkins.

Stevens, B. J. (1979). *Nursing theory: Analysis, application, evaluation.* Boston: Little, Brown.

Walker, L. O., & Avant, K. (1983). *Strategies for theory construction in nursing.* Norwalk, CT: Appleton-Century-Crofts.

Walker, L. O., & Avant, K. (1988). *Strategies for theory construction in nursing* (2nd ed.). Norwalk, CT: Appleton & Lange.

Walker, L. O., & Avant, K. (1995). *Strategies for theory construction in nursing* (3rd ed.). Norwalk, CT: Appleton & Lange.

Walker, L. O., & Avant, K. (2005). *Strategies for theory construction in nursing* (4th ed.). Upper Saddle River, NJ: Prentice-Hall.

Whall, A. L. (2005). The structure of nursing knowledge: Analysis and evaluation of practice, middle range and grand theory. In J. J. Fitzpatrick & A. L. Whall (Eds.), *Conceptual models of nursing: Analysis and application* (3rd ed., pp. 13–51). Upper Saddle River, NJ: Prentice-Hall.

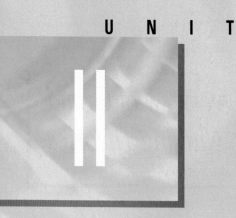

*Nursing Theories*

# 6

# Overview of Grand Nursing Theories

## Evelyn Wills

*J*anet Turner works as a nurse on a postsurgical, cardiovascular floor. Because she desires a broader view of nursing knowledge and wants to become a clinical specialist or acute care nurse practitioner, she recently began a master's degree program. The requirements for a course titled "Theoretical Foundations of Nursing" led Janet to become familiar with the many nursing theories. From her readings she learned about a number of ways to classify theories: grand theory, conceptual model, middle range theory, practice theory, borrowed theory, interactive–integrative model, totality paradigm, and simultaneous action paradigm. She came to the conclusion that there is no cohesion among authors of nursing theory.

A large proportion of Janet's theory course consisted of distance learning methods. To express her frustration and to try to understand the material, she consulted with her theory professor via the web-based live chat room that was part of the course. The entire class eventually logged on to the chat and a long discussion resulted in which students shared interesting ways of conceptualizing grand nursing theories. The chat broke up with the agreement that each student would review the assigned readings and return to next week's live chat ready to discuss the findings.

Janet became frustrated when she concluded that each of the theories was very different and she wondered how she would ever understand them. But, as she continued to study and work with her professor and classmates, she learned that nursing theory has evolved from several schools of philosophical thought and various scientific traditions. To better understand the theories, she looked for ways to group or categorize them based on similarities of perspective. As she studied theories based on similar perspectives, she was able to read and analyze the theories more effectively, and to select three that she intended to examine further.

---

In Chapter 2, the reader was introduced to grand nursing theories and given a brief historical overview of their development. Fawcett (2005) distinguishes between conceptual models and grand theories, and this chapter discusses that differentiation in an effort to assist beginning graduate nursing students to understand the material. According to Fawcett (2005), conceptual models are broad formulations of philosophy that are based on an attempt to include the whole of nursing reality as the scholar understands it. The concepts and propositions are abstract and not likely to be testable in fact. Grand nursing theories, by contrast, may be derived from conceptual models and are the most complex and widest in scope of the levels of theory; they attempt to explain broad issues within the discipline. Grand theories are composed of relatively abstract concepts and typically lack operational definitions; propositions are abstract and are not directly amenable to testing (Fawcett, 2005; Higgins & Moore, 2000). They were developed through thoughtful and insightful appraisal of existing ideas as opposed to empirical research and may incorporate numerous other theories (Figure 6-1).

The grand nursing theories guide research and assist scholars to integrate the results of numerous diverse investigations so that the findings may be applied to education, practice, further research, and administration. Grand theories provide a background of philosophical reasoning that allow nurse scientists to develop an organizing theory for research or practice, sometimes referred to as a middle range theory. (Middle range theories will be discussed in Chapters 10 and 11.) One of the most important benefits of invoking theories in education, administration, research, and practice has been the systematization of those domains of nursing activity.

Practitioners are more likely to succeed in analyzing research into evidence for utility of tested interventions using meta-analysis for evidence-based practice (EBP) when the research fits into a particular theoretical framework. Cody (2003) states that "nursing theory guided practice can be shown to enhance health and quality of life when it is implemented with strong, well-qualified guidance" (p. 167). Mark, Hughes, and Jones (2004) echo his beliefs and posit that theory-guided research results not only in

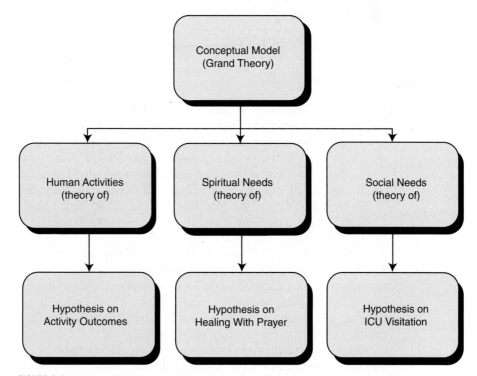

FIGURE 6-1 Relationship of conceptual model, theory, and hypotheses.

greater patient safety, but also in more predictable outcomes. These beliefs among nursing scientists provide clear direction that theory-guided research is necessary in testing implementation of interventions in practice.

Over the last five decades of theory development, review of the health care literature demonstrates that changes in health care, society, and the environment, as well as changes in population demographics (i.e., aging, urbanization, increase in minorities), led to a need to renew or update existing theories and to develop different theories. Health care delivery is a constantly changing process, and to be relevant to health care, theories require constant renewal and reevaluation. Indeed, many established nursing theorists continue to write, reevaluate, and improve their theories in light of these changes. Inspiration for many of the newer theories is linked not only to the changes in the health sciences, but also to changes in society worldwide (Boykin & Schoenhofer, 2001). Such theorists as Roper, Logan, and Tierney (United Kingdom), Ray (Canada), and Martinson (Norway) have achieved worldwide recognition. This chapter introduces conceptual frameworks and grand nursing theories. Chapters 7, 8, and 9 provide additional information about some of the more commonly known and widely recognized nursing frameworks and theories. To better assist the reader in understanding the conceptual frameworks and grand nursing theories, this chapter presents methods for categorizing or classifying them, and describes the criteria that will be used to examine them in the subsequent chapters.

## Categorization of Conceptual Frameworks and Grand Theories

The sheer number and scope of the conceptual frameworks and grand theories are daunting. Students and novice nursing scholars are understandably intimidated when asked to study them, as illustrated in the opening case study. To help understand the formulations, a number of methods categorizing them have been described in the nursing literature. Several are presented in the following sections.

### CATEGORIZATION BASED ON SCOPE

One of the simplest ways to categorize grand nursing theories is by scope. For example, Tomey and Alligood (2006) organized theories according to the scope of the theory. The categories they used were philosophies, nursing models, nursing theories, theories, and middle range nursing theories (pp. xvii–xx). Tomey and Alligood (2006) considered the writings of nursing theorists Wiedenbach, Henderson, Abdellah, Hall, and Roper, Logan, and Tierney as of historical significance. They considered the works of Nightingale, Watson, Ray, Martinson, Benner, and Kari Eriksson to be philosophies, explaining that those theorists had developed philosophies that were derived through "analysis, reasoning and logical arguments . . . [and] form a bases for professional scholarship . . ." (Tomey & Alligood, 2006, p. 69) (Eriksson, Martinson, and Ray are not included in the current volume because of space requirements). This panoply of nursing philosophies guides our understanding of nursing phenomena.

Tomey and Alligood (2006) considered the works of Levine, Rogers, Neuman, Roy, Johnson, and Boykin and Schoenhofer as nursing models. Nursing models "form an organized perspective for viewing phenomena specific to the discipline" (p. 225).

Orlando, Pender, Leininger, Newman, Parse, Helen Erickson, Tomlin, and Swain are classified by Alligood and Tomey (2006) as nursing theories; works that apply to nursing practice and form "ways of looking at a phenomenon to describe, explain, predict or control it" (p. 429). Tomey and Alligood made the point that some of these theories evolved from the more global philosophical frameworks or grand theories.

## CATEGORIZATION BASED ON NURSING DOMAINS

Meleis (2004) did not discriminate according to levels of theory (i.e., grand theory, middle range theory, practice theory), and considered these distinctions a matter of semantics. Rather, she organized a number of theories with reference to nursing's domain concepts, which she stated reflect the current focus of nursing education and practice (Meleis, 2007, p. 275). The organization of theoretical topics used as distinctions in Meleis's work was (1) nursing clients, (2) interactions, (3) human being–environment interactions, and (4) nursing therapeutics.

Theories that Meleis (2007) classified as theories about nursing clients were developed by Johnson, Roy, and Neuman. Meleis distinguished these theories by asking the following questions: "Who is the nursing client? In what ways does a nursing client benefit from nursing care? What is the outcome of care?" (p. 277). She showed that the major influence on each of these theorists was the client and the client's need for nursing.

Meleis's (2007) second classification of theories was nursing as a process of interaction. In this grouping, she included both theorists whose works are often classified by others as grand theories or theoretical or conceptual frameworks, and those whose works are classified as practice and middle range theories. Some of the theories represented in this category included the works of King, Orlando, Patterson and Zderad, Travelbee, and Weidenbach.

The distinction Meleis (2007) made among theories that related to environment was that of client–environment interaction. The major points in this domain were that human beings and environments are unitary, irreducible, and pandimensional energy fields that are identifiable by patterns. Humans and their environment cannot be discussed, considered, or understood in isolation from the other; they are interrelated in an irreducible way. She placed Rogers's work in this category.

Nursing therapeutics is the fourth category of nursing theories in Meleis's (2007) classification of nursing theories. This category is defined by the type of activities and interventions nurses design to assist actual or prospective clients or people who are vulnerable. The stance of the theorist and the substance of the theory dictate the design and type of interventions. The theorists she included in this classification are Levine, whose theory was concerned with the conservation of clients' energy, and Orem, whose theory focused on returning clients to self-care.

Meleis's (2007) categorization of nursing models and theories differs from other categorizations in that nursing's metaparadigm concepts (although expressed in her specific terms)—humans, health, environment, and nursing—were her categorizing principles. The use of the principle concepts of nursing science gives Meleis's categories a focus that is particularly nursing oriented, compared with the philosophically based categorizations found in the next group of categories of nursing theories. Table 6-1 summarizes Meleis's categorization of grand nursing theories.

## CATEGORIZATION BASED ON PARADIGMS

A *paradigm* is a worldview or an overall way of looking at a discipline and its science. It is seen as a universal view of life, rather than just a model or principle of a theory. Kuhn (1962, 1996), a theoretical physicist turned science historian, awakened the scientific community to revolutions in understanding what he called paradigm shifts.

TABLE 6-1 *Categorization of Nursing Theories by Meleis's Domain Concepts*

| Domain Concept | Nursing Theorist/Work |
|---|---|
| Nursing clients | Johnson: *Behavioral System Model for Nursing*<br>Roy: *Roy Adaptation Model*<br>Neuman: *Neuman Systems Model* |
| Human being–environment interactions | Rogers: *Science of Unitary Human Beings* |
| Interactions | King: *Theory of Goal Attainment*<br>Orlando: *Dynamic Nurse–Patient Relationship: Function, Process and Principles*<br>Paterson-Zderad: *Humanistic Nursing*<br>Travelbee: *Interpersonal Aspects of Nursing*<br>Wiedenbach: *Clinical Nursing: A Helping Art* |
| Nursing therapeutics | Levine: *Conservation Principles of Nursing*<br>Orem: *Orem's General Theory of Nursing* |

Paradigm shifts occur when empirical reality no longer fits the existing theories of science. As an example, he cited Einstein's theory of general relativity, which came about when the extant theories no longer fit the evidence that was being generated regarding matter and energy (Kuhn, 1962).

Recent scientific revolutions in health disciplines have changed the way scientists currently view human beings and their health. For example, immunotherapy and gene therapy are currently being studied extensively. Human genes have been mapped and this knowledge has impacted areas of life as varied as ethics, the law, pharmacology, and medicine. The impact of these new ideas and research on health care delivery is, in effect, a paradigm shift.

Nursing scientists are finding that the theories that have guided practice in the past are no longer sufficient to explain, predict, or guide current practice. Further, older theories may not be helpful in developing nursing science because scholars working in nursing's new paradigm are finding evidence that distinguishes nursing science from the sciences that nurses have traditionally consulted to explain the discipline: anthropology, biology, chemistry, physics, psychology, sociology, and the like (Cody, 2000). The following sections outline how three nursing scholars (Parse, Newman, and Fawcett) have categorized nursing theories based on paradigms or worldviews (Figure 6-2).

### Parse's Categorization

Parse (1995) categorized the various nursing theories into two basic paradigms. These she termed the *totality paradigm* and the *simultaneity paradigm*. The totality paradigm includes all theoretical perspectives in which humans are biopsychosocial-spiritual beings, adapting to their environment, in whatever way the theory defines environment. The simultaneity paradigm, on the other hand, includes the theoretical perspectives in which humans are identified as unitary beings, which are energy systems in simultaneous, continuous, mutual process with, and embedded in, the universal energy system. In this classification scheme, the works of Orem, Roy, Johnson, and others would fit within the totality paradigm, and the works of theorists such as herself, Rogers, and Newman would be part of the simultaneity paradigm.

**Three Categories of Theory (Wills, 2002)**

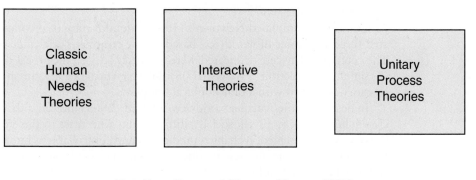

**Two Paradigms of Theory (Parse, 1987)**

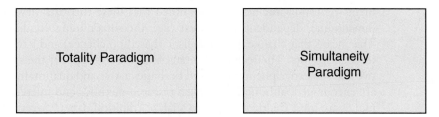

FIGURE 6-2 Comparison of categories (paradigms) of theories.

### Newman's Categorization

Similarly, Newman (1992) classified nursing theories according to existing philosophical schools but found that nursing paradigms did not neatly fit; therefore, she created three categorizations of theories loosely based on the extant philosophies (i.e., positivism, postpositivism, humanism). She named the nursing paradigms: (1) the particulate–deterministic school, (2) the interactive–integrative school, and (3) the unitary–transformative school. In this classification scheme, the first word in the pair indicates the view of the substance of the theory and the second word indicates the way in which change occurs.

To Newman (1992), the *particulate–deterministic* paradigm is characterized by the positivist view of the theory of science and stresses research methods that demanded control in the search for knowledge. Entities (e.g., humans) are viewed as reducible, and change is viewed as linear and causal. Nightingale, Orem, Orlando, and Peplau are representative of theorists in this realm of theoretical thinking.

The *interactive–integrative* paradigm (Newman, 1992) has similarities with the postpositivist school of thought. In this paradigm, objectivity and control are still important, but reality is seen as multidimensional and contextual, and both objectivity and subjectivity are viewed as desirable. Newman lists works of theorists Patterson and Zderad, Roy, Watson, and Erickson, Tomlin, and Swain in this paradigm (Patterson and Zderad are not included in the discussion in Chapters 7, 8, and 9).

Into the *unitary–transformative* category, Newman (1992) places her works and those of Martha E. Rogers and Parse. Each of these theorists views humans as unitary beings, which are self-evolving and self-regulating. Humans are embedded in, and constantly and simultaneously interacting with, a universal, self-evolving energy system. These theorists agree that human beings cannot be known by the sum of their parts; rather, they are known by their patterns of energy and ways of being apart and distinct from others.

### Fawcett's Categorization

Fawcett (2005) simplified Newman's (1992) categorization of theories when she created three categories of worldview based on the treatment of change in each theory. The categories Fawcett delineated were (1) reaction, (2) reciprocal interaction, and (3) simultaneous action (Fawcett, 2005). Like Newman (1992), she showed that each category coincided with a philosophical tradition.

In describing the *reaction* worldview, Fawcett (2005) indicated that these theories classify humans as biopsychosocial-spiritual beings who react to the environment in a causal way. The interaction changes predictably and controllably as humans survive and adapt. She argued that in these theories, phenomena must be objective and observable and may be isolated and measured.

Fawcett (1993) established that in the *reciprocal interaction* worldview, humans are viewed as holistic, active, and interactive with their environments, with the environments returning interactions. She noted that these theorists viewed reality as multidimensional, dependent on context (i.e., the surrounding conditions), and relative. This means that change is probabilistic (based on chance) and a result of multiple antecedent factors. The reciprocal interaction theories support the study of both objective and subjective phenomena, and both qualitative and quantitative research methods are encouraged, although controlled research methods and inferential statistical techniques are most frequently used to analyze empirical data (Fawcett, 2005).

In the third category of grand theories, the *simultaneous action* worldview, Fawcett (2005) reports that human beings are viewed as unitary, are identified by patterns in mutual rhythmical interchange with their environments, are changing continuously, and are evolving as self-organized fields. She states that in the simultaneous action paradigm, change is in a single direction (unidirectional) and is unpredictable in that beings progress through organization to disorganization on the way to more complex organization. In this paradigm, knowledge and pattern recognition are the phenomena of interest.

Fawcett's (2005) categorization explained the major differences among the many current and past nursing theories and conceptual models. Table 6-2 summarizes her grand theory categorization scheme. Table 6-3 compares the classification methods of Fawcett (2005), Meleis (2007), Newman (1995), and Parse (1995).

TABLE 6-2 *Fawcett's Categorization of Nursing Theories*

| Paradigm | Characteristics |
|---|---|
| Reaction | Humans are biopsychosocial-spiritual beings |
| | Humans react to their environment in a causal way |
| | Change is predictable as humans survive and adapt |
| Reciprocal interaction | Humans are holistic beings |
| | Humans interact reciprocally with their environment |
| | Reality is multidimensional, contextual, and relative |
| Simultaneous action | Humans are unitary beings |
| | Humans and their environment are constantly interacting, changing, and evolving |
| | Change is unidirectional and unpredictable |

TABLE 6-3 *Classification of Grand Theories by Current Theory Analysts*

| Theory Analyst | Source | Basis for Typology | Categories |
|---|---|---|---|
| Fawcett | Philosophy | Worldviews | Reaction |
| | | | Reciprocal interaction |
| | | | Simultaneous action |
| Meleis | Patient care | Metaparadigm concepts | Nursing clients |
| | | | Human being–environment interactions |
| | | | Interactions |
| Newman | Paradigm | Philosophical schools | Particulate–deterministic |
| | | | Interactive–integrative |
| | | | Unitary–transformative |
| Parse | Paradigm | Dichotomy between worldviews | Totality |
| | | | Simultaneity |

Sources: Fawcett (2000, 2005); Meleis (2005); Newman (1995); Parse (1995).

## Specific Categories of Models and Theories for This Unit

For this book, the conceptual models and grand nursing theories were categorized based on distinctions that are similar to those presented by Fawcett (2005) and Newman (1992). Chapters 7, 8, and 9 thus present analyses of models and theories according to the following classifications: (1) the human needs theories (which relate to Fawcett's reaction category), (2) the interactive theories, and (3) the unitary process theories.

The theories discussed in Chapter 7 are based on a classical needs perspective and are among the earliest theories and models derived for nursing science. They include the works of Nightingale, Henderson, Johnson, and others. In Chapter 8, each of the perspectives has human interactions as the basis of their content, regardless of the era in which they were developed. The works of Roy, Watson, King, and others are also included in Chapter 8. Finally, the simultaneous process theories (i.e., simultaneity theories) are described in Chapter 9 of this unit. The theorists presented include Rogers, Newman, and Parse. Table 6-4 summarizes the theories that are presented in Chapters 7, 8, and 9.

TABLE 6-4 *Categorization of Grand Nursing Theories for Chapters 7, 8, and 9*

| | Models and Theories | |
|---|---|---|
| **Human Needs** | **Interactive Process** | **Unitary Process** |
| Abdellah | Artinian | Newman |
| Henderson | Erickson, Tomlin, and Swain | Parse |
| Johnson | King | Rogers |
| Nightingale | Levine | |
| Neuman | Roper, Logan, and Tierney | |
| Orem | Roy | |
| | Watson | |

# Analysis Criteria for Grand Nursing Theories

Describing how models and theories can be employed in nursing practice, research, administration/management, and education necessitates a review of selected elements through theory analysis. Seven criteria were selected for description and analysis of grand theories in this unit. As described in Chapter 5, these seven chosen criteria were among the earliest enumerated by Ellis (1968) and Hardy (1978), and promoted by Walker and Avant (2005) and Fawcett (1993, 1995).

Complete analysis of each theory was not performed; instead, the presentation of the models and theories in Chapters 7, 8, and 9 is largely descriptive rather than analytical or evaluative. Each theory's ease of interpretation and application is also briefly critiqued. The criteria used for review of the grand theories in these three chapters are listed in Box 6-1. Each criterion is also discussed briefly in the following sections.

## BACKGROUND OF THE THEORIST

A review of the background of the theorist is likely to reveal the foundations of the theorist's ideas. The individual's educational experiences, in particular, may be relevant to the development of the theory. At one time, higher education, particularly university education, was open only to the children of financially secure families, and often limited to nonminorities. Only in the years after the 1960s were scholarships for students with financial hardships and students of ethnic minorities readily available. In addition, nursing graduate programs were not widely available in most parts of the United States before the creation of federal programs in the late 1960s. Because of the limited availability of graduate nursing programs, the majority of the early nursing scholars who developed conceptual models and grand theories received graduate education in disciplines other than nursing. As a result, the earliest nursing models and theories reflected the paradigms that were accepted in the scholar's educative discipline at the time in which they studied or wrote.

The nurse scholar's experience and specialty also influenced the theoretical perspective. For example, Orlando and Peplau were psychiatric nurses who were educated in the first half of the 20th century. Their graduate education in psychology was tempered by the focus of psychology at that time—that of the logical–positivist era, which emphasized reductionistic principles and was mathematically based. Later scholars (e.g., Fawcett, Parse, Fitzpatrick, and Newman) received their doctoral credentials in the discipline of nursing. The writings of these scholars reflect the scientific thought

---

**BOX 6-1** *Review Criteria for Descriptive Analysis of Grand Nursing Theories*

Background of the theorist
Philosophical underpinnings of the theory
Major assumptions, concepts, and relationships
Usefulness
Testability
Parsimony
Value in extending nursing science

processes, knowledge base, and current thinking of the discipline at the time of their writing, as well as their personal perspectives and experiences.

The placement of the author of the model or theory in historical and conceptual perspective promotes understanding of the extant views of science during the time in which the theorist wrote. Only in the most exceptional of cases are scholars not likely to be influenced by the times in which they formulated their work. One exception to this was Martha Rogers. Interestingly, the discipline of nursing was deep in the positivist era in the 1960s when she began her work; the hard sciences (i.e., physics and chemistry), however, had entered the postpositivist era, which posited the idea that change is inherent in a growing discipline. Rogers' (1970) theory did not fit easily into the concurrent paradigm of nursing science of that time and was rejected by many in favor of more intermediate thinking that corresponded to that of the postpositivist thinkers.

## PHILOSOPHICAL UNDERPINNINGS OF THE THEORY

The background of the scholar most likely contributed heavily to the philosophical basis and paradigmatic origins of the model or theory. Historically, nursing theories of the 1950s and 1960s corresponded to the reaction worldview. In the late 1960s through the early 1980s, the reciprocal interaction worldviews began to take precedence, and by the 1990s the unitary process perspectives began to achieve importance, although the earlier paradigms were still influential (Fawcett, 1993). It is important to note that most of the scholars who adhered to the interaction worldviews were working and writing in the 1950s, before their ideas achieved general recognition in the profession. The simultaneous action scholars, beginning with Rogers and followed by Parse and Newman, developed their ideas in the 1970s and 1980s and continuously grew their theories as each was influenced by modern thinking and technology.

The fundamental philosophies and the disciplines in which the scholars were educated are reflected in their works. Those educated in the social sciences, for example, incorporated some of the characteristics, concepts, and assumptions of those disciplines in their works. Personal philosophies are also reflected in written views on humans, science, environment, and health. Whether written from the positivist philosophy of science or the postpositivist or the modern worldviews, the philosophical viewpoints that form the basis of the works are indicated by the chosen concepts. A component of theory analysis is to point out the underlying philosophy and review the consistency with which the writer demonstrates attention to that background.

## MAJOR ASSUMPTIONS, CONCEPTS, AND RELATIONSHIPS

Examination of the major assumptions, concepts, and relationships of the model or theory is vital because they are the substance of the formulation. These components will direct practice, assist with selection of concepts to be studied, and generate collateral theories for the discipline of nursing. Whether the assumptions are spelled out, or merely inferred, indicates the strength of the theory in elucidating its content. The concepts, carefully defined and explained, along with their derivation, assist the analyst in determining the essence of the model or theory. The relationships between and among the concepts, their strength, and whether they are positive, negative, or neutral indicate the structure of the theory (Walker & Avant, 2005).

## USEFULNESS

Conceptual models and grand theories are reputed not to be particularly useful in directing nursing practice because of their scope and level of abstraction and because they were created through the analytical, logical, and philosophical understandings of a single theorist (Tomey & Alligood, 2002, 2006). The reality is that though many of the conceptual models and grand theories cannot be tested in a single research project, they have been useful in guiding nursing scholarship and practice and in providing the structure from which testable theories may be derived. Grand nursing theories can suggest more concrete theories, with more specifically defined concepts, and more highly derived relationships (Fawcett, 2005) that may be more easily applied in clinical practice, in nursing education, or in nursing administration.

## TESTABILITY

To be useful, theories should be "disprovable"; that is, they can be questioned and tested in the real world through research. Because the major purposes of nursing theory are to guide research, practice, education, and administration, the theory must be subjected to examination. Theories that are capable of being tested make the most reliable guides for scholarly work (Walker & Avant, 2005). Many grand theories are not testable in totality, but they may generate theories that are testable from their conceptual matter, assumptions, or structure. The grand theories that are likely to generate middle range theories and practice theories, as well as theoretical models for research, are those most likely to fulfill the requirement of testability (Kim, 2000).

## PARSIMONY

Parsimony is a criterion that is important because the more complex the theory the less easily it is comprehended. Parsimony does not indicate that a theory is simplistic, in fact, often the more parsimonious the theory, the more depth the theory may have. For example, the standard of parsimony in a theory is Einstein's (1961) theory of relativity, which can be reduced to the formula $E = Mc^2$. Although the theory has a mere four concepts, the explanation of this theory is extremely complicated indeed.

Considering the complexity of nurses' primary subjects of interest, human beings in health and illness, it is unlikely that any of the grand nursing theories could ever approximate the mathematical elegance of Einstein's theory of relativity. Parsimonious theoretical constructions, however, provide nurses in administration, practice, and education with broad general categories into which to conceptualize problems and therefore may assist in the derivation of methods of problem solving. Indeed, the more elegant and universal a conceptual model or grand theory, the more global it is in contributing to the science of nursing.

## VALUE IN EXTENDING NURSING SCIENCE

Ultimately, the value of any nursing theory, not just of grand theory, is its ability to extend the discipline and science of nursing. Understanding the nature of human beings and their interaction with the environment, and the impact of this interaction on their health, will help direct holistic and comprehensive nursing interventions that improve health and well-being. Improvement in nursing care is ultimately the reason for formulating theory. Further, the value of the theory in adding to and elaborating nursing science is an important function of grand theory. Questions to be answered when analyzing any theory include: Does the theory generate new knowledge? Can the theory suggest or support new avenues of knowledge generation beyond those that already exist? Does the theory suggest a disciplinary future that is growing and changing? Can the theory assist nurses to respond to the rapid change and growth of health care?

## The Purpose of Critiquing Theories

Critiquing theory is a necessary part of the process when a scholar is selecting a theory for some disciplinary work. Determining whether a grand theory holds promise or value for the effort at hand, and whether middle range theories, which are useful in research, practice, education, or administration, can be generated from it is a product of critique.

It is likely that a graduate nursing student may find it difficult to critique the work of nursing's grand theorists. Yet determining the usefulness of the theory to a project is important. The user of the theory must comprehend the paradigm of the theory, believe in the concepts and assumptions from which it is built, and be able to internalize the basic philosophy of the theorist. It is hardly beneficial to attempt to use a theory that one cannot accept or understand, or one that seems inappropriate. The choice of a theoretical framework or model must fit with the student's or scholar's personal ideals, and this requires the student or scholar to critique the theory for its value in extending the selected professional work.

One problem that arises among both novice and experienced scholars is combining theories from competing paradigms. Often the work generated from these efforts is confusing and obfuscating; it does not generate clear results that extend the thinking within either paradigm. Therefore the conscientious student or scholar selects theories that relate to the same paradigm in science, philosophy, and nursing when combining theories to guide research or practice. Wide reading in the discipline of nursing and the scientific literature of the disciplines from which the theorist has generated ideas will assist in preventing such errors. Theory review and extraction from the grand theories can result in work that satisfies the scholar, guides the research process, provides structure for safe and effective practice, and extends the science of nursing.

## Summary

Grand theories are global in their application to the discipline of nursing and have been instrumental in helping to develop nursing science. Because of their diversity, their complexity, and their differing worldviews, learning about grand nursing theories can be confusing and frustrating, as illustrated by the experiences of Janet Turner, the student nurse from the opening case study. To help make the study of grand theories more logical and rewarding, this chapter presented several methods for categorizing the grand theories on the basis of scope, basic philosophies, and needs of the discipline. It has also presented the criteria that will be used to describe grand nursing theories in subsequent chapters.

Chapters 7, 8, and 9 discuss many of the grand nursing theories that have been placed into the three defined paradigms of nursing. These analyses are meant to be descriptive to allow the student to choose from different paradigms and the theories contained within them to further their work. The student or scholar must recognize

In an effort to define the uniqueness of nursing and to distinguish it from medicine, nursing scholars from the 1950s through the 1970s developed a number of nursing theories. In addition to medicine, the majority of these early works were strongly influenced by the needs theories of social scientists (e.g., Maslow). In needs-based theories, clients are typically considered to be biopsychosocial beings who are the sum of their parts and who need nursing care. Further, clients are mechanistic beings, and if the correct information can be gathered, the cause or source of their problems can be discerned and measured. At that point, interventions can be prescribed that will be effective in meeting their needs (Dickoff, James, & Wiedenbach, 1968). Evidence-based nursing fits with these theories completely and comfortably.

The grand theories and models of nursing described in this chapter focus on meeting clients' needs for nursing care. These theories and models, like all personal statements of scholars, have continued to grow and develop over the years; therefore, several sources were consulted for each model. The latest writings of and about the theories were consulted and are presented. As much as possible, the description of the model is either quoted or paraphrased from the original texts. Some needs theorists may have maintained their theories over the years with little change; nevertheless, new research has often taken place that extends the original work. Students are advised to consult the literature for the newest research using the needs theory of interest.

It should be noted that a concerted attempt was made to ensure that the presentation of the works of all theorists is balanced. Some theories (e.g., Orem, Neuman) are more complex than others; however, the body of information is greater for some. As a result, the sections dealing with some theorists are a little longer than others. This does not imply that shorter works are inferior or less important to the discipline.

Finally, all theory analysts, whether novice or expert, will comprehend theories and models from their own perspectives. If the reader is interested in using a model, the most recent edition of the work of the theorist should be obtained and used as the primary source for any projects. All further works using the theory or model should come from researchers using the theory in their work. Current research writings are one of the best ways to understand the development of the needs theories.

## Florence Nightingale: Nursing: What It Is and What It Is Not

Nightingale's model of nursing was developed before the general acceptance of modern disease theories (i.e., the germ theory) and other theories of medical science. Nightingale knew the germ theory (Beck, 2005), and prior to its wide publication she had deduced that cleanliness, fresh air, sanitation, comfort, and socialization were necessary to healing. She used her experiences in the Scutari Army Hospital in Turkey and in other hospitals in which she worked to document her ideas on nursing (Beck, 2005; Dossey, 2000; Selanders, 1993; Small, 1998).

Nightingale was from a wealthy family, yet she chose to work in the field of nursing, although it was considered a "lowly" occupation. She believed nursing was her call from God, and she determined that the sick deserved civilized care, regardless of their station in life (Nightingale, 1860/1957/1969).

Through her extensive body of work she changed nursing and health care dramatically. Nightingale's record of letters is voluminous, and several books have been written analyzing them, Dossey, Selanders, Beck, and Attewell (2005a) include many of them in their current publication. She wrote many books and reports to federal and worldwide agencies. Books she wrote that are especially important to nurses and nursing include *Notes on Nursing: What It Is and What It Is Not* (original publication in

1860; reprinted in 1957 and 1969), *Notes on Hospitals* (published in 1863), and *Sick-Nursing and, Health-Nursing* (originally published in Hampton's *Nursing of the Sick*, 1893) (Reed & Zurakowski, 1996) and reprinted *in toto* in Dossey, Selanders, Beck, and Attewell (2005a) to name but a small proportion of her great body of works.

## BACKGROUND OF THE THEORIST

Nightingale was born on May 12, 1820, in Florence, Italy; her birthday is still honored in many places. She was privately educated in the classical tradition of her time by her father, and from an early age, she was inclined to care for the sick and injured (Dossey, 2000, 2005a; Selanders, 1993). Although her mother wished her to lead a life of social grace, Nightingale preferred productivity, choosing to school herself in the care of the sick. She attended nursing programs in Kaiserswerth, Germany, in 1850 and 1851, where she completed what was at that time the only formal nursing education available. She worked as the nursing superintendent at the Institution for Care of Sick Gentlewomen in Distressed Circumstances, where she instituted many changes to improve patient care (Dossey, 2000; Selanders, 1993; Small, 1998).

During the Crimean War, she was urged by Sidney Herbert, Secretary of War for Great Britain, to assist in providing care for wounded soldiers. The dire conditions of British servicemen had resulted in a public outcry that prompted the government to institute changes in the system of medical care (Small, 1998). At Herbert's request, Nightingale and a group of 38 skilled nurses were transported to Turkey to provide nursing care to the soldiers in the hospital at Scutari Army Barracks. There, despite daunting opposition by army physicians, Nightingale instituted a system of care that reportedly cut casualties from 48% to 2% within approximately 2 years (Dossey, 2000, 2005a; Selanders, 1993; Zurakowski, 2005).

Early in her work at the army hospital, Nightingale noted that the majority of soldiers' deaths was caused by transport to the hospital and conditions in the hospital itself. Nightingale found that open sewers and lack of cleanliness, pure water, fresh air, and wholesome food were more often the causes of soldiers' deaths; she implemented changes to address these problems (Small, 1998). Although her recommendations were known to be those that would benefit the soldiers, physicians in charge of the hospitals in the Crimea blocked her efforts. Despite this, by her third trip to the Crimea, Nightingale had been appointed the supervisor of all the nurses (Dossey, 2000).

At Scutari, she became known as the "lady with the lamp" from her nightly excursions through the wards to review the care of the soldiers (Audain, 1998). To prove the value of the work she and the nurses were doing, Nightingale instituted a system of record keeping and adapted a statistical reporting method known as the polar area diagram (Audain, 2007; O'Connor & Robertson, 2003) or Cock's Comb model, to analyze the data she so rigorously collected (Small, 1998). Thus, Nightingale was the first nurse to collect and analyze evidence that her methods were working.

On her return to England from Turkey, she worked to reform the Army Medical School, instituted a program of record keeping for government health statistics and assisted with the public health system in India. The effort for which she is most remembered, however, is the Nightingale School for Nurses at St. Thomas' Hospital. This school was supported by the Nightingale Fund, which had been instituted by grateful British citizens in honor of her work in the Crimea (O'Connor & Robertson, 2003; Selanders, 1993).

## PHILOSOPHICAL UNDERPINNINGS OF THE THEORY

Nightingale's work is considered a broad philosophy. Zurakowski (2005) indicates it is a "perspective" (p. 21). By contrast, Selanders (2005a) states that her work is a foundational philosophy (p. 66). Dossey (2005a) demonstrates that the three tenets of Nightingale's philosophy are "healing, leadership, and global action" (p. 1). Dossey states that "her basic tenet was healing and secondary to it are the tenets of leadership and global action which are necessary to support healing at its deepest level" (p. 1). Nightingale's work has influenced the nursing profession and nursing education for more than 150 years. To Nightingale, nursing was the domain of women, but was an independent practice in its own right. Nurses were, however, to practice in accord with physicians, whose prescriptions nurses were faithfully to carry out (Nightingale, 1893/1954). Nightingale did not believe that nurses were meant to be subservient to physicians. Rather, she believed that nursing was an independent profession or a calling in its own right (Selanders, 1993). Nightingale's educational model is based on anticipating and meeting the needs of patients, and is oriented toward the works a nurse should carry out in meeting those needs. Nightingale's philosophy was inductively derived, abstract yet descriptive in nature, and is classified as a grand theory or philosophy by most nursing writers (Dossey, 2000; Selanders, 1993, 2005a; Tomey & Alligood, 2002, 2006).

## MAJOR ASSUMPTIONS, CONCEPTS, AND RELATIONSHIPS

Nightingale was an educated gentlewoman of the Victorian era. The language she used to write her books—*Notes on Nursing: What It Is and What It Is Not* (1860/1957/1969) and *Sick-Nursing and Health-Nursing* (1893/1954)—was cultured, flowing, logical in format, and elegant in style. She wrote numerous letters many of which are still available. These were topical, direct and yet abstract, and addressed a plethora of topics, such as personal care of patients and sanitation in army hospitals and communities to name only a few (Dossey, 2005b; Selanders, 2005b).

Nightingale (1860/1957/1969) believed that five points were essential in achieving a healthful house: "pure air, pure water, efficient drainage, cleanliness, and light" (p. 24). She thought buildings should be constructed to admit light to every occupant and to allow the flow of fresh air. Further, she wrote that proper household management makes a difference in healing the ill and that nursing care pertained to the house in which the patient lived, and to those who came into contact with the patient, as well as to the care of the patient.

Although the metaparadigm concepts had not been so labeled until over 130 years later, Nightingale (1893/1954) addressed them—human, environment, health, and nursing—specifically in her writings. She believed that a healthy environment was essential for healing. For example, noise was harmful and impeded the need of the person for rest, and noises to avoid included caregivers talking within the hearing of the individual, the rustle of the wide skirts (common at the time), fidgeting, asking unnecessary questions, and a heavy tread while walking. Nutritious food, proper beds and bedding, and personal cleanliness were variables Nightingale deemed essential, and she was convinced that social contact was important to healing. Although the germ theory had been proposed, Nightingale's writings do not specifically refer to it. Her ideals of care, however, indicate that she recognized and agreed that cleanliness prevents morbidity (Nightingale, 1999).

Nightingale believed that nurses must make accurate observations of their patients and report the state of the patient to the physician in an orderly manner (Nightingale,

1860/1957/1969). She explained that nurses should think critically about the care of the patient and do what was appropriate and necessary to assist the patient to heal. Nursing was seen as a way "to put the constitution in such a state as that it will have no disease, or that it can recover from disease" (Nightingale, 1893/1954, p. 3), which will "put us in the best possible conditions for nature to restore or to preserve health—to prevent or to cure disease or injury" (p. 357). She believed that nursing was an art, whereas medicine was a science, and stated that nurses were to be loyal to the medical plan, but not servile. Throughout her writings, Nightingale (1893/1954, 1860/1957/1969) enumerated tasks that nurses should complete to care for ill individuals, and many of the tasks she outlined are still relevant today (Nightingale, 1860/1957/1969).

Health was defined in her treatise, *Sickness-Nursing and Health-Nursing* (1893/1954), as "to be well but to be able to use well every power we have" (p. 357). It is apparent throughout that volume that health meant more than the mere absence of disease, a view that placed Nightingale ahead of her time (Selanders, 1993).

## USEFULNESS

Nightingale wrote on hospitals, nursing, and community health in the 19th and into the 20th century and her works served as the basis of nursing education in Britain and in the United States for over a century. King's College Hospital and St. Thomas' Hospital in London, England, were the initial nursing programs developed by Nightingale, and she maintained a special interest in St. Thomas' Hospital during most of her life (Small, 1998). Nursing programs that used the Nightingale method in the United States included Bellevue Hospital in New York, New Haven Hospital in Connecticut, and Massachusetts Hospital in Boston. Indeed, the influence of Nightingale's methods is felt in nursing programs to the present (Pfettscher, 2006). A resurgence in attention to Nightingale's philosophy is noteworthy. Jacobs (2001) discussed the attribute of human dignity as a central phenomenon uniting nursing theory and practice, two areas that were extensively treated by Nightingale in her own writings.

## TESTABILITY

Nightingale's theory can be the source of testable hypotheses since she treated concrete as well as abstract concepts. Research that is conversant with her ideas of care includes research on noise (Tailor-Ford, Catlin, LaPlant, & Weinke, 2008), environment (Pope, 1995), and spirituality (Tanyi & Werner, 2008).

## PARSIMONY

In her work, Nightingale succinctly stated what she believed was important in caring for ill individuals. Furthermore, in one small volume she includes information about nursing care, patient needs, proper buildings in which the sick are to be treated, and the administration of hospitals.

## VALUE IN EXTENDING NURSING SCIENCE

Nightingale was a noted nurse of her time. She was a consultant who promoted the collection and analyses of health statistics. She was deeply involved in nursing education and promoting the science of public health (Small, 1998), hospital administration, community health, and global health (Dossey, 2005a). Nightingale's legacy continues to be important to nursing scholars and her vast contributions continue to enlighten nursing science. Current Nightingale scholars include Dossey, Selanders, Beck, and Atwell (2005a), Jacobs (2001), and many others who have contributed to the understanding of her multitudinous works. Nightingale's work was revolutionary for its impact on nursing and health care. Furthermore, her many works continue to present effective guidelines for nurses.

# Virginia Henderson: The Principles and Practice of Nursing

Virginia Henderson was a well-known nursing educator and a prolific author. In 1937, Henderson and others created a basic nursing curriculum for the National League for Nursing in which education was "patient centered and organized around nursing problems rather than medical diagnoses" (Henderson, 1991, p. 19). In 1939, she revised Harmer's classic textbook of nursing for its fourth edition, and later wrote the fifth edition, incorporating her personal definition of nursing (Henderson, 1991). Although she was retired, she was a frequent visitor to nursing schools well into her 90s. O'Malley (1996) states that Henderson is known as the modern-day mother of nursing. Her work influenced the nursing profession in America and throughout the world.

## BACKGROUND OF THE THEORIST

Henderson was born in Missouri, but spent her formative years in Virginia. She received a diploma in nursing from the Army School of Nursing at Walter Reed Hospital in 1921, and worked at the Henry Street Visiting Nurse Service for 2 years after graduation. In 1923, she accepted a position teaching nursing at the Norfolk Protestant Hospital in Virginia, where she remained for several years. In 1929, Henderson determined that she needed more education and entered Teachers College at Columbia University where she earned her bachelor's degree in nursing in 1932 and a master's degree in 1934. Subsequently, she joined Columbia as a member of the faculty, where she remained until 1948 (Herrmann, 1998). "Ms. Virginia," as she was known to her friends, died in 1996 at the age of 98 (Allen, 1996). Because of her importance to modern nursing, the Sigma Theta Tau International Nursing Library is named in her honor.

## PHILOSOPHICAL UNDERPINNINGS OF THE THEORY

Henderson was educated during the empiricist era in medicine and nursing, which focused on patient needs, but she believed that her theoretical ideas grew and matured through her experiences (Henderson, 1991). Henderson was introduced to physiologic principles during her graduate education, and the understanding of these principles was the basis for her patient care (Henderson, 1965, 1991). The theory presents the patient as a sum of parts with biopsychosocial needs, and the patient is neither client nor consumer. Henderson stated that "Thorndike's fundamental needs of man" (Henderson, 1991, p. 16) had an influence on her beliefs.

Although her major clinical experiences were in medical-surgical hospitals, she worked as a visiting nurse in New York City. This experience enlarged Henderson's view to recognize the importance of increasing the patient's independence so that progress after hospitalization would not be delayed (Henderson, 1991). Henderson was a nurse educator, and the major thrust of her theory relates to the education of nurses.

## MAJOR ASSUMPTIONS, CONCEPTS, AND RELATIONSHIPS

Henderson's concept of nursing was derived from her practice and education; therefore, her work is inductive. Henderson did not manufacture language to elucidate her theoretical stance; she used correct, scholarly English in all of her writings. She called her definition of nursing her "concept" (Henderson, 1991, pp. 20–21).

### Assumptions

The major assumption of the theory is that nurses care for patients until patients can care for themselves once again (Henderson, 1991). She assumes that patients desire to return to health, but this assumption is not explicitly stated. She also assumes that nurses are willing to serve and that "nurses will devote themselves to the patient day and night" (p. 23). A final assumption is that nurses should be educated at the university level in both arts and sciences.

### Concepts

The major concepts of the theory relate to the metaparadigm (i.e., nursing, health, patient, and environment). Henderson believed that "the unique function of the nurse is to assist the individual, sick or well, in the performance of those activities contributing to health or its recovery (or to a peaceful death) that he would perform unaided if he had the necessary strength, will or knowledge. And to do this in such a way as to help him gain independence as rapidly as possible" (Henderson, 1991, p. 21). She defined the patient as someone who needs nursing care, but did not limit nursing to illness care. She did not define environment, but maintaining a supportive environment is one of the elements of her 14 activities. Health was not explicitly defined, but it is taken to mean balance in all realms of human life. The concept of nursing involved the nurse attending to 14 activities that assist the individual toward independence (Box 7-1).

---

**BOX 7-1** *Henderson's 14 Activities for Client Assistance*

1. Breathe normally
2. Eat and drink adequately
3. Eliminate body wastes
4. Move and maintain desirable postures
5. Sleep and rest
6. Select suitable clothes—dress and undress
7. Maintain body temperature within normal range by adjusting clothing and modifying environment
8. Keep the body clean and well groomed and protect the integument
9. Avoid dangers in the environment and avoid injuring others
10. Communicate with others in expressing emotions, needs, fears, or opinions
11. Worship according to one's faith
12. Work in such a way that there is a sense of accomplishment
13. Play or participate in various forms of recreation
14. Learn, discover, or satisfy the curiosity that leads to normal development and health and use the available health facilities

Source: Henderson (1991, pp. 22–23).

## USEFULNESS

Nursing education has been deeply affected by Henderson's clear vision of the functions of nurses. The principles of Henderson's theory were published in the major nursing textbooks used from the 1930s through the 1960s, and the principles embodied by the 14 activities are still important in evaluating nursing care in the 21st century. Other concepts that Henderson proposed have been used in nursing education from the 1930s until the present (O'Malley, 1996).

## TESTABILITY

Henderson supported nursing research, but believed that it should be clinical research (O'Malley, 1996). Much of the research before her time had been on educational processes and on the profession of nursing itself, rather than on the practice and outcomes of nursing, and she worked to change that.

Each of the 14 activities can be the basis for research. Although the statements are not written in testable terms, they may be reformulated into researchable questions. Further, the theory can guide research in any aspect of the individual's care needs.

## PARSIMONY

Henderson's work is parsimonious in its presentation, but complex in its scope. The 14 statements cover the whole of the practice of nursing, and her vision about the nurse's role in patient care (i.e., that the nurse perform for the patient those activities the patient usually performs independently, until the patient can again adequately perform them) contributes to that complexity.

## VALUE IN EXTENDING NURSING SCIENCE

From an historical standpoint, Henderson's concept of nursing enhanced nursing science; this has been particularly important in the area of nursing education. Her contributions to nursing literature extended from the 1930s through the 1990s. Her work has had an impact on nursing research by strengthening the focus on nursing practice and confirming the value of tested interventions in assisting individuals to regain health.

## Faye G. Abdellah: Patient-Centered Approaches to Nursing

Faye Abdellah was one of the first nursing theorists. In one of her earliest writings (Abdellah, Beland, Martin, & Matheney, 1960), she referred to the model created by her colleagues and herself as a framework. Her writings spanned the period from 1954 to 1992 and include books, monographs, book chapters, articles, reports, forewords to books, and conference proceedings.

## BACKGROUND OF THE THEORIST

Abdellah earned her bachelor's degree in nursing, master's degree, and doctorate from Columbia University, and she completed additional graduate studies in science at Rutgers University. She served as the Chief Nurse Officer and Deputy U.S. Surgeon General, U.S. Public Health Service before retiring in 1993 with the rank of Rear Admiral. She has been awarded many academic honors from both civilian and military sources (Abdellah & Levine, 1994). She retired from her position as dean of the Graduate School of Nursing, Uniformed Services University of the Health Sciences in 2000.

## PHILOSOPHICAL UNDERPINNINGS OF THE THEORY

Abdellah's patient-centered approach to nursing was developed inductively from her practice and is considered a human needs theory (Abdellah et al., 1960). The theory was created to assist with nursing education and is most applicable to education and practice (Abdellah et al., 1960). Although it was intended to guide care of those in the hospital, it also has relevance for nursing care in community settings.

## MAJOR ASSUMPTIONS, CONCEPTS, AND RELATIONSHIPS

The language of Abdellah's framework is readable and clear. Consistent with the decade in which she was writing, she uses the term "she" for nurses, "he" for doctors and patients, and refers to the object of nursing as "patient" rather than client or consumer (Abdellah et al., 1960). Interestingly, she was one of the early writers who referred to "nursing diagnosis" (Abdellah et al., 1960, p. 9) during a time when nurses were taught that diagnosis was not a nurse's prerogative.

### Assumptions

There are no openly stated assumptions in Abdellah's early work (Abdellah et al., 1960), but in a later work she added six assumptions. These relate to change and anticipated changes that affect nursing; the need to appreciate the interconnectedness of social enterprises and social problems; the impact of problems such as poverty, racism, pollution, education, and so forth on health and health care delivery; changing nursing education; continuing education for professional nurses; and development of nursing leaders from underserved groups (Abdellah, Beland, Martin, & Matheney, 1973).

Abdellah and colleagues (1960) developed a list of 21 nursing problems (Box 7-2). They also identified 10 steps to identify the client's problems and 10 nursing skills to be used in developing a treatment typology.

According to Abdellah and coworkers (1960), nurses should do the following:

1. Learn to know the patient
2. Sort out relevant and significant data
3. Make generalizations about available data in relation to similar nursing problems presented by other patients
4. Identify the therapeutic plan
5. Test generalizations with the patient and make additional generalizations
6. Validate the patient's conclusions about his nursing problems
7. Continue to observe and evaluate the patient over a period of time to identify any attitudes and clues affecting his behavior
8. Explore the patient's and family's reaction to the therapeutic plan and involve them in the plan
9. Identify how the nurse feels about the patient's nursing problems
10. Discuss and develop a comprehensive nursing care plan

Abdellah and her colleagues (1960) distinguished between nursing diagnoses and nursing functions. Nursing diagnoses were a determination of the nature and extent

---

**BOX 7-2** *Abdellah's 21 Nursing Problems*

1. To maintain good hygiene and physical comfort
2. To promote optimal activity, exercise, rest, and sleep
3. To promote safety through prevention of accidents, injury, or other trauma and through the prevention of the spread of infection
4. To maintain good body mechanics and prevent and correct deformities
5. To facilitate the maintenance of a supply of oxygen to all body cells
6. To facilitate the maintenance of nutrition of all body cells
7. To facilitate the maintenance of elimination
8. To facilitate the maintenance of fluid and electrolyte balance
9. To recognize the physiologic responses of the body to disease conditions
10. To facilitate the maintenance of regulatory mechanisms and functions
11. To facilitate the maintenance of sensory function
12. To identify and accept positive and negative expressions, feelings, and reactions
13. To identify and accept the interrelatedness of emotions and organic illness
14. To facilitate the maintenance of effective verbal and nonverbal communication
15. To promote the development of productive interpersonal relationships
16. To facilitate progress toward achievement of personal spiritual goals
17. To create and maintain a therapeutic environment
18. To facilitate awareness of self as an individual with varying physical, emotional, and developmental needs
19. To accept the optimum possible goals in light of physical and emotional limitations
20. To use community resources as an aid in resolving problems arising from illness
21. To understand the role of social problems as influencing factors in the cause of illness

Source: Abdellah et al. (1960).

---

of nursing problems presented by individuals receiving nursing care, and nursing functions were nursing activities that contributed to the solution for the same nursing problem. Other concepts central to her work were (1) health care team (a group of health professionals trained at various levels, and often at different institutions, working together to provide health care); (2) professionalization of nursing (requires that nurses identify those nursing problems that depend on the nurse's use of her capacities to conceptualize events and make judgments about them); (3) patient (individual who needs nursing care and is dependent on the health care provider); and (4) nursing (a service to individuals and families and to society, which helps people cope with their health needs) (Abdellah et al., 1960).

## USEFULNESS

The patient-centered approach was constructed to be useful to nursing practice, with the impetus for it being nursing education. Abdellah's publications on nursing education began with her dissertation; her interest in education of nurses continues into the present.

Abdellah has also published on nursing, nursing research, and public policy related to nursing in several international publications. She has been a strong advocate for improving nursing practice through nursing research and has a publication record on nursing research that dates from 1955 to the present. Box 7-3 lists only a few of Abdellah's many publications.

---

**BOX 7-3** *Examples of Abdellah's Publications*

Abdellah, F. G., Beland, I. L, Martin, A., & Matheney, R. V. (1968). *Patient-centered approaches to nursing* (2nd ed.). New York: MacMillan.

Abdellah, F. G. (1972). Evolution of nursing as a profession: Perspective on manpower development. *International Nursing Review, 19,* 3.

Abdellah, F. G. (1986). The nature of nursing science. In L. H. Nicholl (Ed.), *Perspectives on nursing theory.* Boston: Little, Brown.

Abdellah, F. G. (1987). The federal role in nursing education. *Nursing Outlook, 35*(5), 224–225.

Abdellah, F. G. (1991). Public policy impacting on nursing care of older adults. In E. M. Baines (Ed.), *Perspectives on gerontological nursing.* Newbury, CA: Sage Publications.

Abdellah, F. G., & Levine, E. (1994). *Preparing nursing research for the 21st century.* New York: Springer.

---

## TESTABILITY

Abdellah's work is a conceptual model that is not directly testable because there are few stated directional relationships. The model is testable in principle, though, because testable hypotheses can be derived from its conceptual material. One work (Abdellah & Levine, 1957) was identified that described the development of a tool to measure client and personnel satisfaction with nursing care.

## PARSIMONY

Abdellah and colleagues' model (1960, 1973) touches on many factors in nursing, but focuses primarily on the perspective of nursing education. It defines 21 nursing problems, 10 steps to identifying client's problems, and 10 nursing skills. Because of its focus and complexity, it is not particularly parsimonious.

## VALUE IN EXTENDING NURSING SCIENCE

Abdellah's model has contributed to nursing science as an early effort to change nursing education. In the early years of its application, it helped to bring structure and organization to what was often a disorganized collection of lectures and experiences. She categorized nursing problems based on the individual's needs and developed a typology of nursing treatment and nursing skills. Finally, she posited a list of characteristics that described what was distinctly nursing, differentiating the profession from other health professions. Hers was a major contribution to the discipline of nursing, bringing it out of the era of being considered simply an occupation into Nightingale's ideal of becoming a profession.

## Dorothea E. Orem: The Self-Care Deficit Nursing Theory

Dorothea Orem was born in Baltimore, Maryland. She received her diploma in nursing from Providence Hospital School of Nursing in Washington, DC, and her Baccalaureate in Nursing from Catholic University in 1939. In 1945, she also earned her master's degree from Catholic University (Taylor, 2006).

## BACKGROUND OF THE THEORIST

Orem held a number of positions as private duty nurse, hospital staff nurse, and educator. She was the director of both the School of Nursing and Nursing Service at

Detroit's Providence Hospital until 1949, moving from there to Indiana where she served on the Board of Health until 1957. She assumed a role as a faculty member of Catholic University in 1959, later becoming acting dean (Taylor, 2006).

Orem's interest in nursing theory was piqued when she and a group of colleagues were charged with producing a curriculum for practical nursing for the Department of Health, Education, and Welfare in Washington, DC. After publishing the first book on her theory in 1971, she continued working on her concept of nursing and self-care. She had numerous honorary doctorates and other awards as members of the nursing profession have recognized the value of the self-care deficit theory (Taylor, 2006). Dr. Orem died in 2007 after a period of failing health. Nurses will remember her as one of the pioneers of nursing theory (Bekel, 2007).

## PHILOSOPHICAL UNDERPINNINGS OF THE THEORY

Orem (1995) denied that any particular theorist provided the basis for the Self-Care Deficit Nursing Theory (SCDNT). She expressed interest in several theories, although she references only Parsons's structure of social action and von Bertalanfy's system theory (Orem, 1995). Taylor and colleagues (2000), however, stated that the ontology of Orem's SCDNT is the school of moderate realism, and its focus is on the person as agent; the SCDNT is a highly developed formalized theoretical system of nursing.

## MAJOR ASSUMPTIONS, CONCEPTS, AND RELATIONSHIPS

Orem's theory, changed to fit the times, most notably in the concept of the individual and of the nursing system. The original theory, however, remains largely intact.

Orem (2001) delineates three nested theories: theories of self-care, self-care deficit, and nursing systems (Figure 7-1). The theory of nursing systems is the outer or encompassing theory, which contains the theory of self-care deficit. The theory of self-care is a component of the theory of self-care deficit.

### Concepts

Orem (1995, 2001) defined the metaparadigm concepts as follows:

> Nursing is seen as an art through which the practitioner of nursing gives specialized assistance to persons with disabilities which makes more than ordinary assistance necessary to meet needs for self-care. The nurse also intelligently participates in the medical care the individual receives from the physician.
>
> Humans are defined as "men, women, and children cared for either singly or as social units," and are the "material object" (p. 8) of nurses and others who provide direct care.
>
> Environment has physical, chemical, and biological features. It includes the family culture and community.
>
> Health is "being structurally and functionally whole or sound" (p. 96). Also, health is a state that encompasses both the health of individuals and of groups, and human health is the ability to reflect on one's self, to symbolize experience, and to communicate with others.

Numerous additional concepts were formulated for Orem's theory; Table 7-1 lists some of the more significant ones.

### Relationships

An underlying premise of Orem's theory is the belief that humans engage in continuous communication and interchange among themselves and their environments to remain alive and to function. In humans, the power to act deliberately is exercised to

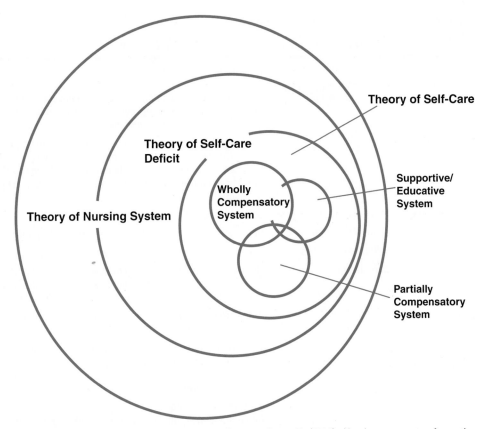

FIGURE 7-1 Self-Care Deficit Nursing Theory. (Source: Orem, D. (2001). *Nursing: concepts of practice* (6th ed.). St. Louis: Mosby.)

identify needs and to make needed judgments. Furthermore, mature human beings experience privations in the form of action in care of self and others involving making life-sustaining and function-regulating actions. Human agency is exercised in discovering, developing, and transmitting to others ways and means to identify needs for, and make inputs into, self and others. Finally, groups of human beings with structured relationships cluster tasks and allocate responsibilities for providing care to group members who experience privations for making required deliberate decisions about self and others (Orem, 1995).

## USEFULNESS

Numerous colleges and schools of nursing base their curricula on the SCDNT. Georgetown University School of Nursing, Oakland University School of Nursing, The University of Missouri, Columbia, and the University of Florida, Gainesville, for example, all have curricula based on Orem's SCDNT (Taylor, 2002, 2006). Hospitals in several areas of the country have based nursing care on Orem's theory, and it has been applied to an ambulatory care setting. Such medical conditions as arthritis or gastrointestinal and renal diseases, and such areas of practice as community nursing, critical care, cultural concepts, maternal–child nursing, medical-surgical nursing, pediatric nursing, perioperative nursing, and renal dialysis, among other specialties have used Orem's theory to structure care (Taylor, 2002, 2006). Orem's SCDNT has

TABLE 7-1 *Concepts in Orem's Self-Care Deficit Theory*

| Concept | Definition |
| --- | --- |
| Self-care | A human regulatory function that is a deliberate action to supply or ensure the supply of necessary materials needed for continued life, growth, and development and maintenance of human integrity. |
| Self-care requisites | Part of self-care and are expressions of action to be performed by or for individuals in the interest of controlling human or environmental factors that affect human functioning or development. There are three types: universal, developmental, and health deviation self-care requisites. |
| Universal self-care requisites | Self-care requisites common to all humans. |
| Developmental self-care requisites | Self-care requisites necessary for growth and development. |
| Health deviation self-care requisites | Self-care requisites associated with health deficits. |
| Therapeutic self-care demand | Nurse's assistance in meeting the client's or client dependent's self-care needs is done therapeutically as a result of the client's inability to calculate or to meet therapeutic self-care needs. |
| Deliberate action | Action knowingly taken with some motivation or some outcome sought by the actor, as self-care or dependent care. |
| Nursing system | The product of a series of relations between the persons: legitimate nurse and legitimate client. This system is activated when the client's therapeutic self-care demand exceeds available self-care agency, leading to the need for nursing. |
| Product of nursing | Nursing has two products: An intellectual product (the design for helping the client). A system of care of long or short duration for persons requiring nursing. |

Source: Orem (1995).

received international interest and has been used in many countries including Great Britain, East Germany, the Netherlands, Norway, Sweden, and New Zealand. Moreover, numerous publications define methods for using Orem's SCDNT in practice, research, and education.

Orem was a prolific author and her writings spanned five decades. In addition to her detailed description of her theory (Orem, 1971, 1985a, 1991, 1995, 2001), she authored an analysis of hospital nursing service (Orem, 1956) and illustrations for self-care for the rehabilitation client (Orem, 1985b). Further evidence of the usefulness of Orem's work is the International Orem Society which celebrates the work of Dr. Orem. Their journal, *Self-Care and Dependent-Care Nursing*, indicates the value to nurses across the globe (Biggs, 2008, p. 6).

## TESTABILITY

Many nursing research studies have used Orem's theory as a conceptual framework or as a source of testable hypotheses. Further, over the years many research studies have tested elements of the theory. The researchers have studied people with diminished self-care agency across age and social groups, in numerous situations, and in many countries. Most research into the SCDNT is descriptive, and the theory has not been subject to testing in its entirety (Taylor, 2002, 2006). Box 7-4 lists some of the recent research studies using the SCDNT.

**BOX 7-4** *Orem's Theory in Nursing Research, Practice, and Education*

Allison, S. E. (2007). Self-care requirements for activity and rest: An Orem nursing focus. *Nursing Science Quarterly, 20*(1), 68–76.

Baldwin, C. M. (2004). Interstitial cystitis and self-care: Bearing the burden. *Urology Nursing, 24*(2), 111–113.

Hines, S. H. (2007). Women's self-care agency to manage urinary incontinence. *Advances in Nursing Science, 30*(2), 175–188.

Kealty, V. M. (2008). Identifying and articulating the characteristics of nursing agency: BSN students' perspective. *Self-Care, Dependent-Care and Nursing, 16*(2), 18–24.

Rafil, F., Shappoorian, F., & Azarbaad, M. (2008). The reality of learning self-care needs during hospitalization: Patients' and nurses' perceptions. *Self-Care, Dependent-Care and Nursing, 16*(2), 34–39.

Matchim, Y., Armer, J. M., & Stewart, B. R. (2008). A qualitative study of participants' perceptions of the effect of mindfulness meditation practice on self-care and overall well being. *Self-Care, Dependent-Care and Nursing, 16*(2), 46–53.

## PARSIMONY

Orem's (2001) SCDNT is complex. It consists of three nested theories, many presuppositions, and propositions in each of the individual theories. Revisions of the theory from the original (1971) have improved the organization; however, its complexity has increased in response to societal needs throughout the several editions.

## VALUE IN EXTENDING NURSING SCIENCE

The SCDNT has been the basis for many college and university nursing curricula (Orem, 1995, 2001). It has been used in practice situations and extensively in research projects, theses, and dissertations (Taylor, 2006). The practical applicability of the theory is attractive to graduate students because it is perceived as a realistic reflection of nursing practice.

## Dorothy Johnson: The Behavioral System Model

Dorothy Johnson began her work on the Behavioral System Model in the late 1950s and wrote into the 1990s. The focus of her model is on needs, the human as a behavioral system, and relief of stress as nursing care.

Johnson (1968, 1990) reported that her work began as a study of the knowledge that identified nursing while synthesizing content for nursing curricula at the graduate and undergraduate levels. She wanted the curricula to be focused on nursing rather than derived from the knowledge bases of other health care disciplines (Johnson, 1959a, 1959b, 1997). Indeed, she believed that nursing, although relying on the contributions of other sciences, is a discrete science and a unique discipline.

Johnson's model was deductively derived through long study of other theories and applying them to nursing (Johnson, 1997). Her goal was to conceptualize nursing for education of nurses at all levels (1990, 1997), and the model emanated from her practice, study, and teaching experiences.

Although Johnson did not write a book on her theory, she did write several chapters and articles that explained her theoretical framework. Box 7-5 lists a sampling of these writings.

| BOX 7-5 | *Examples of Johnson's Writings on Nursing Theory* |

Johnson, D. E. (1959a). A philosophy of nursing. *Nursing Outlook, 7*(4), 198–200.
Johnson, D. E. (1959b). The nature of nursing science. *Nursing Outlook, 7*(5), 291–294.
Johnson, D. E. (1968). Theory in nursing: Borrowed and unique. *Nursing Research, 17*(3), 206–209.
Johnson, D. E. (1974). Development of a theory: A requisite for nursing as a primary health profession. *Nursing Research, 23*(5), 372–377.

Johnson, D. E. (1980). The behavioral system model for nursing. In J. P. Riehl & C. Roy (Eds.), *Conceptual models for nursing practice* (pp. 207–216). New York: Appleton-Century-Crofts.
Johnson, D. E. (1990). The behavioral system model for nursing. In M. E. Parker (Ed.), *Nursing theories in practice* (pp. 23–32). New York: National League for Nursing Press.

## BACKGROUND OF THE THEORIST

Dorothy Johnson was reared in Savannah, Georgia and received a bachelor's degree in nursing from Vanderbilt University. She earned a master's degree in public health from Harvard in 1948, and returned to Vanderbilt to begin her teaching career. In 1949, she joined the nursing faculty of the University of California at Los Angeles (UCLA). She retired from UCLA in 1977 and now lives in Florida.

## PHILOSOPHICAL UNDERPINNINGS OF THE THEORY

Johnson stated that Nightingale's work inspired her model. Nightingale's philosophical leanings prompted Johnson to consider the person experiencing a disease more important than the disease itself (Johnson, 1990). She reported that she derived portions of her theory from the works of Selye on stress, Grinker's theory of human behavior, and Buckley and Chin on systems theories (Johnson, 1980, 1990).

## MAJOR ASSUMPTIONS, CONCEPTS, AND RELATIONSHIPS

### Assumptions

Assumptions of Johnson's model are both stated and derived. There are four assumptions about human behavioral subsystems. First is the belief that drives serve as focal points around which behaviors are organized to achieve specific goals. Second, it is assumed that behavior is differentiated and organized within the prevailing dimensions of set and choice. Third, the specialized parts or subsystems of the behavioral system are structured by dimensions of goal, set, choice, and actions; each has observable behaviors. Finally, interactive and interdependent subsystems tend to achieve and maintain balance between and among subsystems through control and regulatory mechanisms (Grubbs, 1980).

### Concepts

Although she adopted concepts from other disciplines, Johnson modified and defined them to apply specifically to nursing situations. This was an evolving process as shown in her writings (Johnson, 1959a, 1959b, 1968, 1974, 1980, 1990).

The metaparadigm concepts are apparent in Johnson's writings. Nursing is seen as "an external regulatory force which acts to preserve the organization and integration of the patient's behavior at an optimal level under those conditions in which the behavior constitutes a threat to physical or social health, or in which illness is found" (Johnson, 1980, p. 214). The concept of human was defined as a behavioral system that strives to make continual adjustments to achieve, maintain, or regain balance to the steady state that is adaptation (Johnson, 1980).

Health is seen as the opposite of illness, and Johnson (1980) defines it as "some degree of regularity and constancy in behavior, the behavioral system reflects adjustments and adaptations that are successful in some way and to some degree ... adaptation is functionally efficient and effective" (pp. 208, 209). Environment is not directly defined, but it is implied to include all elements of the surroundings of the human system and includes interior stressors. Other concepts defined in Johnson's model are listed in Table 7-2.

### Relationships

Johnson (1980) delineated seven subsystems to which the model applied. These are as follows:

1. Attachment or affiliative subsystem—serves the need for security through social inclusion or intimacy
2. Dependency subsystem—behaviors designed to get attention, recognition, and physical assistance
3. Ingestive subsystem—fulfills the need to supply the biologic requirements for food and fluids
4. Eliminative subsystem—functions to excrete wastes
5. Sexual subsystem—serves the biologic requirements of procreation and reproduction
6. Aggressive subsystem—functions in self and social protection and preservation
7. Achievement system—functions to master and control the self or the environment

TABLE 7-2 *Concepts in Johnson's Behavioral System Theory*

| Concept | Definition |
| --- | --- |
| Behavioral system | Man is a system that indicates the state of the system through behaviors |
| Boundaries | The point that differentiates the interior of the system from the exterior |
| Function | Consequences or purposes of actions |
| Functional requirements | Input that the system must receive to survive and develop |
| Homeostasis | Process of maintaining stability |
| Instability | State in which the system output of energy depletes the energy needed to maintain stability |
| Stability | Balance or steady state in maintaining balance of behavior within an acceptable range |
| Stressor | A stimulus from the internal or external world that results in stress or instability |
| Structure | The parts of the system that make up the whole |
| System | That which functions as a whole by virtue of organized independent interaction of its parts |
| Subsystem | A minisystem maintained in relationship to the entire system when it or the environment is not disturbed |
| Tension | The system's adjustment to demands, change or growth, or to actual disruptions |
| Variables | Factors outside the system that influence the system's behavior, but which the system lacks power to change |

Source: Grubbs (1980).

Finally, there are three functional requirements of humans in Johnson's (1980) model. These are as follows:

1. To be protected from noxious influences with which the person cannot cope
2. To be nurtured through the input of supplies from the environment
3. To be stimulated to enhance growth and prevent stagnation

## USEFULNESS

That Johnson's model is useful for nursing practice and education has been verified in several articles and chapters. Damus (1980), Dee (1990), and Holaday (1980) described situations in which Johnson's model has been used to direct nursing practice. Other authors have used the theory to apply to various aspects of nursing. For example, Benson (1997) used Johnson's model as a framework to describe the impact of fear of crime on an elder person's health, health-seeking behaviors, and quality of life. Fruehwirth (1989) applied Johnson's model to assess and intervene in a group of caregivers for individuals with Alzheimer's disease.

## TESTABILITY

Parts of Johnson's model have been tested or used to direct nursing research. Indeed, more than 20 research studies have been identified using Johnson's model. Turner-Henson (1992), for example, used Johnson's model as a framework to examine how mothers of chronically ill children perceived the environment (i.e., whether it was supportive, safe, and accessible). Poster, Dee, and Randell (1997) used Johnson's theory as a conceptual framework in a study of client outcome evaluation; they found that the nursing theory made it possible to prescribe nursing care and to distinguish it from medical care. Derdiarian and Schobel (1990) used Johnson's model to develop an assessment tool for individuals with acquired immunodeficiency syndrome.

Aspects of Johnson's model have been tested in nursing research. In one study, Derdiarian (1990) examined the relationship between the aggressive/protective subsystem and the other six model subsystems.

## PARSIMONY

Johnson (1980) was able to explicate her entire model in a single short chapter in an edited book. Relatively few concepts are used in the theory, and they are commonly used terms. Additionally, the relationships are clear; therefore, the model is considered to be parsimonious.

## VALUE IN EXTENDING NURSING SCIENCE

Johnson's model has been used in nursing practice and research to a significant extent. In addition, her work has been used as a curriculum guide for a number of schools of nursing (Grubbs, 1980; Johnson, 1980, 1990), and it has been adapted for use in hospital situations (Dee, 1990). Finally, her work inspired the work of at least two other grand nursing theorists, Betty Neuman and Sister Calista Roy, who were her students.

## Betty Neuman: The Neuman Systems Model

Since the 1960s, Betty Neuman has been recognized as a pioneer in the field of nursing, particularly in the area of community mental health. She developed her model while lecturing in community mental health at UCLA and first published it in 1972 under the title, "A Model for Teaching the Total Person Approach to Patient Problems" (Murray, 1999; Neuman & Fawcett, 2002). Since that time, she has been a prolific writer, and her model has been used extensively in colleges of nursing, beginning with Neumann College's baccalaureate nursing program in Aston, Pennsylvania. Numerous other nursing programs have organized their curricula around her model both in the United States and internationally (Neuman & Fawcett, 2002).

The major elements in this review of the Neuman Systems Model are taken from the third and fourth editions of her book (Neuman, 1995; Neuman & Fawcett, 2002), with references to earlier writings to show development of the model over time. The model was deductively derived and emanated from requests of graduate students who wanted assistance with a broad interpretation of nursing (Neuman, 1995).

Neuman's model uses a systems approach that is focused on the human needs of protection or relief from stress. Neuman believed that the causes of stress can be identified and remedied through nursing interventions. She emphasized the need of humans for dynamic balance that the nurse can provide through identification of problems, mutually agreeing on goals, and using the concept of prevention as intervention. Neuman's model is one of only a few considered prescriptive in nature. The model is universal, abstract, and applicable for individuals from many cultures (Neuman, 1995; Neuman & Fawcett, 2002).

## BACKGROUND OF THE THEORIST

Betty Neuman was born in 1924 on a farm near Lowell, Ohio. In 1947, she earned her nursing diploma from People's Hospital School of Nursing, Akron, Ohio, and moved to California shortly thereafter. She earned a bachelor's degree in nursing from UCLA and also studied psychology and public health. In 1966, she earned a master's degree in mental health and public health consultation, also from UCLA, then earned her doctorate in clinical psychology in 1985 from Pacific Western University. She worked as a hospital staff nurse, a head nurse, and an industrial nurse and consultant before becoming a nursing instructor. She has taught medical-surgical nursing, critical care, and communicable disease nursing at the University of Southern California Medical Center in Los Angeles and at other colleges in Ohio and West Virginia (Neuman & Fawcett, 2002).

## PHILOSOPHICAL UNDERPINNINGS OF THE THEORY

Neuman used concepts and theories from a number of disciplines in the development of her theory. In her works, she referred to Chardin and Cornu on wholeness in systems, von Bertalanfy and Lazlo on general systems theory, Selye on stress theory, and Lazarus on stress and coping (Neuman, 1995; Neuman & Fawcett, 2002).

## MAJOR ASSUMPTIONS, CONCEPTS, AND RELATIONSHIPS

### Concepts

Neuman (1995; Neuman & Fawcett, 2002) adhered to the metaparadigm concepts and has developed numerous additional concepts for her model. In her work, she defined human beings as a "client/client system, as a composite of variables (physiological, psychological, sociocultural, developmental, and spiritual), each of which is a subpart of all parts . . . forms the whole of the client . . . a basic structure of protective concentric rings, for retention attainment or maintenance of system stability and integrity" (Neuman & Fawcett, 2002, p. 15). Environment is composed of "both internal and external forces surrounding the client, influencing and being influenced by the client at any point in time, and an open system" (pp. 16–20). Health is defined as "a continuum; wellness and illness are at opposite ends . . . Health for the client is equated with optimal system stability that is the best possible wellness state at any given time" (p. 23). "Variances from wellness or varying degrees of system instability are caused by stressor invasion of the normal line of defense" (p. 24). Finally, in the nursing component, the major concern is to maintain client system stability through accurately assessing environmental and other stressors and assisting in client adjustments to maintain optimal wellness. Table 7-3 lists selected additional concepts from Neuman's model and Figure 7-2 offers a visual representation.

### Relationships

Neuman defined five interacting variables: physiologic, psychological, sociocultural, developmental, and spiritual. These five variables function in time to attain, maintain, or retain system stability. The model is based on the client's reaction to stress as it maintains boundaries to protect client stability.

Neuman (1995; Neuman & Fawcett, 2002) delineated a three-step nursing process model in which nursing diagnosis (the first step) assumes that the nurse collects an adequate database from which to analyze variances from wellness to make the diagnoses. Nursing goals, which are determined by negotiation with the client, are set in the second step. Appropriate prevention as intervention strategies are decided in that step. The third step, nursing outcomes, is the step in which confirmation of prescriptive change or reformulation of nursing goals is evaluated. The nurse links the client, environment, health, and nursing. The findings feed back into the system as applicable. A table of prevention as intervention strategies clarifies what comprises the nursing actions to affect this type of intervention. Neuman outlined 10 propositions or assumptions of the model (Box 7-6).

## USEFULNESS

Neuman's model has been used extensively in nursing education and nursing practice. In her latest work, she provides a number of specific examples of the systems processes (Neuman & Fawcett, 2002). The Neuman Systems Model is in place in numerous states of the United States, and internationally in countries as diverse as Taiwan and the Netherlands. It reportedly has been initiated to guide nursing practice for the management of patient care in the areas of medicine and surgery, mental health, women's health, pediatric nursing, community as client, and gerontology. Some specific conditions described in the literature include depression (Hassell, 1996), lung disease (Narsavage, 1997), and linear scleroderma (Fuller & Hartley, 2000). Graduate students, in particular, find Neuman's model realistic to define their practice.

Because of its utility and popularity as a model, it has been monitored by a group called the Neuman Systems Model Trustees Group, Inc. This group meets periodically to discuss research and practice related to the model and to promote exchange of information and ideas (Neuman & Fawcett, 2002, p. 360).

TABLE 7-3 *Concepts in Neuman's Systems Model*

| Concept | Definition |
|---|---|
| Basic structure | Common client survival factors and unique individual characteristics representing basic system energy resources. |
| Boundary lines | The flexible line of defense is the outer boundary of the client system. |
| Content | The variables of person in interaction with the internal and external environment comprise the whole client system. |
| Degree of reaction | The amount of system instability resulting from stressor invasion of the normal line of defense. |
| Entropy | A process of energy depletion and disorganization moving the system toward illness or possible death. |
| Flexible line of defense | A protective, accordion-like mechanism that surrounds and protects the normal line of defense from invasion by stressors. |
| Goal | Stability for the purpose of client survival and optimal wellness. |
| Input/output | The matter, energy, and information exchanged between client and environment that is entering or leaving the system at any point in time. |
| Lines of resistance | Protection factors activated when stressors have penetrated the normal line of defense, causing a reaction symptomatology. |
| Negentropy | A process of energy conservation that increases organization and complexity, moving the system towards stability or a higher degree of wellness. |
| Normal line of defense | An adaptational level of health developed over time and considered normal for a particular individual client or system; it becomes a standard for wellness–deviance determination. |
| Open system | A system in which there is a continuous flow of input and process, output and feedback. It is a system of organized complexity, where all elements are in interaction. |
| Prevention as intervention | Intervention modes for nursing action and determinants for entry of both client and nurse into the health care system. |
| Reconstitution | The return and maintenance of system stability, following treatment of stressor reaction, which may result in a higher or lower level of wellness. |
| Stability | A state of balance or harmony requiring energy exchanges as the client adequately copes with stressors to retain, attain, or maintain an optimal level of health thus preserving system integrity. |
| Stressors | Environmental factors, intra-, inter-, and extrapersonal in nature, that have potential for disrupting system stability. A stressor is any phenomenon that might penetrate both the flexible and normal lines of defense, resulting in either a positive or negative outcome. |
| Wellness/illness | Wellness is the condition in which all system parts and subparts are in harmony with the whole system of the client. Illness indicates disharmony among the parts and subparts of the client system. |

Source: Neuman (1995).

## TESTABILITY

Although the Neuman model is not testable in its entirety, it gives rise to directional hypotheses that are testable in research. As a result, it has been used as a conceptual framework extensively in nursing research, and aspects of the model have been empirically tested. Intermediate theories using the Neuman System's model have been

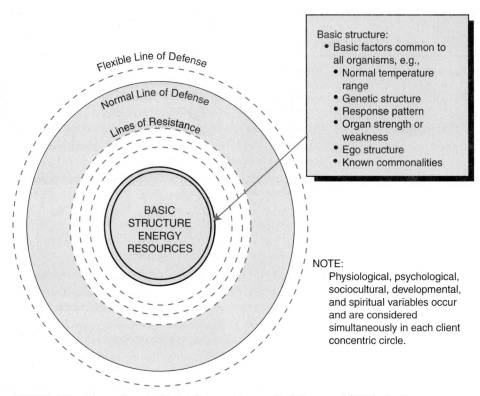

Basic structure:
- Basic factors common to
  all organisms, e.g.,
  - Normal temperature
    range
  - Genetic structure
  - Response pattern
  - Organ strength or
    weakness
  - Ego structure
  - Known commonalities

BASIC
STRUCTURE
ENERGY
RESOURCES

Flexible Line of Defense

Normal Line of Defense

Lines of Resistance

NOTE:
   Physiological, psychological,
   sociocultural, developmental,
   and spiritual variables occur
   and are considered
   simultaneously in each client
   concentric circle.

FIGURE 7-2 The Neuman Systems Model. (Source: Neuman, B., & Fawcett, J. (2002). *The Neuman systems model* (4th ed.). Upper Saddle River, NJ: Pearson Education, Inc.)

developed and are being tested. Box 7-7 lists a few of the many nursing research studies that have used Neuman's Systems Model.

## PARSIMONY

Neuman's model is complex, and many parts of the model function in multiple ways. The description of the model's parts can be confusing; therefore, the model is not considered to be parsimonious. Neuman and Fawcett (2002), however, have developed intermediate diagrams to clarify the interactions among parts of the model and to facilitate its use. The definitions are well developed in the latest edition of the model, and the assumptions (propositions), although multileveled, are well organized.

## VALUE IN EXTENDING NURSING SCIENCE

The Neuman Systems Model has extended nursing science as a needs and causality-focused framework. It appeals to nurses who consider the client to be a holistic individual who reacts to stressors, because it predicts the outcomes of interventions to strengthen the lines of defense against stress, which may destabilize the system. Neuman's model is useful not only in the acute critical care area because of the focus on attaining, regaining, and maintaining system stability (Neuman, 1990), but also in community health situations because of its focus on prevention as intervention (Neuman, 1995; Neuman & Fawcett, 2002).

## BOX 7-6 *Assumptions of Neuman's Systems Model*

1. Each client system is unique, a composite of factors and characteristics within a given range of responses.
2. Many known, unknown, and universal stressors exist. Each differs in its potential for disturbing a client's usual stability level or normal line of defense. The particular interrelationships of client variables at any point in time can affect the degree to which a client is protected by the flexible line of defense against possible reaction to stressors.
3. Each client/client system has evolved a normal range of responses to the environment that is referred to as a normal line of defense. The normal line of defense can be used as a standard from which to measure health deviation.
4. When the flexible line of defense is no longer capable of protecting the client/client system against an environmental stressor, the stressor breaks through the normal line of defense.
5. The client, whether in a state of wellness or illness, is a dynamic composite of the interrelationships of the variables. Wellness is on a continuum of available energy to support the system in an optimal state of system stability.
6. Implicit within each client system are internal resistance factors known as lines of resistance, which function to stabilize and realign the client to the usual wellness state.
7. Primary prevention relates to general knowledge that is applied in client assessment and intervention, in identification and reduction or mitigation of possible or actual risk factors associated with environmental stressors to prevent possible reaction.
8. Secondary prevention relates to symptomatology following a reaction to stressors, appropriate ranking of intervention priorities, and treatment to reduce their noxious effects.
9. Tertiary prevention relates to the adjustive processes taking place as reconstitution begins and maintenance factors move the client back in a circular manner toward primary prevention.
10. The client as a system is in dynamic, constant energy exchange with the environment.

## BOX 7-7 *Examples of Nursing Research Studies Using Neuman's Systems Model*

Cassell, M. (2008). Linking theory, evidence, and practice in assessment of adolescent inhalant use. *Journal of Addictions Nursing, 19*(1), 17–25.

Kubesch, S., Linton, S. M., Hankerson, C., & Wichowski, H. (2008). Holistic intervention protocol for interstitial cystitis symptom control: A case study. *Holistic Nursing Practice, 22*(4), 183–192.

Dunn, K. S. (2007). Predictors of self-reported health among older African-American central city adults. *Holistic Nursing Practice, 21*(5), 237–243.

Bitner, J., Hilde, L., Hall, K., & Duvendack, T. (2007). A team approach to the prevention of unplanned postoperative hypothermia. *Association of peri-Operative Registered Nurses Journal, 85*(5), 921–923.

Gigliotti, E. (2007). Improving external and internal validity of a model of midlife women's maternal–student role stress. *Nursing Science Quarterly, 20*(2), 161–170.

Cooper, S. (2006). The effect of preoperative warming on patients' postoperative temperatures. *Association of periOperative Registered Nurses Journal, 83*(5), 1073–1076.

Ume-Nwagbo, P. N., DeWan, S. A., & Lowry, L.W. (2006). Using the Neuman Systems Model for best practices. *Nursing Science Quarterly, 19*(1), 31–35.

## Summary

The human needs nursing theories discussed in this chapter were among the earliest of the nursing theories. In general, these theories followed the philosophical school of thought of the time by considering the person to be a biopsychosocial being and focusing on meeting the individual's needs.

The opening case study illustrated how one nurse used a human needs-based model to help direct client care through anticipating or predicting client needs and determining desirable outcomes. Many other nurses in a wide variety of settings use these models on an ongoing basis to direct care for many types of clients.

It should be noted that succeeding generations of nursing theorists based their models and theories on the models and theories discussed here. Indeed, they were strong building blocks on which the profession of nursing depended during the last half of the 20th century.

## LEARNING ACTIVITIES

1. Apply one of the above models to the care of a selected client. Write a nursing care plan using the model. Define all elements of the nursing care plan using the language and the assumptions/propositions of the model.

2. Obtain the original work of one of the theorists described. Outline a research study testing components of the model.

   a. Determine what major concepts or propositions of the model can be tested.

   b. Define the elements of the model to be tested in the research project.

   c. Develop a hypothesis statement that examines the model's propositions in a sample from an acute care or community setting.

## INTERNET RESOURCES

A site that has changed venues on several occasions but has been available since about 1998 in some form:

http://www.sandiego.edu/academics/nursing/theory/

Sites devoted to the theorists in this chapter. Nightingale:

http://www.florence-nightingale.co.uk/

http://www.florence-nightingale.co.uk/cms/

http://www.countryjoe.com/nightingale/#contents

http://www.sociology.uoguelph.ca/fnightingale/

http://library.thinkquest.org/20117/nightingale.html

http://www.astr.ua.edu/4000WS/NIGHTINGALE.html

http://clendening.kumc.edu/dc/fn/otherflo.html

Henderson:

http://www.unc.edu/~ehallora/henderson.htm

http://www.stti.org/VirginiaHendersonLibrary/

http://www.sandiego.edu/academics/nursing/theory/henderson.htm

Abdellah:

http://www.nlm.nih.gov/hmd/manuscripts/ead/abdellah.html

http://www.nlm.nih.gov/hmd/manuscripts/ead/abdellah.html

http://www.greatwomen.org/women.php?action=viewone&id=3

http://www.findarticles.com/p/articles/mi_qa3912/is_200411/ai_n9469913

http://www.nurses.info/nursing_theory_person_abdellah_faye.htm

http://www.enursescribe.com/Faye_Abdellah.htm

Johnson:

http://www.nurses.info/nursing_theory_person_johnson_dorothy.htm

http://www.mc.vanderbilt.edu/biolib/hc/biopages/djohnson.html

Orem:

http://www.scdnt.com/download/Vol16_No1_January_2008.pdf

http://www.nurses.info/nursing_theory_person_orem_dorothea.htm

http://www.gfk-pflege.de/Orem.html

Neuman:

http://www.neumann.edu/academics/undergrad/nursing/model.asp/

http://www.neumansystemsmodel.com/news/newspage1.htm#Neuman

Book

http://www.patheyman.com/essays/neuman/

## REFERENCES

Abdellah, F. G., Beland, I. L., Martin, A., & Matheney, R. V. (1960). *Patient-centered approaches to nursing.* New York: MacMillan.

Abdellah, F. G., Beland, I. L., Martin, A., & Matheney, R. V. (1973). *New directions in patient-centered nursing.* New York: MacMillan.

Abdellah, F. G., & Levine, E. (1957). Developing a measure of patient and personnel satisfaction with nursing care. *Nursing Research, 5*(2), 100–108.

Abdellah, F. G., & Levine, E. (1994). *Preparing nursing research for the 21st century.* New York: Springer.

Allen, M. P. (1996). *Tribute to Virginia Avernal Henderson, 1897–1996 from the Interagency Council on Information Resources for Nursing (ICIRN).* Online: http//www.sandiego.edu/nursing/theory/henderson.htm.

Artinian, N. T. (1991). Philosophy of science and family nursing theory development. In A. L. Whall & J. Fawcett (Eds.), *Family theory development in nursing.* Philadelphia: Davis.

Audain, C. (1998). *Florence Nightingale.* Online website: www.scottla.edu/lriddle/women/nitegale.htm.

Audain, C. (2007). *Biographies of women mathematicians: Florence Nightingale.* Agnes Scott College. www.agnesscott.edu/Lriddle/WOMEN/nitegale.htm.

Beck, D. M. (2005). Sick-nursing and health-nursing: Nightingale established our broad scope of practice in 1893. In B. M. Dossey, L. C. Selanders, D. M. Beck, & A. Attewell (Eds.), *Florence Nightingale today: Healing leadership global action.* Silver Spring, MD: American Nurses Association.

Bekel, G. (2007). Dorothea E. Orem—1914– 2007. *Nursing Science Quarterly, 20*(4), 302.

Benson, S. (1997). The older adult and fear of crime. *Journal of Gerontological Nursing, 23*(10), 24–31.

Biggs, A. (2008). "Toast Crumbs"—memories of Dorothea Orem. *Self-Care, Dependant Care & Nursing, 16*(2), 5–6.

Damus, K. (1980). An application of the Johnson behavioral system model for nursing practice. In J. P. Riehl & C. Roy (Eds.), *Conceptual models for nursing practice* (2nd ed., pp. 274–289). New York: Appleton-Century-Crofts.

Dee, V. (1990). Implementation of the Johnson model: One hospital's experience. In M. E. Parker (Ed.), *Nursing theories in practice* (pp. 33–44). New York: National League for Nursing.

Derdiarian, A. K. (1990). The relationships among the subsystems of Johnson's behavioral system model. *Image: Journal of Nursing Scholarship, 22*(4), 219–224.

Derdiarian, A. K., & Schobel, D. (1990). Comprehensive assessment of AIDS patients using the behavioral systems model for nursing practice instrument. *Journal of Advanced Nursing, 15*(4), 436–446.

Dickoff, J., James, P., & Wiedenbach, E. (1968). Theory in a practice discipline. Part 1: Practice-oriented theory. *Nursing Research, 17*(5), 415–435.

Dossey, B. M. (2000). *Florence Nightingale, mystic, visionary, healer.* Springhouse, PA: Springhouse.

Dossey, B. M. (2005a). Florence Nightingale's three tenets: Healing, leadership, global action. In B. M. Dossey, L. C. Selanders, D. M. Beck, & A. Attewell (Eds.), *Florence Nightingale today: Healing leadership global action.* Silver Spring, MD: American Nurses Association.

Dossey, B. M. (2005b). Florence Nightingale's 13 formal letters to her nurses (1872–1900). In B. M. Dossey, L. C. Selanders, D. M. Beck, & A. Attewell (Eds.), *Florence Nightingale today: Healing leadership global action.* Silver Spring, MD: American Nurses Association.

Fruehwirth, S. E. S. (1989). An application of Johnson's behavioral model: A case study. *Journal of Community Health Nursing, 6*(2), 61–71.

Fuller, C. C., & Hartley, B. (2000). Linear scleroderma: A Neuman nursing perspective. *Journal of Pediatric Nursing, 15*(3), 168–174.

Grubbs, J. (1980). The Johnson behavioral system model. In J. P. Riehl & C. Roy (Eds.), *Conceptual models for nursing practice* (2nd ed., pp. 217–254). New York: Appleton-Century-Crofts.

Hassell, J. S. (1996). Improved management of depression through nursing model application and critical thinking. *Journal of the American Academy of Nurse Practitioners, 8*(4), 161–166.

Henderson, V. (1965). The nature of nursing. *International Nursing Review, 12*(1). (Reprinted in E. J. Halloran (Ed.). (1995). *A Virginia Henderson reader: Excellence in nursing* (pp. 213–223). New York: Springer)

Henderson, V. (1991). *The nature of nursing: Reflections after 25 years.* New York: National League for Nursing Press.

Herrmann, E. K. (Ed.). (1998). *Virginia Avenel Henderson: Signature for nursing.* Indianapolis, IN: Sigma Theta Tau International Center Nursing Press.

Holaday, B. (1980). Implementing the Johnson model for nursing practice. In J. P. Riehl & C. Roy (Eds.), *Conceptual models for nursing practice* (2nd ed., pp. 255–263). New York: Appleton-Century-Crofts.

Jacobs, B. B. (2001). Respect for human dignity: A central phenomenon to philosophically unite nursing theory and practice through consilience of knowledge. *Advances in Nursing Science, 24*(1), 17–35.

Johnson, D. E. (1959a). A philosophy of nursing. *Nursing Outlook, 7*(4), 198–200.

Johnson, D. E. (1959b). The nature of nursing science. *Nursing Outlook, 7*(5), 291–294.

Johnson, D. E. (1968). Theory in nursing: Borrowed and unique. *Nursing Research, 17*(3), 206–209.

Johnson, D. E. (1974). Development of a theory: A requisite for nursing as a primary health profession. *Nursing Research, 23*(5), 372–377. (Reprinted in L. H. Nichol (Ed.). (1997). *Perspectives on nursing theory* (3rd ed., pp. 219–225). Philadelphia: Lippincott-Raven)

Johnson, D. E. (1980). The behavioral system model for nursing. In J. P. Riehl & C. Roy (Eds.), *Conceptual models for nursing practice* (pp. 207–216). New York: Appleton-Century-Crofts.

Johnson, D. E. (1990). The behavioral system model for nursing. In M. E. Parker (Ed.), *Nursing theories in practice* (pp. 23–32). New York: National League for Nursing Press.

Johnson, D. E. (1997). Author's comments. In L. H. Nichol (Ed.), *Perspectives on nursing theory* (3rd ed., pp. 225, 405). Philadelphia: Lippincott-Raven.

Murray, P. J. (1999). *Betty Neuman: Biographical details.* Online site: http://www.lemmus.demon.co. uk/neuman1.htm.

Narsavage, G. L. (1997). Promoting function in clients with chronic lung disease by increasing their perception of control. *Holistic Nursing Practice, 12*(1), 17–26.

Neuman, B. M. (1990). The Neuman systems model: A theory for practice. In M. E. Parker (Ed.), *Nursing theories in practice* (pp. 241–261). New York: National League for Nursing Press.

Neuman, B. (1995). *The Neuman systems model* (3rd ed.). Stamford, CT: Appleton & Lange.

Neuman, B., & Fawcett, J. (2002). *The Neuman systems model* (4th ed.). Upper Saddle River, NJ: Prentice-Hall.

Nightingale, F. (1893/1954). Sick-nursing and health-nursing. First printed in A. Burdett-Clouts (Ed.), *Women's mission: A series of congress papers of the philanthropic work of women by eminent writers.* New York: Charles Scribner's Sons (Reprinted in L. R. Seymer (Ed.). (1954). *Selected writings of Florence Nightingale.* New York: MacMillan)

Nightingale, F. (1860/1957/1969). *Notes on nursing: What it is and what it is not.* New York: Dover Publications. (From an original printed in 1860 by D. Appleton)

Nightingale, F. (1999). Online source: http://www.sociology.uoguelph.ca/fnightingale/Introduction/index.htm.

O'Connor, J. J., & Robertson, E. F. (2003). Florence Nightingale. School of Mathematics and Statistics. http://www-history.mcs.st-andrews.ac.uk/Biographies/Nightingale.html.

O'Malley, J. (1996). A nursing legacy: Virginia Henderson. *Advanced Practice Nursing Quarterly, 2*(2), v–vii.

Orem, D. E. (1956). *Hospital nursing service: An analysis.* Indianapolis, IN: Division of Hospital and Institutional Services of the Indiana State Board of Health.

Orem, D. E. (1971). *Nursing: Concepts of practice.* New York: McGraw-Hill.

Orem, D. E. (1985a). *Nursing: Concepts of practice* (3rd ed.). New York: McGraw-Hill.

Orem, D. E. (1985b). A concept of self-care for the rehabilitation client. *Rehabilitation Nurse, 10*, 33–36.

Orem, D. E. (1991). *Nursing: Concepts of practice* (4th ed.). St. Louis: Mosby.

Orem, D. E. (1995). *Nursing: Concepts of practice* (5th ed.). St. Louis: Mosby.

Orem, D. E. (2001). *Nursing: Concepts of practice* (6th ed.). St. Louis: Mosby.

Pfettscher, S. A. (2006). Florence Nightingale: Modern nursing. In A. M. Tomey & M. R. Alligood (Eds.), *Nursing theorists and their work* (6th ed., pp. 71–90). St. Louis: Mosby.

Pope, D. S. (1995). Music, noise, and the human voice in the nurse–patient environment. *Image: Journal of Nursing Scholarship, 27*(4), 291–296.

Poster, E. C., Dee, V., & Randell, B. P. (1997). The Johnson behavioral systems model as a framework for patient outcome evaluation. *Journal of the American Psychiatric Nursing Association, 3*(3), 73–80.

Reed, P. G., & Zurakowski, T. L. (1996). Nightingale: Foundations of nursing. In J. J. Fitzpatrick & A. L. Whall (Eds.), *Conceptual models of nursing: Analysis and application* (3rd ed.). Norwalk, CT: Appleton & Lange.

Selanders, L. C. (1993). *Florence Nightingale: An environmental adaptation theory.* Newbury Park, CA: Sage.

Selanders, L. C. (2005a). Nightingale's foundational philosophy of nursing. In B. M. Dossey, L. C. Selanders, D. M. Beck, & A. Attewell (Eds.), *Florence Nightingale today: Healing leadership global action.* Silver Spring, MD: American Nurses Association.

Selanders, L. C. (2005b). Social change and leadership: Dynamic forces for nursing. In B. M. Dossey, L. C. Selanders, D. M. Beck, & A. Attewell (Eds.), *Florence Nightingale today: Healing leadership global action.* Silver Spring, MD: American Nurses Association.

Small, H. (1998). *Florence Nightingale avenging angel.* New York: St. Martin's Press.

Tailor-Ford, R., Catlin, A., LaPlant, M., & Weinke, C. (2008). Effect of a noise reduction program on a medical-surgical unit. *Clinical Nursing Research, 17*(2), 74–86.

Tanyi, R. A., & Werner, J. S. (2008). Women's experience of spirituality within endstage renal disease and hemodialysis. *Clinical Nursing Research, 17*(1), 32–49.

Taylor, S. G. (2002). Self-care deficit theory of nursing. In A. M. Tomey & M. R. Alligood (Eds.), *Nursing theorists and their work* (pp. 189–211). St Louis: Mosby.

Taylor, S. G. (2006). Self-care deficit theory of nursing. In A. M. Tomey & M. R. Alligood (Eds.), *Nursing theorists and their work* (6th ed., pp. 267–296). St Louis: Mosby.

Taylor, S. G., Geden, E., Isaramalai, S., & Wongvatunyu, S. (2000). Orem's self-care deficit nursing theory: Its philosophic foundation and the state of the science. *Nursing Science Quarterly, 13*(2), 104–110.

Tomey, A. M., & Alligood, M. R. (2002). *Nursing theorists and their work* (5th ed.). St. Louis: Mosby.

Tomey, A. M., & Alligood, M. R. (2006). *Nursing theorists and their work* (6th ed.). St. Louis: Mosby.

Turner-Henson, A. (1992). Chronically ill children's mothers' perceptions of environmental variables. Doctoral dissertation, University of Alabama at Birmingham.

Zurakowski, T. L. (2005). Florence Nightingale: Pioneer in nursing knowledge development. In J. J. Fitzpatrick & A. L. Whall (Eds.), *Conceptual models of nursing: Analysis and application* (4th ed.). Upper Saddle River, NJ: Pearson.

# 8

# Grand Nursing Theories Based on Interactive Process

## Evelyn Wills

*J* ean Willowby is a student in a master's of nursing program. She is working to become
a pediatric nurse practitioner. For one of her practicum assignments, she must
incorporate a nursing theory into her clinical work using the theory as a guide. During
an earlier course on theory, Jean read several nursing theories that focused on interactions
between the client and the nurse and between the client and the health care system. She
remembered that in the interaction models and theories, human beings are viewed as
interacting wholes and client problems are seen as multifactorial.

*The theories that stressed human interactions best fit Jean's personal philosophy of
nursing because they take into account the multitude of factors she believed to be part of
clinical nursing practice. Like the perspective taken by interaction model theorists, Jean
understood that at times the results of interventions are unpredictable and that many
elements in the client's background and environment have an effect on the outcomes of
interventions. She also acknowledged that there are many interactions between clients and
their environments, both internal and external, some of which cannot be measured.*

*To better prepare for the assignment, Jean studied several of the human interaction
models and theories, focusing most of her attention on the works of Roy and King. But after
discussing her thoughts with her professor, she was referred to the Intersystem Model, a
relatively new model by Artinian. After reviewing some of the precepts of the model, she
thought that it seemed to best fit her pediatrics practice and was determined to learn more
about it.*

As discussed in Chapter 6, interactive process nursing theories occupy a place between
the needs-based theories of the 1950s and 1960s, most of which were philosophically
grounded in the positivist school of thought, and the unitary process models, which
are grounded in humanist philosophy, which expresses the belief that humans are unitary beings and energy fields in constant interaction with the universal energy field.

The theorists presented in this chapter believe that humans are holistic beings who interact with and adapt to situations in which they find themselves. These theorists ascribe to systems theory and agree that there is constant interaction between humans and their environments. In general, human interaction theorists believe that health is a value and that a continuum of health ranges from high-level wellness to illness. They acknowledge, however, that people with chronic illnesses may have healthy lives and live well despite their illnesses.

Nursing models that can be described as interactive process theories include: Levine's Conservation Model; Artinian's Intersystem Model; Erickson, Tomlin, and Swain's Modeling and Role-Modeling; King's Systems Framework and Theory of Goal Attainment; Roper, Logan, and Tierney's Model of Nursing Based on Activities of Living; Roy's Adaptation Model; and Watson's Philosophy and Science of Caring. Each is discussed in this chapter. The models treated in this chapter are not arranged historically; some date back to the 1960s, whereas some are relatively new. Levine's model is placed early in the chapter because it is one of the earlier models.

An attempt was made to ensure that a balanced approach was used in presenting the works of these theorists. However, some of the theories (e.g., Erickson, Tomlin, and Swain; and King) are quite complex, whereas others are quite parsimonious (e.g., Levine; Roper, Logan, and Tierney; and Watson). Additionally, some of the models have been revised repeatedly (e.g., King, Roy, and Watson). As a result, the sections dealing with some models are longer or more involved than others, but this does not imply that the works of any of the theorists discussed are more or less important to the discipline than others.

## Myra Estrin Levine: The Conservation Model

The ideal of conservation pervades the background of some nurses' ideas (Mefford, 2004). Myra Levine (1973) stated that "nursing is a human interaction" (p. 237). Her model deals with the interactions of nurse and client. It considers multiple factorial interactions, which may produce predictable effects using probability as the reality.

### BACKGROUND OF THE THEORIST

Myra Levine earned a diploma in nursing from Cook County School of Nursing in Chicago, Illinois, in 1944, a bachelor's degree in science at the University of Chicago in 1949, and a master of science in nursing from Wayne State University in Detroit, Michigan, in 1962. She held numerous clinical and education positions during her long career (Schaefer, 2002). She published *An Introduction to Clinical Nursing* in 1969; this work was revised in 1973 and again in 1989 (Levine, 1989). Levine enjoyed a long and productive career, which included a distinguished publication record. She died in 1996, at age 75, leaving a legacy to nursing of education, administration, and scholarship (Schaefer, 2002).

### PHILOSOPHICAL UNDERPINNINGS OF THE THEORY

Levine (1973) based the Conservation Model on Nightingale's idea that "the nurse created an environment in which healing could occur" (p. 239). She drew from the works of Tillich on the unity principle of life, Bernard on internal environment, Cannon on the theory of homeostasis, and Waddington on the concept of homeorrhesis. The works of other scientists were also used. Four conservation principles form the basis of the model; these were synthesized from her scientific study and practice (Levine, 1990).

## MAJOR ASSUMPTIONS, CONCEPTS, AND RELATIONSHIPS

The following four conservation principles are the major principles around which the model is constructed:

- The principle of the conservation of energy
- The principle of the conservation of structural integrity
- The principle of the conservation of personal integrity
- The principle of the conservation of social integrity (Levine, 1973, p. 244; 1990, p. 331).

According to Levine's model, nursing interventions are based on conservation of the client's integrity in each of the conservation domains. The nurse is seen as a part of the environment and shares the repertoire of skill, knowledge, and compassion, assisting each client to confront environmental challenges in resolving the problems encountered in the client's own unique way. The effectiveness of the interventions is measured by the maintenance of client integrity (Levine, 1973, 1990).

### Assumptions About Individuals

Each individual "is an active participant in interactions with the environment constantly seeking information from it" (Levine, 1969, p. 6).

The individual "is a sentient being and the ability to interact with the environment seems ineluctably tied to his sensory organs" (Levine, 1973, p. 450).

"Change is the essence of life and it is unceasing as long as life goes on. Change is characteristic of life" (Levine, 1973, p. 10).

### Assumptions About Nursing

"Ultimately the decisions for nursing intervention must be based on the unique behavior of the individual patient" (Levine, 1973, p. 6).

"Patient centered nursing care means individualized nursing care. It is predicated on the reality of common experience: every man is a unique individual, and as such he requires a unique constellation of skills, techniques and ideas designed specifically for him" (p. 23).

### Concepts

Many concepts are used in the model. Major concepts are listed in Table 8-1.

### Relationships

Relationships are not specifically stated but can be extracted from the descriptions given by Levine (1973). The relationships serve as the basis for nursing interventions and include:

1. Conservation of energy is based on nursing interventions to conserve energy through a deliberate decision as to the balance between activity and the person's available energy.
2. Conservation of structural integrity is the basis for nursing interventions to limit the amount of tissue involvement.
3. Conservation of personal integrity is based on nursing interventions that permit the individual to make decisions for himself or participate in the decisions.

TABLE 8-1 *Major Concepts of the Conservation Model*

| Concept | Definition |
|---|---|
| Environment | Includes both the internal and external environment. |
| Person | The unique individual in unity and integrity, feeling, believing, thinking, and whole. |
| Health | Patterns of adaptive change of the whole being. |
| Nursing | The human interaction relying on communication, rooted in the organic dependency of the individual human being in his [sic] relationships with other human beings. |
| Adaptation | The process of change and integration of the organism in which the individual retains integrity or wholeness. It is possible to have degrees of adaptation. |
| Conceptual environment | The part of the person's environment that includes ideas, symbolic exchange, belief, tradition, and judgment. |
| Conservation | Includes joining together and is the product of adaptation including nursing intervention and patient participation to maintain a safe balance. |
| Energy conservation | Nursing interventions based on the conservation of the patient's energy. |
| Holism | The singular, yet integrated response of the individual to forces in the environment. |
| Homeostasis | Stable state normal alterations in physiologic parameters in response to environmental changes; an energy-sparing state, a state of conservation. |
| Modes of communication | The many ways in which information, needs, and feelings are transmitted among the patient, family, nurses, and other health care workers. |
| Personal integrity | A person's sense of identity and self-definition. Nursing intervention is based on the conservation of the individual's personal integrity. |
| Social integrity | Life's meaning gained through interactions with others. Nurses intervene to maintain relationships. |
| Structural integrity | Healing is a process of restoring structural integrity through nursing interventions that promote healing and maintain structural integrity. |
| Therapeutic interventions | Interventions that influence adaptation in a favorable way, enhancing the adaptive responses available to the person. |

Source: Adapted from Levine (1973).

4. Conservation of social integrity is based on nursing interventions to preserve the client's interactions with family and the social system to which they belong.
5. All nursing interventions are based on careful and continued observation over time (abstracted from Levine, 1973).

## USEFULNESS

Levine's (1973) model has been useful in nursing education. For example, it was used to develop a nursing undergraduate program at Allentown College of Saint Francis de Sales in Center Valley, Pennsylvania, where it was deemed to be compatible with the mission and philosophy of the college (Grindley & Paradowski, 1991). It was also used in the graduate program at the same school as the framework for development of the content of the graduate nursing courses (Schaefer, 1991a).

The emergency department at the Hospital of the University of Pennsylvania used the four conservation principles of Levine's model as an organizing framework for nursing practice (Pond & Taney, 1991). It was believed that use of the model strengthened communication and improved nursing care in the hospital through an atmosphere of collaboration among disciplines. The conservation principles were also found to be useful in directing nursing practice in the care of children (Dever, 1991). The concept of adaptation and the four conservation principles were particularly relevant, and conservation of personal and social integrity was especially important to the healing of the ill child. A concept analysis was published using Levine's conservation model to refine the concept of creativity for nursing practice (Fasnacht, 2003). Mefford (2004) based her theory of health promotion for preterm infants on Levine's conservation model.

Neswick (1997) suggested Levine's model as the theoretic basis for enterostomal therapy (ET) nursing. She integrated the four conservation principles into wound and ostomy care. The principles that she found useful are energy, structure, personal integrity, and social integrity. She found Levine's framework useful because of its holistic approach (Neswick, 1997).

## TESTABILITY

Levine's (1990) Conservation Model has guided research studies *internationally*. Piccoli and Galvao (2005) investigated methods of assessing and preparing perioperative *nursing patients*, focusing on Levine's four conservation principles. Leach (2006) studied wound management in Australia using Levine's four principles and found that the model contributed to health and wholeness of the client, and assisted in cost-effective care. Mock et al. (2007) stated that the model "provided a useful framework" (p. 509) for their investigation of nursing interventions to manage fatigue in cancer patients. The Canadian Association of Critical Care Nursing, which published the abstract of Vandall-Walker, Jensen, and Oberle (2006), cited Levine in their investigation of nursing support of family members of critically ill adults.

Conserving the cognitive integrity of hospitalized elderly was the focus of a research study by Foreman (1991). In that study, 71 participants were administered several cognitive measures by an interview process. The researchers stated that the four conservation principles were supported in their study. The model has been the guide for qualitative studies to understand clients in their whole state. Schaefer (1991b) reported a case study of a patient with congestive heart failure and found the model "pragmatic and parsimonious in studying the subject" (p. 130). Schaefer and Potylycki (1993) used Levine's model to study fatigue in patients with congestive heart failure with a focus on client adaptation.

## PARSIMONY

The model is fairly parsimonious; however, there are a great many concepts with comparatively unspecified relationships and unstated assumptions. Four conservation principles comprise the model; these principles are succinctly stated. According to Levine (1991), redundancy of the domains allows multiple means of configuring interventions. When domain redundancy is lost by the seriousness of disease, the options for intervention are limited. Practitioners and researchers using the model have considerable latitude to configure ways in which the model will be used or studied and to derive the theoretical structures that proceed from the model.

## VALUE IN EXTENDING NURSING SCIENCE

Levine's (1973) Conservation Model has impacted the discipline of nursing in education, practice, and research, providing four defining principles that are sufficiently universal to allow research and practice in a large number of situations. The concept of holism, although not unique to this model, was proposed at an early stage in nursing's scientific history and has made an important difference in the care of clients.

## Barbara M. Artinian: The Intersystem Model

The Intersystem Model was first published in 1983 as the Intersystem Patient-Care Model (Artinian, 1983), and was later expanded to the Intersystem Model (Artinian, 1991). It is currently in its third iteration and following refinement and revision, it became the basis for the curriculum at Azusa Pacific University in Azusa, California (Wood, 1997).

### BACKGROUND OF THE THEORIST

Barbara Artinian received her bachelor's degree from Wheaton (IL) College; master's degrees from Case Western Reserve University in Cleveland, Ohio, and the University of California, Los Angeles (UCLA); and her doctorate from the University of Southern California. Influenced by her education as a sociologist, Artinian developed a nursing model that used an intersystems approach and focused on the interactions between client and nurse. She is currently professor emeritus of the School of Nursing at Azusa Pacific University having taught graduate and undergraduate students in the areas of community health nursing, family theory, nursing theory, and qualitative research methods.

### PHILOSOPHIC UNDERPINNINGS OF THE THEORY

The Intersystem Model supplanted Chrisman and Riehl's (1974, 1989) systems model at the School of Nursing at Azusa Pacific University. Several works were used in developing the components of the model. For example, *sense of coherence* (SOC), a social science construct proposed by Antonofsky, provided grounding for the concept *situational sense of coherence* (SSOC). The SSOC serves as a measure of the integrative potential of clients within the context of situations (Artinian, 1997a) (see Table 8-2 and Figure 8-1).

TABLE 8-2 *Relationship Between SOC and SSOC in Artinian's Model*

| Term | Definition |
| --- | --- |
| *SOC (sense of coherence)* | The progenitor to the SSOC. |
| *SSOC (situational sense of coherence)* | The analytic structure for evaluating the effectiveness of interventions in the plan of care, and the current level of health. |
| Comprehensibility | The extent to which one perceives the stimuli present in the situational environment deriving from the internal and external environments as making cognitive sense, in that information is ordered, consistent, structured, and clear, versus disordered random or inexplicable. |
| Meaningfulness | The extent to which one feels that the problem demands posed by the situation are worth investing energy in, and are challenges for which meaning or purpose is sought rather than burdens. |
| Manageability | The extent to which one perceives that resources at one's disposal are adequate to meet the demands posed by stimuli present in the situation. |

Source: Antonofski (1987) as cited in Artinian (1991, p. 199); Erdmann (2003, p. 336).

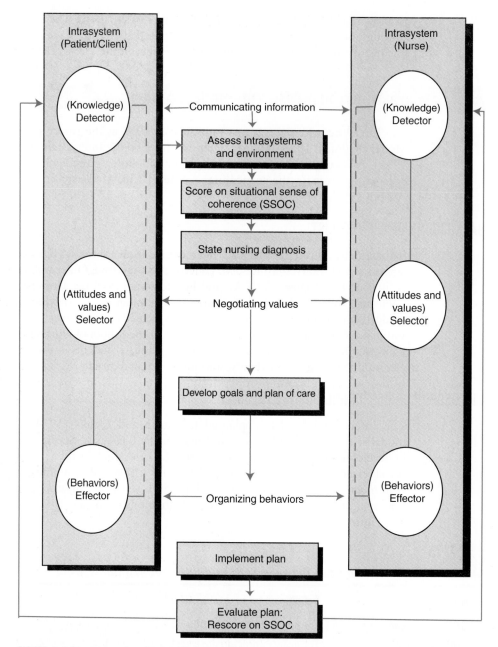

FIGURE 8-1 The Intersystem Model. (Source: Artinian, B. M. (1991). *Journal of Advanced Nursing*, p. 201 [Reprinted with permission].)

Additionally, the model of intrasystem analysis and intersystem interaction developed by Alfred Kuhn was refined by Artinian to explain client–nurse interaction processes in health care situations and for use in developing the nursing plan of care. Finally, the work of Maturana and Varela provided the conceptualization of the person as a perceiving, self-determining, self-regulating human system and explains the patient/client concept of the model (Artinian, 1997a).

## MAJOR ASSUMPTIONS, CONCEPTS, AND RELATIONSHIPS

In the Intersystem Model, there is a differentiation between the human as a system (the intrasystem) and the interactive systems of individuals or groups, known as the intersystem. The language of the Intersystem Model is scholarly English, and non-sexist language is used throughout.

### Assumptions

A number of major assumptions of the model (Artinian, 1997a) are listed in Box 8-1.

### Concepts

The Intersystem Model incorporates nursing's metaparadigm concepts of person, environment, and health, and specifies the concept nursing action. Definitions for these concepts are presented in Table 8-3. Person is viewed as a "coherent being who continually strives to make sense of his or her world" (Artinian, 1991, p. 3). The person as an individual has biological, psychosocial, and spiritual subsystems (Artinian, 1997a). Person may also be an aggregate meaning a group of people, such as a family, community, or other aggregates. Environment includes internal and external environments and specifies developmental environment and situational environment as important to the interaction.

Health is viewed on a multidimensional continuum involving health/disease. The focus is on stability and adaptation, and Artinian developed the concept of SSOC, to measure adaptation. Health is considered to be "a dynamic state of functioning within the limitations of the person" (Artinian, 1991, p. 10), and includes the element of effective adaptation that occurs through strengthening the SSOC. As a result, the model defines health as "a strong SSOC."

Nursing is specified as "nursing action," which is identified by the mutual communication, negotiation, organization, and priorities of both the client and nurse intrasystems. This is accomplished through intersystem interaction; feedback loops are necessary to produce a mutually determined plan of care (Artinian, 1991). One major innovation of this model is that client spirituality and values are important in the assessment of client needs and within the resulting nursing process.

---

**BOX 8-1** *Assumptions of Artinian's Intersystem Model*

1. The human being exists within a framework of development and change, which is inherent to life
2. The human's life is a unit of interrelated systems that is viewed as past and potential future
3. Persons interact with the environment on the biological level, and the senses are the mode of input from the environment; bodily functions are the mode for output
4. The person's present can be seen in terms of his past and future
5. The human spirit is at the center of the person's being, transcending time and affecting all aspects of life
6. The nurse focuses on all aspects of the total person, systematically noting the interrelations of the systems and the relationships of the systems to time and environment
7. The nursing process can take place only in the present

Source: Artinian (1997a).

TABLE 8-3 *Concepts of the Intersystem Model*

| Concept | Definition |
| --- | --- |
| Person | A coherent being who continually strives to make sense of his or her world. The person is a system, the subsystems of which are biological, psychosocial, and spiritual. Subsystem configuration is such that "transactions among the subsystems result in emergent properties at the systemic level" (Artinian, 1997a, p. 3). |
| Environment | The environment has two dimensions, developmental and situational. The developmental environment is "all the events, factors, and influences that affect the system as it passes through its developmental stages" (p. 8). This developmental environment provides the context for other developmental arenas such as the healing environment. Situational environment occurs when the nurse and client interact, and this includes all the details of the encounter. |
| Health | Health is considered to be a multidimensional continuum. The client's situational sense of coherence (SSOC) is a reflection of the client's adaptation to crisis and is the factor that the nurse assesses, and to which the nurse ministers, in assisting the client to adapt. In the Intersystem Model health is defined as having a strong SSOC, illness has a low SSOC, and adaptation moves the SSOC toward a higher level. |
| Nursing | Those actions (interventions) that are needed when the client enters the hospital environment. It is the goal of both the nurse and client to move the client to a higher SSOC. The nurse assesses the client's knowledge (comprehensibility of the problem), the available resources needed to manage the problem (manageability), and the client's motivation to meet the challenges posed by the problem (meaningfulness). |

Source: Artinian (1997a).

### Relationships

The Intersystem Model consists of two levels: the *intrasystem* and the *intersystem*. The intrasystem applies both to the client and to the nurse, and focuses on the individual. The intersystem, by contrast, focuses on the interactions between the nurse and client.

In the intrasystem model, three basic components comprise each intrasystem: the detector, selector, and effector. The detector processes information, the selector compares the situation with the attitudes and values of the individual, and the effector identifies behaviors relevant to the situation (Artinian, 1991, 1997a).

The first step in an interaction in the intrasystem is to evaluate the detector domain, each person's knowledge of the problem. The detector incorporates knowledge about the internal environment (physical symptoms), social situations, the condition, treatment, and available resources. The selector allows the client and nurse to examine their attitudes and values in choosing a course of action that fits both patient/client and nurse. The effector is the behavioral level in which a response is selected from the repertoire of the behaviors available. This intrasystem level of the model provides the nurse with the capability of progressively clarifying with the client to bring about a mutual plan of care (Artinian, 1997a).

The intersystem (Artinian, 1991, 1997a) is seen when client and nurse interact, which occurs when nursing assistance is required. Communication and negotiation between nurse and client lead to development of a plan of care. If the planned intervention is not effective, the determination is made that further assessment is necessary.

SOC and SSOC are the concepts that relate to health. In the intervention phase of the process, "input is the nurse–client interaction to change the SSOC if it is judged to be low" (Artinian, 1997a, p. 13). Outcomes are scored on the SSOC by changes in knowledge, values and beliefs, and behaviors.

## USEFULNESS

The Intersystem Model is relatively new; examples in nursing literature describing its use in practice and education are available. Online searches indicate that Artinian's qualitative research method is being used in Europe and the United States. A recent investigation by Giske and Artinian (2008) used classical grounded theory and studied adults aged 80 and older in a Norwegian hospital who were undergoing gastro-enterologic studies. Findings indicate that participants were concerned with preparing themselves for life after their diagnosis, a difficult period for the participants.

Research on educational issues includes that by Cason et al. (2008), who studied perceived barriers and supports for nursing students as seen by successful Hispanic health care professionals. They found that multiple barriers deter Hispanic students from success. Bond et al. (2008), followed up with a study of Hispanic students in baccalaureate nursing programs, and found multiple barriers and supports. Critchley and Ball (2007) studied rheumatology patients using Artinian's (1998) descriptive qualitative method. Dover and Pfieffer (2006) studied spiritual care of Christian clients of parish nurses. They developed a theory of spirituality for work in parish nursing. Vukovitch and Artinian (2005) investigated mental health nurses who administered medications to psychiatric patients and their methods of avoiding coercion.

## TESTABILITY

The Intersystem Model has not been fully tested. Research studies applying the model primarily involve using grounded theory methodology to examine the meanings of events and the person's reactions to those events in the effort to formulate theories and hypotheses (Artinian, personal communication, May 30, 2003).

The SSOC instrument has been used in research as a self-report instrument (Artinian, 1997b). Major themes that emerged from a study of patients with chronic obstructive pulmonary disease (COPD) by Milligan-Hecox (Artinian, 1997c) were "pacing, depending on others, clarifying values, maintaining independence, maintaining the struggle and accepting ambiguity" (p. 259). Other research efforts using the model included caring for cancer patients, COPD patients, and patients experiencing difficulties in managing illness situations (Artinian, 1997d).

## PARSIMONY

The model developed by Artinian (1997a) is parsimonious and is explained in a logical and coherent way using two simple diagrams. It is not simplistic, however, and has multiple interacting elements.

## VALUE IN EXTENDING NURSING SCIENCE

The Intersystem Model has value in guiding education and in implementing practice. Its innovation is attention to the spirituality, goals, and values of both the client and nurse. Nurses use it in diverse clinical settings, such as psychiatric, acute care, and community nursing. Several chapters, a book by the author, and numerous journal articles have been generated by this model (Artinian, 1998; Giske & Artinian, 2008; Treolar & Artinian, 2001; Vukovitch & Artinian, 2005).

## Helen C. Erickson, Evelyn M. Tomlin, and Mary Ann P. Swain: Modeling and Role-Modeling

Modeling and role-modeling (MRM) is considered by its authors to be a theory and a paradigm. They constructed the theory from a multiplicity of resources that explain nurses' interactions with clients.

## BACKGROUND OF THE THEORISTS

Helen Erickson earned a diploma in nursing from Saginaw General Hospital in Saginaw, Michigan. She earned a bachelor's degree in nursing, master's degree in psychiatric nursing, and a doctorate in educational psychology from the University of Michigan. Her career spans positions in nursing practice and education, both in the United States and abroad. She chaired the adult health nursing curriculum in the graduate program at the University of Texas at Austin, and was a Special Assistant to the Dean for Graduate Studies. She is professor emeritus of the University of Texas at Austin (Erickson Biosketch 2008), chairs the board of directors of the American Holistic Nurses' Certification Corporation, and is active in the Society for the Advancement of Modeling and Role-Modeling (SAMRM) (Erickson, 2008). *Modeling and Role-Modeling: A Theory and Paradigm for Nursing* has been the life work of Dr. Erickson and is now in its third printing (Erickson, 2008).

Evelyn M. Tomlin was educated at Pasadena City College in southern California and Los Angeles General Hospital School of Nursing. She received her bachelor's degree in nursing from the University of Southern California and her master's degree from the University of Michigan. She has had varied experiences in practice and education including medical-surgical nursing, maternity, and pediatric nursing. Tomlin was a member of the faculty at the University of Michigan. In semiretirement from active nursing, she counsels homeless mothers in a religious-based environment (Erickson, 2006).

Mary Ann P. Swain was educated in psychology at DePauw University in Greencastle, Indiana, and earned master's and doctoral degrees from the University of Michigan. She taught research methods in psychology at DePauw University and at the University of Michigan. She also served as the director of the doctoral program in nursing at the University of Michigan for a year and assumed the role of chairperson of nursing research from 1977 to 1982. Later she was professor of nursing research at the University of Michigan, and, in 1983, was appointed the Associate Vice President for Academic Affairs at the same university. Swain currently resides in New York State and is a provost for the New York State University system (Erickson, 2006).

## PHILOSOPHICAL UNDERPINNINGS OF THE THEORY

A number of theoretical works served as the foundation for MRM. Indeed, MRM is a synthesis of the foundational works of Maslow, Milton Erickson, Piaget, Bowlby, Winnicott, Engel, Lindemann, Selye, Lazarus, and Seligman (Erickson, 2006).

Philosophically, Erickson, Tomlin, and Swain (1983) believe "that nursing is a process between the nurse and client and requires an interpersonal and interactive nurse-client relationship" (p. 43). For this reason, their work is considered to be human interaction theory.

## MAJOR ASSUMPTIONS, CONCEPTS, AND RELATIONSHIPS

### Assumptions

Assumptions about adaptation and nursing are proposed in the MRM theory; the authors state that adaptation "is an innate drive toward holistic health, growth, and development. Self-healing, recovery and renewal, and adaptation are all instinctual despite the aging process or inherent malformations" (Erickson et al., 1983, p. 47).

When describing nursing, it is assumed that (1) "nursing is the nurturance of holistic self-care"; (2) "nursing is assisting persons holistically to use their adaptive strengths to attain and maintain optimum biopsychosocial-spiritual functioning"; (3) "nursing is helping with self-care to gain optimum health"; and (4) "nursing is an integrated and integrative helping of persons to better care for themselves" (Erickson et al., 1983, p. 50).

### Concepts

The MRM theory contains a detailed set of concepts, and a glossary is provided in their work that assists in its comprehension. Table 8-4 provides definitions for some of the major concepts.

### Relationships

The active potential assessment model (APAM) directs nursing assessment in the MRM theory. The APAM is a synthesis of Selye's general adaptation syndrome and

TABLE 8-4 *Major Concepts of the Modeling and Role-Modeling Theory*

| Concept | Definition |
|---|---|
| Holism | The idea that "human beings have multiple interacting subsystems including genetic make up and spiritual drive, body, mind, emotion, and spirit are a total unit and act together, affecting and controlling one another interactively" (Erickson et al., 1983, p. 44). |
| Health | "The state of physical, mental, and social well-being, not merely the absence of disease or infirmity" (p. 46). |
| Lifetime growth and development | Lifetime growth and development are continuous processes. When needs are met, growth and development promote health. |
| Affiliated-individuation | The dependence on support systems while maintaining the independence of the individual. |
| Adaptation | The individual's response to external and internal stressors in a health-and growth-directed manner. The opposite is maladaptation, which is the taxing of the system when the individual is "unable to engage constructive coping methods or mobilize appropriate resources to contend with the stressor(s)" (p. 47). |
| Self-care | Knowledge, resources, and action of the client, knowledge considers what has made the client sick, what will make him or her well, and "the mobilization of internal resources, and acquisition of additional resources to gain, maintain, or promote an optimal level of holistic health" (p. 48). |
| Nursing | "The holistic helping of persons with their self-care activities in relation to their health—an interactive, interpersonal process that nurtures strengths to achieve a state of perceived holistic health" (p. 49). |
| Modeling | The process by which the nurse seeks to understand the client's unique model of the world. |
| Role-modeling | The process by which the nurse understands the client's unique model within the context of scientific theories and uses the model to plan interventions that promote health for the client. |

Source: Erickson et al. (1983).

Engles' response to stressors (Erickson et al., 1983). The APAM assists the nurse in predicting a client's potential to cope and is used to assess three states: equilibrium, arousal, and impoverishment. Equilibrium has two facets: adaptive and maladaptive. People in equilibrium have potential for mobilizing resources; those in maladaptive equilibrium have fewer resources.

Both arousal and impoverishment are considered to be states of stress in which mobilizing resources are expected. Persons in impoverishment have diminished or depleted abilities for mobilizing resources. People move between the states as their capacities to meet stress change. The APAM is considered dynamic rather than unidirectional and depends on the person's abilities to mobilize resources. Nursing interventions influence the person's ability to mobilize resources and move from impoverishment to equilibrium within the APAM (Erickson et al., 1983).

From the data collected, a client model is developed, with a description of the functional relationship among the factors. Etiologic factors are analyzed, and possible therapeutic interventions are devised recognizing possible conflicts with treatment plans of other health professionals. Diagnoses and goals are established to complete the planning process (Erickson et al., 1983).

The success of the process is predicated on nurse's coming to know client. The five aims of nursing interventions are building trust, promoting the client's positive orientation, promoting the client's control, affirming and promoting the client's strength, and setting health-directed mutual goals while meeting the client's needs (e.g., biophysical, safety and security, love and belonging, esteem and self-esteem) (Erickson et al., 1983; Erickson, 2006).

## USEFULNESS

Currently the model is the basis for a series of conferences incorporating MRM into research, practice settings, and curricula. Adherents of the theory state that it is used in courses or in the curricula of several universities. These include Humboldt State University School of Nursing in Arcata, California; Metropolitan State University in St. Paul, Minnesota; and the University of Texas at Austin, Alternate Entry Program where graduate nursing students use MRM as a unifying model (MRM website, 2008); St. Catherine's University, Associate Degree Program Minneapolis, MN; Washetnaw Community College AD-N Program, Ypsilanti MI; Portland Health Science Center, Portland, OR; Harding University, Search, AR; and East Carolina University, Greensboro, NC (retrieved December 30, 2008 from http://www.mrmnursingtheory.org).

Several institutions use the model for practice. The University of Texas Medical Branch at Galveston uses the model to structure the academic/service model. The University of Michigan Medical Center, Brigham and Women's Hospital in Boston, and the University of Pittsburgh (PA) hospitals all used the MRM as a theoretical basis for practice (Erickson et al., 1998). Several examples demonstrate how MRM has been applied in nursing practice. One in particular, Baldwin (2004), used the model to describe effective nursing interventions to promote independence for clients with interstitial cystitis.

## TESTABILITY

Modeling and role-modeling provides assumptions and relationships that are amenable to testing and have been and continue to be tested in research. The model has been used by nurses who have studied with Erickson, Tomlin, and Swain, and many theses and dissertations have incorporated elements of the model. Box 8-2 lists some of the current works using MRM in research.

| BOX 8-2 | *Examples of Research Studies Using Modeling and Role-Modeling Theory* |
|---|---|

Beery, T., Baas, L. S., & Henthorn, C. (2007). Self reported adjustment to implanted cardiac devices. *Journal of Cardiovascular Nursing, 22*(6), 516–524.

Beery, T., Baas, L. S., Mathews, H., Burrough, J., & Henthorn, R. (2005). Development of the implanted devices adjustment scale. *Dimensions of Critical Care Nursing, 24*(50), 242–248.

Nash, K. (2007). Evaluation of the empower peer support and education program for middle school-aged adolescents. *Journal of Holistic Nursing, 25*(1), 26–36.

Mitchel, J. B. (2007). Enhancing patient connectedness: Understanding the nurse–patient relationship. International *Journal for Human Caring, 11*(4), 79–82.

## PARSIMONY

The MRM theory is not parsimonious. Its complexity, however, reflects human beings, to whom it applies. MRM incorporates several borrowed theories that are synthesized for use in nursing science. The many linkages among the concepts and multiple levels need to be addressed, and considerable explanation is needed to enhance understanding of the tenets of the theory for nursing practice and for client care activities.

## VALUE IN EXTENDING NURSING SCIENCE

In addition to the uses of MRM in nursing education, practice, and research, three middle range nursing theories have been based on MRM. Acton (1997) developed a model describing affiliated-individuation, Irvin and Acton (1996) described caregiver stress, and Rogers (1996) discussed the concept of facilitative affiliation.

MRM theory is used in education, practice, and research. The Society for Promoting MRM Theory has been formed to promote understanding and use of the theory. This group meets annually and maintains a website at http://www.mrmnursingtheory.org. Research has been completed with people of all ages and with those who are suffering from many different health problems. According to those who espouse the theory, its major attraction is that it is practical, reflects the domain of nursing, and is a realistic model for guiding research, practice, and education.

## Imogene M. King: King's Conceptual System and Theory of Goal Attainment and Transactional Process

King's theory evolved from early writings about theory development. In her first book in 1971, she synthesized scholarship from nursing and related disciplines into a theory for nursing (King, 1971). She wrote the Theory of Goal Attainment in 1980. The most recent edition (King, 1995a) contains further refinements and more detailed explanation of the general nursing framework and the theory.

### BACKGROUND OF THE THEORIST

Imogene King graduated from St. John's Hospital School of Nursing in St. Louis, Missouri, with a diploma in nursing in 1945. She received a bachelor of science in nursing education from St. Louis University in 1948, and a master of science in nursing from the same school in 1957. In 1961, she received the doctor of education degree from Teacher's College, Columbia University, in New York (Sieloff, 2006). She held a variety of staff nursing, educational, research, and administrative roles throughout her professional life. She worked as a research consultant for the Division of Nursing in the Department of Health, Education, and Welfare from 1964 to 1966 (King, personal communication, October, 2005). King moved to Tampa, Florida in 1980, assuming the position of professor at the University of South Florida College of Nursing (Sieloff, 2006). She remained active in professional organizations for many years. She died in 2008 and has been celebrated by a plethora of her colleagues (Mensik, 2008; Mitchell, 2008; Smith, Wright, & Fawcet, 2008; Stevens & Messmer, 2008).

## PHILOSOPHICAL UNDERPINNINGS OF THE THEORY

The von Bertalanffy General Systems Model is acknowledged to be the basis for King's work. She stated that the science of wholeness elucidated in that model gave her hope that the complexity of nursing could be studied "as an organized whole" (King, 1995b, p. 23).

## MAJOR ASSUMPTIONS, CONCEPTS, AND RELATIONSHIPS

King's conceptual system and theory contain many concepts and multiple assumptions and relationships. A few of the assumptions, concepts, and relationships are presented in the following sections. The scholar wishing to use King's model or theory is referred to the original writings as both the model and theory are complex (Figure 8-2).

### Assumptions

The Theory of Goal Attainment lists several assumptions relating to individuals, nurse–client interactions, and nursing. When describing individuals, the model shows that (1) individuals are social, sentient, rational, reacting beings and (2) are controlling, purposeful, action oriented, and time oriented in their behavior (King, 1995b).

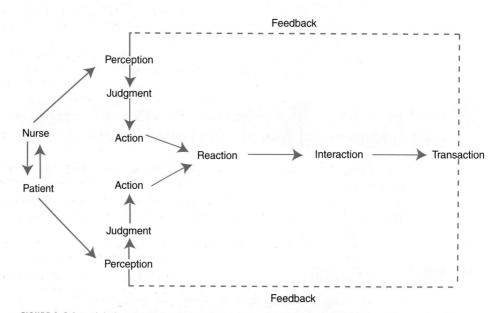

FIGURE 8-2 A model of nurse–patient interactions. (Source: King, I. M. (1981). *A theory for nursing: Systems, concepts, process*, p. 61 [Reprinted with permission of Sage Publications, Inc.].)

Regarding nurse–client interactions, King (1981) believed that (1) perceptions of the nurse and client influence the interaction process; (2) goals, needs, and values of the nurse and client influence the interaction process; (3) individuals have a right to knowledge about themselves; (4) individuals have a right to participate in decisions that influence their lives, health, and community services; (5) individuals have a right to accept or reject care; and (6) goals of health professionals and goals of recipients of health care may not be congruent.

With regard to nursing, King (1981, 1995b) wrote that (1) nursing is the care of human beings; (2) nursing is perceiving, thinking, relating, judging, and acting *vis-a-vis* the behavior of individuals who come to a health care system; (3) a nursing situation is the immediate environment in which two individuals establish a relationship to cope with situational events; and (4) the goal of nursing is to help individuals and groups attain, maintain, and restore health. If this is not possible, nurses help individuals die with dignity.

### Concepts

King's Theory of Goal Attainment defines the metaparadigm concepts of nursing as well as a number of additional concepts. Table 8-5 lists some of the major concepts.

### Relationships

The Theory of Goal Attainment encompasses a great many relationships, many of them complex. King organized them into useful propositions that enhance the understanding

TABLE 8-5 *Major Concepts of the Theory of Goal Attainment*

| Concept | Definition |
| --- | --- |
| Nursing | A process of action, reaction, and interaction whereby nurse and client share information about their perceptions in the nursing situation. The nurse and client share specific goals, problems, and concerns and explore means to achieve a goal. |
| Health | A dynamic life experience of a human being, which implies continuous adjustment to stressors in the internal and external environment through optimum use of one's resources to achieve maximum potential for daily living. |
| Individuals | Social beings who are rational and sentient. Humans communicate their thoughts, actions, customs, and beliefs through language. Persons exhibit common characteristics such as the ability to perceive, to think, to feel, to choose between alternative courses of action, to set goals, to select the means to achieve goals, and to make decisions. |
| Environment | The background for human interactions. It is both external to, and internal to, the individual. |
| Perception | The process of human transactions with environment. It involves organizing, interpreting, and transforming information from sensory data and memory. |
| Communication | A process by which information is given from one person to another either directly in face-to-face meetings or indirectly. It involves intrapersonal and interpersonal exchanges. |
| Interaction | A process of perception and communication between person and environment and between person and person represented by verbal and nonverbal behaviors that are goal-directed. |
| Transaction | A process of interactions in which human beings communicate with the environment to achieve goals that are valued; transactions are goal-directed human behaviors. |
| Stress | A dynamic state in which a human interacts with the environment to maintain balance for growth, development, and performance; it is the exchange of information between human and environment for regulation and control of stressors. |

Source: King (1981).

of the relationships of the theory. A review of some relationships among the theory's concepts follows:

- Nurse and client are purposeful interacting systems.
- Nurse and client perceptions, judgments, and actions, if congruent, lead to goal directed transactions.
- If perceptual accuracy is present in nurse–client interactions, transactions will occur.
- If nurse and client make transactions, goals will be attained.
- If goals are attained, satisfaction will occur.
- If goals are attained, effective nursing care will occur.
- If transactions are made in nurse–client interactions, growth and development will be enhanced.
- If role expectations and role performance as perceived by nurse and client are congruent, transactions will occur.
- If role conflict is experienced by nurse or client or both, stress in nurse–client interactions will occur.
- If nurses with special knowledge and skills communicate appropriate information to clients, mutual goal setting and goal attainment will occur (King, 1981, pp. 61, 149).

## USEFULNESS

King's Theory of Goal Attainment has enhanced nursing education. For example, it served as a framework for the baccalaureate program at the Ohio State University School of Nursing, where it determined the content and processes taught at each level of the program (Daubenmire, 1989). Similarly, in Sweden, King's model was used to organize nursing education (Frey, Rooke, Sieloff, Messmer, & Kameoka, 1995). In more recent years King's model has been useful in nursing education programs in Sweden, Portugal, Canada, and Japan (Sieloff, 2002, 2006).

King's conceptual system is an organizing guide for nursing practice. Palmer (2006) found King's model important to educating older adult clients in a plastic surgery practice, noting that anxiety and disruption may affect their ability to recall information. Similarly, Page (2008) found the theory of goal attainment assisted clients with sarcoidosis to cope and to remain strong in the face of this debilitating immune system disease.

Hughes, Lloyd, and Clarke (2008) found King's model "a radical approach to process of nursing . . . in the United Kingdom" (p. 48). They found King's transaction process especially suited to nursing information systems.

## TESTABILITY

Parts of the Theory of Goal Attainment have been tested, and a number of research studies reported in the literature used the model as a conceptual framework. For example, recent research by Falcao, Guedes, and da Silva (2006), who employed the theory of goal attainment, studied arterial hypertension and adherence to prescribed therapy in Brazil. Khowaja (2006) tested clinical pathways in transurethral resection of the prostate at Aga Khan University Hospital in Karachi, Pakistan. Findings indicated a significant improvement in outcomes with the clinical pathway using King's interacting systems framework. A study in South America by Souza, De Martino, and Lopes (2007) identified nursing diagnoses of hemodialysis patients with King's conceptual system as the referent. The results of the sample of 20 patients with chronic renal disease in dialysis centers indicated three nursing diagnoses were most prevalent: risk of infection, altered protection, and altered comfort.

## PARSIMONY

The conceptual system and theory were presented together in several versions of King's writings and remain largely as written in 1981. The theory is not parsimonious, having numerous concepts, multiple assumptions, many statements, and many relationships on a number of levels. This complexity, however, mirrors the complexity of human transactions for goal attainment. The model is general and universal and can be the umbrella for many midrange and practice theories.

## VALUE IN EXTENDING NURSING SCIENCE

In addition to application in practice and research described previously, King's work has been the basis for development of several middle range nursing theories. For example, the Theory of Goal Attainment was used by Rooda (1992) to develop a model for multicultural nursing practice. King's Systems Framework was reportedly used by Alligood and May (2000) to develop a theory of personal system empathy, and by Doornbos (2000) to derive a middle range theory of family health. Several Magnet status hospitals in the United States are using King's conceptual system in practice (King, personal communication, October, 2005).

King's conceptual system and theory have been used internationally in Australia, Brazil, Canada, Pakistan, and Sweden, as well as in numerous university nursing programs in the United States and have provided a foundation for many research studies. Her work has extended nursing science by its usefulness in education, practice, and research across international boundaries (King, 2001; Sieloff, 2006).

# Roper, Logan, and Tierney: Model of Nursing Based on Activities of Living

The Activities of Living (ALs) Model as initially described by Roper in the mid-1970s has been revised several times. The model was developed from the nursing education experiences of the authors as they analyzed data from numerous hospitals and other clinical practicum locations to identify a core of nursing knowledge across specialties (Roper, Logan, & Tierney, 2000).

## BACKGROUND OF THE THEORISTS

Nancy Roper spent 15 years as a principal tutor at a school of nursing in England. In the 1960s, she moved to Edinburgh, Scotland, where she was also an editor for Churchill-Livingstone Publishers. In the early 1970s she studied and achieved the M.Phil degree. Her thesis, "Clinical Experience on Nurse Education," became the basis for her later work on the model (Roper et al., 2000, p. v). Roper has worked as a nursing research officer for the Scottish Home and Health Department and carried out assignments for the World Health Organization (WHO) European Office. She has had a distinguished career as a nurse educator and speaker.

Winifred Logan began her nursing education in Edinburgh, and she earned an M.A. in Nursing from Columbia University in 1966. She held a high-level position in the Department of Nursing Studies at the University of Edinburgh for 12 years in the

1960s and 1970s, and was then appointed as Nurse Education Officer at the Scottish Office. Among other accomplishments, Logan was the executive director of the International Council of Nurses, a consultant for WHO in Malaysia, Iraq, and Europe, and directed nursing services in Abu Dhabi. She is now retired (Roper et al., 2000).

Alison Tierney was one of the first nurses to earn a PhD in the United Kingdom. She held the position of Director of Nursing Research based in the Department of Nursing Studies at the University of Edinburgh for 10 years, after which she was promoted to a Personal Chair in Nursing Research. Her work in nursing education early in her career prompted her to join Roper and Logan as they began to develop, refine, and publish the ALs Model. Tierney has contributed to the development of research in nursing in the United Kingdom and throughout Europe (Roper et al., 2000).

## PHILOSOPHICAL UNDERPINNINGS OF THE THEORY

Roper, Logan, and Tierney (R-L-T) (2000) explained that the ALs Model was created for educational purposes following an extensive literature review of the care of patients in hospitals and other situations. The data they gathered from clinical areas were analyzed, and they determined that there was a core of common, everyday living activities. Thus, the model was inductively formulated. The language of the model is a universally recognized, modern scholarly English.

## MAJOR ASSUMPTIONS, CONCEPTS, AND RELATIONSHIPS

### Assumptions

The major assumptions that Roper et al. (2000) list are included in Box 8-3.

---

**BOX 8-3** *Major Assumptions of the Roper, Logan, and Tierney Model*

Living can be described as an amalgam of activities of living (ALs).

The way ALs are carried out by each person contributes to individuality in living.

The individual is valued at all stages of the lifespan.

Through the lifespan until adulthood, the majority of individuals tend to become increasingly independent in the ALs.

While independence in the ALs is valued, dependence should not diminish the dignity of the individual.

An individual's knowledge about, attitudes to, and behavior related to the ALs are influenced by a variety of factors that can be categorized broadly as biological, psychological, sociocultural, environmental, and politico-economic factors.

The way in which an individual carries out the ALs can fluctuate within a range of normal for that person.

When the individual is "ill," there may be problems (actual or potential) with ALs.

During the lifespan, most individuals experience significant life events or untoward events which can affect the way they carry out ALs, and may lead to problems, actual or potential.

The concept of potential problems incorporates the promotion and maintenance of health and the prevention of disease and also identifies the role of the nurse as a health teacher, even in illness settings.

Within a health care context, nurses and patients/clients enter into a professional relationship whereby, whenever possible, the patient/client continues to be an autonomous, decision-making individual.

Nurses are part of a multiprofessional health care team; they work in partnership for the benefit of the client/patient, and for the health of the community.

The specific function of nursing is to assist the individual to prevent, alleviate, solve, or cope positively with problems (actual or potential) related to ALs.

Source: Roper et al. (2000, pp. 79–80).

## Concepts

The major concepts of the model are ALs, lifespan, and dependence/independence continuum. Five factors influence the ALs; these are the biological factors, psychological factors, sociocultural factors, environmental factors, and politico-economic factors (Table 8-6). The ALs are divided into 12 categories; these are then assessed within each of the five factors, along the continuum from dependence to independence, and across the lifespan of the person (Roper et al., 2000). Roper et al. (2000) do not explicitly define the metaparadigm concepts of nursing: human, health, nursing, and environment. However, descriptions of these concepts are found throughout the model, defined by context.

In the ALs model, humans are called "persons." Nurses are also persons, and they live the ALs along with other persons. Nursing is defined by what nursing is, rather than by what nurses do. The nursing process is defined as assessing, diagnosing, treating, and evaluating. Health refers to how the individual carries out the ALs in interaction with the five factors on the dependence/independence continuum (Holland, Jenkins, Solomon, & Whittam, 2003; Roper et al., 2000).

Environment is one of the five influencing factors of the model. The environment interacts with the 12 ALs, lifespan, dependence/independence continuum leading to individuality in living and in the nursing model, to individualized nursing.

Two models comprise Roper et al.'s (2000) work: the living model and the nursing model. Both models are based on the core ALs; the patient's model of living leads

TABLE 8-6 *Major Concepts of the Model of Nursing Based on Activities of Living*

| Concept | Definition |
| --- | --- |
| Activities of living | A complex interaction of factors that people are involved in every day and are largely performed "without much conscious deliberation but which contribute to the complex process of living" (p. 22). |
| Lifespan | The progression from birth through death that influences the health of a person or population and affects most aspects of health, including health of populations. |
| Dependence/independence continuum | The ability to perform those activities of living (ALs) throughout the lifespan; place on continuum depends on the health of the individual. |
| Factors influencing ALs | Individual differences that influence the ALs and how individuals carry out the ALs; all are interrelated. |
| Biological | The human body's anatomical and physiological performance. |
| Psychological | Elements of the person including intellectual and emotional aspects. |
| Sociocultural | Factors including culture, religion, spirituality, ethics, role, relationships, and status in the community. |
| Environmental | Factors physically external to the individual that affect all other factors. |
| Politico-economic | Legal, political, and/or economic factors that may be reflected in legislation. |
| Individuality in living | The product of the interaction of the ALs with the influencing factors, dependence/independence continuum, and lifespan. |
| Individualizing nursing | The process of nursing based on the assessment of the concepts in the patient model and individualization of nursing based on logical use of the process; assessing, planning, implementing, and evaluating. As much as possible, the patient should be involved in each phase of the process. |

Source: Roper et al. (2000).

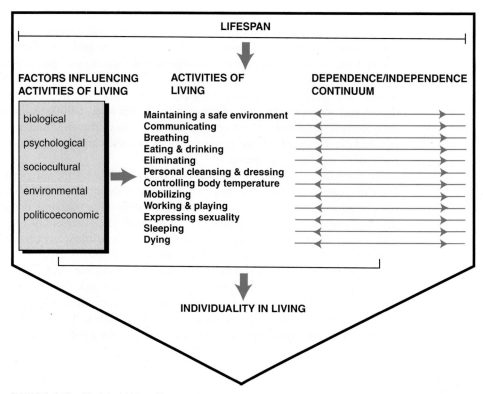

FIGURE 8-3 The Model of Living. (Source: Roper, N., Logan, W., & Tierney, A. J. (2000). *The Roper, Logan, Tierney model of nursing based on activities of living* (p. 14). London: Churchill Livingstone [Reprinted with permission].)

to "individualized living" (p. 78) and the nursing model leads to "individualizing nursing" (p. 152) (Figures 8-3 and 8-4).

## USEFULNESS

The R-L-T model of nursing has been shown to be useful in many ways. Several recent articles in the nursing literature describe its use in nursing practice. Kara (2007) used the R-L-T model in care of people suffering from COPD, as did Barnette (2007) who applied the principles of the model to assist clients to maintain quality of life by maintaining their independence (p. 10). Mantzoukas and Zoi (2008) found the R-L-T model useful in practice in Greece. They assert that this model more clearly assists with nursing practice in Europe than do the abstract nursing theories from the United States, which relate better to the U.S. health system.

In education, the R-L-T model has been widely used in the United Kingdom and throughout Europe; nurse educators in the United States are also interested in its applicability to the profession and to nursing education (Roper et al., 2000). Holland and colleagues (2003) authored a workbook to assist students and practicing nurses in applying the model.

## TESTABILITY

The R-L-T model is testable. Indeed, as mentioned, it was the product of testing in relation to the "core" of living (Roper et al., 2000). Because of its universality, it is

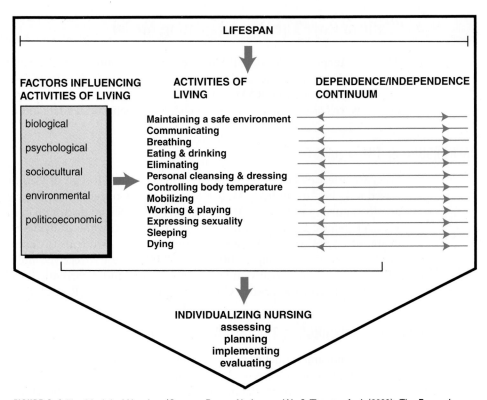

FIGURE 8-4 The Model of Nursing. (Source: Roper, N., Logan, W., & Tierney, A. J. (2000). *The Roper, Logan, Tierney model of nursing based on activities of living* (p. 78). London: Churchill Livingstone [Reprinted with permission].)

capable of generating middle range research theories and testable hypotheses. Several research projects were identified in the nursing literature. Kacmaz and Kasikci (2007) tested the effectiveness of bran supplementation in elderly orthopedic patients with constipation, finding that nursing intervention with bran supplementation was more effective than nursing interventions alone. Dewey and Dean (2007) interviewed nurses on their assessments of nutrition in patients with extreme weight loss as a result of cancer. Most of the nurses did not screen for weight loss, but were most interested in learning more about it (p. 265).

## PARSIMONY

The R-L-T model of nursing based on ALs has logical, parsimonious construction in which two parallel models—that of living and that of nursing—were developed simultaneously. The models seem simple on the surface, but the reality is that the model is quite complex.

## VALUE IN EXTENDING NURSING SCIENCE

Roper et al. (2000) state they hope that nurses using the model "will go on to refine the model further or to adapt it or even incorporate it" into their own practice (p. 12). With the current effort of the theorists and future work by others, the R-L-T model can be used to generate both middle range theories and practice models, and useful research.

# Sister Callista Roy: The Roy Adaptation Model

The Roy Adaptation Model (RAM) focuses on the interrelatedness of four adaptive systems. Like many of the models/theories in this unit, it is a deductive theory based on nursing practice. The RAM guides the nurse who is interested in physiologic adaptation, as well as the nurse who is interested in psychosocial adaptation.

## BACKGROUND OF THE THEORIST

Sister Callista Roy is a member of the Sisters of Saint Joseph of Carondelet. She received a BS in nursing from Mount Saint Mary's College in Los Angeles, California, an MS in nursing from UCLA, and a master's degree and doctorate in sociology from UCLA (Phillips, 2006). Roy first proposed the RAM while studying for her master's degree at UCLA, where Dorothy Johnson challenged students to develop conceptual models of nursing (Phillips, 2006; Roy, 2009). She has received numerous honors and awards for her scholarly and professional work and is currently the Graduate Faculty Nurse Theorist at Boston College School of Nursing (Roy, 2009).

## PHILOSOPHICAL UNDERPINNINGS OF THE THEORY

Johnson's nursing model was the impetus for the development of the RAM. Roy also incorporated concepts from Helson's adaptation theory, von Bertalanffy's system model, Rapoport's system definition, the stress and adaptation theories of Dohrenrend and Selye, and the coping model of Lazarus (Phillips, 2002).

## MAJOR ASSUMPTIONS, CONCEPTS, AND RELATIONSHIPS

### Assumptions

In the RAM, assumptions are specified as, philosophical, scientific, and cultural (Roy, 2009, p. 31). Philosophical assumptions include:

- Persons have mutual relationships with the world and God.
- Human meaning is rooted in the omega point convergence of the universe.
- God is intimately revealed in the diversity of creation.
- Persons use human creative abilities of awareness, enlightenment, and faith.
- Persons are accountable for sustaining, and transforming the universe (Roy, 2009, p. 31).

Scientific assumptions of the RAM for the 21st century include:

- Systems of matter and energy progress to higher levels of complex self-organization.
- Consciousness and meaning constitute person and environment integration.
- Self and environmental awareness is rooted in thinking and feeling.
- Human decisions account for integration of creative processes.
- Thinking and feeling mediate human action.
- System relationships include acceptance, protection, and fostering interdependence.
- Persons and the earth have common patterns and integral relationships.
- Person and environment transformations are created in human consciousness.
- Integration of human and environment results in adaptation (Roy, 2009, p. 1).

Cultural assumptions include:

- Cultural experiences influence how RAM is expressed.
- A concept central to the culture may influence the RAM to some extent.
- Cultural expressions of the RAM may lead to changes in practice activities such as nursing assessment (Roy, 2009, p. 31).
- As RAM evolves within a culture implications for nursing may differ from experience in the original culture (Roy, 2009, p. 31).

All elements of the model are part of the care of clients and groups. The nurse undertakes a bi-level assessment to accurately define the problem and come to decisions on the plan of care. The process in formulating the nursing plan is intricate and is prescriptive in its objectives.

### Concepts

The RAM contains many defined concepts, including the metaparadigm concepts. Table 8-7 lists some of these.

### Relationships

Roy's model is composed of four adaptive modes that constitute the specific categories that serve as framework for assessment (Figure 8-5). Through the four modes

TABLE 8-7 *Major Concepts of the Roy Adaptation Model*

| Concept | Definition |
| --- | --- |
| Environment | Conditions, circumstances, and influences that affect the development and behavior of humans as adaptive systems. |
| Health | A state and process of being and becoming integrated and whole. |
| Person | "The human adaptive system" and defined as "a whole with parts that function as a unity for some purpose. Human systems include people groups organizations, communities, and society as a whole" (Roy & Andrews, 1999, p. 31). |
| Goal of nursing | The "promotion of adaptation in each of the four modes" (p. 31). |
| Adaptation | The "process and outcome whereby thinking and feeling persons as individuals or in groups use conscious awareness and choice to create human and environmental integration" (p. 30). |
| Focal stimuli | Those stimuli that are the proximate causes of the situation. |
| Contextual stimuli | All other stimuli in the internal or external environment, which may or may not affect the situation. |
| Residual stimuli | Those immeasurable and unknowable stimuli that also exist and may affect the situation. |
| Cognator subsystem | "A major coping process involving four cognitive-emotive channels: perceptual and information processing, learning, judgment, and emotion" (p. 31). |
| Regulator subsystem | A basic type of adapttive process that responds automatically through neural, chemical, and endocrine coping channels (p. 46). |
| Stabilizer control processes | The structures and processes aimed at system maintenance and involving values and daily activities whereby participants accomplish the primary purpose of the group and contribute to the common purposes of the society. |
| Innovator control processes | The internal subsystem that involves structures and processes for growth. |

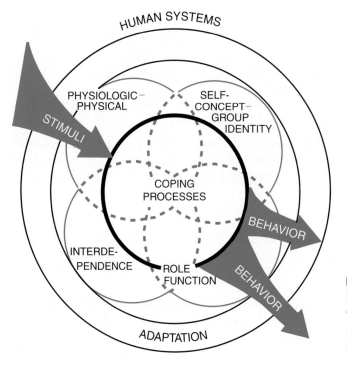

FIGURE 8-5 Diagrammatic representation of human adaptive systems. (Source: Roy, C., & Andrews, H. A. (1999). *The Roy adaptation model* (2nd ed.). Stamford, CT: Appleton & Lange [Reprinted with permission of Pearson Education, Inc, Upper Saddle River, NJ].)

"responses to and interaction with the client's environment are carried out and adaptation can be observed" (Roy, 2009, pp. 69–72). They are the:

1. *Physiologic-physical mode:* Physical and chemical processes involved in the function and activities of living organisms; the underlying need is physiologic integrity: the degree of wholeness achieved through adaptation to changes in needs. In groups, this is the manner in which human systems manifest adaptation to basic operating resources (Roy, 2009, pp. 69–70).
2. *Self-concept-group identity mode:* Focuses on psychological and spiritual integrity and a sense of unity, meaning, purposefulness in the universe (p. 70).
3. *Role function mode:* Refers to the roles that individuals occupy in society fulfilling the need for social integrity; it is knowing who one is, in relation to others (p. 70).
4. *Interdependence mode:* The close relationships of people and their purpose, structure, and development, individually and in groups and the adaptation potential of these relationships (Roy, 2009, p. 71).

Two subsystems require assessment in the RAM: the regulator and the cognator. These are coping subsystems that allow the client to adapt and make changes when stressed. The regulator is the physiologic coping subsystem and the cognator is the cognitive-emotive coping subsystem (Roy, 2009).

## USEFULNESS

The RAM has been used extensively to guide practice and to organize nursing education. International conferences on the RAM have been conducted across the United States and abroad (Roy, 2009). The RAM was adopted as a component of the curricular framework of such widely diverse colleges and departments of nursing as Mount Saint Mary's College, Department of Nursing; the University of Texas at Austin

School of Nursing; Boston College School of Nursing; and the nurse practitioner program at the University of Miami in Florida. The RAM has also been implemented internationally at the University of Ottawa School of Nursing and in university schools of nursing in Japan and France (Phillips, 2002).

Among middle range nursing theories derived from the RAM are a longitudinal model of psychosocial determinants of adaptation (Ducharme, Richard, Duquette, Levesque, & Lachance, 1998); a middle range theory of psychological adaptation (Levesque, Ricard, Ducharme, Duquette, & Bonin, 1998); and another middle range nursing theory, the Urine Control Theory, by Jirovec, Jenkins, Isenberg, and Baiardi (1999). The RAM has also been tested and applied to practice in Latin America (Moreno-Fergusen, 2007).

## TESTABILITY

The RAM is testable. Indeed, the Boston Based Adaptation Research in Nursing Society (BBARNS, 1999) reported that, since the 1970s, 163 studies had been conducted using the model. *Note*: An international nursing society specifically focused on researching adaptation nursing, Roy Adaptation Association (RAA), supplanted the BBARNS organization which was based in Boston College School of Nursing (Roy, 2009). Box 8-4 lists a few recent examples of nursing research using aspects of the RAM.

## PARSIMONY

The RAM is not parsimonious because of its many elements, systems, structures, and concepts. It is complete and comprehensive, and it attempts to explain the reality of the clients so that nursing interventions can be specifically targeted. The nursing assessment is conducted on two levels and is extensive and complex. It requires assessment of the stimuli to which the client is responding and of the coping subsystems. It targets the client in the four adaptive modes, and an assessment must be made to determine how effectively the subsystems (i.e., cognator and regulator) are working.

---

**BOX 8-4** *Examples of Studies Using the Roy Adaptation Model*

Barone, S. H., Roy, C. L., & Fredrickson, K. C. (2008). Instruments used in Roy adaptation model-based research: Review, critique, and future directions. *Nursing Science Quarterly, 21*(4), 353–362.

Black, K. D. (2008). Stress, symptoms, self-monitoring confidence, well-being, and social support in the progression of pre-eclampsia/gestational hypertension. *Journal of Obstetric, Gynecologic, and Neonatal Nursing, 36*(5), 419–429.

Chen, Y., & Tsai, H. (2008). The nursing experience of caring for a sexual assault victim [Chinese]. *Journal of Nursing (China), 55*(1), 99–104.

Cheng, C. H., Qin, L. X., & Tee, H. K. (2008). An exploratory study on the isolation experience of patients with haematological disorders. *Singapore Nursing Journal, 35*(1), 15–23.

Evans, L. A. (2008). Feasibility of family member presence in the OR during breast biopsy procedures. *Association of periOperative Registered Nurses Journal, 88*(4), 568, 570, 573–578.

Flood, M., & Boyd, M. (2008). Successful aging in a southern older adult sample. *Southern Online Journal of Nursing Research, 8*(3), 12 pp. Retrieved on August 20, 2008.

Narsavage, G. L., & Chen, K. (2008). Factors related to depressed mood in adults with chronic obstructive pulmonary disease after hospitalization. *Home Healthcare Nurse, 26*(8), 474–482.

Roper, K., Cooley, M., Powell, M., McDermott, K., Coakley, C., Boyd, K., & Fawcett, J. (2008). Health-related quality of life after treatment for Hodgkin disease. *Oncology Nursing Forum, 35*(3), 547–548.

## VALUE IN EXTENDING NURSING SCIENCE

The RAM has been a valuable asset in extending nursing science. Dunn and Dunn (1997) summarized the impact of the RAM on nursing practice, education, and administration, stating that it has contributed significantly to the science and practice of nursing. Indeed, the RAM has generated hundreds of research studies and has contributed to nursing education for more than 35 years (Roy, 2009).

## Jean Watson: Caring Science as Sacred Science

Jean Watson's (2008) *Philosophy and Science of Caring*, a recent publication, builds on her previous work, *Nursing: Human Science and, Human Care: A Theory of Nursing*. This theory is one of the newest of nursing's grand theories, having only been completely codified in 1979, revised in 1985 (Watson, 1988), and broadened and advanced more recently (Watson, 2005, 2008). Watson called her earlier work a descriptive theory of caring and stated that it was the only theory of nursing to incorporate the spiritual dimension of nursing at the time it was first conceptualized. The theory was both deductive and inductive in its origins and was written at an abstract level of discourse.

It is somewhat difficult to categorize Watson's work with the works of other nursing theorists. It has many characteristics of a human interaction model, although it also incorporates many ideals of the unitary process theories, which are discussed in Chapter 9. Watson (2005) has always described the human as a holistic, interactive being, and is now explicit in describing the human as an energy field and in explaining health and illness as manifestations of the human pattern, two tenets of the unitary process theories. Parse (2004) points out, however, that although theorists profess belief in unitary human beings, other definitions and relationships still separate theories from the interactive process paradigms and the unitary process nursing paradigms. Based on overall considerations, the philosophy and science of caring reflects the interactive process nursing theories.

## BACKGROUND OF THE THEORIST

Jean Watson was born in West Virginia and attended Lewis Gale School of Nursing in Roanoke, Virginia. She earned a bachelor's degree in nursing, a master of science degree in psychiatric-mental health nursing, and a doctorate in educational psychology and counseling, all from the University of Colorado (Neill, 2002). Watson is an internationally published author, having written many books, book chapters, and articles about the science of human caring (Watson, 1994, 1996, 1999, 2005, 2008).

Watson is the former Dean of the School of Nursing at the University of Colorado, and she founded and directed the Center for Human Caring at the Health Sciences Center in Denver. She has received numerous awards and honors and is currently Distinguished Professor of Nursing at the University of Colorado (Neill, 2002). Her work is well known worldwide (Watson, vitae, 2008).

## PHILOSOPHICAL UNDERPINNINGS OF THE THEORY

Watson (1988) noted that she drew parts of her theory from nursing writers, including Nightingale and Rogers. She also used concepts from the works of psychologists Giorgi,

Johnson, and Koch, as well as concepts from philosophy. She reported being widely read in these disciplines and synthesized a number of diverse concepts from them into nursing as a science of human caring. In a recent work, Watson (2005) continues to "bridge paradigms and point toward transformative models for the 21st century" (p. 2).

## MAJOR ASSUMPTIONS, CONCEPTS, AND RELATIONSHIPS

The value system that permeates Watson's (1988, 2008) theory of human caring includes a "deep respect for the wonders and mysteries of life" (1988, p. 34) and recognition that spiritual and ethical dimensions are major elements of the human care process. A number of assumptions are both stated and implicit in her theory. Additionally, several concepts were defined, refined, and adapted for it. From this, 10 carative factors were developed (Box 8-5; Watson, 1985, 2008).

### Assumptions

Watson (2008) describes the tenets of caring science and sacred science. She proposed that caring and love are universal and mysterious "cosmic forces" that comprise the primal and universal psychic energy. Further, she believes that health professionals make social, moral, and scientific contributions to humankind and that nurses' caring ideal can affect human development. Further, she believes that it is critical in today's society to sustain human caring ideals and a caring ideology in practice, as there has been a proliferation of radical treatment and "cure techniques," often without regard to costs or human considerations.

Explicit assumptions that were derived for Watson's (2005) work include:

- An ontological assumption of oneness, wholeness, unity, relatedness, and connectedness.
- An epistemological assumption that there are multiple ways of knowing.
- Diversity of knowing assumes all, and various forms of evidence can be included.
- A Caring Science model makes these diverse perspectives explicitly and directly.
- Moral-metaphysical integration with science evokes spirit; this orientation is not only possible but also necessary for our science, humanity, society-civilization, and world-planet.
- A Caring Science emergence, founded on new assumptions makes explicit an expanding unitary, energetic worldview with a relational human caring ethic and ontology as its starting point (Watson, 2005, p. 28).

---

**BOX 8-5** | *Watson's 10 Carative Factors*

1. Humanistic-altruistic system of values
2. Faith–hope
3. Sensitivity to self and others
4. Developing helping–trusting, caring relationship
5. Expressing positive and negative feelings and emotions
6. Creative, individualized, problem-solving caring process
7. Transpersonal teaching–learning
8. Supportive, protective, and/or corrective, mental, physical, societal, and spiritual environment
9. Human needs assistance
10. Existential-phenomenological and spiritual forces

Source: Watson (1999, 2005).

TABLE 8-8 *Major Concepts of the Science of Human Caring*

| Concept | Definition |
|---|---|
| Human being | A valued person to be cared for, respected, nurtured, understood, and assisted. |
| Health | Unity and harmony within the mind, body, and soul; health is associated with the degree of congruence between the self as perceived and the self as experienced. |
| Nursing | A human science of persons and human health—illness experiences that are mediated by professional, personal, scientific, esthetic, and ethical human care transactions. |
| Actual caring occasion | Involves actions and choices by the nurse and the individual .The moment of coming together in a caring occasion presents the two persons with the opportunity to decide how to be in the relationship—what to do with the moment. |
| Transpersonal | An intersubjective human-to-human relationship in which the nurse affects and is affected by the person of the other. Both are fully present in the moment and feel a union with the other; they share a phenomenal field that becomes part of the life history of both. |
| Phenomenal field | The totality of human experience of one's being in the world. This refers to the individual's frame of reference that can only be known to that person. |
| Self | The organized conceptual gestalt composed of perceptions of the characteristics of the "I" or "ME" and the perceptions of the relationship of the "I" or "ME" to others and to various aspects of life. |
| Time | The present is more subjectively real and the past is more objectively real. The past is prior to, or in a different mode of being than the present, but it is not clearly distinguishable. Past, present, and future incidents merge and fuse. |

Sources: Watson (1999); online site: http://www.uchsc.edu/ctrsinst/chc/index.html.

### Concepts

Watson (1988) defined three of the four metaparadigm concepts (human being, health, and nursing). She coined several other concepts and terms that are integral to understanding the science of human caring (Table 8-8). Her 10 carative factors are caring needs specific to human experiences that should be addressed by nurses with their clients in the caring role. She continues to value those carative factors (Watson, 2008). The carative factors are listed in Box 8-5.

### Relationships

Watson has refined and updated the relationships of the theory, bringing them closer to her current way of understanding human caring and spirituality. Her continued study has involved lengthy examination of her beliefs about caring, spirituality, and human and energy fields (Watson, 2005, 2008). The following are some of the relationships of the theory:

- A transpersonal caring field resides within a unitary field of consciousness and energy that transcends time, space, and physicality.
- A transpersonal caring relationship connotes a spirit-to-spirit unitary connection within a caring moment, honoring the embodied spirit of both practitioner and patient, within a unitary field of consciousness.
- A transpersonal caring relationship transcends the ego level of both practitioner and patient, creating a caring field with new possibilities for how to be in the moment.

- The practitioner's authentic intentionality and consciousness of caring has a higher frequency of energy than noncaring consciousness, opening up connections to the universal field of consciousness and greater access to one's inner healer.
- Transpersonal caring is communicated via the practitioner's energetic patterns of consciousness, intentionality, and authentic presence in a caring relationship.
- Caring-healing modalities are often noninvasive, nonintrusive, natural-human, energetic environmental field modalities.
- Transpersonal caring promotes self-knowledge, self-control, and self-healing patterns and possibilities.
- Advanced transpersonal caring modalities draw upon multiple ways of knowing and being; they encompass ethical and relational caring, along with those intentional consciousness modalities that are energetic in nature (e.g., form, color, light, sound, touch, vision, scent) that honor wholeness, healing, comfort, balance, harmony, and well-being (Watson, 2005, p. 6).

## USEFULNESS

Watson's works on the Theory of Human Caring and the Art and Science of Human Caring are used by nurses in diverse settings; for example, Drake et al. (2008) found the model important in caring for the morbidly obese in several practice settings. Pipe (2008) wrote about inner leadership as a journey in practice focusing on intentionality and mindfulness. Caring science concepts have also been applied to various groups, including people with human immunodeficiency virus/acquired immunodeficiency syndrome, with elderly people, and with people suffering from wounds as a result of recent military duty (Baldwin et al., 2008).

The University of Colorado School of Nursing implemented the model not only in its education programs (BSN, MSN, and PhD), but also in clinical practice at the Center for Human Caring (Watson, 1988). In addition, the School of Nursing at Georgia Southern University in Statesboro taught both undergraduate courses and the nurse practitioner program from the human caring philosophy (Watson, 1988). Writings that detail how Watson's work is used in nursing education include Bevis and Watson (1989), Leininger and Watson (1990), and Watson (1994).

## TESTABILITY

Testing of Watson's theory and dissemination of findings are progressing. The science allows both quantitative and qualitative research methods. For example, Watson's work was used as the framework for a study by Pipe et al. (2008) who used descriptive methods to explore the constructs of hope, spiritual well-being, and quality of life in hospitalized patients. Delaney and Barrere (2008) studied the influence of blessings, a spiritual intervention, on psychosocial outcomes in cardiac patients; and Persky, Nelson, Watson, and Bent (2008) examined profile characteristics of caritas nurses and effectiveness of practice within that model. Watson's Science of Caring has been researched by an extremely large number of nurses recently. Additional research articles are listed in Box 8-6.

## PARSIMONY

Watson's theory is comparatively parsimonious. Although a number of new concepts and terms are defined, there are only 10 carative factors or areas to be addressed by

| BOX 8-6 | *Examples of Research Using Watson's Model* |

Adegbola, M. (2006). Spirituality and quality of life in chronic illness. *Journal of Theory Construction and Testing, 10*(2), 42–46.

Baldwin, C. M., Grant, M., Wendel, C., Rawl, S., Schmidt, C. M., Lo, C., & Krouse, R. S. (2008). Influence of intestinal stoma on spiritual quality of life of US Veterans. *Journal of Holistic Nursing, 26*(3), 185–194.

Cossette, S., Pepin, J., Cote, J. K., & deCourval, F. P. (2008). The multidimensionality of caring: A confirmatory factor analysis of the Caring Nurse–Patient Interaction Short Scale. *Journal of Advanced Nursing, 61*(6), 699–710.

Pipe, T. B., Kelly, A., LeBrun, G., Atherton, P., & Robinson, C. (2008). A prospective descriptive study exploring hope, spiritual well-being, and quality of life in hospitalized patients. *MEDSURG Nursing, 17*(4), 247–253.

Porcel, M. A. (2008). Nursing care adopted for use in homes for the elderly based on Watson model (Spanish). *Gerokomos, 18*(4), 18–22.

Tan, J., Low, J. A., Yap, P., Lee, A., Pang, W. S., & Wu, Y. (2006). Multicultural aging, caring for dying patients and those facing death in an acute-care hospital in Singapore: A nurse's perspective. *Journal of Gerontological Nursing, 17*(5), 17–24.

Wade, G. H., & Kasper, N. (2006). Nursing students' perceptions of instructor caring: An instrument based on Watson's theory of transpersonal caring. *Journal of Nursing Education, 45*(5), 162–168.

nurses. In addition, there are six "working assumptions" (Watson, 2005, p. 28) and three considerations as to how to frame caring science.

## VALUE IN EXTENDING NURSING SCIENCE

*The Philosophy and Science of Caring* (Watson, 2008) explicitly describes the connection between nursing and caring. It is used in education and in practice internationally, and in numerous research studies. Collectively, findings present impressive indicators of the value of Watson's theory of caring, to the discipline of nursing.

## Summary

The models presented in this chapter all focus on human interactive processes as the basis for nursing care, research, and education. Some of the theories described (e.g., King and Levine) are among the oldest of the grand nursing theories, whereas others (e.g., Watson, Artinian, and Roper et al.) are among the most recently developed. There is a wide variety of complexity among the models, but each has demonstrated applicability to the discipline, and all are currently used in schools of nursing, clinical settings, and nursing research. Like Jean, the nurse in the opening case study, nurses in all settings will be able to relate to the perspective described by these theorists. Indeed, the premise that humans are adaptive, holistic beings, in constant interaction with their environment, is easily applied in nursing practice. Some philosophical bases, concepts, assumptions, and relationships (e.g., systems focus, adaptation, goal of nursing, ALs) are relatively consistently held within the works of this group of theorists, whereas others (e.g., situational sense of coherence [Artinian], conservation principles [Levine], cognator and regulator subsystems [Roy]) are unique to just one theory.

Nurses, particularly those in advanced practice, studying this group of theories will become aware of how they present and prescribe nursing practice. Many will undoubtedly consider adopting one as a basis for their own professional practice.

## LEARNING ACTIVITIES

1. Compare and contrast two of the models or theories presented in this chapter considering their usefulness in practice, research, education, and administration. Share findings with classmates.

2. Select one of the models from this chapter and obtain the original work(s) of the theorist. From the work(s), outline a plan for a research study either using the work as the conceptual framework or testing components of the work.

   a. What concepts, assumptions, or relationships can be studied?

   b. To what population(s) can the work be applied?

   c. What concepts can be used as study variables?

3. Explain how a model of your choice can be used to guide evidence gathering through research for evidence-based practice.

## INTERNET RESOURCES

Artinian:

http://www.nc.bin.lm.nihgov/pubmed/2013662

Erickson:

http://unicornsunlimited.com/modeling_and_rolemodeling.htm

Roper, Logan, Tierney:

http://www.nursesinfo/nursing_theory_person_roper_logan_tierney.htm

Roy:

http://www.bc.edu/schools/son/faculty/theorist/Roy_Adaptation_Association.html

Watson:

http://www.nursing.ucdenver.edu/faculty/jw_connections.htm
http://www.nursing.ucdenver.edu/faculty/j_watson_about.htm

## REFERENCES

Acton, G. J. (1997). Affiliated-individuation as a mediator of stress and burden in caregivers of adults with dementia. *Journal of Holistic Nursing, 15*(4), 336–357.

Alligood, M. R., & May, B. A. (2000). A nursing theory of personal system empathy: Interpreting a conceptualization of empathy in King's interacting systems. *Nursing Science Quarterly, 13*(3), 243–247.

Antonofski, A. (1987). *Unraveling the mystery of health: How people manage stress and stay well.* San Francisco: Jossey-Bass (as cited in Artinian, 1991).

Artinian, B. M. (1983). Implementation of the intersystem patient-care model in clinical practice. *Journal of Advanced Nursing, 8*(2), 117–124.

Artinian, B. M. (1991). The development of the intersystem model. *Journal of Advanced Nursing, 16*, 164–205.

Artinian, B. M. (1997a). Overview of the intersystem model. In B. M. Artinian & M. M. Conger (Eds.), *The intersystem model: Integrating theory and practice* (pp. 1–17). Thousand Oaks, CA: Sage.

Artinian, B. M. (1997b). Situational sense of coherence. In B. M. Artinian & M. M. Conger (Eds.), *The intersystem model: Integrating theory and practice* (pp. 18–30). Thousand Oaks, CA: Sage.

Artinian, B. M. (1997c). Research: Refining and testing the theoretical constructs of the intersystem model. In B. M. Artinian & M. M. Conger (Eds.), *The intersystem model: Integrating theory and practice* (pp. 225–269). Thousand Oaks, CA: Sage.

Artinian, B. M. (1997d). The nursing assessment decision grid. In B. M. Artinian & M. M. Conger (Eds.), *The intersystem model: Integrating theory and practice* (pp. 269–280). Thousand Oaks, CA: Sage.

Artinian, B. M. (1998). Grounded theory research: Its value for nursing. *Nursing Science Quarterly, 11*(1), 5–6.

Baldwin, C. M. (2004). Interstitial cystitis and self-care: Bearing the burden. *Urologic Nursing, 24*(2), 111–112.

Baldwin, C. M., Grant, M., Wendel, C., Rawl, S., Schmidt, C. M., Ko, C., & Krouse, R. S. (2008). Influence of intesinal stoma on spiritual quality of life of US Veterans. *Journal of Holistic Nursing, 26*(3), 185–194.

Barnette, M. (2007). Using a model in the assessment and management of COPD. *Journal of Community Nursing, 21*(11), 4, 6, 8, 10.

Bevis, E. O., & Watson, J. (1989). *Toward a caring curriculum: A new pedagogy for nursing.* New York: National League for Nursing Press.

Bond, M. L., Gray, J. R., Baxley, S., Cason, C. L., Denke, L., & Moon, M. (2008). Voices of Hispanic students in baccalaureate nursing programs: Are we listening? *Nursing Education Perspectives, 29*(3), 136–142.

Boston Based Adaptation Research in Nursing Society (BBARNS). (1999). *Roy Adaptation Model-based research: 25 years of contributions to nursing science.* Indianapolis, IN: Center Nursing Press, Sigma Theta Tau International.

Cason, C., Bond, M. L., Gleason-Wynn, P., Coggin, C., Trevino, E., & Lopez, M. (2008). Perceived barriers and needed supports for today's Hispanic students in the health professions: Voices of seasoned Hispanic health care professionals. *Hispanic Care International, 6*(1), 41–50.

Chrisman, M., & Riehl, J. (1974). The systems-developmental stress model. In J. Riehl & C. Roy (Eds.), *Conceptual models for nursing practice* (pp. 247–266). New York: Appleton-Century-Crofts.

Chrisman, M., & Riehl, J. (1989). The systems-developmental stress model. In J. Riehl & C. Roy (Eds.), *Conceptual models for nursing practice* (3rd ed., pp. 247–268). New York: Appleton-Century-Crofts.

Critchley, S., & Ball, E. (2007). Evaluation of the primary/secondary care interface in relation to primary care rheumatology service. *Quality in Primary Care, 15*(1), 33–36.

Daubenmire, M. J. (1989). A baccalaureate curriculum based on King's conceptual framework. In J. Riehl-Siska (Ed.), *Conceptual models for nursing practice* (3rd ed., pp. 167–178). Norwalk, CT: Appleton & Lange.

Delaney, C., & Barrere, C. (2008). Blessings: The influence of a spirituality-based intervention on psychosocial outcomes in a cardiac population. *Holistic Nursing Practice, 22*(4), 210–219.

Dever, M. (1991). Care of children. In K. M. Schaefer & J. B. Pond (Eds.), *Levine's conservation model: A framework for nursing practice* (pp. 71–82). Philadelphia: Davis.

Dewey, A., & Dean, T. (2007). Assessment and monitoring of nutritional status in patients with advanced cancer: Part 1. *International Journal of Palliative Nursing, 13*(6), 258–265.

Doornbos, M. M. (2000). King's systems framework and family health: The derivation and testing of a theory. *Journal of Theory Construction and Testing, 4*(1), 20–26.

Dover, L., & Pfieffer, J. B. (2006). Spiritual care in Christian parish nursing. *Journal of Advanced Nursing, 57*(2), 213–221

Drake, D. J., Baker, G., Engelke, M. K., McAuliffe, M., Pokorny, M., Swanson, M., Waters, W., Watkins, F. R., Jr., & Rose, M. A. (2008). Challenges in caring for the morbidly obese: Differences by practice settings. *Southern Online Journal of Nursing Research, 8*(3), 13pp.

Ducharme, F., Richard, N., Duquette, A., Levesque, L., & Lachance, L. (1998). Empirical testing of a longitudinal model derived from the Roy Adaptation Model. *Nursing Science Quarterly, 119*(4), 149–159.

Dunn, H. C., & Dunn, D. G. (1997). The Roy Adaptation Model and its application to clinical nursing practice. *Journal of Ophthalmic Nursing and Technology, 16*(2), 74–78.

Erdmann, C. M. (2003). The value of the Intersystem Model for cosmetic nursing practice. *Dermatology Nursing, 15*(4), 335–339.

Erickson, H. C., Tomlin, E. M., & Swain, M. A. P. (1983). *Modeling and role-modeling: A theory and paradigm for nursing.* Englewood Cliffs, NJ: Prentice-Hall.

Erickson, H. L. (2008). Biosketch. Available on: http://www.unicornsunlimited.com. Retrieved on December, 30, 2008.

Erickson, M. E., Caldwell-Gwin, J. A., Carr, L. A., Harmon, B. K., Hartman, K., Jarlsberg, C. R., et al. (1998). Helen C. Erickson, Evelyn M. Tomlin, Mary Ann P. Swain: Modeling and role-modeling. In A. M. Tomey & M. R. Alligood (Eds.), *Nursing theorists and their work* (pp. 387–406). St. Louis: Mosby.

Erickson, M. E. (2006). Modeling and role-modeling. In A. M. Tomey & M. R. Alligood (Eds.), *Nursing theorists and their work* (6th ed., pp. 560–581). St. Louis: Mosby.

Falcao, L. M., Guedes, M. V. C., & da Silva, L. F. (2006). Arterial hypertension bearer: Comprehension based on Imogene King's personal system. *Revista Paulista de Enfermagem, 44*(1), 44–50.

Fasnacht, P. H. (2003). Creativity: A refinement of the concept for nursing practice. *Journal of Advanced Nursing, 41*(2), 195–202.

Foreman, M. D. (1991). Conserving cognitive integrity of hospitalized elderly. In K. M. Schaefer & J. B. Pond (Eds.), *Levine's conservation model: A framework for nursing practice* (pp. 134–149). Philadelphia: Davis.

Frey, M. A., Rooke, L., Seiloff, C., Messmer, P. R., & Kameoka, T. (1995). King's framework and theory in Japan, Sweden, and the United States. *Image: Journal of Nursing Scholarship, 27*(2), 127–130.

Giske, T., & Artinian, B. (2008). Patterns of "balancing between hope and despair" in the diagnostic phase: A grounded theory study of patients on a gastroenterology ward. *Journal of Advanced Nursing, 62*(1), 22–31.

Grindley, J., & Paradowski, M. B. (1991). Developing an undergraduate program using Levine's model. In K. M. Schaefer & J. B. Pond (Eds.), *Levine's conservation model: A framework for nursing practice* (pp. 199–208). Philadelphia: Davis.

Holland, K., Jenkins, J., Solomon, J., & Whittam, S. (2003). *Applying the Roper-Logan-Tierney model in practice.* London: Churchill Livingstone.

Hughes, R., Lloyd, D., & Clarke, J. (2008). A conceptual model for nursing information. *International Journal of Nursing Technologies and Classifications, 29*(2), 48–56.

Irvin, B. L., & Acton, G. J. (1996). Stress mediation in caregivers of cognitively impaired adults: Theoretical model testing. *Nursing Research, 45*(3), 160–166.

Jirovec, M. M., Jenkins, J., Isenberg, M., & Baiardi, J. (1999). Urine control theory derived from Roy's conceptual framework. *Nursing Science Quarterly, 12*(3), 251–255.

Kacmaz, Z., & Kasikci, M. (2007). Effectiveness of bran supplement in older orthopaedic patients with constipation. *Journal of Clinical Nursing, 16*(11), 928–936. [Turkish, translator unknown.]

Kara, M. (2007). Using the Roper, Logan and Tierney model in care of people with COPD. *Journal of Nursing and Healthcare of Chronic Illnesses, 16*(7b Suppl.), 223–233.

Khowaja, K. (2006). Utilization of King's interacting systems framework and theory of goal attainment with new multidisciplinary model: Clinical Pathway. *Australian Journal of Advanced Nursing, 24*(2) 44–50.

King, I. (1971). *Toward a theory for nursing.* New York: Wiley.

King, I. (1981). *A theory for nursing, systems, concepts, process.* New York: Wiley.

King, I. M. (1995a). A systems framework for nursing. In M. A. Frey & C. L. Sieloff (Eds.), *Advancing King's systems framework and theory of nursing* (pp. 13–22). Thousand Oaks, CA: Sage.

King, I. M. (1995b). The theory of goal attainment. In M. A. Frey & C. L. Sieloff (Eds.), *Advancing King's systems framework and theory of nursing* (pp. 23–33). Thousand Oaks, CA: Sage.

King, I. M. (2001). Theory of goal attainment. In M. Parker (Ed.), *Nursing theories and nursing practice* (pp. 275–286). Philadelphia: Davis.

Leach, M. J. (2006). Wound management: Using Levine's conservation model to guide practice. *Ostomy Wound Management, 52*(8), 74–76, 78–80.

Leininger, M., & Watson, J. (Eds.). (1990). *The caring imperative in education.* New York: National League for Nursing Press.

Levesque, L., Ricard, N., Ducharme, F., Duquette, A., & Bonin, J. (1998). Empirical verification of a theoretical model derived from the Roy adaptation model: Findings from five studies. *Nursing Science Quarterly, 11*(1), 31–39.

Levine, M. E. (1969). Introduction *to clinical nursing.* Philadelphia: Davis.

Levine, M. E. (1973). Introduction to patient-centered nursing care. (Reprinted in K. M. Schafer & J. B. Pond. (1991). *Levine's conservation model* (pp. 237–259). Philadelphia: Davis)

Levine, M. E. (1989). The conservation principles of nursing: Twenty years later. In J. P. Riehl-Siska (Ed.),

*Conceptual models for nursing practice* (3rd ed., pp. 325–337). Norwalk, CT: Appleton & Lange.

Levine, M. E. (1990). Conservation and integrity. In M. E. Parker (Ed.), *Nursing theories in practice* (pp. 189–201). New York: National League for Nursing Press.

Levine, M. E. (1991). The conservation principles: A model for health. In K. M. Schaefer & J. B. Pond (Eds.). *Levine's conservation model: A framework for nursing practice* (pp. 1–11). Philadelphia: Davis.

Mantzoukas, S., & Zoi, L. (2008) The Roper-Logan-Tierney nursing model and its implementation in practice [Greek] *Nosileftiki, 47*(1), 21–36 [Translator unknown].

Mefford, L. C. (2004). A theory of health promotion for preterm infants based on Levine's conservation model of nursing. *Nursing Science Quarterly, 17*(3), 260–266.

Mensik, J. (2008, May). Nurses make a difference every day. *Arizona Nurse,* p. 2.

Mitchell, P. H. (2008). President's message: Legends and legacies . . . M. Elizabeth Carnegie, Imogene King and Marie J. Cowan. *Nursing Outlook, 56*(3), 97–98.

Mock, V., Ours, C., Hall, S., Bositis, A., Tillery, M., Belcher, A., Krumm, S., & Mccorkle, R. (2007). Using a conceptual model in nursing research—mitigating fatigue in cancer patients. *Journal of Advanced Nursing, 58*(3), 503–512.

Moreno-Fergusen, M. E. (2007). Application of the Roy adaptation model in Latin America, Literature review. *Roy Adaptation Association Conference,* Los Angeles, CA.

MRM website (2008). http://unicornsunlimited.com/modeling_and_rolemodeling.htm.

Neill, R. M. (2002). Jean Watson: Philosophy and science of caring. In A. M. Tomey & M. R. Alligood (Eds.), *Nursing theorists and their work* (5th ed., pp. 144–164). St. Louis: Mosby.

Neswick, R. S. (1997). Myra E. Levine: A theoretic basis for ET nursing. *Journal of Wound Ostomy Continence Nursing, 24*(1), 6–9.

Page, M. (2008). Nursing care and management of patients with sarcoidosis. *British Journal of Nursing, 17*(4), 252–257.

Palmer, J. A. (2006). Nursing implications for older adult patient education. *Plastic Surgical Nursing, 26*(4), 189–194.

Parse, R. R. (2004). Editorial: The many meanings of unitary: A plea for clarity. *Nursing Science Quarterly, 17*(4), 293.

Persky, G. J., Nelson, J. W., Watson, J., & Bent, K. (2008). Creating a profile of a nurse effective in caring. *Nursing Administration Quarterly, 32*(1), 15–20.

Phillips, K. D. (2002). Sister Callista Roy: Adaptation model. In A. M. Tomey & M. R. Alligood (Eds.), *Nursing theorists and their work* (5th ed., pp. 269–298). St. Louis: Mosby.

Phillips, K. D. (2006). Sister Callista Roy: Adaptation model. In A. M. Tomey & M. R. Alligood (Eds.), *Nursing theorists and their work* (6th ed., pp. 355–385). St. Louis: Mosby.

Piccoli, M., & Galvao, C. M. (2005). Pre-operative nursing visit: Methodological proposal based on Levine's conceptual model. *Revista Electronica de enfermagem, 7*(3), 365–371 (Portuguese).

Pipe, T. B. (2008). Illuminating the inner leadership journey by engaging intention and mindfulness as guided by caring theory. *Nursing Administration Quarterly, 32*(2), 117–125.

Pipe, T. B., Kelly, A., LeBrun, G., Atherton, P., & Robinson, C. (2008). A prospective descriptive study exploring hope, spiritual well-being, and quality of life in hospitalized patients. *MEDSURG Nursing, 17*(4), 247–253.

Pond, J. B., & Taney, G. (1991). Emergency care in a large university emergency department. In K. M. Schaefer & J. B. Pond (Eds.), *Levine's conservation model: A framework for nursing practice* (pp. 151–166). Philadelphia: Davis.

Rogers, S. (1996). Facilitative affiliation: Nurse–client interactions that enhance healing. *Issues in Mental Health Nursing, 17*(3), 171–184.

Rooda, L. A. (1992). The development of a conceptual model for multicultural nursing. *Journal of Holistic Nursing, 10*(4), 337–347.

Roper, N., Logan, W., & Tierney, A. J. (2000). *The Roper, Logan, Tierney model of nursing based on activities of living.* London: Churchill Livingstone.

Roy, C. (2009). *The Roy adaptation model* (3rd ed.). Upper Saddle River, NJ: Pearson.

Schaefer, K. M. (1991a). Developing a graduate program in nursing. In K. M. Schaefer & J. B. Pond (Eds.), *Levine's conservation model: A framework for nursing practice* (pp. 209–217). Philadelphia: Davis.

Schaefer, K. M. (1991b). Care of the patient with congestive heart failure. In K. M. Schaefer & J. B. Pond (Eds.), *Levine's conservation model: A framework for nursing practice* (pp. 119–130). Philadelphia: Davis.

Schaefer, K. M. (2002). Myra Estrin Levine: The conservation model. In A. M. Tomey & M. R. Alligood (Eds.), *Nursing theorists and their work* (5th ed., pp. 212–225). St. Louis: Mosby.

Schaefer, K. M., & Potylycki, M. J. S. (1993). Fatigue associated with congestive heart failure: Use of Levine's conservation model. *Journal of Advanced Nursing, 18*(2), 260–268.

Seiloff, C. L. (2002). Imogene King: Interacting systems framework and theory of goal attainment. In A. M. Tomey & M. R. Alligood (Eds.), *Nursing theorists and their work.* (pp. 336–355). St. Louis: Mosby.

Sieloff, C. L. (2006). Imogene King: Interacting systems framework and middle range theory of goal attainment. In A. M. Tomey & M. R. Alligood (Eds.), *Nursing theorists and their work* (pp. 297–317). St. Louis: Mosby.

Smith, M., Wright, B. W., & Fawcet, J. (2008). In Memory: A tribute to two giants of nursing conceptual models and theories. *Visions: Journal of Rogerian Nursing Science, 15*(1), 65–66.

Souza, E. F., De Martino, M. M. F., & Lopes, M. H. B. (2007). Nursing diagnoses in chronic renal patients using Imogene King's conceptual system as reference (Portuguese). *Revista da Escola de Emfermagem, 41*(4), 629–634.

Stevens, K. R., & Messmer, P. R. (2008). In remembrance of Imogene King, January 30, 1923–December 24, 2007: Imogene, a pioneer and dear colleague. *Nursing Outlook, 56*(3), 100–101.

Treolar, L., & Artinian, B. M. (2001). Populations affected by disability. In M. Neis & M. McEwen (Eds.), *Community health nursing.* Philadelphia: Saunders.

Vandall-Walker, V., Jensen, L., & Oberle, K. (2006). Lightening the load: Nursing support with family members of critically ill adults. *Dynamics of Critical Care: Canadian Association of Critical Care Nurses, 17*(2), 43–44.

Vukovitch, P. K., & Artinian, B. M. (2005). Justifying coercion. *Nursing Ethics, 12*(4), 370–380.

Watson, J. (1985). The *philosophy and science of caring* (pp. 9–10). Revised 1995. Boulder: Colorado Associated University Press.

Watson, J. (1988). *Nursing: Human science and human care: A theory of nursing.* New York: National League for Nursing Press.

Watson, J. (Ed.). (1994). *Applying the art and science of human caring.* New York: National League for Nursing Press.

Watson, J. (1996). Nursing, caring-healing paradigm. In Pesat, D. (Ed.), *Capsules of comments in psychiatric nursing.* Chicago: Mosby-Year Book.

Watson, J. (1999). *Postmodern nursing and beyond.* London: Churchill Livingstone.

Watson, J. (2005). *Caring science as sacred science.* Philadelphia: Davis.

Watson, J. (2008). *The philosophy and science of caring.* Boulder, CO: University Press of Colorado.

Wood, M. J. (1997). Foreword. In B. M. Artinian & M. M. Conger (Eds.), *The intersystem model* (pp. vii–viii). Thousand Oaks: Sage.

# 9

# Grand Nursing Theories Based on Unitary Process

## Evelyn Wills

*K*ristin Kowalski is a hospice nurse who wishes to expand the scope of her therapeutic practice. She desires to delve more deeply into holistic health care and nursing, having recently completed courses of study in herbal medicine, touch therapy, and holistic nursing. Kristin was aware that to practice independently she needs professional credentials that would be widely accepted; therefore, she applied to the graduate program of a nationally ranked nursing school at a large state university.

Because Kristin believes strongly in holistic nursing practice, for her master's degree she focused her study of nursing theories on those that look at the whole person and have a broad, nontraditional view of health. She was particularly interested in Rosemarie Parse's Human Becoming perspective because this viewpoint stresses the individual's way of being and becoming healthy.

Kristin was attracted to Parse's idea of true presence and wished to explore this concept as well as the rest of the perspective further. She hoped to eventually apply it to her practice and use it as the research framework for her thesis. For her thesis, Kristin wants to examine the experiences of nurses who practice therapeutic touch. She desires to learn their perceptions of how therapeutic touch interventions help their clients. She also wants to learn more about Parse's research method and hopes to use it for her study.

The term *simultaneity paradigm* was first coined by nursing theorist Rosemarie Parse (1987) to describe a group of theories that adhered to a unitary process perception of human beings. This group of theorists believed that humans are unitary beings: energy systems embedded in the universal energy system. Within this group of theories, human beings are seen as unitary, "whole, open and free to choose ways of becoming" (Parse, 1998, p. 6); and health is described as continuous human environmental interchanges (Newman, 1994).

The unitary process nursing model and two corollary theories are described in this chapter: Science of Unitary Human Beings (Rogers, 1994), Health as Expanding

Consciousness (Newman, 1999), and Human Becoming School of Thought (Parse, 1998). The three are grouped together because they are significantly different in their concepts, assumptions, and propositions when compared to the theories described in Chapters 7 and 8. They are universal in scope and relatively abstract.

## Martha Rogers: The Science of Unitary and Irreducible Human Beings

Martha E. Rogers first described her Theory of Unitary Man in 1961, and almost from the first there has been widespread controversy and debate among nursing theorists and scholars regarding her work (Phillips, 1994). Prior to Rogers, it was rare that anyone in nursing viewed human beings as anything other than the receivers of care by nurses and physicians. Furthermore, the health care system was organized by specialization in which health providers focused on discrete areas or functions (e.g., a dressing change, medication administration, health teaching), rather than on the whole person. As a result, it took many professionals working in isolation, none of whom knew the whole person, to care for patients. Rogers' (1970) insistence that the person was a "unitary energy system" in "continuous mutual interaction with the universal energy system," dramatically influenced nursing by encouraging nurses to consider the person as a whole entity (a unity) when planning and delivering care.

### BACKGROUND OF THE THEORIST

Martha Rogers was born on May 12, 1914 (the anniversary of Florence Nightingale's birth) (Dossey, 2000) in Dallas, Texas. She earned a diploma in nursing from Knoxville General Hospital in 1936 and a bachelor's degree from George Peabody College in Nashville, Tennessee in 1937. She later received a master's degree in public health nursing from Teachers College, Columbia University in New York, and a master's degree in public health and a Doctor of Science from The Johns Hopkins University in Baltimore, Maryland (Gunther, 2006).

Rogers became the head of the Division of Nursing of New York University (NYU) in 1954, where she focused on teaching and formulating and elaborating her theory (Hektor, 1989). She was teacher and mentor to an impressive list of nursing scholars and theorists, including Parse and Newman, whose works are described later in the chapter. Rogers continued her work and writing until her death in March 1994.

### PHILOSOPHICAL UNDERPINNINGS OF THE THEORY

The Science of Unitary and Irreducible Human Beings started as an abstract theory that was synthesized from theories of numerous sciences; therefore, it was deductively derived. Of particular importance was von Bertalanffy's theory on general systems that contributed the concepts of entropy and negentropy and posited that open systems are characterized by constant interaction with the environment. The work of Rapoport provided a background on open systems, and the work of Herrick contributed to the premise of evolution of human nature (Rogers, 1994).

Rogers' synthesis of the works of these scientists formed the basis of her proposition that human systems are open systems, embedded in larger, open environmental systems. She also brought in other concepts, including the idea that time is unidirectional, that living systems have pattern and organization, and that man is a sentient, thinking being, capable of awareness, feeling, and choosing. From all these theories, and from her personal study of nature, Rogers (1970) developed her original Theory of Unitary Man. She continuously refined and elaborated her theory, which she retitled Science of Unitary Humans (Rogers, 1990) and finally, shortly before her death, the Science of Unitary and Irreducible Human Beings (Rogers, 1994).

## MAJOR ASSUMPTIONS, CONCEPTS, AND RELATIONSHIPS

### Assumptions

Rogers presented several assumptions about man. These are as follows:

> Man is a unified whole possessing integrity and manifesting characteristics that are more than and different from the sum of his parts (Rogers, 1970, p. 47).
> Man and environment are continuously exchanging matter and energy with one another (Rogers, 1970, p. 54).
> The life process evolves irreversibly and unidirectionally along the space–time continuum (Rogers, 1970, p. 59).
> Pattern and organization identify man and reflect his innovative wholeness (Rogers, 1970, p. 65).
> Man is characterized by the capacity for abstraction and imagery, language and thought, sensation, and emotion (Rogers, 1970, p. 73).

Rogers (1990) later revised the term *man* to *human being* to coincide with the request for gender-neutral language in the social sciences and nursing science.

### Concepts

In Rogers' work, the unitary human being and the environment are the focus of nursing practice. Other central components are energy fields, openness, pandimensionality, and pattern; these she identified as the "building blocks" (Rogers, 1970, p. 226) of her system. Rogers also derived three other components for the model, which served as a basis of her work. These were based on principles of homeodynamics and were termed resonancy, helicy, and integrality (Rogers, 1990) (Box 9-1). Definitions of the nursing metaparadigm concepts and other important concepts in Rogers' work are listed in Table 9-1.

### Relationships

The Science of Unitary and Irreducible Human Beings is fundamentally abstract; therefore, specifically defined relationships differ from those in more linear theories. The major components of Rogers' model revolve around the building blocks (energy fields, openness, pattern, and pandimensionality) and the principles of homeodynamics (resonancy, helicy, and integrality). These explain the nature of, and direction of, the interactions between unitary human beings and the environment.

---

**BOX 9-1** *Principles of Homeodynamics Applied in Rogers' Theory*

1. Resonancy is continuous change from lower to higher frequency wave patterns in human and environmental fields.
2. Helicy is continuous innovative, unpredictable, increasing diversity of human and environmental field patterns.
3. Integrality is continuous mutual human and environmental field processes.

Source: Rogers (1990, p. 8).

TABLE 9-1 *Central Concepts of Rogers' Science of Unitary Human Beings*

| Concept | Definition |
|---------|-----------|
| Human–unitary human beings | "Irreducible, indivisible, multidimensional energy fields identified by pattern and manifesting characteristics that are specific to the whole and which cannot be predicted from the knowledge of the partns" (p. 7). |
| Health | "Unitary human health signifies an irreducible human field manifestation. It cannot be measured by the parameters of biology or physics or of the social sciences" (p. 10). |
| Nursing | "The study of unitary, irreducible, indivisible human and environmental fields: people and their world" (p. 6). Nursing is a learned profession that is both a science and an art. |
| Environmental field | "An irreducible, indivisible, pandimensional energy field identified by pattern and integral with the human field" (p. 7). |
| Energy field | "The fundamental unit of the living and the non-living. Field is a unifying concept. Energy signifies the dynamic nature of the field; a field is in continuous motion and is infinite" (p. 7). |
| Openness | Refers to qualities exhibited by open systems; human beings and their environment are open systems. |
| Pandimensional | "A nonlinear domain without spatial or temporal attributes" (p. 28). |
| Pattern | "The distinguishing characteristic of an energy field perceived as a single wave" (p. 7). |

Source: Rogers (1990).

Among the relationships that Rogers posited are that all things are integral in that their energy fields are in continuous mutual process and that pattern is the manifestation of the integrality of each entity and of the environmental energy field (Rogers, 1986). Other major relationships within Rogers' work are contained in the following statements:

> Humans and environment are interrelated in that neither "has an energy field," both are integral energy fields (Rogers, 1990, pp. 6–7).
>
> Manifestations of pattern emerge out of the human/environmental field mutual process and are continuously innovative (Rogers, 1990, p. 8).
>
> The group field is irreducible and indivisible to itself and integral with its own environmental field (Rogers, 1990, p. 8).

Nursing is concerned with maintaining and promoting health, preventing illness, and caring for the sick and the disabled. The purpose of nursing for Rogers (1986) is to help human beings achieve well-being within the potential of each individual, family, or group. Because human energy fields are complex, individualizing nursing services supports simultaneous human and environmental exchange, encouraging health (Rogers, 1990).

## USEFULNESS

Rogers' theory is a synthesis of phenomena that are important to nursing. It is an abstract, unified, and highly derived framework and does not define particular hypotheses or theories. Rather, it provides a worldview from which nurses may derive theories and hypotheses and propose relationships specific to different situations. In essence, the theory allows many options for studying humans as individuals and groups and for studying various situations in health as manifestations of pattern and innovation. Rogers' model stresses the unitary experience and provides an abstract philosophical framework that can guide nursing practice.

Rogers' theory has been evident in nursing education, scholarship, and practice for more than three decades. In education, among other programs, it has guided the nursing curriculum at NYU, where Rogers was head of the Division of Nursing in the 1970s. This resulted in the education of numerous nurses who use her theory in practice internationally (Hektor, 1989). In the area of nursing scholarship, several noted nursing theorists (i.e., Fitzpatrick, 1989; Newman, 1994; Parse, 1998) derived theories from Rogers' work.

In other scholarly works, Barrett (1989) derived a theory of power for nursing practice from Rogers' theory. She used several of Rogers' concepts (i.e., energy fields, openness, pattern, and four-dimensionality [now *pandimensionality*]) and the principles of resonancy, helicy, and integrality to form the theory of power. The theory of power as knowing participation in change consisted of awareness, choices, freedom to act intentionally, and involvement in creating changes, and was tested in research using Barrett's Power as Knowing Participation in Change test. Barrett's (1986) theory has recently been used in research on patterning of pain and power with guided imagery by Lewandowski (2004), who found that guided imagery was effective in reducing pain for chronic pain sufferers.

In practice settings, Rogerian practitioners employ the visible manifestations of Rogers' science. Barrett's (2004) practice in health patterning modalities is an example. Imagery is one repatterning modality she employs in assisting her clients with healing. She has written and presented her experiences with these modalities (Barrett, 2003, 2004). In other examples, Epstein (2003) created a program of audiotapes and CDs to assist people in self-healing through the use of imagery. Barnes and Adair (2002) found parallels with Rogers' Science of Unitary Human Beings in their work with their cognition-sensitive approach to dementia. Rogers' model, along with other theories, enhances a client-centered, family-focused, school-based family planning program (Porter, 1998).

Reed (2008) wrote about nursing time as a dimension of practice, research, and theory. Heggie, Garon, Kodiath, and Kelly (1994) discussed the process of integrating Rogers' theory into nursing practice at the San Diego Veterans Affairs Medical Center. These nurses found implementing the model in practice settings to be challenging and complex, but initial evaluations were positive.

## TESTABILITY

Because of the model's abstractness, Rogers' (1990) work is not directly testable, but it is testable in principle. Theories are being derived from the Science of Unitary Man and hypotheses to test those theories (Barrett, 1989; Cody, 1991; Kwekkeboom, Huseby-Moore, & Ward, 1998; Phillips, 1990).

Numerous research studies using Rogers' model have been completed and reported in the nursing literature. A plethora of these studies can be found in *Visions: The Journal of Rogerian Nursing Science*. In addition, a book, *Patterns of Rogerian Knowing* (Madrid, 1997) was published detailing a number of research studies. Madrid and Winstead-Fry (2001) found in a focused review of literature that from 1990 through 2000, twenty-eight research studies on therapeutic touch were published in peer-reviewed journals and nine of them were based on the Science of Unitary Human Beings. Nine additional research studies included Rogers' model as explanation for the underlying processes of therapeutic touch and its relation to energy fields and energy transfer. Examples of some recent nursing studies using Rogers' theory are listed in Box 9-2.

## PARSIMONY

This theory is relatively parsimonious. The model has five key definitions. These, combined with the three principles of homeodynamics and the six assumptions about

**BOX 9-2** *Examples of Research Studies Using Rogers' Theory*

Cowling, W. R., & Shattell, M. M. (2007). Research as the researchers story. *Nursing Science Quarterly, 20*(4), 315–320.

Davis, L. (2006). The experience of time and nursing practice. *Journal of Rogerian Nursing Science, 14*(1), 36–44.

Kim, T. S., Kim, C., Park, K. M., Park, Y. S., & Lee, B. S. (2008). The relation of power and well-being in Korean adults. *Nursing Science quarterly, 21*(3), 247–254.

Mahoney, J. (2006). Do you feel like you belong? An online versus face to face pilot study.

*Journal of Rogerian Nursing Science, 14*(1), 16–26.

Rushing, A. M. (2008). The unitary life pattern of persons experiencing serenity in recovery from alcohol and drug addiction. *Advances in Nursing Science, 31*(3), 198–210.

Todaro-Francesci, V. (2006). Studying synchronicity related to dead loved ones AKA after-death communication: Martha, what do you think? *Nursing Science Quarterly, 19*(3), 297–298.

human beings, are the major elements of the work. Despite its simplicity, however, it is difficult for many nurses to comprehend because the concepts are extremely abstract. Nurses who wish their research and practice to be guided by Rogers' model will benefit from studying with a Rogerian scholar who uses the model regularly.

## VALUE IN EXTENDING NURSING SCIENCE

Rogers' contributions to nursing have been noted in the nursing literature and she has had a significant influence on scientific inquiry in professional nursing practice. The major value of Rogers' work has been extending nursing science by challenging traditional ways of thinking about the world and nursing. She moved beyond a focus on such concepts and principles as adaptation, biopsychosocial beings, causal/probabilistic views, and the human-as-sum-of-parts thinking that had been common in nursing science (Parse, 2003; Phillips, 1990; Rogers, 1990). The contribution to nursing science of the Science of Unitary and Irreducible Human Beings theory is that it carries nursing into areas that are impossible to study using linear, three-dimensional, and reductionistic methods.

## Margaret Newman: Health as Expanding Consciousness

Margaret Newman reported that she became interested in theory when asked to speak at a nursing conference in 1978 (George, 2002). She published a theory of health a year later (Newman, 1979) and *Health as Expanding Consciousness* in 1986. She revised this work in 1994 and 1999. Newman has published extensively on her theory and theoretical issues in books, book chapters, and articles (Newman, 1990a, 1990b, 1994, 1995, 1999, 2005, 2008a, 2008b).

Newman's *Health as Expanding Consciousness* is one of the most recent nursing theories; her work builds on the work of Rogers and others. Because of its similarity to Rogers' theory, particularly with regard to its conceptualizations of person, nursing, and the environment, it is included here among the unitary process theories. In 2008, Newman brought out a new book which she titled *Transforming Presence: The Difference Nursing Makes* (Newman, 2008a).

## BACKGROUND OF THE THEORIST

As a young woman, Margaret Newman was involved in caring for her mother, who suffered from amyotrophic lateral sclerosis. She explained that it was during this period that she came to know her mother in ways that would have been impossible otherwise (Newman, 1986). This experience led Newman to study nursing, and she enrolled at the University of Tennessee where she completed her bachelor's degree in 1962. She received a master's degree from the University of California, San Francisco, in 1964, and a doctorate from NYU in 1971 (Brown, 2006).

Newman has served on the faculty at the University of Tennessee (which named her an outstanding alumnus), NYU, Pennsylvania State University, and the University of Minnesota. She is currently professor emeritus at the University of Minnesota, Minneapolis. Her work has been recognized internationally, and she has received numerous awards and honors both in the United States and abroad (Jones, 2007b).

## PHILOSOPHICAL UNDERPINNINGS OF THE THEORY

While at NYU, Newman attended seminars taught by Martha Rogers, and she stated that Rogers' Science of Unitary Human Beings was the basis of her theory of Health as Expanding Consciousness. She also noted that, among others, Itzhak Bentov's explanation of the concept of evolution of consciousness, Arthur Young's work on pattern recognition, and David Bohm's theory of implicate order brought perspective to her thoughts and ideas (Newman, 1986).

## MAJOR ASSUMPTIONS, CONCEPTS, AND RELATIONSHIPS

### Assumptions

As a student of Rogers, Newman believed that "the human is unitary, that is, cannot be divided into parts, and is inseparable from the larger unitary field" (Newman, 1994, p. xviii). She saw humans as open energy systems in continual contact with a universe of open systems (i.e., the environment). Additionally, humans are continuously active in evolving their own pattern of the whole (i.e., health) and are intuitive as well as cognitive and affective beings (Marchione, 1995). She further posited that "persons as individuals, and human beings as a species, are identified by their patterns of consciousness" and that "the person does not possess consciousness—the person is consciousness" (Newman, 1999, p. 33).

In describing health, Newman (1994) explained that health encompasses illness or pathology and that pathologic conditions can be considered manifestations of the pattern of the individual. In addition, the pattern of the individual that eventually manifests itself as pathology is primary and exists prior to structural or functional changes; removal of the pathology in itself will not change the pattern of the individual. Finally, she noted an assumption that changes occur simultaneously and not in linear fashion (Newman, 1994).

### Concepts

Newman built on Rogers' definitions for human and environment, but she redefined nursing and health. Health is an essential component of the theory of Health as Expanding Consciousness and is seen as a process of developing awareness of self and the environment together with increasing the ability to perceive alternatives and respond in a variety of ways (Newman, 1986). Nursing is described as "caring in the human health experience" (Newman, 1994, p. 139). Other central concepts in Newman's

## TABLE 9-2 *Central Concepts of Newman's Health as Expanding Consciousness*

| Concept | Definition |
| --- | --- |
| Nursing | The act of assisting people to use the power within them to evolve toward higher levels of consciousness. Nursing is directed towards recognizing the patterns of the person in interaction with the environment and accepting the interaction as a process of evolving consciousness. Nursing facilitates the process of pattern recognition by a rhythmic connecting of the nurse with the client for the purpose of illuminating the pattern and discovering the rules of a higher level of organization. |
| Health | The expanding of consciousness; an evolving pattern of the whole of life. A unitary process, a fluctuating pattern of rhythmic phenomena that includes illness within the pattern of energy. Sickness can "be the shock that reorganizes the relationships of the person's pattern in a more harmonious way" (Newman, 1999, p. 11). |
| Person | A dynamic pattern of energy and an open system in interaction with the environment. Persons can be defined by their patterns of consciousness. |
| Consciousness | The information of the system; consciousness refers to the capacity of the system to interact with the environment, and includes thinking, feeling, and processing the information embedded in physiologic systems. |
| Expanding consciousness | The evolving pattern of the whole. Expanding consciousness is the increasing complexity of the living system and is characterized by illumination and pattern recognition resulting in transformation and discovery. Expanding consciousness is health. |
| Integration via movement | The natural condition of living creatures. Consciousness is expressed in movement, which is the way that the organism interacts with the environment and exerts control over it. Movement patterns reflect and communicate the person's inner pattern and organization. Changes in the person's health patterns may be reflected in changes in their movement rhythms. |
| Pattern | Relatedness, which is characterized by movement, diversity, and rhythm. Pattern is a scheme, design, or framework and is seen in person–environment interactions. Pattern is recognized on the basis of variation and may not be seen all at once. It is manifest in the way one moves, speaks, talks, and relates with others. |
| Pattern recognition | The insight or recognition of a principle, realization of a truth, or reconciliation of a duality. Pattern recognition illuminates the possibilities for action and is the key to the process of evolving to a higher level of consciousness. |
| Time and space | Temporal patterns that are specific to individuals and define their ways of being within their world. Patterns of health may be detected in temporal patterns. |

Sources: Marchione (1995); Newman (1999).

theory are pattern, pattern recognition, movement, and time and space. Definitions for these and other concepts specific to the theory are presented in Table 9-2.

### Relationships

A fundamental proposition in Newman's model is the idea that health and illness are synthesized as "health." Indeed, the fusion of one state of being (disease) with its opposite (nondisease) results in what can be regarded as health (Newman, 1979, 2008a).

To Newman, health is pattern. *Pattern* is information that depicts the whole and pattern recognition is essential. Pattern recognition involves moving from looking at parts to looking at patterns. Expanding consciousness occurs as a process of pattern recognition (insight) following a synthesis of contradictory events or disturbances in the flow of daily living. Pattern recognition comes from within the observer, and patterns unfold over time and cannot be predicted with certainty. Understanding the meaning of relationships through pattern recognition is important in providing care because patterns are the essence of a unitary view of health.

Newman (1979) also wrote of the interrelatedness of time, space, and movement. She explained that time and space have a complementary relationship, and movement is the means by which space and time become reality. Movement is seen as a reflection of consciousness; time is a function of movement; and time is a measure of consciousness (Newman, 2008b). Man is in a constant state of motion and is constantly changing; movement through time and space gives man his unique perception of reality. Constant change is visible currently as technology, such as iphones and Blackberries, that give individuals immediate, conscious, and unrestricted access to information; and MP3 players that provide immediate access to music and other entertainment.

## USEFULNESS

Newman (1994) believed that theory must be derived from practice and theory must inform practice. To illustrate this relationship, she proposed a model for practice that she derived from her theory (Newman, 1990b).

Her work has been used by nurses in a number of settings, providing care for different types of clients, and for a variety of interventions. For example, Newman (1995) reported that her theory guided her nursing practice with families. In another instance, her work was selected to direct practice among case managers at Tucson, Arizona's, Carondelet, St. Mary's Hospital (Ethridge, 1991; Ethridge & Lamb, 1989). In describing the application of the theory in case management, Newman, Lamb, and Michaels (1991) explained that the theory–practice link helped facilitate the complementary link between nursing and medicine.

Pharris and Endo (2007) described the nature of Health as Expanding Consciousness with ill elders, groups and communities, and systems. They look forward to nursing in 2050 using the Health as Expanding Consciousness theory. Brown, Chen, Mitchell, and Province (2007) studied help-seeking by older husbands who were caring for wives with dementia using a grounded theory approach. They found that help-seeking for the sample was complex and gender-specific. They came to understand that interventions to assist the male caregivers must be gender-specific and complement their help-seeking patterns.

In the recent past, Neill (2005) completed an investigation into patterns of lives of women with multiple sclerosis. Jones (2007a) discussed Newman's theory in knowledge development for nursing practice, and in 2008, Musker published her work on life transitions in menopausal women. These studies indicate that the ideal of health as expanding consciousness continues to generate caring interventions in numerous populations.

## TESTABILITY

Newman's theory has been the basis for an impressive number of doctoral dissertations. Other research projects have tested parts of the theory (i.e., time and movement) or used it as a framework. Most of the nursing studies using Newman's theory found in recent literature were qualitative in nature. Pickard (2000), for example, expanded Newman's praxis method, a hermeneutic dialectic process, "to include

---

**BOX 9-3** *Examples of Research Studies Using Newman's Health as Expanding Consciousness*

Brown, J. W., Chen, S., Mitchell, C., & Province, A. (2007). Help-seeking by older husbands caring for wives with dementia. *Journal of Advanced Nursing, 59*(4), 352–360.

Hayes, M. O., & Jones, D. (2007). Health as expanding consciousness: Pattern recognition and incarcerated mothers, a transforming experience. *Journal of Forensic Nursing, 3*(2), 61–66.

McCarthy, C. A. (2007). The evolving pattern of urban African American adolescents during pregnancy. Doctoral Dissertation Weidner University. UMI Order AA13290060.

Neill, J. (2005). Health as expanding consciousness: Seven women living with multiple sclerosis or rheumatoid arthritis. *Nursing Science Quarterly, 18*(4), 334–343.

Peters-Lewis, A. (2006). How the strong survive: Health as expanding consciousness and the life experiences of black Caribbean women. Dissertation, Boston College. UMI Order AA31209829.

Zust, B. L. (2006). Death as a transformation of wholeness: An "aha" experience of health as expanding consciousness. *Nursing Science Quarterly, 19*(1), 57–60.

---

creative movement as a mode of expression" (p. 150). Findings indicated that movement supported women's self-awareness and expanding consciousness at midlife. The author also described activities of consciousness as choosing, balancing, accepting, and letting go. Pickard (2002) studied family reflections of living through sudden death of a child; Endo, Miyahara, Suzuki, and Ohmasa (2005) studied the process of partnering a researcher with a practicing nurse at a Japanese cancer center. They found that the nurses encountered a transformative experience with patients when the nursing interventions in everyday practice were enacted in the unitary perspective.

In other studies, Karian, Jankowski, and Beal (1998) examined the lived experience of survivors of childhood cancer by studying their patterns of interaction with family members and the environment. The researchers concluded that pattern recognition and insight into the meaning of the family pattern assisted in a process of transformation; most families found meaning in their patterns. Berry (2004) found a link between theory, research, and practice in her research with women maintaining weight loss. She found that a model of change supported the understanding of lifestyle change. Box 9-3 lists recent research studies that were conducted using Newman's model.

## PARSIMONYS

Newman's model consists of two major concepts, health and consciousness, and thus it seems parsimonious. Despite this seeming simplicity, however, the theory is one of great complexity (George, 2002). Those who do not comprehend the simultaneity paradigm may wander in its enfolded relationships. The real complexity relates to the nature of the relationships between and among the concepts and to its abstractness.

## VALUE IN EXTENDING NURSING SCIENCE

The focus of Newman's work is on the person, client, individual, and family. It places the client and nurse as integrated actors in understanding the client's health as consciousness. It also requires the understanding that health and disease are the same and not separate in the life of the individual (Newman, 1994).

As illustrated by the examples from the literature presented, Newman's model has been successfully used in nursing practice and research. Newman's view can be applied in any setting, and research and practice application are underway to further verify its importance to the discipline (Jones, 2007b).

## Rosemarie Parse: The Theory of Human Becoming

Rosemarie Parse is a noted nursing scholar and prolific author. She first published her theory of nursing, *Man-Living-Health*, in 1981, and has continually revised the work. In 1992, Parse changed the name to the Theory of Human Becoming. She is the author of at least eight books and numerous articles. Her works have been translated into Danish, Finnish, French, German, Japanese, Korean, and other languages.

## BACKGROUND OF THE THEORIST

Parse was educated at Duquesne University in Pittsburgh, Pennsylvania, and earned her master's and doctoral degrees from the University of Pittsburgh. Some years later, she became dean of the College of Nursing at Duquesne, and is currently Professor and Niehoff Chair at Loyola University in Chicago, Illinois. She is the founder and editor of *Nursing Science Quarterly*, and president of Discovery International, which sponsors international nursing theory conferences. She is also the founder of the Institute of Human Becoming, where she teaches the ontologic, epistemologic, and methodologic aspects of the Human Becoming school of thought. The Human Becoming perspective is honored and acknowledged in colleges of nursing worldwide.

## PHILOSOPHICAL UNDERPINNINGS OF THE THEORY

Parse synthesized the Theory of Human Becoming from principles and concepts from Rogers' work. She also incorporated concepts and principles from existential phenomenological thought as expressed by Heidegger, Sartre, and Merleau-Ponty (Parse, 1981). The theory comes from her experience in nursing and from a synthesis of theoretical principles of human sciences.

## MAJOR ASSUMPTIONS, CONCEPTS, AND RELATIONSHIPS

### Assumptions

As with many of the major concepts, the major assumptions of Parse's theory come from Rogers' Science of Unitary Human Beings and from existential phenomenology. Assumptions about humans and becoming are shown in Box 9-4.

Parse synthesized the nine assumptions of humans and becoming into three broad statements:

1. Human becoming is freely choosing personal meaning in situations in the intersubjective process of living value priorities.
2. Human becoming is cocreating rhythmical patterns of relating in mutual process with the universe.
3. Human becoming is cotranscending multidimensionally with the emerging possibles (Parse, 1998, pp. 19–20, 29).

### Concepts

A number of concepts from Rogers' theory and from existential phenomenalism are inherent in Parse's theory. Concepts from Rogers' work include energy field, openness, pattern, and pandimensionality (Parse, 1998). From existential phenomenalism

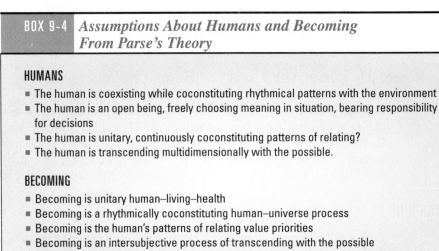

**BOX 9-4** *Assumptions About Humans and Becoming From Parse's Theory*

**HUMANS**

- The human is coexisting while coconstituting rhythmical patterns with the environment
- The human is an open being, freely choosing meaning in situation, bearing responsibility for decisions
- The human is unitary, continuously coconstituting patterns of relating?
- The human is transcending multidimensionally with the possible.

**BECOMING**

- Becoming is unitary human–living–health
- Becoming is a rhythmically coconstituting human–universe process
- Becoming is the human's patterns of relating value priorities
- Becoming is an intersubjective process of transcending with the possible
- Becoming is unitary human's emerging

Source: Parse (1998, pp. 19–20).

Parse (1998) drew coconstitution, which explains that the "meaning in any situation is related to the particular constituents of that situation" (p. 17). Additionally, she identified and defined a number of concepts that are unique to the theory. Table 9-3 presents definitions of nursing's metaparadigm concepts and other significant concepts from Parse's theory.

**Relationships**

From the major concepts, Parse (1987) outlined three principles in the theory:

1. Structuring meaning multidimensionality is cocreating reality through the languaging of valuing and imaging.
2. Cocreating rhythmical patterns of relating is living the paradoxical unity of revealing–concealing and enabling–limiting while connecting–separating.
3. Cotranscending with the possibles is powering the unique ways of originating in the process of transforming (Parse, 1987).

Additionally, there are three theoretical structures that are designed to guide practice and research:

1. Powering is a way of revealing–concealing imaging.
2. Originating is a manifestation of enabling–limiting valuing.
3. Transforming unfolds in the languaging of connecting–separating (Parse, 1981).

Nurses guide individuals and families in choosing possibilities in changing the health process; this is accomplished by intersubjective participation with the clients. Practice focuses on illuminating meaning, and the nurse acts as a guide to choose possibilities in the changing health experiences (Parse, 1981, 2001, 2002).

Practitioners using Parse's method do not focus on changing an individual's behavior to fit a defined nursing process and do not attempt to label them with possibly erroneous nursing diagnoses. Rather, they practice from the understanding that the human–universe process involves the nurse's true presence with the person and the family. The nurse "dwells with the rhythms of the person and family" (Parse, 1995, p. 83) as they move through the experience.

TABLE 9-3 *Central Concepts of Parse's Theory of Human Becoming*

| Concept | Definition |
|---|---|
| Humans | Intentional beings involved with their world, having a fundamental nature of knowing, being present, and open to their world (Parse, 1998). The unitary human is one who coparticipates in the universe in creating becoming and who is whole, open, and free to choose ways of becoming. |
| Health | A way of being in the world; it is not a continuum of healthy to ill, nor is it a dichotomy of health or illness, rather it is the living of day-to-day ways of being. |
| Nursing | Grounded in the view that the human is a unitary being who is free to choose in situations, nursing is guiding humans toward ways of being, finding meaning in situations, choosing ways of cocreating their own health, and living true presence in the day-to-dayness of the person's life. |
| Environment | The world, the universe, and those who occupy spaces along with others who freely choose to be in the situation. |
| Meaning | An ever-changing interpretation one gives to what is valued and the ways in which these interpretations reflect the person's reality. |
| Rhythmicity | The cadent, mutual patterning of the human–universe mutual process. |
| Transcendence | Reaching beyond the possibles–the hopes and dreams envisioned in multidimensional experiences. |
| Imaging | Picturing meanings from both concrete experience and from imagined experience; this imaging is both spontaneous to and personal to each individual's worldview. |
| Valuing | A person's choosing, prizing, and acting on those symbols that have meaning in the person's life. |
| Languaging | Sharing valued images through symbols of words, gestures, gaze, touch, and posture; the way human beings represent personal structures of reality. |
| Powering | The pushing–resisting process of affirming–not affirming in the light of nonbeing. |
| Originating | Inventing new ways of conforming–nonconforming in the certainty–uncertainty of living. |
| Transforming | Shifting the view of the familiar–unfamiliar, the changing of change in coconstituting anew in a deliberate way. |

Sources: Parse (1995, 1998, 2007).

## USEFULNESS

Parse's theory has been a guide for practice in health care settings in Canada, Finland, South Korea, Sweden, the United States, and other countries. Additionally, Parse's method for research, a qualitative method of inquiry, titled "the human becoming hermeneutic method" (Barrett, 2002, p. 53), has been selected by nurse scholars in Australia, Canada, Denmark, Finland, Greece, Italy, Japan, South Korea, Sweden, the United Kingdom, and the United States. Legault and Ferguson-Pare (1999) discussed application of Parse's theory to guide practice in an acute care surgical setting. The authors concluded that there were positive patterns of change in nursing practice after implementing the guidelines; nursing care was more client-centered and more considerate of the individual and family experiences. Similarly, Kelley (1999) used Parse's theory to evaluate the practice of advanced practice nurses and found it to be beneficial. Practice regulation in one state, South Dakota, has adopted a decisioning model based on human becoming (Benedict, Bunkers, Damgaard, Hohman, & Vander Woude, 2000). This is the first theory-based model of this sort in the nation (Bournes, Bunkers, & Welch, 2004).

| BOX 9-5 | *Examples of Current Research Studies Using Parse's Human Becoming Theory* |

Baumann, S. (2008). Wisdom, compassion, and courage in the *Wizard of Oz:* A humanbecoming hermeneutic study. *Nursing Science Quarterly, 21*(4), 322–329.

Dempsey, L. F. (2008). A qualitative descriptive exploratory study of feeling confined using Parse's humanbecoming school of thought. *Nursing Science Quarterly, 21*(2), 140–149.

Doucet, T. J. (2008). Having faith: A Parse research method study. *Nursing Science Quarterly, 21*(4), 343–352.

Hayden, S. J. (2007). Laughing: A Parse research method study. Dissertation, Ph.D., University of Chicago. UMI Order AAI3295453.

Kostas-Poulson, E. A. (2007). Persisting while wanting to change: A Parse method research study. Dissertation, Ph.D., Loyola University of Chicago. UMI order AAI3295462.

Parse, R. R. (2007). Hope in "Rita Hayworth and Shawshank Redemption": A human becoming hermeneutic study. *Nursing Science Quarterly, 20*(2), 148–154.

Welch, A. J. (2007). The phenomenon of taking life day by day: Using Parse's method. *Nursing Science Quarterly, 20*(3), 265–272.

In describing this group, the authors concluded that "health is an abiding vitality emanating through moments of rhapsodic reverie in generating fulfillment" (Wondoloski & Davis, 1991, p. 113).

Researchers studying within the Parse method viewed hope from the perspective of persons worldwide, and a significant amount of their research has been published. Bunkers and Daly (1999) examined the lived experience of hope for families living with coronary disease in Australia. Hope was also described in persons from Wales (Pilkington & Millar, 1999) and persons in Finland (Toikkanen & Muurinen, 1999). In more recent works, Milton (2004) brings out the importance of patient's stories as referents of their lived experiences as they heal. Noh (2004) studied quality of life for persons living with serious mental illness. Their research involved the lived experience of the person with mental illness and was conducted within the Parse method (based on existential phenomenology). Noh (2004) found that the meanings uncovered in the analysis were the paradoxes of living. A small sample of the numerous current studies of other aspects of human experience within Parse's human becoming perspective are listed in Box 9-5.

## PARSIMONY

Parse's model is comparatively parsimonious. Although the theory has many concepts, assumptions, and principles, they are organized together in a logical, balanced way to explain human ways of being. With careful study, the theory lends itself to scholarly comprehension. The theory is abstract and complex, however, and much of the terminology is unfamiliar to most nurses. As a result, the theory requires careful study by those who wish to study human ways of being and becoming (Hickman, 2002). Students who want this model to guide their research and practice might consider contacting Parse and or one of her students for assistance to fully understand this perspective.

## VALUE IN EXTENDING NURSING SCIENCE

The principal value of the human becoming perspective is the worldview that sees humans as intentional beings, freely choosing to live within paradoxical ways of being. It is a unique way to view health and gives insight into how individuals create their own destiny.

Practice and research in the human becoming perspective are quite different from those espoused in the other nursing perspectives. By living true presence with their clients, nurses guide and cocreate ways of being that enable choosing health. The amount of literature depicting use of Parse's work is multiplying rapidly and support for the human becoming perspective is growing. It has become evident that time and continued research is having a significant effect on the adoption of the perspective to the discipline of nursing.

## Summary

The models presented in this chapter are considerably different from those described in the previous chapters. Additionally, significant similarities and differences are evident among these three models. Table 9-5 summarizes some of these by comparing definitions of the metaparadigm concepts. As Table 9-5 shows, the conceptualization of human beings is similar because Rogers heavily influenced both Newman and Parse. On the other hand, Parse was more specific when describing the environment and

TABLE 9-5 *Comparison of Concepts Common to the Unitary Process Nursing Theories*

| Author and Model | Human | Health | Environment | Nursing |
|---|---|---|---|---|
| Rogers: Unitary Human Beings (Rogers, 1990) | A sentient, unitary being; a multidimensional irreducible energy field known by pattern manifestation, and who cannot be known by the sum of parts. | Signifies an irreducible human field manifestation. | "An irreducible, indivisible, multidimensional energy field identified by pattern … integral with the human field" (p. 7). | A learned profession, a science and an art, whose uniqueness lies in concern for human beings. |
| Newman: Health as Expanding Consciousness (Newman, 1999) | Accepts the definition of human as stated by Rogers. | Health is a unitary process, a fluctuating pattern of rhythmic phenomena. Health includes illness within the pattern of energy. | Universal energy system as in Rogers' Science of Unitary Human Beings. | Assist persons to use innate power to evolve toward a higher level of consciousness. Nurses facilitate pattern recognition in this process. |
| Parse: Human Becoming (Parse, 1998) | Intentional beings involved with their world, having a fundamental nature of knowing, being present, and open to their world. The unitary human is one who "coparticipates in the universe in creating becoming and who is whole, open, free to choose ways of becoming" (p. 6). | A way of being in the world; it is not a continuum of healthy to ill, nor is it a dichotomy of health or illness, rather it is the living of day-to-day ways of being. | The world, the universe, and those who occupy spaces along with others who freely choose to be in the situation. | Guides humans toward ways of being, finding meaning in situations, and choosing ways of cocreating their own health. Nurses live true presence in the day-to-dayness of the person's life. |

Newman was much more explicit in her discussions of health. Perhaps the greatest difference, however, relates to how they view nurses and nursing. Those wishing to use these theories should study these concepts closely and seek to apply them in their practice and research. When employing the research methods, which are unique, close work with the researchers or their former students will assist the novice researcher to develop the depth of effort that is required (Welch, 2004).

Nurses, such as Kristin from the opening case study, who prefer to view the person as a unitary being and who have a comprehensive view of health, often find the theories from the simultaneity paradigm fascinating and helpful. These works have been extremely enlightening and helpful for the discipline of nursing, and all three have many adherents worldwide. A large and growing body of research explores patterns of lived experiences, and health perspectives based on them, and the expanding topics of study currently enhance nursing science and will continue to do so into the future.

## LEARNING ACTIVITIES

1. Select one of the theories described and apply it in developing comprehensive patterns of nursing care for young teenagers who are becoming first-time mothers. Consider all of the issues they encounter as they prepare for the birth of their babies. Share findings with classmates.

2. Select a different theory from the one used in the above case and apply it in developing comprehensive patterns of nursing care for the family of an elderly client with Alzheimer's disease. Compare the two models for ease of application.

3. Reflect on a case or situation from your personal practice or experience. Apply one of the theories to the situation. How does the perspective from the theory alter how you view the situation? Are nursing interventions the same? Why or why not?

4. Construct a research question that fits one of the theories in this chapter. How will you name the research and construct the question? What would be a likely method of study in the theoretical perspective you have chosen?

## INTERNET RESOURCES

Newman:

http://www.healthasexpandingconsciousness.org/index.html

http://www.healthasexpandingconsciousness.org/biography/biography.html

http://www.healthasexpandingconsciousness.org/overview/overview.html

Parse:

http://www.humanbecoming.org/index.html

http://www.humanbecoming.org/site/default.html

Rogers:

http://www.societyofrogerianscholars.org/biography_mer.html

http://www.societyofrogerianscholars.org/news.html

## REFERENCES

Barnes, S. J., & Adair, B. (2002). The cognition-sensitive approach to dementia. Parallels with the science of unitary human beings. *Journal of Psychosocial Nursing and Mental Health Services, 40*(11), 30–37.

Barrett, E. A. M. (1986). Investigation of the principle of helicy: The relationship of human field motion and power. In V. M. Malinski (Ed.), *Explorations in Martha Rogers' Science of Unitary Human Beings* (pp. 173–188). Norwalk, CT: Appleton-Century-Crofts.

Barrett, E. A. M. (1989). A nursing theory of power for nursing practice. In J. Riehl-Siska (Ed.), *Conceptual models for nursing practice* (3rd ed., pp. 207–217). Norwalk, CT: Appleton & Lange.

Barrett, E. A. M. (2002). What is nursing science? *Nursing Science Quarterly, 15*(1), 51–60.

Barrett, E. A. M. (November 15, 2003). *Imagery: Experiencing pandimensional awareness*. Proceedings of Conference of the Society of Rogerian Scholars, Emerging Pattern in a Changing World, Savannah, GA.

Barrett, E. A. M. (2004). *Imagery: Experiencing pandimensional awareness*. Retrieved from http://medweb.uwcm.ac.uk/martha/barrettpaper.htm.

Benedict, L., Bunkers, S. S., Damgaard, G., Hohman, M., & Vander Woude, D. (2000). The South Dakota theory-based regulatory decisioning model. *Nursing Science Quarterly, 13*(2), 167–171.

Berry, D. (2004). An emerging model of behavior change in women maintaining weight loss. *Nursing Science Quarterly, 17*(3), 242–252.

Bournes, E. A., Bunkers, S. S., & Welch, A. J. (2004). Human becoming: Scope and challenge. *Nursing Science Quarterly, 17*(3), 227–232.

Brown, J. W. (2006). Margaret A. Newman: Model of Health. In A. M. Tomey & M. R. Alligood (Eds.), *Nursing theorists and their work* (6th ed., pp. 497–521). St. Louis: Mosby.

Brown, J. W., Chen, S., Mitchell, C., & Province, A. (2007). Help-seeking by older husbands caring for wives with dementia. *Journal of Advanced Nursing, 59*(4), 352–360.

Bunkers, S. S. (2004). Socrates' questions: A focus for nursing. *Nursing Science Quarterly, 17*(3), 212–218.

Bunkers, S. S., & Daly, J. (1999). The lived experience of hope for Australian families living with coronary disease. In R. R. Parse (Ed.). *Hope: An international perspective* (pp. 45–61). Sudbury, MA: Jones & Bartlett and National League for Nursing Press.

Cody, W. K. (1991). Multidimensionality, its meaning and significance. *Nursing Science Quarterly, 4*, 140–141.

Cody, W. K. (1999). True presence with families living with HIV disease. In R. R. Parse (Ed.), *Illuminations: The human becoming theory in practice and research* (pp. 115–133). New York: National League for Nursing Press.

Cody, W. K., Hudepol, J. H., & Brinkman, K. S. (1999). True presence with a child and his family. In R. R. Parse (Ed.), *Illuminations: The human becoming theory in practice and research* (pp. 135–146). New York: National League for Nursing Press.

Dossey, B. M. (2000). *Florence Nightingale: Mystic, visionary, healer*. Springhouse, PA: Springhouse.

Endo, E., Miyahara, T., Suzuki, S., & Ohmasa, T. (2005). Partnering of researcher and practicing nurses for transformative nursing. *Nursing Science Quarterly, 18*(2), 138–145.

Epstein, G. (2003). The natural laws of self healing: Harnessing your inner imaging power to restore health and reach spirit. Audiotapes and CDs. Niles, IL: Nightingale-Conant.

Ethridge, P. (1991). A nursing HMO: Carondelet St. Mary's experience. *Nursing Management, 22*(7), 22–27.

Ethridge, P., & Lamb, G. S. (1989). Professional nursing case management improves quality, access and costs. *Nursing Management, 20*(3), 30–35.

Fitzpatrick, J. J. (1989). A life perspective rhythm model. In J. J. Fitzpatrick & A. L. Whall (Eds.), *Conceptual model of nursing: Analysis and application* (2nd ed., pp. 401–407). Princeton, NJ: Appleton-Century-Crofts.

Futrell, M., Wondolowski, C., & Mitchell, G. (1993). Aging in the oldest old living in Scotland: A phenomenological study. *Nursing Science Quarterly, 6*(4), 189–194.

George, J. B. (2002). Health as expanding consciousness: Margaret Newman. In J. B. George (Ed.), *Nursing theories: The base for professional nursing practice* (5th ed., pp. 519–538). Upper Saddle River, NJ: Prentice-Hall.

Gunther, M. E. (2006). Martha E. Rogers. In A. M. Tomey and M. R. Alligood (Eds.), *Nursing theorists and their work* (5th ed., pp. 244–266). St. Louis: Mosby.

Heggie, J., Garon, M., Kodiath, M., & Kelly, A. (1994). Implementing the science of unitary human beings at the San Diego Veterans Affairs medical Center. In M. Madrid & E. A. M. Barrett (Eds.), *Rogers' scientific art of nursing practice* (pp. 285–304). New York: National League for Nursing Press.

Hektor, L. M. (1989). Martha E. Rogers: A life history. *Nursing Science Quarterly, 2*(2), 63–73.

Hickman, J. S. (2002). Theory of Human Becoming: Rosemarie Rizzo Parse. In J. B. George (Ed.), *Nursing theories: The base for professional nursing practice* (5th ed., pp. 427–462). Upper Saddle River, NJ: Prentice-Hall.

Jonas, C. (1999). True presence through music for persons living with their dying. In R. R. Parse (Ed.), *Illuminations: The human becoming theory in practice and research* (pp. 97–104). New York: National League for Nursing Press.

Jones, D. A. (2007a). Newman's health as expanding consciousness. *Nursing Science Quarterly, 19*(4), 330–332.

Jones, D. (2007b). Margaret A. Newman over the years. *Nursing Science Quarterly, 20*(4), 306.

Karian, V. E., Jankowski, S. M., & Beal, J. A. (1998). Exploring the lived-experience of childhood cancer survivors. *Journal of Pediatric Oncology Nursing, 15*(3), 153–162.

Kelley, L. S. (1999). Evaluating change in quality of life from the perspective of the person: Advanced practice nursing and Parse's goal of nursing. *Holistic Nursing Practice, 13*(4), 61–70.

Kwekkeboom, K., Huseby-Moore, K., & Ward, S. (1998). Imagining ability and effective use of guided imagery. *Research in Nursing and Health, 21*(3), 189–198.

Legault, F., & Ferguson-Pare, M. (1999). Advancing nursing practice: An evaluation study of Parse's theory of human becoming. *Canadian Journal of Nursing Leadership, 12*(1), 30–35.

Lewandowski, W. A. (2004). Patterning of pain and power with guided imagery. *Nursing Science Quarterly, 17*(3), 233–241.

Madrid, M. (1997). Patterns *of Rogerian knowing*. New York: National League for Nursing Press.

Madrid, M., & Winstead-Fry, P. (2001). Nursing research on the health patterning modalities of therapeutic touch and imagery. *Nursing Science Quarterly, 14*(3), 187–194.

Marchione, J. (1995). Margaret Newman: Health as expanding consciousness. In C. M. McQuiston & A. A. Webb (Eds.), *Foundations of nursing theory: Contributions of 12 key theorists* (pp. 261–316). Thousand Oaks, CA: Sage.

Milton, C. L. (2004). Stories: Implications for nursing ethics and respect for another. *Nursing Science Quarterly, 21*(4), 330–342.

Musker, K. M. (2008). Life patterns of women transitioning through menopause. *Nursing Science Quarterly, 17*(3), 208–211.

Neill, J. (2005). Recognizing patterns in the lives of women with multiple sclerosis. In C. Picard and D. Jones (Eds.), *Giving voice to what we know: Margaret Newman's theory of health as expanding consciousness in nursing practice, research, and education* (pp. 153–165). Sudbury, MA: Jones & Bartlett.

Newman, M. A. (1979). *Theory development in nursing*. Philadelphia: Davis.

Newman, M. A. (1986). *Health as expanding consciousness*. St. Louis: Mosby.

Newman, M. A. (1990a). Newman's theory of health as praxis. *Nursing Science Quarterly, 3*(1), 37–41.

Newman, M. A. (1990b). Toward an integrative model of professional practice. *Journal of Professional Nursing, 6,* 167–173.

Newman, M. A. (1994). *Health as expanding consciousness*. New York: National League for Nursing Press.

Newman, M. A. (1995). *A developing discipline: Selected works of Margaret Newman*. New York: National League for Nursing Press.

Newman, M. A. (1999). *Health as expanding consciousness* (2nd ed.). New York: National League for Nursing Press.

Newman, M. A. (2005). Caring in the human health experience. In C. Picard & D. Jones (Eds.), *Giving voice to what we know: Margaret Newman's Theory of health as expanding consciousness in nursing practice, research, and education* (pp. 3–9). Sudbury, MA: Jones & Bartlett.

Newman, M. A. (2008a). Transforming presence: The difference that nursing makes. Philadelphia: Davis.

Newman, M. A. (2008b). It's about time. *Nursing Science Quarterly, 21*(3), 225–229.

Newman, M. A., Lamb, G. S., & Michaels, C. (1991). Nurse case management: The coming together of theory and practice. *Nursing and Health Care, 12*(8), 404–408. (Reprinted in M. A. Newman (Ed.). (1995). *A developing discipline: Selected works of Margaret Newman* (pp. 249–263). New York: National League for Nursing Press).

Noh, C. H. (2004). Meaning of the quality of life for persons living with serious mental illness: Human becoming practice with groups. *Nursing Science Quarterly, 17*(3), 220–225.

Parse, R. R. (1981). *Man-living-health: A theory of nursing*. New York: Wiley.

Parse, R. R. (1987). *Nursing science: Major paradigms and theories and critiques*. Philadelphia: Saunders.

Parse, R. R. (1995). *Illuminations: The human becoming theory in practice and research*. New York: National League for Nursing Press.

Parse, R. R. (1998). *The human becoming school of thought: A perspective for nurses and other health professionals*. Thousand Oaks, CA: Sage.

Parse, R. R. (2001). The human becoming school of thought. In M. Parker (Ed.), *Nursing theories and nursing practice* (pp. 227–238). Philadelphia: Davis.

Parse, R. R. (2002). Transforming healthcare with a unitary view of the human. *Nursing Science Quarterly, 15*(1), 46–50.

Parse, R. R. (2003). *Community: A human becoming perspective*. Sudbury, MA: Jones & Bartlett.

Pharris, M. D., & Endo, E. (2007). Flying free: The evolving nature of nursing practice guided by the theory of health as expanding consciousness. *Nursing Science Quarterly, 20*(2), 136–140.

Phillips, J. R. (1990). Changing human potentials and future visions of nursing: A human field image perspective. In E. A. M. Barrett (Ed.), *Visions of Rogers' science-based nursing* (pp. 13–25). New York: National League for Nursing Press.

Phillips, J. R. (1994). Foreword. In V. M. Malinski, E. A. M. Barrett, & J. R. Phillips (Eds.), *Martha E. Rogers: Her life and her work* (pp. v–ix). Philadelphia: Davis.

Pickard, C. (2000). Pattern of expanding consciousness in midlife women: Creative movement and the narrative as modes of expression. *Nursing Science Quarterly, 13*(2), 150–157.

Pickard, C. (2002). Family reflections on living through sudden death of a child: Cooperative inquiry grounded in Newman's health as expanding consciousness. *Nursing Science Quarterly, 15*(3), 242–250.

Pilkington, F. B., & Millar, B. (1999). The lived experience of hope with persons from Wales, UK. In R. R. Parse (Ed.), *Hope: An international human becoming perspective* (pp. 163–189). Sudbury, MA: Jones & Bartlett and National League for Nursing Press.

Porter, L. S. (1998). Reducing teenage and unintended pregnancies through client-centered and family-focused school-based family planning programs. *Journal of Pediatric Nursing, 13*(3), 158–163.

Reed, P. (2008). Nursing time: Research, practice, and theory dimensions. *Nursing Science Quarterly, 21*(3), 222–223.

Rogers, M. E. (1970). *An introduction to the theoretical basis of nursing.* Philadelphia: Davis.

Rogers, M. E. (1986). Science of unitary human beings. In V. M. Malinski (Ed.), *Explorations on Martha Rogers' science of unitary human beings* (pp. 3–8). Norwalk, CT: Appleton-Century-Crofts. (Reprinted in V. M. Malinski, E. A. M. Barrett, & J. R. Phillips (Eds.). (1994). *Martha E. Rogers: Her life and her work* (pp. 233–238). Philadelphia: Davis).

Rogers, M. E. (1990). Nursing: The science of unitary, irreducible, human beings: Update 1990. In E. A. M. Barrett (Ed.), *Visions of Rogers' science-based nursing* (pp. 5–11). New York: National League for Nursing Press.

Rogers, M. E. (1994). Nursing science evolves. In M. Madrid & E. A. M. Barrett (Eds.), *Rogers' scientific art of nursing practice* (pp. 3–10). New York: National League for Nursing Press.

Toikkanen, T., & Muurinen, E. (1999). Tiovo: Hope for persons in Finland. In R. R. Parse (Ed.), *Hope: An international human becoming perspective* (pp. 79–96). Sudbury, MA: Jones & Bartlett and National League for Nursing Press.

Welch, A. J. (2004). The researcher's reflections on the research process. *Nursing Science Quarterly, 17*(3), 201–207.

Wondoloski, C., & Davis, D. K. (1991). The lived experience of health in the oldest old: A phenomenological study. *Nursing Science Quarterly, 4*(3), 113–118.

# 10

# Introduction to Middle Range Nursing Theories

## Melanie McEwen

*A*nnette Cohen is a second-year graduate nursing student interested in starting her
major research/scholarship project. For this project, she would like to develop some of
her experiences in hospice nursing into a preliminary middle range theory of spiritual
health. Annette has studied spiritual needs and spiritual care for many years but believes
that the construct of spiritual health is not well understood. She views spiritual health as the
result of the interaction of multiple intrinsic values and external variables within a client's
experiences, and she believes that it is a significant contributing factor to overall health and
well-being.

   After reviewing theoretical writings dealing with spiritual nursing care, Annette found a
starting point for her work in Jean Watson's Theory of Human Caring because of its
emphasis on spirituality and faith. From Watson's work, she was particularly interested in
applying the concepts of "actual caring occasion" and "transpersonal" care. To develop the
theory, Annette obtained a copy of Watson's most recent work and performed a comprehensive
review of the literature covering theory development and the Theory of Human Caring. She
then did an analysis of the concept of spiritual health. Combining the concept analysis and
the literature review of Watson's work led to the development of assumptions and formal
definitions of related concepts and empirical indicators. After conversing with her instructor,
she concluded that her next steps were to construct relational statements and then draw a
model depicting the relationships among the components of spiritual health.

---

As discussed in Chapter 2, middle range nursing theories lie between the most
abstract theories (grand nursing theories, models, or conceptual frameworks) and
more circumscribed, concrete theories (practice theories, situation-specific theories,
or microtheories). Compared to grand theories, middle range theories are more specific, have fewer concepts, and encompass a more limited aspect of the real world.
Concepts are relatively concrete and can be operationally defined. Propositions are
also relatively concrete and may be empirically tested.

The discipline of nursing recognizes middle range theory as one of the latest steps in knowledge development, and there is broad acceptance of the need to develop middle range theories to support nursing practice (Blegen & Tripp-Reimer, 1997; Chinn, 1997; Fitzpatrick, 2003; Morris, 1996). According to Morris (1996) and Suppe (1996), this call to develop middle range theory is consistent with the third stage of legitimizing the discipline of nursing. The first stage focuses on differentiation of the perspective of the emerging discipline, which is characterized by separation from antecedent disciplines (i.e., medicine) and the establishment of university-based education, which in nursing occurred during the 1950s and 1960s. The second stage is marked by the quest to secure institutional legitimacy and academic autonomy. This stage characterized nursing during the 1970s and through the 1980s, when pursuit of nursing's unique perspective on and clarification of the phenomena of interest to the discipline were stressed. The third stage is distinguished by increased attention to substantive knowledge development, which includes development and testing of middle range theories.

Middle range theories are also increasingly being used in nursing research studies. Many researchers prefer to work with middle range theories rather than grand theories or conceptual frameworks because they provide a better basis for generating testable hypotheses and addressing particular client populations. A review of nursing research journals and dissertation abstracts indicates that nursing research is currently being used in the development and testing of a number of middle range theories, and middle range theories are frequently being used as frameworks for investigation. Furthermore, middle range theories are presently being refined on the basis of research results.

Despite the promotion of middle range theories in recent years, there is a lack of clarity regarding what constitutes middle range theory in nursing. According to Cody (1999), "It appears that almost any theoretical entity that is more concrete than the broadest of grand theories is considered middle range by someone" (p. 10). It has been noted that nursing theory textbooks (e.g., Alligood, 2006; Chinn & Kramer, 2008; Fawcett, 1993, 1995, 1999, 2000, 2005) disagree to some degree on which theories should be labeled as middle range. Indeed, some authors list a few of the readily accepted grand theories (e.g., Parse, Newman, Peplau, and Orlando) as middle range. Others consider somewhat more circumscribed theories (e.g., Leininger, Pender, Benner and Erickson, Tomlin, and Swain) to be middle range, although the theory's authors may not agree. In essence, there has been a paucity of discussion on the subject and therefore there is little consensus. This issue is discussed in more detail later in the chapter.

## Purposes of Middle Range Theory

Middle range theories were first suggested in the discipline of sociology in the 1960s and were introduced to nursing in 1974. At that time, it was observed that middle range theories were useful for emerging disciplines because they are more readily operationalized and addressed through research than are grand theories. More than 15 years elapsed, however, before there was a concerted call for middle range theory development in nursing (Blegen & Tripp-Reimer, 1997; Meleis, 2007).

Development of middle range theories is supported by the frequent critique of the abstract nature of grand theories and the difficulty of their application to practice and research. The function of middle range theories is to describe, explain, or predict phenomena, and, unlike grand theory, they must be explicit and testable. Thus, they are easier to apply in practice situations and use as frameworks for research studies. In addition, middle range theories have the potential to guide nursing interventions and change conditions of a situation to enhance nursing care (Morris, 1996). Finally, a major role of middle range theory is to define or refine the substantive component of nursing science and practice (Higgins & Moore, 2000). Indeed, Lenz (1996) noted that practicing nurses are actually using middle range theories but are not consciously aware that they are doing so.

Each middle range theory addresses relatively concrete and specific phenomena by stating what the phenomena are, why they occur, and how they occur. In addition, middle range theories can provide structure for the interpretation of behavior, situations, and events. They support understanding of the connections between diagnosis and outcomes, and between interventions and outcomes (Fawcett, 2005).

Enhancing the focus on middle range theories in nursing is supported by several factors. These include the observations that middle range theories

- are more useful in research than grand theories because of their low level of abstraction and ease of operationalization.
- tend to support prediction better than grand theories due to circumscribed range and specificity of the concepts.
- are more likely to be adopted in practice because their relative simplicity eases the process of developing interventions for identified health problems (Cody, 1999; Peterson, 2009).

Further, middle range theories offer a level of theory that provides a basis for deliberative, knowledgeable, clinical problem solving (Morris, 1996).

Like theory in general, middle range theory has three functions in nursing knowledge development. First, middle range theories are used as theoretical frameworks for research studies. Second, middle range theories are open to use in practice and should be tested by research. Finally, middle range theories can be the scientific end product that expresses nursing knowledge (Suppe, 1996).

## Characteristics of Middle Range Theory

Several characteristics identify nursing theories as middle range. First, the principal ideas of middle range theories are relatively simple, straightforward, and general. Second, middle range theories consider a limited number of variables or concepts; they have a particular substantive focus and consider a limited aspect of reality. In addition, they are receptive to empirical testing and can be consolidated into more wide-ranging theories. Third, middle range theories focus primarily on client problems and likely outcomes, as well as the effects of nursing interventions on client outcomes (Blegen & Tripp-Reimer, 1997). Finally, middle range theories are specific to nursing and may specify an area of practice, age range of the client, nursing actions or interventions, and proposed outcomes (Liehr & Smith, 1999).

The more frequently cited middle range theories tend to be those that are clearly stated, easy to understand, internally consistent, and coherent. They deal with current nursing perspectives and address socially relevant topics that solve meaningful and persistent problems (Lenz, 1996). In summary, middle range theories for nursing combine postulated relationships between specific, well-defined concepts with the ability to measure or objectively code concepts (Good & Moore, 1996). Thus, middle range theories contain concepts and statements from which hypotheses may be logically derived and

TABLE 10-1 *Characteristics of Grand, Middle Range, and Practice Theories*

| | Grand Theories | Middle Range Theories | Practice Theories |
|---|---|---|---|
| **Characteristic** | | | |
| Complexity/abstractness, scope | Comprehensive, global viewpoint (all aspects of human experience) | Less comprehensive than grand theories, middle view of reality | Focused on a narrow view of reality, simple and straightforward |
| Generalizability/specificity | Nonspecific, general application to the discipline irrespective of setting or specialty area | Some generalizablity across settings and specialties, but more specific than grand theories | Linked to special populations or an identified field of practice |
| Characteristics of concepts | Concepts abstract and not operationally defined | Limited number of concepts that are fairly concrete and may be operationally defined | Single, concrete concept that is operationalized |
| Characteristics of propositions | Propositions not always explicit | Propositions are clearly stated | Propositions defined |
| Testability | Not generally testable | May generate testable hypotheses | Goals or outcomes defined and testable |
| Source of development | Developed through thoughtful appraisal and careful consideration over many years | Evolve from grand theories, clinical practice, literature review, practice guidelines | Derived from practice or deduced from middle range or grand theory |

empirically tested, and they can be easily adopted to guide nursing practice. Table 10-1 compares characteristics of grand theory, middle range theory, and practice theory, and characteristics of middle range theory are summarized in Box 10-1.

## Concepts and Relationships for Middle Range Theory

Middle range theories consist of two or more concepts and a specified relationship between the concepts. Middle range theories address phenomena (concepts) that are toward the middle of a continuum of scope with the metaparadigm concepts (nursing, person, health, environment) at one end and specific concrete actions or events (medication administration, preoperative teaching, electrolyte management, fall prevention) at the other. The concepts should be discrete, observable, and sufficiently abstract to be applied across multiple settings and used with clients with differing problems (Blegen & Tripp-Reimer, 1997). Examples from the nursing literature include theories describing

---

**BOX 10-1** *Characteristics of Middle Range Nursing Theory*

Not comprehensive, but not narrowly focused
Some generalizations across settings and specialities
Limited number of concepts
Propositions that are clearly stated
May generate testable hypotheses

health promotion, comfort, coping, resilience, uncertainty, pain, grief, fatigue, self-care, adaptation, self-transcendence, and transitions (Acton, Irvin, Jensen, Hopkins, & Miller, 1997; Chinn & Kramer, 2008; Peterson, 2009; Smith, 2008).

Middle range theories link discrete and observable phenomena or concepts in relationships statements. In middle range theory relationships are explicitly stated and, preferably, they are unidirectional. Relationships can be of several types. The most common are causal relationships that state that a change in the value of one variable or concept is associated with a change in the value of another variable or concept (Blegen & Tripp-Reimer, 1997).

## Categorizing Middle Range Theory

The question as to which nursing theories are middle range is not clear-cut. Middle range theory is more specific than grand theory but abstract enough to support both generalization and operationalization across a range of populations; this sets it apart from practice theory.

In a well-researched effort to describe the place of middle range theory in nursing, Liehr and Smith (1999) analyzed 22 middle range theories published during the previous decade. These theories were categorized as "high-middle," "middle," and "low-middle" based on their level of abstraction or degree of specificity. In the review, high-middle theories included concepts such as caring, growth and development, self-transcendence, resilience, and psychological adaptation. Middle theories included concepts such as uncertainty in illness, unpleasant symptoms, chronic sorrow, peaceful end of life, cultural brokering, and nurse-expressed empathy. Low-middle theories, those that are closer to practice or situation-specific theories, included hazardous secrets, women's anger, nurse midwifery care, acute pain management, helplessness, and intervention for postsurgical pain.

As mentioned, there is some debate on which theories should be considered middle range. Indeed, some theories *not* termed middle range more appropriately fit the criteria of middle range theory than a grand theory, and some theories that are labeled middle range better fit the criteria of practice theory. Chapter 11 presents a number of middle range nursing theories recently described in the literature, organized as high, middle, and low theories. It should be noted that the designations are arguably arbitrary and that one theory that is listed here as high-middle may be considered by others to be a grand theory. Likewise, another theory listed here as middle might be considered by others to be high-middle and so forth.

## Development of Middle Range Theory

Several methods for development of middle range theories have been identified in the nursing literature. Middle range theories emerge from combining research and practice and building on the work of others. Sources used to generate middle range theory include literature reviews, qualitative research, field studies, conceptual models, taxonomies of nursing diagnoses and interventions, clinical practice guidelines, theories from other disciplines, and statistical analysis of empirical data (Good & Moore, 1996; Peterson, 2009). Five approaches for middle range theory generation were identified by Liehr and Smith (1999) (Box 10-2). The following sections present examples describing the source and development process of middle range theories from each of the five approaches listed in Box 10-2.

**BOX 10-2**  *Approaches for Middle Range Theory Generation*

1. Induction through research and practice
2. Deduction from research and practice or application of grand theories
3. Combination of existing nursing and nonnursing middle range theories
4. Derivation from theories of other disciplines that relate to nursing
5. Derivation from practice guidelines and standards rooted in research

## MIDDLE RANGE THEORIES DERIVED FROM RESEARCH AND/OR PRACTICE

One of the most common sources for development of middle range nursing theories and models is nursing research or nursing practice. Grounded theory research and other qualitative methods in particular are frequently noted as sources for middle range theory development. Examples of middle range theories derived from qualitative research include the Theory of Normalizing Risky Sexual Behaviors (Weiss, Jampol, Lievano, Smith, & Wurster, 2008), a theory for nursing care for patients at risk of suicide (Sun, Long, Boore, & Tsao, 2006), Beck's (1993) work on postpartum depression, and a theory describing the phenomena of Keeping the Spirit Alive (Woodgate & Degner, 2003).

Variations of the idea of development of middle range theory from research are fairly common. Theorists report combining qualitative research with literature review, concept analysis, concept synthesis, and other techniques in the process of developing middle range theory. For example, Bu and Jezewski (2006) used concept analysis to develop a middle range theory of patient advocacy, and Covell (2008) used concept analysis and theory derivation methods to develop a middle range theory of nursing intellectual capital. The Chronic Illness Trajectory Framework (Corbin & Strauss, 1991, 1992) was developed from a series of studies related to management of chronic illness, combined with numerous accounts of practice experiences by nurses. Similarly, Eakes, Burke, and Hainsworth (1998) developed the middle range Theory of Chronic Sorrow from an extensive review of the literature and data gathered through 10 qualitative research studies.

Identification of middle range theories and models derived primarily from practice is more difficult. One example is the Theory of Unpleasant Symptoms (Lenz, Pugh, Milligan, Gift, & Suppe, 1997; Lenz, Suppe, Gift, Pugh, & Milligan, 1995), which was reportedly developed by integrating or melding existing practice and research information about a variety of symptoms. Some models that describe areas of specialty nursing practice report being developed from combination of practice and another source, typically research or standards. The Omaha System, which is a model for community and home health nursing practice, is an example. Martin (2005) explained that the conceptual framework for the Omaha System was a combination of practice, research, and literature review (see Chapter 11 for more detail on these theories).

Another example of theory development combining practice with other elements is Rogers' (1994) model for occupational health nursing practice, which combined practice experiences with standards. Lastly, Purnell (2000) explained that his Model for Cultural Competence was "developed from practice and working with staff and students in culturally diverse clinical settings" (p. 40). In addition to using practice experiences, he also detailed how concepts from many theories from other disciplines (e.g., organization/administration, anthropology, sociology, psychology, religion, and history) were incorporated into the model's development.

## EXEMPLAR 1–MIDDLE RANGE THEORY DERIVED FROM RESEARCH/PRACTICE

The process used to develop a middle range theory of caring was described by Swanson (1991). Her purpose was to provide a definition of caring and describe its characteristics, and to outline caring processes used by nurses.

*Theory Development Process:* The Theory of Caring was derived from three phenomenological studies in perinatal nursing. The focus was on experiences of women who had miscarried, with an emphasis on patients and professionals in the newborn intensive care unit (NICU). In the first study, women who had recently miscarried were interviewed to learn about their perception of caring behaviors of others. Five caring processes (knowing, being with, doing for, enabling, and maintaining belief) were derived from this study and preliminary definitions were proposed.

A second study involved interviews and observation of care providers in an NICU. This study confirmed the five caring processes and allowed for refinement of the theoretical definitions. In the final study, interviews with 68 pregnant women who were considered to be at high risk from a social perspective were conducted. In that study, the five caring processes were reconfirmed, then slightly refined. Following that, subdimensions of each caring process were identified, the concept of caring was defined, and the theory fully delineated.

## MIDDLE RANGE THEORY DERIVED FROM A GRAND THEORY

As described previously, many nursing theorists and scholars agree that grand theories are difficult to apply in research and practice and suggest development of middle range theories derived from them. During the last 15 years, a number of theories developed from grand theories have been published in the nursing literature. One example is a middle range theory of nurse-expressed empathy (Olson & Hanchett, 1997), which was derived from three relational statements taken from Orlando's model. These statements were developed into theoretical propositions focusing on nurse-expressed empathy. In other examples, Rew (2003) developed a theory of self-care from experiences of homeless youth based on Orem's theory, and Hastings-Tolsma (2006) developed the Theory of Diversity of Human Field Pattern from Martha Rogers' Science of Unitary Human Beings. August-Brady (2000) employed the Neuman Systems Model as a basis for the middle range theory of prevention as intervention, and in another work, Polk (1997) cited the work of both Margaret Newman and Martha Rogers as being sources contributing to her middle range theory of resilience.

Several middle range theories were found which were developed from Roy's Adaptation Model (RAM). Hamilton and Bowers (2007) developed the Theory of Genetic Vulnerability from Roy's work. Similarly, Smith, Pace, Kochinda, Kleinbeck, Koehler, and Popkess-Vawter (2002) developed a theory describing caregiving effectiveness based on the structure and concepts from the RAM; Jirovec and colleagues (1999) used it to develop the Urine Control Theory; and Whittemore and Roy (2002) used concept syntheses to integrate concepts and assumptions from the RAM to theoretically describe "adapting to diabetes mellitus." Finally, Roy's model was also used in the development of a middle range theory of caregiver stress (Tsai, 2003).

## EXEMPLAR 2–MIDDLE RANGE THEORY DERIVED FROM A GRAND THEORY

In a well-written report, Mefford (2004) used Levine's Conservation Model of Nursing to develop a Theory of Health Promotion for Preterm Infants. In this case, Levine's theory was used as a framework for development of a framework for nursing practice for the NICU to ensure that needs of both the infant and family are addressed.

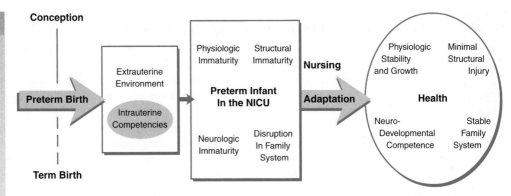

FIGURE 10-1 Conceptual diagram of Levine's Conservation Model of Nursing. (From Mefford, L. C. (2004). A theory of health promotion for preterm infants based on Levine's Conservation Model of Nursing. *Nursing Science Quarterly, 17*(3), p. 261.)

*Theory Development Process:* To develop the Theory of Health Promotion for Preterm Infants, the theorist first described elements of Levine's Conservation Model internal and external environments, wholeness and conservation principles (conservation of energy, structural integrity, personal integrity, and social integrity) and applied these concepts in the NICU. She determined a "goal of restoring a state of wholeness, or health" (p. 260) (Figure 10-1).

Following initial development of the theory, its validity was tested in a retrospective study of 235 preterm infants. This study was designed to examine the influence of "consistency nursing care" on the health outcomes of the infants at discharge. Structural equation modeling demonstrated "strong support for the utility of this theory of health promotion … as a guide for nursing practice in the NICU" (p. 266). It was noted that the derived middle range theory validated Levine's work.

## MIDDLE RANGE THEORY COMBINING EXISTING NURSING AND NONNURSING THEORIES

Combining concepts or elements of multiple theories is common in middle range theory development. In many cases found in recent nursing literature, the author(s) of a middle range theory reported that they had derived their theory from both nursing and nonnursing theories. For example, Sousa and Zauszniewski (2005) used Orem's Self-Care Theory and Bandura's Self-Efficacy Theory to develop a theory of diabetes self-care management. Similarly, Ulbrich (1999) developed the Theory of Exercise as Self-Care through "triangulation of Orem's self-care deficit theory of nursing, the transtheoretical model of exercise behavior, and characteristics of a population at risk for cardiovascular disease" (p. 65). In another example, Reed (1991) used elements of Rogers' Science of Unitary Human Beings work as the "nursing perspective of human development for … self-transcendence" (p. 65). For this theory, Rogers' work was used as a framework and it was reportedly combined with concepts and elements from developmental psychologists including Piaget and Fagin.

## EXEMPLAR 3–MIDDLE RANGE THEORY COMBINING EXISTING NURSING AND NONNURSING THEORIES

Dunn (2004) provided an excellent example of combining existing nursing and nonnursing theories in development of a middle range Theory of Adaptation to Chronic Pain. Her intention was to describe coping and pain control in elders with the purpose of maintaining their quality of life and functional ability.

*Theory Development Process:* Dunn wrote that the first step in developing her theory was to review and synthesize the theoretical knowledge related to pain in elders, coping with pain, religious coping, and spirituality. She reported identification of three theoretical models that addressed concepts related to pain control and coping in elders. These were Melzak and Wall's (1992) gate control theory of pain, Lazarus and Folkman's (1984) stress and coping theory, and Wallace, Benson, and Wilson's (1971) relaxation response. To ensure that the final model was applicable to nursing, she selected the Roy Adaptation Model to guide the theory development process.

The second step reported by Dunn was to define assumptions for the theory; these were reportedly based on the assumptions from the four models from which the theory was drawn. Using the process of theoretical substruction, she then took concepts, relational statements and propositions from the existing theories, and arranged them into a diagram to represent the theoretical and operational systems. Finally, the concepts from the Adaptation to Chronic Pain model were linked to empirical indicators to provide a logical and consistent connection.

## MIDDLE RANGE THEORY DERIVED FROM NONNURSING DISCIPLINES

A very significant number of middle range nursing theories are developed from one or more nonnursing theories. Indeed, nonnursing theories, including those from the behavioral sciences, sociology, physiology, and anthropology, appear to be the most common source for theory development, and many examples are evident. Kolcaba's (1994) Theory of Comfort, for example, was reportedly derived from a review of literature from medicine, psychiatry, ergonomics, and psychology, as well as from nursing literature and history. Benner (2001) explained that the Dreyfus model of skill acquisition, developed by a mathematician and a philosopher, was the primary source for her work. Mishel's Uncertainty in Illness Theory incorporated elements of chaos theory (Mishel & Clayton, 2003) and Mercer (1985) used role theory as the framework for her theory describing maternal role attainment.

Several middle range nursing theories have been derived from theories or models of behavioral change. Frequently cited are the Health Belief Model (Becker & Maiman, 1975; Rosenstock, 1990), the Theory of Reasoned Action (Ajzen & Fishbein, 1980), and Social Learning/Social Cognitive Theory (Bandura, 1977, 1986), along with others. Table 10-2 lists some of these middle range theories and gives sources from which the theorist claims derivation of portions of their work.

TABLE 10-2 *Middle Range Nursing Theories Derived From Behavioral Theories*

| Theory | Nonnursing Theory Source(s) |
| --- | --- |
| Commitment to Health Theory (Kelly, 2008) | Transtheoretical Model of Behavior Change |
| Recovery Alliance Theory of Mental Health Nursing (Shanley & Jubb-Shanley, 2007) | Humanistic Philosophy |
| Health Promotion Model (Pender, 1996) | Social Learning Theory and Expectancy-Value Theory |
| Theory of Care-Seeking Behavior (Lauver, 1992) | Health Belief Model and the Theory of Reasoned Action |
| Medication Adherence Model (Johnson, 2002) | Health Belief Model, Social Learning Theory, the Theory of Reasoned Action, and the Self-Regulation Model |
| Self-Efficacy in Nursing Theory (Lenz & Shortridge-Baggett, 2002) | Social Learning Theory |
| Health Behavior Self-Determinism (Cox, 1985) | Health Belief Model, Schuman Model |
| Cues to Participation in Prostate Screening (Nivens, Herman, Weinrich, & Weinrich, 2001) | Health Belief Model, Social Learning Theory |
| Model for Cross-Cultural Research (Poss, 2001) | Health Belief Model, Theory of Reasoned Action |

## EXEMPLAR 4–MIDDLE RANGE THEORY DERIVED FROM A NONNURSING DISCIPLINE

McGahee, Kemp, and Tingen (2000) developed a theoretical model to study smoking behaviors and prevention interventions among preteens. They stated that the "theoretical framework was derived from the literature linking different concepts to smoking behaviors and from literature that supports recommended intervention methods" (p. 135). The theorists reportedly used Social Cognitive Theory and the Theory of Reasoned Action in designing their model.

*Theory Development Process*: In developing the model to study smoking behaviors, the theorists described a detailed study of the concepts and components of the two theories mentioned. They determined that Social Cognitive Theory helped explain the psychosocial dynamics underlying individual behaviors. It also described how behavior is determined by expectancies and incentives as perceived by the individual and the importance of self-efficacy beliefs in influencing behavior. From the Theory of Reasoned Action, the theorists learned the importance of intention, which is described as a function of attitudes and subjective norms. From this, they recognized the significance of measuring an individual's intention to perform a behavior rather than the behavior itself.

Four major concepts affecting smoking prevention intervention were identified and defined in the theory. The first concept is sociodemographics, which includes gender, ethnicity, and household composition. The second concept is internal factors, which includes subjective personal variables (e.g., attitude toward smoking), subjective norms (e.g., beliefs about whether others think the individual should smoke and motivation to comply with the opinions of others), and perception of refusal skills (self-reported judgment of how well the individual can successfully refuse offers to smoke). The third concept is external factors, which involves parental attitudes toward smoking and preteens' perceptions of how much others smoke. The final variable identified is outcome behaviors. This includes smoking behaviors, which includes both self-reported intentional smoking (whether or not the preteen thinks he/she will smoke before the end of the current school year) and self-reported actual smoking (frequency and amount of smoking). Figure 10-2 depicts the theoretical model.

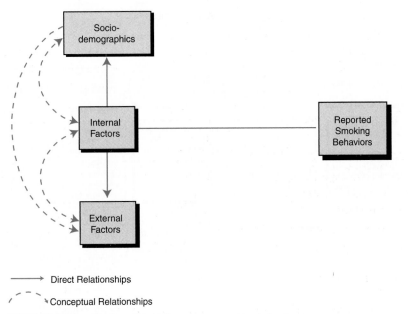

→ Direct Relationships

╱ ⌐ ╲ Conceptual Relationships

FIGURE 10-2 Theoretical model of influences on smoking behaviors.

**Note:** The solid lines indicate direct relationships that can be tested. The broken lines represent conceptual relationships that are supported by the literature. (From McGahee, T. W., Kemp, V., & Tingen, M. (2000). A theoretical model for smoking prevention studies in preteen children. *Pediatric Nursing, 26*(2), 137.)

# MIDDLE RANGE THEORY DERIVED FROM PRACTICE GUIDELINES OR STANDARD OF CARE

Practice guidelines or standards of care appear to be the least common source for middle range theory development, as only a few examples could be found. In one example, the Public Health Nursing Practice Model (Smith & Bazini-Barakat, 2003) was developed by "melding of nationally recognized components" (p. 44) of public health nursing practice (PHN). The identified components were the Standards of PHN practice, the 10 Essential Services of Public Health, *Healthy People 2010*'s 10 Leading Health Indicators, and Minnesota's Public Health Interventions Model. In other examples, Good (1998) used clinical guidelines for management of postoperative pain to develop a middle range theory of acute pain management, and Huth and Moore (1998) used practice standards to develop a theory of acute pain management in infants and children. Finally, Ruland and Moore (1998) used standards of care to develop the Theory of the Peaceful End of Life from standards of care for terminally ill patients.

## EXEMPLAR 5–MIDDLE RANGE THEORY DERIVED FROM PRACTICE GUIDELINES OR STANDARD OF CARE

Ruland and Moore (1998) developed the Theory of the Peaceful End of Life from standards of care for terminally ill patients. In this work, the theorists observed that relational statements of the standards needed to be more specifically defined to make them applicable for empirical testing. Because the standards were too specific, they were too detailed to illustrate the major themes succinctly.

*Theory Development Process:* The first step of the theory development process was to define the theory's assumptions based on the standards of care. The second step was to perform a "statement synthesis," whereby five outcome criteria were developed that contributed to a peaceful end of life (not being in pain, experiencing comfort, experiencing dignity and respect, being at peace and closeness to significant others or another caring person). For the third step, conceptual definitions for each of the outcome indicators

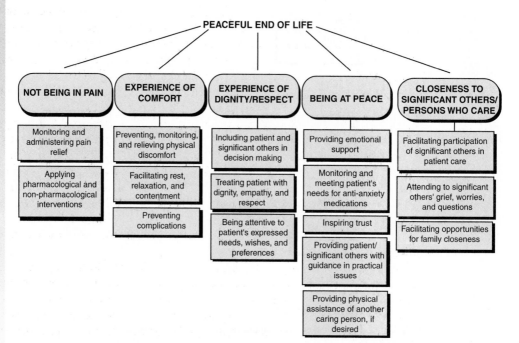

FIGURE 10-3 Theory of Peaceful End of Life: Relationships between the concepts of the theory. (From Ruland, C. M., & Moore, S. M. (1998). Theory construction based on standards of care: A proposed theory of the peaceful end of life. *Nursing Outlook, 46,* 174.)

were determined, and the fourth step involved defining relational statements between the outcome indicators and the nursing interventions. In this step all process criteria from the standard were examined and combined into "prescriptors" to facilitate the desired outcome. The process of theory synthesis was then used to combine the relational statements into an integrated structure or theory. The final step was to draw a diagram of the relationships as a model (Figure 10-3).

## FINAL THOUGHTS ON MIDDLE RANGE THEORY DEVELOPMENT

In short, middle range theories should be "user-friendly" in language and style. They need to be described with practice implications in journals that practicing nurses are likely to read, and the theorists need to identify implications and specific interventions suggested by the theory (Lenz, 1996). To enhance understanding and use, several factors should be considered when developing middle range theory. Liehr and Smith's (1999) specific recommendations to enhance development and use of middle range theory follow:

- Clearly articulate the theory name.
- Succinctly describe approaches used for generating the theory.
- Clarify the conceptual linkages of the theory in a diagrammed model.
- Elucidate the research–practice links of the theory.
- Explain the association between the theory and the discipline of nursing.

## Analysis and Evaluation of Middle Range Theory

The move to enhance middle range theory development and use in nursing practice and research necessitates corresponding analysis and critique. Like grand theories and conceptual frameworks, middle range theories should be subject to evaluation. In addition, research guided by middle range theory should be congruent with the philosophical underpinnings of the theory and should be critiqued with regard to more than just the statistical significance of the findings (Cody, 1999).

Whall (2005) specifically addressed analysis and evaluation of middle range theory. Her criteria modified the guidelines she used for analysis and evaluation of grand nursing theories. The modifications removed explicit review of the metaparadigm concepts, which are assumed to be more implicit than explicit in middle range theory, and added questions regarding the "fit of the middle range theory with the existing nursing perspective and domains" (p. 14). Further, Whall explained that middle range theories should provide specific empirical referents for defined concepts. The ability to operationalize and measure aspects of the theory is extremely important in middle range theory, and operational definitions should be evaluated. Finally, she suggested analysis of middle range theories to assess their congruence with grand theories.

Smith (2008) also proposed a format for evaluation of middle range theories. She suggested evaluation based on three categories: substantive foundations, structural integrity, and functional adequacy. When evaluating substantive foundations, one would determine whether the theory was within the focus of nursing, whether assumptions are specified and congruent with the focus, if the theory provides substantive description, explanation, or interpretation of a phenomenon that would be considered middle range, and whether the theory is rooted in practice or research experience. Evaluation of structural integrity would determine whether concepts are clearly defined and at the middle range of abstraction, whether the number of concepts is appropriate, and whether the concepts and relationship are logically represented with a model. Evaluation of functional adequacy examines whether the theory can be applied in practice or with various client groups, if empirical indicators have been identified for theoretical concepts, and if there are published examples of use of the theory in practice or research.

Chapter 5 includes a more detailed discussion of analysis and evaluation of middle range theories. In addition, the synthesized method for theory evaluation (see Box 5-3) can be used as a guide for analysis and evaluation of middle range theory.

## Summary

This chapter has described the current emphasis of nursing theory development which focuses on efforts to construct, test, refine, and evaluate middle range theories. To help advance the discipline, nurses should be encouraged to write and publish papers that describe middle range theories and report research studies in which a middle range theory has been used. This process of middle range theory generation and refinement will further develop the discipline's substantive knowledge base.

Annette Cohen, the graduate student in the opening case study, who was working toward development of a theory of spiritual health related it to the practice of hospice nursing. Like Annette, nurses in all settings should strive to learn about existing or emerging middle range theories or seek to develop and describe theories that will explain phenomena they observe in practice.

Nursing has the knowledge, skills, manpower, and resources to move beyond delineation of conceptual models and domain concepts to emphasize development and application of middle range theory (Morris, 1996). Middle range theory holds much promise for the evolution of the discipline's science and practice. But, as Liehr and Smith (1999) pointed out, the challenge is to develop middle range theories that are empirically sound, coherent, meaningful, useful, and illuminating.

## LEARNING ACTIVITIES

1. Search current nursing journals for examples of the development, analysis, or use of middle range theories in the discipline of nursing. Can any trends be identified?

2. Select one of the middle range theories derived from a grand nursing theory and one derived from a nonnursing theory. Analyze both for ease of application to research and practice.

3. Identify a concept of interest or one relevant to your practice. For a major paper or thesis, develop the concept into a preliminary middle range theory following the process presented in the case study.

## INTERNET RESOURCE

General information on middle range theory:

http://www.nurses.info/nursing_theory_midrange_theories.htm

# REFERENCES

Acton, G. J., Irvin, B. L., Jensen, B. A., Hopkins, B. A., & Miller, E. W. (1997). Explicating middle range theory through methodological diversity. *Advances in Nursing Science, 19*(3), 78–86.

Ajzen, I., & Fishbein, M. (1980). *Understanding attitudes and predicting social behavior.* Englewood Cliffs, NJ: Prentice-Hall.

Alligood, M. R. (2006). Introduction to nursing theory: History, terminology and analysis. In A. M. Tomey & M. R. Alligood (Eds.), *Nursing theorists and their work* (6th ed., pp. 3–15). St. Louis: Mosby.

August-Brady, M. (2000). Prevention as intervention. *Journal of Advanced Nursing, 31*(6), 1304–1308.

Bandura, A. (1977). *Social learning theory.* Englewood Cliffs, NJ: Prentice-Hall.

Bandura, A. (1986). *Social foundations of thought and action: A social cognitive theory.* Englewood Cliffs, NJ: Prentice-Hall.

Beck, C. T. (1993). Teetering on the edge: A substantive theory of postpartum depression. *Nursing Research, 42*(1), 42–48.

Becker, M. H., & Maiman, L. A. (1975). Socio behavioral determinates of compliance with health and medical care recommendations. *Medical Care, 13,* 10–24.

Benner, P. (2001). *From novice to expert: Excellence and power in clinical nursing practice* (commemorative edition). Englewood Cliffs, NJ: Prentice-Hall.

Blegen, M. A., & Tripp-Reimer, T. (1997). Implications of nursing taxonomies for middle range theory development. *Advances in Nursing Science, 19*(3), 37–50.

Bu, X., & Jezewski, M. A. (2006). Developing a mid-range theory of patient advocacy through concept analysis. *Journal of Advanced Nursing, 57*(1), 101–110.

Chinn, P. L. (1997). Why middle range theory? *Advances in Nursing Science, 19*(3), viii.

Chinn, P. L., & Kramer, M. K. (2008). *Theory and nursing: Integrated knowledge development* (7th ed.). St. Louis: Mosby.

Cody, W. K. (1999). Middle range theories: Do they foster the development of nursing science? *Nursing Science Quarterly, 12*(1), 9–14.

Corbin, J. M., & Strauss, A. (1991). A nursing model for chronic illness management based upon the trajectory framework. *Scholarly Inquiry for Nursing Practice, 5*(3), 155–174.

Corbin, J. M., & Strauss, A. (1992). A nursing model for chronic illness management based upon the trajectory framework. In P. Woog (Ed.), *The chronic illness trajectory framework: The Corbin and Strauss nursing model* (pp. 9–28). New York: Springer Publishing Company.

Covell, C. L. (2008). The middle-range theory of nursing intellectual capital. *Journal of Advanced Nursing, 63*(1), 94–103.

Cox, C. (1985). The self-determinism index. *Nursing Research, 34,* 177–183.

Dunn, K. S. (2004). Toward a middle range theory of adaptation to chronic pain. *Nursing Science Quarterly, 17*(1), 78–84.

Eakes, G., Burke, M. L., & Hainsworth, M. A. (1998). Middle range theory of chronic sorrow. *Image: Journal of Nursing Scholarship, 30*(2), 179–185.

Fawcett, J. (1993). *Analysis and evaluation of nursing theories.* Philadelphia: Davis.

Fawcett, J. (1995). *Analysis and evaluation of conceptual frameworks.* Philadelphia: Davis.

Fawcett, J. (1999). *The relationship of theory and research* (3rd ed.). Philadelphia: Davis.

Fawcett, J. (2000). *Analysis and evaluation of contemporary nursing knowledge: Nursing models and theories.* Philadelphia: Davis.

Fawcett, J. (2005). *Contemporary nursing knowledge: Analysis and evaluation of nursing models and theories* (2nd ed.). Philadelphia: Davis.

Fitzpatrick, J. J. (2003). Foreword. In M. J. Smith & P. R. Liehr (Eds.), *Middle range theory for nursing* (pp. ix–x). New York: Springer Publishing Company.

Good, M. (1998). A middle range theory of acute pain management: Use in research. *Nursing Outlook, 46*(3), 120–124.

Good, M., & Moore, S. M. (1996). Clinical practice guidelines as a new source of middle range theory: Focus on acute pain. *Nursing Outlook, 44*(2), 74–79.

Hamilton, R. J., & Bowers, B. J. (2007). The theory of genetic vulnerability: A Roy model exemplar. *Nursing Science Quarterly, 20*(3), 254–264.

Hastings-Tolsma, M. (2006). Toward a theory of diversity of human field pattern. *Visions: The Journal of Rogerian Nursing Science, 14*(2), 34–46.

Higgins, P. A., & Moore, S. M. (2000). Levels of theoretical thinking in nursing. *Nursing Outlook, 48*(4), 179–183.

Huth, M. M., & Moore, S. M. (1998). Prescriptive theory of acute pain management in infants and children. *Journal of the Society of Pediatric Nurses, 3*(1), 23–32.

Jirovec, M. M., Jenkins, J., Isenberg, M., & Baiardi, J. (1999). Urine control theory derived from Roy's conceptual framework. *Nursing Science Quarterly, 12*(3), 251–255.

Johnson, M. J. (2002). The medication adherence model: A guide for assessing medication taking. *Research and Theory for Nursing Practice, 16*(3), 179–192.

Kelly, C. W. (2008). Commitment to health theory. *Research and Theory for Nursing Practice: An International Journal, 22*(2), 148–158.

Kolcaba, K. (1994). A theory of holistic comfort for nursing. *Journal of Advanced Nursing, 19,* 1178–1184.

Lauver, D. (1992). A theory of care-seeking behavior. *Image: Journal of Nursing Scholarship, 24*(4), 281–287.

Lazarus, R. S., & Folkman, S. (1984). *Stress, appraisal and coping.* New York: Springer.

Lenz, E. R. (1996, May). *Middle range theory: Role in research and practice.* Conference Proceedings, Sixth Rosemary Ellis Scholar's Retreat: Nursing Science: Implications for the 21st Century, Cleveland, OH.

Lenz, E. R., Pugh, L. C., Milligan, R. A., Gift, A., & Suppe, F. (1997). The middle range. *Advances in Nursing Science, 19*(3), 14–27.

Lenz, E. R., & Shortridge-Baggett, L. (Eds.). (2002). *Self-efficacy and nursing.* New York: Springer.

Lenz, E. R., Suppe, F., Gift, A. G., Pugh, L. C., & Milligan, R. A. (1995). Collaborative development of middle range nursing theories: Toward a theory of unpleasant symptoms. *Advances in Nursing Science, 17*(3), 1–13.

Liehr, P., & Smith, M. J. (1999). Middle range theory: Spinning research and practice to create knowledge for the new millennium. *Advances in Nursing Science, 21*(4), 81–91.

Martin, K. S. (2005). *The Omaha system: A key to practice, documentation and information management.* St. Louis: Elsevier.

McGahee, T. W., Kemp, V., & Tingen, M. (2000). A theoretical model for smoking prevention studies in preteen children. *Pediatric Nursing, 26*(2), 135–140.

Mefford, L. C. (2004). A theory of health promotion for preterm infants based on Levine's Conservation Model of Nursing. *Nursing Science Quarterly, 17*(3), 260–266.

Meleis, A. I. (2007). *Theoretical nursing: Development and progress* (4th ed.). Philadelphia: Lippincott Williams & Wilkins.

Melzak, R., & Wall, P. D. (1992). Psychophysiology of pain. In D. C. Turk & R. Melzak (Eds.), *Handbook of pain and assessment* (pp. 3–25). New York: Guilford Press.

Mercer, R. T. (1985). The process of maternal role attainment over the first year. *Nursing Research, 34*(4), 198–204.

Mishel, M. H., & Clayton, M. F. (2003). Theories of uncertainty in illness. In M. J. Smith & P. R. Liehr (Eds.), *Middle range theory for nursing* (pp. 25–48). New York: Springer.

Morris, D. L. (1996, May). *Middle range theory: Role in education.* Conference Proceedings, Sixth Rosemary Ellis Scholar's Retreat: Nursing Science: Implications for the 21st Century, Cleveland, OH.

Nivens, A. S., Herman, J., Weinrich, S. P., & Weinrich, M. C. (2001). Cues to participation in prostate cancer screening: A theory for practice. *Oncology Nursing Forum, 28*(9), 1449–1456.

Olson, J., & Hanchett, E. (1997). Nurse-expressed empathy, patient outcomes and development of a middle range theory. *Image: Journal of Nursing Scholarship, 29*(1), 71–76.

Pender, N. J. (1996). *Health promotion in nursing practice* (3rd ed.). Stamford, CT: Appleton & Lange.

Peterson, S. J. (2009). Introduction to the nature of nursing knowledge. In S. J. Peterson & T. S. Bredow (Eds.), *Middle range theories: Application to nursing research* (2nd ed., pp. 3–45). Philadelphia: Lippincott Williams & Wilkins.

Polk, L. V. (1997). Toward a middle range theory of resilience. *Advances in Nursing Science, 19*(3), 1–13.

Poss, J. E. (2001). Developing a new model for cross-cultural research: Synthesizing the health belief model and the theory of reasoned action. *Advances in Nursing Science, 23*(4), 1–15.

Purnell, L. (2000). A description of the Purnell model for cultural competence. *Journal of Transcultural Nursing, 11*(1), 40–46.

Reed, P. G. (1991). Toward a nursing theory of self-transcendence: Deductive reformulation using developmental theories. *Advances in Nursing Science, 13*(4), 64–77.

Rew, L. (2003). A theory of taking care of oneself grounded in experiences of homeless youth. *Nursing Research, 52*(4), 234–241.

Rogers, B. (1994). *Occupational health nursing: Concepts and practice.* Philadelphia: Saunders.

Rosenstock, I. (1990). The health belief model: Explaining health behavior through expectancies. In K. Glanz, F. Lewis, & B. Rimer (Eds.), *Health behavior and health education* (pp. 39–62). San Francisco, CA: Jossey-Bass.

Ruland, C. M., & Moore, S. M. (1998). Theory construction based on standards of care: A proposed theory of the peaceful end of life. *Nursing Outlook, 46*(4), 169–175.

Shanley, E., & Jubb-Shanley, M. (2007). The recovery alliance theory of mental health nursing. *Journal of Psychiatric and Mental Health Nursing, 14*(8), 734–743.

Smith, C. E., Pace, K., Kochinda, C., Kleinbeck, S. V. M., Koehler, J., & Popkess-Vawter, S. (2002). Caregiving effectiveness model evaluation to a midrange theory of home care: A process for critique and replication. *Advances in Nursing Science, 25*(1), 50–64.

Smith, K., & Bazini-Barakat, N. (2003). A public health nursing practice model: Melding public health principles with the nursing process. *Public Health Nursing, 20*(1), 42–48.

Smith, M. C. (2008). Evaluation of middle range theories for the discipline of nursing. In M. J. Smith & P. R. Liehr (Eds.), *Middle range theory for nursing* (2nd ed., pp. 293–306). New York: Springer.

Sousa, V. D., & Zauszniewski, J. A. (2005). Toward a theory of diabetes self-care management. *Journal of Theory Construction and Testing, 9*(2), 61–67.

Sun, F. K., Long, A., Boore, J., & Tsao, L. I. (2006). A theory for the nursing care of patients at risk of suicide. *Journal of Advanced Nursing, 53*(6), 680–690.

Suppe, F. (1996, May). *Middle range theory: Nursing theory and knowledge development.* Conference Proceedings, Sixth Rosemary Ellis Scholar's Retreat: Nursing Science: Implications for the 21st Century, Cleveland, OH.

Swanson, K. M. (1991). Empirical development of a middle range theory of caring. *Nursing Research, 40*(3), 161–166.

Tsai, P. F. (2003). A middle range theory of caregiver stress. *Nursing Science Quarterly, 16*(2), 137–145.

Ulbrich, S. L. (1999). Nursing practice theory of exercise as self-care. *Image: The Journal of Nursing Scholarship, 31*(1), 65–70.

Wallace, R., Benson, H., & Wilson, A. F. (1971). A wakeful hypometabolic physiologic state. *American Journal of Physiology, 221*(3), 795–799.

Weiss, J. A., Jampol, M. L., Lievano, J. A., Smith, S. M., & Wurster, J. L. (2008). Normalizing risky sexual behaviours: A grounded theory study. *Pediatric Nursing, 34*(2), 163–169.

Whall, A. L. (2005). The structure of nursing knowledge: Analysis and evaluation of practice, middle range and grand theory. In J. J. Fitzpatrick & A. L. Whall (Eds.), *Conceptual models of nursing: Analysis and application* (4th ed., pp. 5–20). Upper Saddle River, NJ: Prentice-Hall.

Whittemore, R., & Roy, C. (2002). Adapting to diabetes mellitus: A theory synthesis. *Nursing Science Quarterly, 15*(4), 311–317.

Woodgate, R. L., & Degner, L. F. (2003). A substantive theory of keeping the spirit alive: The spirit within children with cancer and their families. *Journal of Pediatric Oncology Nursing, 20*(3), 103–119.

# 11

# Overview of Selected Middle Range Nursing Theories

## Melanie McEwen

*E*laine Chavez is employed as a nurse at a public health clinic in an urban area. She is also in her second semester of a graduate nursing program preparing to become a mental health nurse practitioner. In her practice, Elaine has worked with a number of women who have been abused by their partners, and she has observed a pattern of comorbidities in these women, including depression, alcoholism, substance abuse, and suicide attempts. Over the last few months Elaine has reviewed the literature and identified several intervention strategies that have been effective in working with women who have been victims of domestic violence. Using this information, she would like to implement a program to promote early identification and multiple-level intervention. This is a project that will work well with one of her master's portfolio assignments.

From her literature review, Elaine identified several theories related to her study. She was particularly interested in examining the set of circumstances that would cause the women to seek help. For this she performed a more detailed literature review and identified Kolcaba's (1994, 2003, 2009) Theory of Comfort, which helped her conceptualize many of the issues that the women faced. Indeed, the theory described individual characteristics that contributed to health-seeking behavior. These were stimulus situations, which can cause negative tension. By providing comfort measures, the nurse can help decrease negative tensions and promote positive tension. Elaine wanted to work to identify comfort measures that would encourage the women to seek care for their problems.

For the next phase of her project, Elaine collected all of the information she could on Kolcaba's theory. This included studies that had used the model as a conceptual framework and studies that had tested the model. From that information and the articles she had gathered previously about issues related to domestic violence, she was able to draft a set of interventions that she hoped to implement at the clinic following approval by her supervisor.

Previous chapters have described the growing emphasis on the development and testing of middle range theories in nursing. As a result, during the last decade a significant number of these theories have been presented. The purpose of this chapter is to introduce some of the commonly used middle range nursing theories as well as some of the recently published ones to familiarize readers with these works and direct them to resources for more information. An attempt was made to include works from a variety of areas and from many scholars, but by no means is the list presented here exhaustive. Nor does inclusion or exclusion relate to the quality or significance of the theory or its usefulness in research or practice.

To assist with organization of the chapter, the theories are divided into sections based on whether they appear to be "high," "middle," or "low" middle range theories. As explained in Chapter 10, the high/middle/low distinction relates to the level of abstraction as posed by Liehr and Smith (1999), with the "high" middle range theories being the most abstract and nearest to the grand theories. The "low" middle range theories, on the other hand, are the least abstract, and they are similar to practice theories. It is noted that these designations are arguably arbitrary and that one theory that is listed here as "high middle" may be considered by others to be a grand theory. Likewise another theory listed here as "middle middle" might be considered by others to be a high middle range theory and so forth.

Elements of theory description and theory analysis as explained in Chapter 5 serve as the basis for the more detailed discussions of selected theories. Each will include a brief overview, an outline of the purpose and major concepts of the theory, followed by context for use, and nursing implications. Finally, evidence of empirical testing is described.

## High Middle Range Theories

The high middle range theories presented here are some of the more well-known and most-used theories in nursing and include the works of Benner, Leininger, and Pender. These theories may be considered grand theories or conceptual frameworks by other nursing scholars and possibly by the author of the theory. These theories, however, do not totally fit with the criteria for grand theories as outlined in this text and, therefore, are not covered in the chapters dealing with that content. In addition, the Omaha System and the Synergy Model are two newer nursing models that are relatively widely used. These can also be considered high middle range theories and will be discussed in more depth. Table 11-1 lists other high middle range theories or conceptual models, their purposes, and major concepts.

### BENNER'S MODEL OF SKILL ACQUISITION IN NURSING

Patricia Benner's work, which applies the Dreyfus model of skill acquisition to nursing, was first published in 1984. The model outlines five stages of skill acquisition: novice, advanced beginner, competent, proficient, and expert. Although her work is much more encompassing in regard to nursing domains and specific functions and interventions, it is the five stages of skill acquisition that has received the most attention with regard to application in administration, education, practice, and research.

#### Purpose and Major Concepts

Benner's work delineates the importance of retaining and rewarding nurse clinicians for their clinical expertise in practice settings, because it describes the evolution of "excellent caring practices." She notes that research demonstrates that practice grows "through experiential learning and through transmitting that learning in practical settings"

## TABLE 11-1 *High Middle Range Nursing Theories*

| Theory/Model | Purpose | Major Concepts |
|---|---|---|
| Tidal model (psychiatric and mental health nursing) (Baker, 2001a, 2001b) | Describes psychiatric nursing practice focusing on three care processes; emphasizes the fluid nature of human experience characterized by change and unpredictability | Personhood (dimensions—world, self, others), discrete holistic (exploratory) assessment; focused (risk) assessment empowerment, narrative as the medium of self |
| Parish nursing (Bergquist & King, 1994) | Describes the integration of physical, emotional, and spiritual components in provision of holistic health care in a faith community | Client (spiritual, physical, emotional components), parish nurse (spiritual maturity, pastoral team member, autonomy, caring, effective communication), health (physical, emotional, and spiritual wellness and wholeness), environment (faith community) |
| Parish nursing (Miller, 1997) | Integrates the concepts of evangelical Christianity with application of parish nursing interventions | Person/parishioner, health, nurse/parish nurse, community/parish, the triune God |
| Neal theory of home health nursing (Neal, 1999a, 1999b) | Describes the practice of home health nurses as they use process of adaptation to attain autonomy | Autonomy, three stages (dependence, moderate dependence, and autonomy), logistics, client's home, client's resources, client's needs, and learning capacity |
| Occupational health nursing (Rogers, 1994) | Shows how the occupational health nurse works to improve, protect, maintain, and restore the health of the worker/workforce, and depicts how practice is affected by both external and internal work setting influences | Work setting influences (corporate culture/mission, resources, work hazards, workforce characteristics), external factors (economics, population/health trends, legislation/politics, technology), occupational health nursing practice (health promotion, workplace hazard detection, case management/primary care, counseling, management, research, legal/ethical monitoring, community orientation) |
| Public health nursing practice (Smith & Bazini-Barakat, 2003) | Guides public health nurses to improve the health of communities and target populations | Interdisciplinary public health team, standards of public health nursing practice, essential public health services, health indicators, population-based practice (systems, community, individual, and family focus), healthy people in health communities |
| Rural nursing (Weinert & Long, 1991) | Guides rural nursing practice, research, and education by understanding and addressing the unique health care needs and preferences of rural persons | Health (health as ability to work), environment (distance and isolation), person (self-reliance and independence), nursing (lack of anonymity, outsider/insider, and old-timer/newcomer) |

(Benner, 2001, p. vi). Expertise develops when the clinician tests and refines propositions, hypotheses, and principle-based expectations in actual practice situations. Finally, the model seeks to describe clinical expertise including six areas of practical knowledge (e.g., graded qualitative distinctions; common meanings; assumptions, expectations, and sets; paradigm cases and personal knowledge; maxims; and unplanned practices).

The central concepts of Benner's model are those of competence, skill acquisition, experience, clinical knowledge, and practical knowledge. She also identifies the following seven domains of nursing practice:

- Helping role
- Teaching or coaching function
- Diagnostic client-monitoring function
- Effective management of rapidly changing situations
- Administering and monitoring therapeutic interventions and regimens
- Monitoring and ensuring quality of health care practices
- Organizational and work-role competencies (Benner, 2001)

### Context for Use and Nursing Implications

The Benner model has been used extensively as rationale for career development and continuing education in nursing. Areas specifically cited for utilization include nursing management, career development, clinical specialization, staff development programs, staffing, evaluation, clinical internships, and precepting students and novice nurses (Benner, 2001).

### Evidence of Empirical Testing

A Cumulative Index of Nursing and Allied Health Literature (CINAHL) search covering a period between 1999 through 2008 revealed 82 English language listings of articles in nursing journals citing Benner's model; a number of these were research-based studies. For example, Altier and Krsek (2006) used Benner's work as a conceptual framework in a study of the effect of a residency program on job satisfaction and retention among new nursing graduates. In other works, Standing (2007) used Benner's model to frame a longitudinal study to determine acquisition of clinical decision-making skills; and Rischel, Larsen, and Jackson (2008) used Benner's model to examine and categorize nurses' competence in admission assessment.

Nonresearch-based articles included a report by Cathcart (2008), which explained the role of the chief nursing officer based on tenet's of Benner's work and a personal account of a nurse (Dest, 2008) describing the importance of mentors during her professional transition to an expert in oncology nursing. A fairly common theme was noted as several writers discussed Benner's applicability in development of procedures and protocols for orientation of new nurses and new graduates. For example, Morris and others (2007) provided a detailed description of the development of a critical care orientation program designed from Benner's criteria explaining the development of "expert" practitioners; and Wilgis and McConnell (2008) described the process of development of an educational program designed to improve graduate nurses' critical thinking skills. Likewise, Benner's work was used in several articles (e.g., Cote & Burwell, 2007; Kanaskie, Felmlee, & Shay, 2008; Storey, Crist, Nelis, Murphy, & Fisher, 2007) to discuss the development or updating of career enhancement or clinical ladder programs.

## LEININGER'S CULTURAL CARE DIVERSITY AND UNIVERSALITY THEORY

Madeline Leininger has been instrumental in demonstrating to nurses the importance of considering the impact of culture on health and healing (Leininger, 2002). She has been a prolific nursing scholar and is credited with starting the specialty of transcultural nursing. In addition, she is a leading proponent of the idea that nursing is synonymous with caring.

Leininger reported that she conceptualized transcultural nursing as a distinct area of nursing practice in the late 1950s during her doctoral work in anthropology; she continued to study and develop a transcultural nursing conceptual framework throughout the 1960s. In the mid-1970s, she presented a "transcultural health model" that was expanded in 1978 and 1980. The Leininger Sunrise Model was first described as such in 1984 and depicts the transcultural dimensions of culturologic interviews, assessments, and therapies (Leininger & McFarland, 2006; McFarland, 2006).

### Purpose and Major Concepts

The purpose of Leininger's theory is to generate knowledge related to the nursing care of people who value their cultural heritage and lifeways. Major concepts of the model are culture, culture care, and culture care differences (diversities) and similarities (universals) pertaining to transcultural human care. Other major concepts are care and caring, emic view (language expressions, perceptions, beliefs, and practice of individuals or groups of a particular culture in regard to certain phenomena), etic view (universal language expression beliefs and practices in regard to certain phenomena that pertain to several cultures or groups), lay system of health care, professional system of health care, and culturally congruent nursing care (Leininger, 2007; Leininger & McFarland, 2006).

### Context for Use and Nursing Implications

The goal for application of Leininger's theory is to provide culturally congruent nursing care to persons of diverse cultures. A central tenet of the theory is that it is important for the nurse to understand the individual's view of illness. Also, the focus is on recognizing and understanding cultural similarities and differences and using this information to positively influence nursing care and health (Leininger & McFarland, 2006). Because the theory has been widely used for research, findings are appropriate for nurses in any setting who work with individuals, families, and groups from a cultural group different from the nurse's.

### Evidence of Empirical Testing

Leininger (2007) reported that the theory was derived and refined through a number of years of study. Over the past 2 decades, research on various groups was conducted, and she listed cultural values and culture care meanings and action modes for 23 cultural groups in her book. Many graduate students and nursing scholars have used Leininger's theory as a basis for research, and a CINAHL search conducted between 1999 and 2008 produced more than 200 citations of articles using Leininger's theory. Many of these used Leininger's work as a conceptual framework to study cultural implications of a variety of health problems. For example, Plowden (2006) examined the decision-making process of African-American men regarding whether and when they were screened for prostate cancer; and Anderson, Jun, and Choi (2007) looked at Korean women's choices to undergo breast cancer screening. In other studies, Jones (2008) reported on Mexican American's use of emergency departments and Evans and Crogan (2006) looked at nutrition among Hispanic nursing home residents.

Leininger's model has also been used by many authors to identify variables or characteristics of cultural groups or subcultures that might influence health. For example, Thibodeaux and Deatrick (2007) identified the effect of cultural values and beliefs on the management of childhood cancer and Munoz and Hilgenberg (2005) reported on "ethnopharmacology," explaining the importance of recognizing how ethnicity can influence drug use (i.e., patient adherence to a medication regimen) and physiologic response (i.e., absorption, metabolism, and elimination).

A number of nonresearch articles describing aspects of transcultural nursing, focusing on Leininger's works have also been published in recent years. These include

| BOX 11-1 | *Research Studies Using Leininger's Theory of Cultural Care Diversity and Universality* |

Anuforo, P. O., Oyedele, L., & Pacquiao, D. F. (2004). Comparative study of meanings, beliefs, and practices of female circumcision among three Nigerian tribes in the United States and Nigeria. *Journal of Transcultural Nursing, 15*(2), 103–113.

Evanson, T. A., & Zust, B. L. (2006). "Bittersweet Knowledge": The long-term effects of an international experience. *Journal of Nursing Education, 45*(1), 412–417.

Martin, M. L., Jensen, E., Coatsworth-Puspoky, C. F., et al. (2007). Integrating an evidence-based research intervention in the discharge of mental health clients. *Archives of Psychiatric Nursing, 21*(2), 101–111.

Plowden, K. O., John, W., Vasquez, E., & Kimani, J. (2006). Reaching African American men: A qualitative analysis. *Journal of Community Health Nursing, 23*(3), 147–158.

Running, A., Martin, K., & Tolle, L. W. (2007). An innovative model for conducting a participatory community health assessment. *Journal of Community Health Nursing, 24*(4), 203–213.

Torsvik, M., & Hedlund, M. (2008). Cultural encounters in reflective dialogue about nursing care: A qualitative study. *Journal of Advanced Nursing, 63*(4), 389–396.

a review of cultural education in nursing (Campesino, 2008), a report on how to enhance awareness of diversity and racism in nursing education (Lancellotti, 2008), and the description of a model to teach nursing students about cultural influences on health (Kleiman, Frederickson, & Lundy, 2004). Other examples of research studies using Leininger's model are listed in Box 11-1. See the list of websites at the end of the chapter for additional information.

## PENDER'S HEALTH PROMOTION MODEL

Nola Pender began studying health-promoting behavior in the mid-1970s and first published the Health Promotion Model (HPM) in 1982. She reported that the model was constructed from expectancy-value theory and social cognitive theory using a nursing perspective. The model was modified slightly in the late 1980s, again in 1996 (Pender, 1996; Pender, Murdaugh, & Parsons, 2006).

### Purpose and Major Concepts

The HPM was proposed as a framework for integrating nursing and behavioral science perspectives on factors that influence health behaviors. The model is to be used as a guide to explore the biopsychosocial processes that motivate individuals to engage in behaviors directed toward health enhancement (Pender et al., 2006). The model has been used extensively as a framework for research aimed at predicting health-promoting lifestyles as well as specific behaviors.

Major concepts of the HPM are individual characteristics and experiences (prior related behavior and personal factors), behavior-specific cognitions and affect (perceived benefits of action, perceived barriers to action, perceived self-efficacy, activity-related affect, interpersonal influences, and situational influences), and behavioral outcomes (commitment to a plan of action, immediate competing demands and preferences, and health-promoting behavior). Figure 11-1 shows the Health Promotion Model.

### Context for Use and Nursing Implications

Health promotion services are essential for improving the health of populations everywhere. It is noted that people of all ages can benefit from health promotion care, which should be delivered at sites where people spend much of their time (e.g., schools and

Individual
Characteristics
and Experiences

Behavior-Specific
Cognitions
and Affect

Behavioral
Outcome

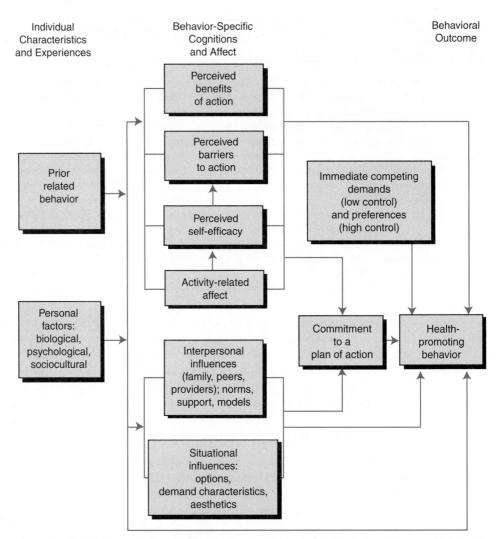

FIGURE 11-1 Health Promotion Model. (Adapted from Pender, N. J., Murdaugh, C. L., & Parsons, M. A. (2002). *Health promotion in nursing practice* (4th ed.). Upper Saddle River, NJ: Prentice-Hall.)

workplaces). Nurses can develop and execute health-promoting interventions to individuals, groups, and families in schools, nursing centers, occupational health settings, and the community at large. Nurses should work toward empowerment for self-care and enhancing the client's capacity for self-care through education and personal development.

### Evidence of Empirical Testing

Pender and colleagues (2006) wrote that the model has been used by numerous nursing scholars and researchers, and has been useful in explaining and predicting specific health behaviors. A CINAHL search in late 2008 produced listings for 235 English language articles that reported using or applying Pender's HPM during the previous decade.

Most research studies used Pender's work as one component of a conceptual framework for study. For example, Smith and Bashore (2006) used the HPM to explain health perceptions and health-promoting behaviors among young cancer survivors; and Mendias and Paar (2007) used the model to study perceptions of health and self-care strategies of persons with HIV/AIDS. Similarly, Eschiti (2008) used

BOX 11-2 *Research Studies Using Pender's Health Promotion Model*

Allen, K. N., Taylor, J. S., & Kuiper, R. (2007). Effectiveness of nutrition education on fast food choices in adolescents. *The Journal of School Nursing, 23*(6), 337–342.

Calvert, W. J., & Bucholz, K. K. (2008). Adolescent risky behaviours and alcohol use. *Western Journal of Nursing Research, 30*(1), 147–148.

Gallagher, M. R., Gill, S., & Reifsnider, E. (2008). Child health promotion and protection among Mexican mothers. *Western Journal of Nursing Research, 30*(5), 588–605.

Kwong, E. W., & Kwan, A. Y. (2007). Participation in health-promoting behaviour: Influences on

community-dwelling older Chinese people. *Journal of Advanced Nursing, 57*(5), 522–534.

Shin, K. R., Kang, Y., Park, H. J., et al. (2008). Testing and developing the Health Promotion Model in low-income, Korean elderly women. *Nursing Science Quarterly, 21*(2), 173–178.

Skybo, T., & Polivka, B. (2006). Health promotion model for childhood violence prevention and exposure. *Journal of Clinical Nursing, 16*(1), 38–45.

Taylor, E. J. (2008). Promoting spiritual health in home health care. *Home Heathcare Nurse, 26*(6), 367–373.

Pender's concepts to examine use of complementary and alternative modalities by women who had experienced breast and gynecological cancers.

Other studies use health promotion as an outcome or to predict behaviors. Conway, McClune, and Nosel (2007), for example, used the model to identify how primary care practitioners provided "anticipatory guidance" to prevent farm accidents. And, in other research, Wood (2008) used the HPM to study the motivation for exercise to reduce breast cancer risk and Esperat and others (2007) used it to study and then predict health-promoting behaviours of low-income pregnant women. Additional examples of recent research studies using Pender's HPM are listed in Box 11-2. For more information on Pender and the HPM, see the Internet Resources section at the end of this chapter.

# THE OMAHA SYSTEM

The Omaha System is described as a research-based, comprehensive classification system that promotes documentation of client care. The origins of the Omaha System date to the early 1970s. The system was led by efforts of the nurses of the Visiting Nurses Association (VNA) of Omaha, Nebraska. Martin (2005) reported that it "was developed and revised during four federally funded research projects that were conducted from 1975 to 1993" (p. 18).

## Purpose and Major Concepts

The Omaha System is developed to guide community health nursing practice and serve as a method for documentation of care and data management. Martin and Scheet (1992) list its "capabilities and characteristics":

- Advances the scientific practice of nursing
- Offers capabilities to quantify community health nursing
- Is practical for general community health application
- Is congruent with the nursing process
- Minimizes redundancies in the client record
- Limits documentation time (p. 20)

In the Omaha System model, the client is central to the model and can be an individual, family, or community. The practitioner–client relationship encompasses the core of the model, which depicts the steps of the nursing process in a circular rather than linear format, indicating that decisions made by the nurse are cyclic and ongoing. The specific terms used for the nursing process are "collect and assess data, state problems, identify admission problem rating, plan and intervene, identify interim/dismissal problem rating, and evaluate problem outcomes" (Martin, 2005).

### Context for Use and Nursing Implications

The Omaha System is a tool or method for nurses working in community settings that provide a framework for provision and documentation of care. The system can be used to facilitate evidence-based, multidisciplinary practice, documentation, and information management through using a standardized taxonomy of client problems, interventions, and client outcomes.

The Omaha System is intended for use in community health and home health nursing settings. It is assumed that the nurse in these settings will begin service to a client following an intake or referral process. During the initial visit and throughout care provision, the importance of establishing and maintaining a positive nurse–client relationship is stressed. Initial activities include data collection and analysis. Planning and intervention involve setting priorities and determining a course of action. Identification of admission, interim, and dismissal ratings relate to the evaluation process. Each rating is based on criteria within the Omaha System that allows the nurse to compare the client health status at different points in time to determine nursing effectiveness (Martin, 2005).

### Evidence of Empirical Testing

The Omaha System has been used in home health nursing since the early 1990s and numerous articles on it have been published. A CINAHL search listed 93 English language articles between 1999 and late 2008. Many of these articles describe practice applications of the model. Some articles reported on research studies that used data gathered through employing the Omaha System in practice. For example, McEwen and Slack (2005) studied various types of health problems—identified using the Omaha System—among persons of Mexican origin living in Arizona. In another work, Wong, Chow, and Chung (2008) compared data from more than 330 clients to assess whether home health nursing visits reduced hospital readmissions.

Although the Omaha System was developed to guide community and home health nursing, it has been used in other settings. For example, several articles (Barkauskas et al., 2006; Connolly, Mao, Yoder, & Canham, 2006; Neff, Kinion, & Cardina, 2007) described its utility in providing care in nurse managed centers. In another work, Yu and Lang (2008) used the model to describe care for patients in an outpatient rehabilitation setting. Also, use of the Omaha System in nursing education was described by Barton, Clark, and Baramee (2004) and Elfrink and Davis (2004). More information about the Omaha System can be found at the website listed in the Internet Resources section at the end of this chapter.

## THE SYNERGY MODEL

The Synergy Model for Patient Care was developed in the mid-1990s by a panel of nurses of the American Association of Critical-Care Nurses (AACN) Certification Corporation as a framework for certified practice. The initial model was revised somewhat and the revised version was then used as the basis for the AACN's certification examination (Hardin, 2005).

> **BOX 11-3** *The Synergy Model: Patient Characteristics and Nurse Competencies*
>
> | PATIENT CHARACTERISTICS | NURSE COMPETENCIES |
> |---|---|
> | Resiliency | Clinical judgment |
> | Vulnerability | Clinical inquiry |
> | Stability | Facilitation of learning |
> | Complexity | Collaboration |
> | Resource availability | Systems thinking |
> | Participation in care | Advocacy and moral agency |
> | Participation in decision making | Caring practices |
> | Predictability | Response to diversity |
>
> Source: AACN (2004).

### Purpose and Major Concepts

The purpose of the Synergy Model is to articulate nurses' contributions, activities, and outcomes with regard to caring for critically ill patients. The model identifies eight patient needs or characteristics and eight competencies of nurses in critical care situations (Box 11-3) (AACN, 2008). "According to the model, each patient brings a unique set of characteristics to the health care situation" (Hardin, 2005, p. 4). Of the many unique characteristics nurses assess, the eight most consistently observed are listed in Box 11-3. The nursing competencies denote how knowledge, skills, and experience are integrated within nursing care.

The Synergy Model also describes three levels of outcomes—those relating to the patient, the nurse, and the system. Patient outcomes include functional and behavioral change, trust, satisfaction, comfort, and quality of life. Nurse outcomes include physiological changes, presence or absence of complications, and extent to which care objectives were attained. System outcomes include recidivism, costs, and resource utilization (Curley, 1998). Figure 11-2 depicts the Synergy Model.

### Context for Use and Nursing Implications

As mentioned, originally the Synergy Model was developed to structure the AACN's certification examination by identifying nursing competencies that are essential for those providing care to the critically ill. In 2002, assumptions of the model were expanded to establish the model as a conceptual framework for designing practice and developing competencies required to care for critically ill patients. Use of the Synergy Model in practice is designed to optimize patient outcomes. When patient characteristics and nurse competencies match and synergize, outcomes for the patient are optimal (Curley, 1998; Hardin, 2009). In addition, the model can be used for developing nursing curricula and for conducting research (Hardin, 2005).

### Evidence of Empirical Testing

Although the Synergy Model is relatively new, a significant number of articles have been published describing its use in practice and education. Indeed, a CINAHL search in late 2008 indicated almost 90 notations related to it. Identified were two articles that tested application of the model. Brewer and colleagues (2007) described the large scale testing of an assessment tool developed from the Synergy Model that showed effectiveness for

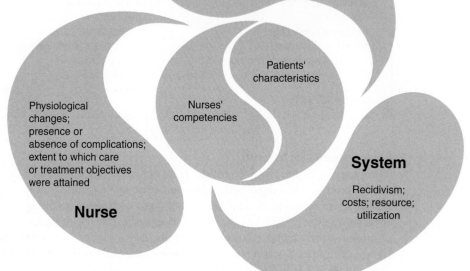

FIGURE 11-2 The Synergy Model delineates three levels of outcomes: Those derived from the patient, those derived from the nurse, and those derived from the health care system. (From Curley, M. A. Q. (1998). Patient–nurse synergy: Optimizing patients' outcomes. *American Journal of Critical Care, 7*(1), 69.)

both adult and pediatric patients. Another article (Sechrist, Berlin, & Biel, 2000) explained the process of testing and validating the model. A few works (Becker, Kaplow, Muenzen, & Hartigan, 2006; Brewer, 2006; Brewer et al., 2007; Cox, 2003) described research studies using the Synergy Model as a framework. Box 11-4 shows several examples of articles describing the model's use in leadership/administration, practice, and education.

---

**BOX 11-4** *The Synergy Model in Practice and Education*

Collins, A. S., & Strother, D. (2008). Synergy and competence: Tools of the trade. *Journal for Nurses in Staff Development, 24*(4), E1–8.

Freyling, M. E., Kesten, K. S., & Heath, J. (2008). The Synergy Model at work in a military ICU in Iraq. *Critical Care Nursing Clinics of North America, 20*(1), 23–29.

Graham-Garcia, J., George-Gay, B., Heater, D., Butts, A., & Heath, J. (2006). Application of the Synergy Model with the surgical care of smokers. *Critical Care Nursing Clinics of North America, 18*(1), 29–38.

Green, D. A. (2006). A Synergy Model of nursing education. *Journal for Nurses in Staff Development, 22*(6), 277–285.

Kaplow, R., & Reed, K. D. (2008). The AACN Synergy Model for Patient Care: A nursing model as a force of magnetism. *Nursing Economics, 26*(1), 17–25.

Reilly, T., & Humbrecht, D. (2007). Fostering Synergy: A nurse-managed remote telemetry model. *Critical Care Nurse, 27*(3), 22–28.

Smith, A. R. (2006). Using the Synergy Model to provide spiritual nursing care in critical care settings. *Critical Care Nurse, 26*(4), 41–50.

## Middle Middle Range Theories

A number of nursing theories may be categorized as middle middle range. Four theories that have been cited in a considerable number of nursing studies are discussed in the following sections. They are Mishel's (1984) Uncertainty in Illness Theory; Kolcaba's (1994) Theory of Comfort; Lenz, Suppe, Gift, Pugh, and Milligan's (1995; Lenz, Pugh, Milligan, Gift, & Suppe, 1997) Theory of Unpleasant Symptoms; and Reed's (1991a) Self-Transcendence Theory. Table 11-2 lists other middle middle range theories that have been used in nursing practice and research.

TABLE 11-2 *Middle Middle Range Nursing Theories*

| Theory/Model | Purpose | Major Concepts |
|---|---|---|
| Self-help (Braden, 1990) | Describes a process of factors that decrease self and life quality and factors that increase learning a self-help response and thus a greater quality of life | Disease characteristics, background inducements, monitoring (level of information about illness), severity of illness, dependency, uncertainty, enabling skill, self-help, life quality |
| Chronic illness trajectory framework (Corbin & Strauss, 1991, 1992) | Describes a view of chronic illness with eight phases, from pretrajectory to dying, with each possessing the possibilities of reversals, plateaus and upward or downward movement; allows for conceptualization of the course of illness to comprehensively direct care and conduct research | Trajectory, trajectory phases (pretrajectory, trajectory onset, crisis, acute, stable, unstable, downward, dying), trajectory projection, trajectory scheme (shape illness course, control symptoms, and handle disability) |
| Motivation in health behavior (health behavior, self-determinism) (Cox, 1985) | Describes intrinsic motivation in health behavior | Individual's self-determined health judgments, self-determined health behavior, perceived competency in health matters, internal–external cue responsiveness |
| Theory of care-seeking behavior (Lauver, 1992) | Explains the probability of engaging in health behavior as a function of psychosocial variables and facilitating conditions regarding the behavior | Clinical and sociodemographic variables, affect (feelings associated with care-seeking behavior), utility (expectations and values about outcomes), normative influences, habits, care-seeking behavior |
| Self-efficacy (Lenz & Shortridge-Baggett, 2002) | Applies of Bandura's work in nursing to assist people to be as independent as possible in managing their health | Person (perception, self-referent), behavior (initiation, effort, persistence), efficacy-expectation (magnitude, strength, generality), information sources (performance, vicarious experiences, verbal persuasion, physiological information), and outcome expectations |
| Experiencing transitions (Meleis, 1994; Meleis, Sawyer, Im, Messias, & Schumacher, 2000; Schumacher & Meleis, 1994) | Explains the process of transition in a client following changes in health and illness; nurses may help prepare clients for impending transitions by uncovering associated risks | Types of transitions (developmental, situational, health/illness, and organizational), patterns of transitions (single, multiple, sequential, simultaneous, related, and unrelated), transition experiences, transition conditions, process indicators, outcome indicators, and nursing therapeutics |

*(Continued)*

TABLE 11-2 *Middle Middle Range Nursing Theories (Continued)*

| Theory/Model | Purpose | Major Concepts |
|---|---|---|
| Model for social support (Norbeck, 1981) | Outlines the elements and relationships that must be studied to incorporate social support into nursing practice; emphasis placed on developing the environment | Properties of the person (age, demographic characteristics, needs), properties of the situation (role demands, resources, stressors), need for social support, available social support |
| Theory of resilience (Polk, 1997) | Proposes interrelatedness of dispositional, relational, situational and philosophical patterns to describe concept of resilience to guide generation of nursing interventions to assess and strengthen resilience | Dispositional pattern (pattern of physical and ego-related psychosocial attributes that contribute to manifestation of resilience), relational pattern (roles and relationships that influence resilience), situational pattern (characteristic approach to situations or stressors), philosophical pattern (personal beliefs) |
| Theory of caring (Swanson, 1991) | Proposes a definition of caring and the five essential categories or processes that characterize caring | Knowing, being with, doing for, enabling, and maintaining belief |

## MISHEL'S UNCERTAINTY IN ILLNESS THEORY

Mishel began studying the concept of uncertainty in illness in the early 1980s when she desired to explain the stress that results from hospitalization (Mishel, 1981, 1984). She developed the Mishel Uncertainty in Illness Scale to better examine the concept, and since that time her model and instrument have been used in numerous nursing studies (Bailey & Stewart, 2006; Mishel, 1984, 1988). In the late 1980s she formally developed the theory, which she then revised in the early 1990s (Mishel, 1988, 1990).

### Purpose and Major Concepts

According to Mishel (1988, 1999), the Uncertainty in Illness Theory explains how clients cognitively process illness-related stimuli and construct meaning in these events. Uncertainty is seen as the inability to structure meaning and may develop if the person does not form a "cognitive schema for illness events" (Mishel, 1988, p. 225).

The early iteration of the model (Mishel, 1988) described the concepts of "stimuli frame" (symptom pattern, event familiarity, event congruency), "cognitive capacities," and "structure providers" (credible authority, social support, education) that may lead to uncertainty. Other concepts include appraisal, inference, illusion, and opportunity, as well as coping mechanisms; these may lead to adaptation. In 1990, the process of theory derivation was used to update and revise the theory to address issues related to chronic uncertainty. Interestingly, chaos theory was used in this process (Mishel, 1990). Figure 11-3 shows the Uncertainty in Illness Theory.

### Context for Use and Nursing Implications

The Uncertainty in Illness Theory explains how individuals cognitively process illness-related stimuli and how they structure meaning for those events. In the theory, adaptation is the desirable end-state achieved after coping with the uncertainty. Nurses may develop nursing interventions that attempt to influence the person's cognitive process to address the uncertainty. This, in turn, should produce positive coping and adaptation (Mishel, 1984, 1999).

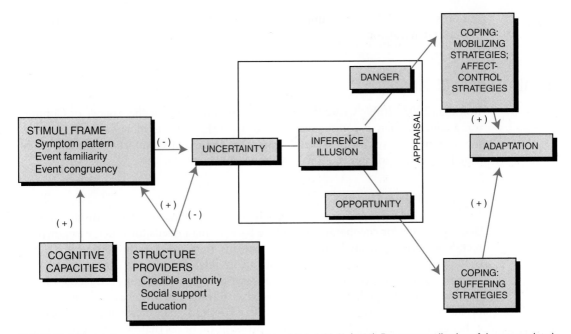

FIGURE 11-3 Model of perceived uncertainty in illness. (From Mishel, M. H. (1990). Reconceptualization of the uncertainty in illness theory. *Image: Journal of Nursing Scholarship, 22*(4), 256–262.)

### Evidence of Empirical Testing

During the process of theory development and refinement, Mishel developed and tested several research instruments. These are the Adult Uncertainty in Illness Scale and the Adult Uncertainty in Illness Scale—community form; the Parents' Perception of Uncertainty in Illness Scale and the Parents' Perception of Uncertainty in Illness Scale—Family Member (Mishel, 2008). These have been used by Mishel and her colleagues as well as a number of additional nursing researchers in various studies. In early works testing the theory, Mishel (1984) showed that perceived uncertainty about symptoms, treatment, and outcomes was a major predictor of stress. And, Mishel and Sorenson (1991) tested a portion of the model and concluded that uncertainty significantly predicted "mastery" and that coping strategies could influence the variable of danger.

The Uncertainty in Illness model is becoming increasingly recognized in nursing literature as a resource for research and practice. Based on a CINAHL search, in recent years (1999–2008), 46 articles were published involving Mishel's work, and a number of research studies were identified using Mishel's theory or instrument or both in addressing health issues among a wide variety of groups and covering many different health problems. For example, while studying elders who had survived breast cancer, Clayton, Mishel and Belyea (2006) determined that symptom clusters, age, and uncertainty strongly influenced well-being and that communication with providers can reduce emotional distress. Also working with oncology patients, Decker and colleagues (2007) examined the concept of uncertainty among adolescents and young adults with cancer and reported significant differences in several measures comparing newly diagnosed patients with those who were 1–5 years post-diagnosis. In other studies, Kloos and Daly (2008) used Mishel's work to study the effect of journaling on anxiety levels of family members of critically ill patients; Eastwood and others (2008) examined uncertainty and quality of life among patients 1 year after undergoing cardiac angiography;

and Sossong (2007) studied uncertainty in individuals living with an implantable cardioverter defibrillator.

## KOLCABA'S THEORY OF COMFORT

Kolcaba (2003, 2009) wrote that the first step in developing the Theory of Comfort was a concept analysis conducted in 1988 while she was a graduate student. Following a number of steps over several years, the Theory of Comfort was initially published in 1994, and later modified (Kolcaba, 1994, 2001).

### Purpose and Major Concepts

Kolcaba (1994) defined comfort within nursing practice as "the satisfaction (actively, passively, or co-operatively) of the basic human needs for relief, ease, or transcendence arising from health care situations that are stressful" (p. 1178). She explained that a client's needs arise from a stimulus situation and can cause negative tension. Increasing comfort can result in having negative tensions reduced and positive tensions engaged. Comfort is viewed as an outcome of care that can promote or facilitate health-seeking behaviors. It is posited that increasing comfort can enhance health-seeking behaviors. One proposition notes that "if enhanced comfort is achieved, patients, family members and/or nurses are strengthened to engage in HSBs [health-seeking behaviors], which further enhances comfort" (Kolcaba, 2009, p. 260).

Major concepts described in the theory of comfort include comfort, comfort care, comfort measures, comfort needs, health-seeking behaviors, institutional integrity, and intervening variables. There are also eight defined propositions that link the defined concepts (Box 11-5) (Kolcaba, 2001, 2009). Figure 11-4 presents the Theory of Comfort.

---

**BOX 11-5** | *Propositions of Comfort Theory*

1. Nurses and members of the health care team identify comfort needs of patients and family members
2. Nurses design and coordinate interventions to address comfort needs
3. Intervening variables are considered when designing interventions
4. When interventions are delivered in a caring manner and are effective, the outcome of enhanced comfort is attained
5. Patients, nurses and other health care team members agree on desirable and realistic health-seeking behaviors
6. If enhanced comfort is achieved, patients, family members and/or nurses are more likely to engage in health-seeking behaviors; these further enhance comfort
7. When patients and family members are given comfort care and engage in health-seeking behaviors, they are more satisfied with health care and have better health-related outcomes
8. When patients, families, and nurses are satisfied with health care in an institution, public acknowledgment about that institution's contributions to health care will help the institution remain viable and flourish. Evidence-based practice or policy improvements may be guided by these propositions and the theoretical framework

Adapted from Kolcaba (2001, 2009).

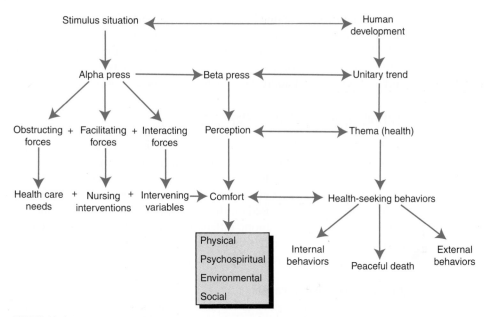

FIGURE 11-4 The conceptual framework for the Theory of Comfort. (From Kolcaba, K. (2001). Evolution of the middle range Theory of Comfort for outcomes research. *Nursing Outlook, 49*(2), 86–92.)

### Context for Use and Nursing Implications

Comfort Theory observes that patients experience needs for comfort in stressful health care situations. Some of these needs are identified by the nurse who then implements interventions to meet the needs (Kolcaba, 1995). Kolcaba (2009) stated that "Comfort Theory can be adapted to any health care setting or age group … " (p. 260). Understanding of comfort can promote nursing care that is holistic and inclusive of physical, psychospiritual, social, and environmental interventions. It is noted that any actual unhappy, unhealthy, or unwell patients can be made more comfortable (Kolcaba, 1994). Finally, outcomes of comfort can be measurable, holistic, positive, and nurse-sensitive.

### Evidence of Empirical Testing

The General Comfort questionnaire (GCQ) is a 48-item Likert-type scale that was developed to measure concepts and propositions described in the theory (Kolcaba, 2009). The GCQ has been modified to be used for different populations in a number of studies, and a shortened GCQ (28 items) is also in use (Kolcaba, 2009).

Kolcaba (2009) described development of other tools to assist in research and practice application for the Theory of Comfort. These include the visual analog scale (VAS), which was developed to measure the three subscales of comfort (relief, ease, and transcendence), and the Comfort Behaviors Checklist, which was developed to measure comfort in patient who can't use traditional questionnaires or other instrument.

A number of research studies have been conducted by Kolcaba and colleagues using the instruments described above. For example, Dowd and others (2007) reported on using Kolcaba's instruments to study reduction of stress among college students combining healing touch and coaching, and Wagner, Byrne, and Kolcaba (2006) studied how comfort measures (e.g., warming) positively affected preoperative patients.

Kolcaba, Tilton, and Drouin (2006) described how Comfort Theory can be used to provide consistency and coherence to enhance nursing care, promote professional practice, and serve as a unifying framework to support magnet recognition status. In another work, Kolcaba and DiMarco (2005) showed how the theory can be used to provide "proactive" and "multifaceted" nursing care for pediatric patients. For more information about Comfort Theory and the use of the various instruments, see Kolcaba's website (the internet address can be found at the end of the chapter).

# LENZ ET AL.'S THEORY OF UNPLEASANT SYMPTOMS

The Theory of Unpleasant Symptoms was developed by a group of nurses interested in a variety of nursing issues including symptom management, theory development, and nursing science (Gift, 2009). The theory was initially published in the nursing literature in the mid-1990s (Lenz et al., 1995) and then updated a few years later (Lenz et al., 1997). The theory was based on the premise that there are commonalities in experiencing different symptoms among different groups and in different situations. The theory was developed to integrate existing knowledge about a variety of symptoms to better prepare nurses in symptom management.

### Purpose and Major Concepts
The purpose of the Theory of Unpleasant Symptoms is "to improve understanding of the symptom experience in various contexts and to provide information useful for designing effective means to prevent, ameliorate, or manage unpleasant symptoms and their negative effects" (Lenz & Pugh, 2008, p. 160). Lenz and colleagues (1997) reported that the theory has three major components: (1) the symptoms that the individual is experiencing; (2) influencing factors that produce or affect the symptom experience; and (3) the consequences of the symptom experience.

Within the theory, symptoms are described in terms of duration, intensity, distress, and quality. Influencing factors can be physiologic factors, psychological factors, and/or situational factors. Performance is described in terms of functional status, cognitive functioning, or physical performance (Lenz et al., 1997). Figure 11-5 depicts the Theory of Unpleasant Symptoms.

### Context for Use and Nursing Implications
Gift (2009) explained that the Theory of Unpleasant Symptoms helps nurses recognize the need to assess multiple aspects of symptoms including characteristics of the symptom(s) itself, the underlying disease or other cause, as well as the frequency, intensity, duration, quality, and distress felt by the patient due to the symptom(s). The developers of the Theory of Unpleasant Symptoms note that it is clinically applicable to multiple client situations, as it should stimulate nurses to consider factors that might influence more than one symptom and the ways in which symptoms interact with each other (Lenz et al., 1997). The theory's developers mentioned that it has been used in an emergency department to develop a symptom assessment scale for cardiac patients and has been useful in predicting the need for hospitalization among patients with chronic obstructive pulmonary disease (COPD).

### Evidence of Empirical Testing
A growing number of research studies using the Theory of Unpleasant Symptoms as a conceptual or organizing framework have been conducted. One study by Huth and Broome (2007) used the theory to examine the collection of postoperative symptoms of children undergoing tonsillectomy. Another study (Rychnovsky, 2007) examined postpartum fatigue among military women and correlated findings with other symptoms including depression, anxiety, sleep patterns, and functional status. Corwin and

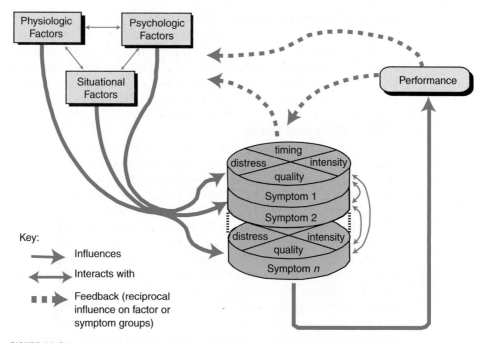

FIGURE 11-5 Updated version of the middle range Theory of Unpleasant Symptoms. (From Lenz, E. R., Pugh, L. C., Milligan, R. A., Gift, A., & Suppe, F. (1997). The middle range Theory of Unpleasant Symptoms: An update. *Advances in Nursing Science, 19*(3), 14–27.)

colleagues (2005) also studied postpartum fatigue, analyzing its correlation with development of postpartum depression. Finally, Liu (2006) studied symptoms associated with fatigue among patients undergoing hemodialysis.

## REED'S SELF-TRANSCENDENCE THEORY

Pamela Reed first wrote about the concept of self-transcendence in 1983, and formally outlined her theory in 1991 (Reed, 1991a). She reported that she used "deductive reformulation" of theories of lifespan development in constructing the theory. These she integrated with Rogers' conceptual system, clinical experience, and empirical work (Reed, 1991a). Self-transcendence is developed by introspective activities and concerns about the welfare of others and by integrating perceptions of one's past and future to enhance the present (Reed, 1991b).

### Purpose and Major Concepts

Self-transcendence is considered to be a "characteristic of developmental maturity whereby there is an expansion of self-boundaries and orientation toward broadened life perspectives and purposes" (Reed, 1991a, p. 64). Self-transcendence moves the individual beyond the immediate or constricted view of self and the world (Reed, 1996). Within self-transcendence there is "an expansion of personal boundaries outwardly (toward others and the environment), inwardly (toward greater awareness of beliefs, values, and dreams), and temporally (toward integration of past and future in the present)" (Reed, 1996, p. 3). Other central concepts of the theory include well-being (a sense of wholeness and health) and vulnerability (awareness of personal mortality) (Reed, 2008).

### Context for Use and Nursing Implications

Reed (1991a) reported that a theory of self-transcendence may be used by nurses to attend to spiritual and psychosocial expressions of self-transcendence in clients who are confronted with end-of-life issues. To promote self-transcendence, nurses may use interventions such as meditation, self-reflection, visualization, religious expression, counseling, and journaling to expand the individual's boundaries.

### Evidence of Empirical Testing

A number of nursing research studies have used the theory of self-transcendence. In an early work, Reed (1991b) found support for the theory in an examination of the mental health of elders. In the study she also found that there was a relationship between self-transcendence and mental health and an inverse relationship between self-transcendence and depression. More recently, Coward and Kahn (2005) and Coward (2003) reported on efforts to facilitate self-transcendence among breast cancer patients, and Ellermann and Reed (2001) examined self-transcendence and depression in middle-aged adults.

Several current projects have looked at self-transcendence among nurses and/or nursing students. For example, Hunnibell and others (2008) studied differences in self-transcendence between hospice and oncology nurses, analyzing how it influenced burnout in those groups. In similar works, Gottlieb (2007) studied self-transcendence and well-being in newly graduated RNs, and Walsh and colleagues (2008) examined whether student nurses' self-transcendence could positively influence their attitudes toward caring for elders.

## Low Middle Range Theories

The number of low middle range theories appears to be growing as nursing researchers and nursing scholars describe phenomena directly related to practice. Three theories are examined in the following sections. They are Eakes, Burke, and Hainsworth's (1998) Theory of Chronic Sorrow; Beck's (1993) Postpartum Depression Theory; and Mercer's (1983) Conceptualization of Maternal Role Attainment/Becoming a Mother. Table 11-3 lists other low middle range theories.

## EAKES, BURKE, AND HAINSWORTH'S THEORY OF CHRONIC SORROW

The concept of chronic sorrow was introduced in the early 1960s to describe grief observed in the parents of children with mental deficiencies. Subsequent research indicated similar patterns of chronic sorrow in parents of mentally or physically disabled children. The Nursing Consortium for Research on Chronic Sorrow expanded the concept to include individuals who experience a variety of loss situations and to their family caregivers (Eakes, 2009; Eakes et al., 1998).

The middle range Theory of Chronic Sorrow was formalized in 1998. The theory was inductively derived and validated through a series of studies and a critical review of the existing research. Chronic sorrow is defined as the "periodic recurrence of permanent, pervasive sadness or other grief related feelings associated with a significant loss" (Eakes et al., 1998, p. 179), which was described as a normal response to ongoing disparity associated with loss.

### Purpose and Major Concepts

The Theory of Chronic Sorrow was developed to help analyze individual responses of people experiencing ongoing disparity due to chronic illness, caregiving responsibilities,

TABLE 11-3 *Low Middle Range Nursing Theories*

| Theory/Model | Purpose | Major Concepts |
|---|---|---|
| Theory of adaptation to chronic pain (Dunn, 2004) | Describes the process and outcome of adaptation to chronic pain through use of religious and nonreligious coping to create human and environmental integration that promotes survival, growth, and integrity | Stimuli (background contextual variables, total pain intensity), compensatory life process (religious and nonreligious coping), adaptive modes (functional ability, psychological and spiritual well-being) |
| Acute pain management (Good, 1998; Good & Moore, 1996) | Proposes prescriptions for nursing activities to reduce pain after surgery or trauma to ensure that clients have less intense pain with minimal side effects of medications | Potent pain medication, pharmacologic adjuvant, nonpharmacologic adjuvant, assessment of pain and side effects, goal setting, and balance between analgesia and side effects |
| Theory of suffering (Morse, 2001) | Describes phases of suffering and relationship between states of enduring suffering and caregiver response | Enduring (emotional suppression) and emotional suffering, outcomes (recognition, acknowledgments, acceptance) |
| Theory of the peaceful end of life (Ruland & Moore, 1998) | Directs care necessary for terminally ill clients, enhances nursing care by combining the dimensions that are important to dying in a unifying whole | Not being in pain, experience of comfort, experience of dignity and respect, being at peace, closeness to significant others and people who care |
| Caregiving effectiveness model (Smith, Pace, Kochinda, Kleinbeck, Koehler, & Popkess-Vawter, 2002) | Explains and predicts outcomes of technology-based home caregiving provided by family members | Caregiving context (caregiving characteristics, caregiving/care-receiving interactions, patient education), adaptive context (family economic stability, caregiver health status, family adaptation, reactions to caregiving), caregiving effectiveness outcomes (patient quality of life, caregiver quality of life, patient condition, technological side effects) |
| Theory of caregiver stress (Tsai, 2003) | Predicts caregiver stress and its outcomes from demographic characteristics, burden in care giving, stressful life events, social support, and social roles | Caregiver adaptation, input (objective burden, stressful life events, social support, social roles, demographic information), control process (perceived caregiver stress and depression), output (physical function, self-esteem, role enjoyment, marital satisfaction) |
| Theory of keeping the spirit alive: the spirit within children with cancer and their families (Woodgate & Degner, 2003) | Describes how children and their families use the core process of keeping the spirit alive in response to cancer | Core phenomenon: "keeping the spirit alive" (basic psychosocial process), "getting through all the rough spots" (basic psychosocial phenomenon), "way of being in the world" (living through it, sense of self, sense of well-being) |

loss of the "perfect" child, or bereavement. Chronic sorrow was characterized as pervasive, permanent, periodic, and potentially progressive in nature. The person has a perception of sadness or sorrow over time in a situation with no predictable end. The sadness or sorrow is cyclic or recurrent and brings to mind a person's losses, disappointments, or fears (Eakes, 2009).

The primary antecedent to chronic sorrow is involvement in an experience of significant loss. The loss is ongoing with no predictable end. Disparity is a second antecedent and is created by loss experiences when the individual's current reality differs from the idealized. Trigger events (e.g., milestones, circumstances, situations, and conditions that create negative disparity resulting from the loss experience) focus or exacerbate the experience of disparity (Eakes, 2009).

### Context for Use and Nursing Implications

Chronic sorrow is commonly experienced by individuals across the lifespan who have encountered significant loss or experience ongoing loss. Nurses need to view chronic sorrow as a normal response to loss and provide support by fostering positive coping strategies and encouraging activities that increase comfort.

Interventions that demonstrate an empathic presence and a caring professional are helpful. These include taking time to listen, offering support and reassurance, recognizing and focusing on feelings, and appreciating the uniqueness of each individual. Other interventions include providing information in a manner that can be understood and offering practical tips for dealing with the challenges of caregiving.

### Evidence of Empirical Testing

Eakes and colleagues (1998) reported that a number of research studies were used to develop and support the theory. One research study using the theory was found. In that study, Burke, Eakes, and Hainsworth (1999) examined chronically ill and bereaved persons and their caregivers. Several recent research studies were identified using the Theory of Chronic Sorrow as a conceptual framework. These include Isaksson and Ahlstrom's (2008) examination of the experiences of patients with multiple sclerosis, Hobdell's (2004) report on chronic sorrow and depression in parents of children with neural tube defects, and a case study depicting a mother's experiences while having two children with lissencephaly (Scornaienchi, 2003).

## BECK'S POSTPARTUM DEPRESSION THEORY

Building on a background of research on postpartum depression (Beck, Reynolds, & Rutowski, 1992), Cheryl Beck (1993) developed a theory regarding postpartum depression. A grounded theory approach was used to formulate the theory, which she described as a four-stage process of "teetering on the edge" into postpartum depression.

### Purpose and Major Concepts

The purpose of the theory was to provide insight into the experience of postpartum depression. The concepts or stages in Beck's (1993) theory were defined as encountering terror (horrifying anxiety attacks, obsessive thinking, enveloping fogginess), dying of self (alarming "unrealness," isolation of self, contemplating self-destruction), struggling to survive (battling the system, praying for relief, seeking solace), and regaining control (making transitions, mounting lost time, and attaining a guarded recovery). A meta-synthesis of postpartum depression by Beck (2002a) produced a list of predictors or risk factors including prenatal depression, child care stress, life stress, social support, prenatal anxiety, marital satisfaction, history of depression, infant temperament, maternity blues, self-esteem, socioeconomic status, marital status, and if the pregnancy was planned.

### Context for Use and Nursing Implications

The model proposed nursing interventions to alert nurses to the incidence and impact of postpartum depression. Beck stressed the importance of identifying new mothers who might be suffering from postpartum depression and suggested interventions such as referral to postpartum depression support groups (Beck et al., 1992).

### Evidence of Empirical Testing

Beck's theory is relatively new, but it has been used in a significant number of nursing studies. To further examine the concept of postpartum depression, Beck (1995, 1998) performed a meta-analysis to document its effects. Based on the information from a meta-analysis, Beck and Gable (2000) developed the Postpartum Depression Screening Scale to improve detection of the disorder. The tool was revised in 2002 (Beck, 2002b) and later translated into Spanish (Beck and Gable, 2003), and revised further in 2006 (Beck, Records, & Rice, 2006). These tools have been validated (Beck et al., 2006; Clemmens, Driscoll, & Beck, 2004) and been used by nurses in a growing list of research studies. For example, Olshansky and Sereika (2005) used the Beck Depression Inventory to assess previously infertile mothers' vulnerability to depression, and McCarter-Spaulding and Horowitz (2007) looked at how postpartum depression effects breastfeeding. Also, Ugarriza and Schmidt (2006) cited Beck's work as a basis for development and evaluation of a "telecare" program for women with postpartum depression.

## MERCER'S CONCEPTUALIZATION OF MATERNAL ROLE ATTAINMENT/BECOMING A MOTHER

Ramona Mercer first described a theoretical framework for the maternal role in the early 1980s; she expanded on the process in a subsequent publication in 1985. She reported that the theory was based on role theory, knowledge of the infant's traits, and a review of the literature to identify variables that influence or are influenced by maternal roles. She defined maternal role attainment as a process "in which the mother achieves competence in the role and integrates the mothering behaviors into her established role set so that she is comfortable with her identity as a mother" (Mercer, 1985, p. 198).

Following a review and synthesis of research related to the concept of "maternal role attainment," Mercer (2004) proposed changing the name of her theory to "Becoming a Mother." This change was later expanded upon (Mercer, 2006) and a number of related nursing interventions were identified supporting the change (Mercer & Walker, 2006).

### Purpose and Major Concepts

Mercer attempted to identify the "form and strength of the relationships between key maternal and infant variables and maternal role attainment" as well as "other factors that appear to influence maternal role attainment" (Mercer, 1983, p. 73). She proposed that the variables of age, perception of the birth experience, early maternal–infant separation, social stress, support system, self-concept and personality traits, maternal illness, child-rearing attitudes, infant temperament, infant illness, culture, and socioeconomic level affect the maternal role.

In the more recent iteration of her theory, Mercer (2004) explains that the process of establishing maternal identity in becoming a mother were (1) commitment, attachment, and preparation (during pregnancy); (2) acquaintance, learning, and physical restoration (in the first 2–6 weeks following birth); (3) moving toward a new normal (2 weeks to 4 months); and (4) achievement of the maternal identity (around 4 months). She noted that these stages may overlap and may be highly variable, due to maternal and infant variables as well as the social/environmental context.

### Context for Use and Nursing Implications

Nurses in postpartum situations should recognize that competency in the maternal role toward "becoming a mother" increases with age and experience. Also, the demands on first-time mothers challenge the nurse to be active in anticipatory socialization and guidance to prepare for the realities of the maternal role. Interventions suggested in Mercer's works include promoting parenting groups to highlight maternal needs during the first months.

### Evidence of Empirical Testing

In early works, Mercer (1985) reported that mothering over the first year presents similar challenges for all groups, and a study by Fowles (1994) used Mercer's work as part of her conceptual framework to examine the relationship between maternal attachment, postpartum depression, and maternal role attainment. More recently, using the updated version of Mercer's work, Gaffney (2006) examined how "becoming a mother" influenced postpartum smoking relapse.

## Summary

This chapter has presented a wide variety of middle range nursing theories. Because of space limitations, the descriptions are very brief and are intended to merely introduce the theories. The reader is directed to original and supporting sources for more information.

Elaine Chavez, the graduate student from the opening case study, saw how one of the numerous middle range nursing theories that have been published in recent years could be used to develop interventions in her practice. All nurses should likewise continue to review current nursing literature for new theories and ideas that are being presented to remain current and knowledgeable about nursing practice.

It must be mentioned that the high, middle, and low range theories described here are by no means an exhaustive display of the growing number that have been presented in the nursing literature. Indeed, it was remarkable to observe the growth in middle range theory development since the first edition of this book was published 8 years ago, and it is anticipated that this emphasis will continue well into the future.

## LEARNING ACTIVITIES

1. Select one of the middle range theories discussed in this chapter. Obtain a copy of the original work(s) and perform an analysis/evaluation using the criteria presented in Chapter 5.

2. Select one of the high middle range theories covered in this chapter and obtain a copy of the original work. Review three or four of the research studies cited for that theory that either study relationships of the theory or use it as a conceptual framework. While reviewing these works, consider the following questions: Do the studies appear to use the theory appropriately? Are the works consistent in their use of the theory? Do the studies contribute to knowledge base of the theory? How? Write a paper describing your findings.

3. Search current nursing journals for examples of the development, analysis, or use of middle range theories in the discipline of nursing. Debate trends with classmates or develop your analysis into a paper.

## INTERNET RESOURCES

The Transcultural Nursing Society provides information about transcultural nursing and links to find out more about Dr. Leininger's theory:

http://www.tcns.org

Website for Nola Pender and the Health Promotion Model:

http://www.nursing.umich.edu/faculty/pender-nola.html

Provides information for using the Omaha System:

http://www.omahasystem.org/

Contains information about Kolcaba's Theory of Comfort:

http://www.thecomfortline.com

## REFERENCES

Altier, M. E., & Krsek, C. A. (2006). Effects of a 1-year residency program on job stratification and retention of new graduate nurses. *Journal for Nurses in Staff Development, 22*(2), 70–77.

American Association of Critical-Care Nurses (AACN). (2008). The AACN Model for Patient Care. Retrieved December 4, 2008 from http://www.aacn.org/WD/Certifications/content/synmodel.pcms?pid=1&&menu=#Patient

Anderson, G., Jun, M., & Choi, K. (2007). Breast cancer screening for Korean women must consider traditional risks as well as two genetic risk factors. *Cancer Nursing, 30*(3), 213–219.

Bailey, D. E., & Stewart, J. L. (2006). Uncertainty in illness theory. In A. M. Tomey & M. R. Alligood (Eds.), *Nursing theorists and their work* (6th ed., pp. 623–642). St. Louis: Mosby.

Baker, P. (2001a). The Tidal Model: Developing a person-centered approach to psychiatric and mental health nursing. *Perspectives in Psychiatric Care, 37*(3), 79–87.

Baker, P. (2001b). The Tidal Model: Developing an empowering, person-centered approach to recovery within psychiatric and mental health nursing. *Journal of Psychiatric and Mental Health Nursing, 8*, 233–240.

Barkauskas, V. H., Schafer, P., Sebastian, J. G., Pohl, J. M., et al. (2006). Clients served and services provided by academic nurse-managed centers. *Journal of Professional Nursing, 22*(6), 331–338.

Barton, A. J., Clark, L., & Baramee, J. (2004). Tracking outcomes in community-based care. *Home Health Care Management and Practice, 16*(3), 171–176.

Beck, C. T. (1993). Teetering on the edge: A substantive theory of postpartum depression. *Nursing Research, 42*(1), 42–48.

Beck, C. T. (1995). The effects of postpartum depression on maternal–infant interaction: A meta-analysis. *Nursing Research, 44*(5), 298–304.

Beck, C. T. (1998). The effects of postpartum depression on child development: A meta-analysis. *Archives of Psychiatric Nursing, 12*(1), 12–20.

Beck, C. T. (2002a). A meta-synthesis of qualitative research. MCN: T*he American Journal of Maternal Child Nursing, 27*(4), 214–221.

Beck, C. T. (2002b). Revision of the postpartum depression predictors inventory. *Journal of Obstetric, Gynecologic, and Neonatal Nursing, 31*(4), 394–402.

Beck, C. T., & Gable, R. K. (2000). Postpartum depression screening scale: Development and psychometric testing. *Nursing Research, 49*(5), 272–281.

Beck, C. T., & Gable, R. K. (2003). Postpartum depression screening scale: Spanish version. *Nursing Research, 52*(5), 296–306.

Beck, C. T., Records, K., & Rice, M. (2006). Further development of the postpartum depression predictors inventory-revised. *AWHONN: The Association of Women's Health, Obstetrics and Neonatal Nurses, 35*(6), 735–742.

Beck, C. T., Reynolds, M. A., & Rutowski, P. (1992). Maternity blues and postpartum depression. *Journal of Obstetric, Gynecologic, and Neonatal Nursing, 21*(4), 287–293.

Becker, D., Kaplow, R., Muenzen, P. M., & Hartigan, C. (2006). Activities performed by acute and critical care advance practice nurses: American Association of Critical-Care Nurses Study of practice. *American Journal of Critical Care, 15*(2), 130–141.

Benner, P. (1984). *From novice to expert: Excellence and power in clinical nursing practice.* Menlo Park, CA: Addison Wesley.

Benner, P. (2001). *From novice to expert: Excellence and power in clinical nursing practice* (commemorative edition). Englewood Cliffs, NJ: Prentice-Hall.

Bergquist, S., & King, J. (1994). Parish nursing: A conceptual framework. *Journal of Holistic Nursing, 12*(2), 155–170.

Braden, C. J. (1990). A test of the self-help model: Learned response to chronic illness experience. *Nursing Research, 39*(1), 42–47.

Brewer, B. B. (2006). Is patient acuity a proxy for patient characteristics of the AACN Synergy Model for Patient Care? *Nursing Administration Quarterly, 30*(4), 351–357.

Brewer, B. B., Wojner-Alexandrov, A. W., Triola, N., Pacini, C., Cline, M., Rust, J. E., & Kerfoot, K. (2007). AACN Synergy Model's characteristics of patients: Psychometric analyses in a tertiary care health system. *American Journal of Critical Care, 16*(2), 158–165.

Burke, M. L., Eakes, G. G., & Hainsworth, M. A. (1999). Milestones of chronic sorrow: Perspectives of chronically ill and bereaved persons and family care-givers. *Journal of Family Nursing, 5*(4), 374–387.

Campesino, M. (2008). Beyond transculturalism: Critiques of cultural education in nursing. *Journal of Nursing Education, 47*(7), 298–304.

Cathcart, E. B. (2008). The role of the chief nursing officer in leading the practice: Lessons from the Benner tradition. *Nursing Administration Quarterly, 32*(2), 87–91.

Clayton, M. F., Mishel, M. H., & Belyea, M. (2006). Testing a model of symptoms, communication, uncertainty and well-being in older breast cancer survivors. *Research in Nursing and Health, 29*(1), 18–39.

Clemmens, D., Driscoll, J. W., & Beck, C. T. (2004). Postpartum depression as profiled through the postpartum depression screening scale. *The American Journal of Maternal Child Nursing, 29*(3), 180–185.

Connolly, P. M., Mao, C., Yoder, M., & Canham, D. (2006). Evaluation of the Omaha System in an academic nurse managed center. *Online Journal of Nursing Informatics, 10*(3), 14.

Conway, A. E., McClune, A. J., & Nosel, P. (2007). Down on the farm: Preventing farm accidents in children. *Pediatric Nursing, 33*(1), 45–52.

Corbin, J. M., & Strauss, A. (1991). A nursing model for chronic illness management based upon the trajectory framework. *Scholarly Inquiry for Nursing Practice, 5*(3), 155–174.

Corbin, J. M., & Strauss, A. (1992). A nursing model for chronic illness management based upon the trajectory framework. In P. Woog (Ed.), *The chronic illness trajectory framework: The Corbin and Strauss nursing model* (pp. 9–28). New York: Springer.

Corwin, E. J., Brownstead, J., Barton, N., Heckard, S., & Morin, K. (2005). The impact of fatigue on the development of postpartum depression. *Journal of Obstetric, Gynecologic, and Neonatal Nursing, 34*(5), 577–586.

Cote, D. A., & Burwell, K. T. (2007). A revised nephrology nurses' clinical ladder. *Nephrology Nursing Journal, 34*(2), 243–238.

Coward, D. D. (2003). Facilitation of self-transcendence in a breast cancer support group. *Oncology Nursing Forum, 30*(2), 291–300.

Coward, D. D., & Kahn, D. L. (2005). Transcending breast cancer: Making meaning from diagnosis and treatment. *Journal of Holistic Nursing, 23*(3), 264–283.

Cox, C. (1985). The self-determinism index. *Nursing Research, 34*(3), 177–183.

Cox, E. (2003). Synergy in practice: Caring for victims of intimate partner violence. *Critical Care Nursing Quarterly, 26*(4), 323–330.

Curley, M. A. Q. (1998). Patient–nurse synergy: Optimizing patient's outcomes. *American Journal of Critical Care, 7*(1), 64–72.

Decker, C. L., Haase, J. E., & Bell, C. J. (2007). Uncertainty in adolescents and young adults with cancer. *Oncology Nursing Forum, 34*(3), 681–690.

Dest, V. M. (2008). From novice to expert. *RN, 71*(6), 7.

Dowd, T., Kolcaba, K., Steiner, R., & Fashinpaur, D. (2007). Comparison of a healing touch, coaching, and a combined intervention on comfort and stress in younger college students. *Holistic Nursing Practice, 21*(4), 194–202.

Dunn, K. S. (2004). Toward a middle range theory of adaptation to chronic pain. *Nursing Science Quarterly, 17*(1), 78–84.

Eakes, G. (2009). Chronic sorrow. In S. J. Peterson & T. S. Bredow (Eds.), *Middle range theories: Application to nursing research* (2nd ed., pp. 149–160). Philadelphia: Lippincott Williams & Wilkins.

Eakes, G., Burke, M. L., & Hainsworth, M. A. (1998). Middle range theory of chronic sorrow. *Image: Journal of Nursing Scholarship, 30*(2), 179–185.

Eastwood, J. A., Doering, L., Rober, J., & Hays, R. D. (2008). Uncertainty and health-related quality of life 1 year after coronary angiography. *American Journal of Critical Care, 17*(3), 232–238.

Elfrink, V. L., & Davis, L. S. (2004). Using Omaha System data to improve the clinical education experiences of nursing students: The University of Cincinnati project. *Home Health Care Management and Practice, 16*(3), 185–191.

Ellermann, C. R., & Reed, P. G. (2001). Self-transcendence and depression in middle age adults. *Western Journal of Nursing Research, 23*(7), 698–713.

Eschiti, V. S. (2008). Complementary and alternative modalities used by women with female-specific cancers. *Holistic Nursing Practice, 22*(3), 127–140.

Esperat, C., Feng, D., Zang, Y., & Owen, D. (2007). Health behaviors of low-income pregnant minority women. *Western Journal of Nursing Research, 20*(3), 284–300.

Evans, B. C., & Crogan, N. L. (2006). Building a scientific base for nutrition care of Hispanic nursing home residents. *Geriatric Nursing, 27*(5), 273–279.

Fowles, E. R. (1994). *The relationship between prenatal maternal attachment, postpartum depressive symptoms and maternal role attainment.* Chicago: Loyola University of Chicago.

Gaffney, K. F. (2006). Postpartum smoking relapse and becoming a mother. *Journal of Nursing Scholarship, 38*(1), 26–30.

Gift, A. (2009). Unpleasant symptoms. In S. J. Peterson & T. S. Bredow (Eds.), *Middle range theories: Application to nursing research* (2nd ed., pp. 82–98). Philadelphia: Lippincott Williams & Wilkins.

Good, M. (1998). A middle range theory of acute pain management: Use in research. *Nursing Outlook, 46*(3), 120–124.

Good, M., & Moore, S. M. (1996). Clinical practice guidelines as a new source of middle range theory: Focus on acute pain. *Nursing Outlook, 44*(2), 74–79.

Gottlieb, J. A. K. (2007). Vulnerability, self-transcendence and the professional well-being of new graduate registered nurses. Doctoral Dissertation, Barry University School of Nursing.

Hardin, S. R. (2005). Introduction to the AACN Synergy Model for patient care. In S. R. Hardin & R. Kaplow (Eds.), *Synergy for clinical excellence: The AACN Synergy Model for patient care* (pp. 3–10). Sudbury MA: Jones & Bartlett Publishers.

Hardin, S. R. (2009). The AACN Synergy Model. In S. J. Peterson & T. S. Bredow (Eds.), *Middle range theories: Application to nursing research* (2nd ed., pp. 99–114). Philadelphia: Lippincott Williams & Wilkins.

Hobdell, E. (2004). Chronic sorrow and depression in parents of children with neural tube defects. *Journal of Neuroscience Nursing, 6*(2), 82–88.

Hunnibell, L. S., Reed, P. G., Qunn-Griffin, M., & Fitzpatrick, J. J. (2008). Self-transcendence and burnout in hospice and oncology nurses. *Journal of Hospice and Palliative Nursing, 10*(3), 172–179.

Huth, M. M., & Broome, M. E. (2007). A snapshot of children's postoperative tonsillectomy outcomes at home. *Journal of Specialists in Pediatric Nursing, 12*(3), 186–195.

Isaksson, A., & Ahlstrom, G. (2008). Managing chronic sorrow: Experiences of patients with multiple sclerosis. *Journal of Neuroscience Nursing, 40*(3), 180–191.

Jones, S. M. (2008). Emergency nurses' caring experiences with Mexican American patients. *Journal of Emergency Nursing, 34*(3), 199–204.

Kanaskie, M. L., Felmlee, M., & Shay, M. L. (2008). A peer review model for clinical ladder programs across all practice settings. *Oncology Nursing Forum, 35*(3), 540.

Kleiman, S., Frederickson, K., & Lundy, T. (2004). Using an eclectic model to educate students about cultural influences in the nurse–patient relationship. *Nursing Education Perspectives, 25*(5), 249–256.

Kloos, J. A., & Daly, B. J. (2008). Effect of a family-maintained progress journal on anxiety of families of critically ill patients. *Critical Care Nursing Quarterly, 31*(3), 96–107.

Kolcaba, K. Y. (1994). A theory of holistic comfort for nursing. *Journal of Advanced Nursing, 19*(6), 1178–1184.

Kolcaba, K. Y. (1995). The art of comfort care. *Image: Journal of Nursing Scholarship, 27*(4), 287–289.

Kolcaba, K. (2001). Evolution of the middle range: Theory of Comfort for outcomes research. *Nursing Outlook, 49*(2), 86–92.

Kolcaba, K. (2003). *Comfort theory and practice: A vision for holistic health care and research.* New York: Springer.

Kolcaba, K. (2009). Comfort. In S. J. Peterson & T. S. Bredow (Eds.), *Middle range theories: Application to nursing research* (2nd ed., pp. 254–272). Philadelphia: Lippincott Williams & Wilkins.

Kolcaba, K., & DiMarco, M. A. (2005). Comfort theory and its application to pediatric nursing. *Pediatric Nursing, 31*(3), 187–193.

Kolcaba, K., Tilton, C., & Drouin, C. (2006). Comfort theory: A unifying framework to enhance the practice environment. *Journal of Nursing Administration, 36*(11), 538–544.

Lancellotti, K. (2008). Culture care theory: A framework for expanding awareness of diversity and racism in nursing education. *Journal of Professional Nursing, 24*(3), 179–183.

Lauver, D. (1992). A theory of care-seeking behavior. *Image: Journal of Nursing Scholarship, 24*(4), 281–287.

Leininger, M. M. (2002). Culture care theory: A major contribution to advance transcultural nursing knowledge and practices. *Journal of Transcultural Nursing, 13*(3), 189–192.

Leininger, M. M. (2007). Theoretical questions and concerns: Response from the Theory of Culture Care Diversity and Universality perspective. *Nursing Science Quarterly, 20*(1), 9–15.

Leininger, M. M., & McFarland, M. (2006). *Culture care diversity and universality: A worldwide nursing theory* (2nd ed.). Sudbury, MA: Jones & Bartlett.

Lenz, E. R., & Pugh, L. C. (2008). Theory of unpleasant symptoms. In M. J. Smith & P. R. Liehr (Eds.), *Middle range theory for nursing* (2nd ed., pp. 159–181). New York: Springer.

Lenz, E. R., Pugh, L. C., Milligan, R. A., Gift, A., & Suppe, F. (1997). The middle range theory of unpleasant symptoms: An update. *Advances in Nursing Science, 19*(3), 14–27.

Lenz, E. R., & Shortridge-Baggett, L. M. (2002). *Self-efficacy in nursing: Research and measurement perspectives.* New York: Springer.

Lenz, E. R., Suppe, F., Gift, A. G., Pugh, L. C., & Milligan R. A. (1995). Collaborative development of middle range nursing theories: Toward a theory of unpleasant symptoms. *Advance in Nursing Science, 17*(3), 1–13.

Liehr, P., & Smith, M. J. (1999). Middle range theory: Spinning research and practice to create knowledge for the new millennium. *Advances in Nursing Science, 21*(4), 81–91.

Liu, H. (2006). Fatigue and associated factors in hemodialysis patients in Taiwan. *Research in Nursing and Health, 29*(1), 40–50.

Martin, K. S. (2005). *The Omaha System: A key to practice, documentation and information management* (2nd ed.). Philadelphia: Elsevier.

Martin, K. S., & Scheet, N. J. (1992). *The Omaha System: Applications for community health nursing.* Philadelphia: Saunders.

McCarter-Spaulding, D., & Horowitz, J. A. (2007). How does postpartum depression affect breastfeeding? *The American Journal of Maternal Child Nursing, 32*(1), 10–17.

McEwen, M. M., & Slack, M. K. (2005). Factors associated with health-related behaviors in Latinos with or at risk of diabetes. *Hispanic Health Care International, 3*(3), 143–151.

McFarland, M. (2006). Madeleine Leininger: Culture care Theory of Diversity and Universality. In A. M. Tomey & M. R. Alligood (Eds.), *Nursing theorists and their work* (6th ed., pp. 472–496). St. Louis: Mosby.

Meleis, A. I., Sawyer, L. M., Im, E. O., Messias, D. D. H., & Schumacher, K. (2000). Experiencing transitions: An emerging middle range theory. *Advances in Nursing Science, 23*(1), 12–28.

Mendias, E. P., & Paar, D. P. (2007). Perceptions of health and self-care learning needs of outpatients with HIV/AIDS. *Journal of Community Health Nursing, 24*(1), 49–64.

Mercer, R. T. (1983). A theoretical framework for studying factors that impact on the maternal role. *Nursing Research, 30*(2), 73–77.

Mercer, R. T. (1985). The process of maternal role attainment over the first year. *Nursing Research, 34*(4), 198–204.

Mercer, R. T. (2004). Becoming a mother versus maternal role attainment. *Journal of Nursing Scholarship, 36*(3), 226–232.

Mercer, R. T. (2006). Nursing support of the process of becoming a mother. *AWHONN: The Association of Women's Health, Obstetrics and Neonatal Nurses, 35*(5), 649–651.

Mercer, R. T., & Walker, L. O. (2006). A review of nursing interventions to foster becoming a mother. *AWHONN: The Association of Women's Health, Obstetrics and Neonatal Nurses, 35*(5), 568–582.

Miller, L. W. (1997). Nursing through the lens of faith: A conceptual model. *Journal of Christian Nursing, 14*(1), 17–21.

Mishel, M. H. (1981). The measurement of uncertainty in illness. *Nursing Research, 30*(5), 258–263.

Mishel, M. H. (1984). Perceived uncertainty and stress in illness. *Research in Nursing and Health, 7,* 163–171.

Mishel, M. H. (1988). Uncertainty in illness. *Image: Journal of Nursing Scholarship, 20*(4), 225–232.

Mishel, M. H. (1990). Reconceptualization of the uncertainty in illness theory. *Image: Journal of Nursing Scholarship, 22*(4), 256–262.

Mishel, M. H. (1999). Uncertainty in chronic illness. *Annual Review of Nursing Research, 17,* 269–294.

Mishel, M. H. (2008). Managing uncertainty in cancer: How to request Dr. Mishel's scales. Retreived December 3, 2008 from http://nursing.unc.edu/muic/instruments.html.

Mishel, M. H., & Sorenson, D. S. (1991). Uncertainty in gynecological cancer: A test of the mediating functions of mastery and coping. *Nursing Research, 40*(3), 167–171.

Morris, L. L., Pfeiffer, P. B., Catalano, R., Fortney, R., et al. (2007). Designing a comprehensive model for critical care orientation. *Critical Care Nurse, 27*(6), 37–57.

Morse, J. (2001). Toward a praxis theory of suffering. *Advances in Nursing Science, 24*(1), 47–59.

Munoz, C., & Hilgenberg, C. (2005). Ethnopharmacology: Understanding how ethnicity can affect drug response is essential to providing culturally competent care. *The American Journal of Nursing, 105*(8), 40–52.

Neal, L. J. (1999a). Neal theory of home health nursing practice. *Image: Journal of Nursing Scholarship, 31*(3), 251.

Neal, L. J. (1999b). The Neal theory: Implications for practice and administration. *Home Health Care Nurse, 17*(3), 181–187.

Neff, D. F., Kinion, E. S., & Cardina, C. (2007). Nurse managed center: Access to primary health care for urban Native Americans. *Journal of Community Health Nursing, 24*(10), 19–30.

Norbeck, J. S. (1981). Social support: A model for clinical research and application. *Advances in Nursing Science, 3*(4), 43–59.

Olshansky, E., & Sereika, S. (2005). The transition from pregnancy to postpartum in previously infertile women: A focus on depression. *Archives in Psychiatric Nursing, 19*(6), 273–280.

Pender, N. J. (1996). *Health promotion in nursing practice* (3rd ed.). Stamford, CT: Appleton & Lange.

Pender, N. J., Murdaugh, C. L., & Parsons, M. A. (2006) *Health promotion in nursing practice* (5th ed.). Upper Saddle River, NJ: Prentice-Hall.

Plowden, K. O. (2006). To screen or not to screen: Factors influencing the decision to participate in prostate cancer screening among urban African-American men. *Urologic Nursing, 26*(6), 477–483.

Polk, L. V. (1997). Toward a middle range theory of resilience. *Advances in Nursing Science, 19*(3), 1–13.

Reed, P. G. (1991a). Toward a nursing theory of self-transcendence: Deductive reformulation using developmental theories. *Advances in Nursing Science, 13*(4), 64–77.

Reed, P. G. (1991b). Self-transcendence and mental health in oldest-old adults. *Nursing Research, 40*(1), 5–11.

Reed, P. G. (1996). Transcendence: Formulating nursing perspectives. *Nursing Science Quarterly, 9*(1), 2–3.

Reed, P. G. (2008). Theory of self-transcendence. In M. J. Smith & P. R. Liehr (Eds.), *Middle range theory for nursing* (2nd ed., pp. 105–129). New York: Springer.

Rischel, V., Larsen, K., & Jackson, K. (2008). Embodied dispositions or experience? Identifying new patterns of professional competence. *Journal of Advanced Nursing, 61*(5), 512–521.

Rogers, B. (1994). *Occupational health nursing: Concepts and practice.* Philadelphia: Saunders.

Ruland, C. M., & Moore, S. M. (1998). Theory construction based on standards of care: A proposed theory of the peaceful end of life. *Nursing Outlook, 46*(4), 169–175.

Rychnovsky, J. D. (2007). Postpartum fatigue in the active-duty military woman. *Journal of Obstetric, Gynecologic, and Neonatal Nursing, 36*(1), 38–46.

Schumacher, K. L., & Meleis, A. I. (1994). Transitions: A central concept in nursing. *Image: Journal of Nursing Scholarship, 26*(2), 119–127.

Scornaienchi, J. M. (2003). Chronic sorrow: One mother's experience with two children with lissencephaly. *Journal of Paediatric Health Care, 17*(6), 290–294.

Sechrist, K. R., Berlin, L. E., & Biel, M. (2000). The Synergy Model: Overview of the theoretical review process. *Critical Care Nurse, 20*(1), 85–86.

Smith, A. B., & Bashore, L. (2006). The effect of clinic-based health promotion education on perceived health status and health promotion behaviors of adolescent and young adult cancer survivors. *Journal of Pediatric Oncology, 23*(6), 326–335.

Smith, K., & Bazini-Barakat, N. (2003). A public health nursing practice model: Melding public health principles with the nursing process. *Public Health Nursing, 20*(1), 42–48.

Smith, C. E., Pace, K., Kochinda, C., Kleinbeck, S. V. M., Koehler, J., & Popkess-Vawter, S. (2002). Caregiving effectiveness model evolution to a midrange theory of home care: A process for critique and replication. *Advances in Nursing Science, 25*(1), 50–64.

Sossong, A. (2007). Living with an implantable cardioverter defibrillator. *Journal of Cardiovascular Nursing, 22*(2), 99–104.

Standing, M. (2007). Clinical decision-making skills on the developmental journey from student to Registered Nurse: A longitudinal inquiry. *Journal of Advanced Nursing, 60*(3), 257–269.

Storey, S., Crist, L., Nelis, D. A., Murphy, L., & Fisher, M. L. (2007). Creation of a career enhancement program for a hospital-based education and development department. *Journal for Nurses in Staff Development, 23*(2), 55–63.

Swanson, K. M. (1991). Empirical development of a middle range theory of caring. *Nursing Research, 40*(3), 161–166.

Thibodeaux, A. G., & Deatrick, J. A. (2007). Cultural influence on family management of children with cancer. *Journal of Pediatric Oncology Nursing, 24*(4), 227–233.

Tsai, P. F. (2003). A middle range theory of caregiver stress. *Nursing Science Quarterly, 16*(2), 137–145.

Ugarriza, D. N., & Schmidt, L. (2006). Telecare for women with postpartum depression. *Journal of Psychosocial Nursing and Mental Health Services, 44*(1), 37–47.

Wagner, D., Byrne, M., & Kolcaba, K. (2006). Effect of comfort warming on preoperative patients. *Association of periOperative Registered Nurses Journal, 84*(3), 1–13.

Walsh, S. M., Chen, S., Hacker, M., & Broschard, D. (2008). A creative-bonding intervention and a friendly visit approach to promote nursing students' self-transcendence and positive attitudes toward elders: A pilot study. *Nurse Education Today, 28*(3), 363–370.

Weinert, C., & Long, K. A. (1991). The theory and research base for rural nursing practice. In A. Bush (Ed.), *Rural nursing* (pp. 21–38). Newbury Park, CA: Sage.

Wilgis, M., & McConnell, J. (2008). Concept mapping: An educational strategy to improve graduate nurses' critical thinking skills during a hospital orientation program. *Journal of Continuing Education in Nursing, 39*(3), 119–126.

Wong, F. K. Y., Chow, S., Chung, L., et al. (2008). Can home visits help reduce readmissions? Randomized controlled trial. *Journal of Advanced Nursing, 62*(5), 585–595.

Wood, M. E. (2008). Theoretical framework to study exercise motivation for breast cancer risk reduction. *Oncology Nursing Forum, 35*(1), 89–95.

Woodgate, R. L., & Degner, L. F. (2003). A substantive theory of keeping the spirit alive: The spirit within children with cancer and their families. *Journal of Pediatric Oncology Nursing, 20*(3), 103–119.

Yu, F., & Lang, N. M. (2008). Using the Omaha System to examine outpatient rehabilitation problems, interventions and outcomes between clients with and without cognitive impairment. *Rehabilitation Nursing, 33*(3), 124–134.

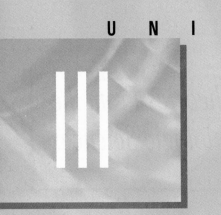

# Borrowed Theories
# Used by Nurses

# 12

# Theories From the Sociologic Sciences

## Grace M. Bielkiewicz

*S*  *imon Brown is a school nurse who is currently working in a school-based clinic located within a high school in a disadvantaged, inner-city neighborhood. In his practice, Simon sees a number of students who are sexually active, as well as some who are already parents. Although teen pregnancy and childbearing rates have dramatically dropped over the last few years elsewhere, they have remained disproportionately high at his school. Simon has conducted sex education classes, but he speculates that the key to a more effective intervention lies elsewhere.*

*A literature review reinforced what Simon suspected—that abstinence and contraception-focused programs for adolescents have had only modest results in reducing teen pregnancy rates and minimal impact on teens in disadvantaged inner-city communities. He confirmed that patterns of adolescent sexual-risk behavior are shaped by social class, position, race, and gender. He also learned that in the United States, young motherhood is increasingly concentrated in disadvantaged groups, both white and nonwhite, but that the role of mother is not the typical first choice of young women who perceive themselves as having options.*

*From his review of the literature, Simon identified a sociologic perspective, role theory, which he believes will help him develop a relevant and culturally sensitive intervention model for the adolescents in his school. He understood that roles are deeply embedded in social structures and are not easily changed. Inner-city neighborhoods typically have a scarcity of role models and often lack appropriate adult supervision and meaningful job networks.*

*The reproductive role is one area over which poor, inner-city adolescents have control. Young men can validate their masculine role by biologically fathering a child, and young women can demonstrate their capacity for love in the maternal role. It is sometimes perceived that postponing childbearing will not improve their circumstances and becoming a parent may elevate their personal status.*

*Armed with the information gathered from his literature searches, Simon is seeking to learn even more about cultural variations in role expectations. His goal is to use this knowledge to develop interventions that will promote adolescent health and facilitate developmentally appropriate and productive role behaviors among the students in his school.*

Historically, nursing has been responsive to society's needs. Early nurse leaders such as Nightingale, Barton, Wald, Sanger, and Staupers were, to varying degrees, social activists. They observed and understood the historical and social forces that affected large aggregates of individuals. Their understanding was demonstrated through their population-focused nursing interventions. C. Wright Mills (1959) coined the term *sociological imagination* to refer to this process of looking at social phenomena to discover the unseen and repetitive patterns that govern individuals' social existence.

Beginning in the early 1900s, as Americans became increasingly focused on the ideology of individualism, and as cures were discovered for dreaded infectious diseases, the emphasis of health care shifted from populations and social factors that affect health, to the individual and personal lifestyles. Consideration of the influences of social forces became almost obsolete. An understanding of theories from sociology and related disciplines that focus on the interaction between human society and individuals is important for nurses, however, because sociologic issues have a dramatic impact on the health and well-being of individuals, families, groups, and society. Thus, advanced nursing practice and research must consider the social factors and issues that constrain and shape health behaviors.

This chapter reviews selected sociologic concepts, theories, and frameworks for their relevance to nursing practice, research, administration, and education. Three major sections are presented: exchange theories, interaction theories, and conflict theories. These are followed by an overview of chaos theory. Each section begins with a brief historical overview, which is followed by a discussion of basic assumptions, central concepts, and differing theoretical viewpoints. Examples of nursing practice or research application of the theory are included.

# Exchange Theories

What have become known as exchange theories have their basis in the philosophical perspective called *utilitarianism*. Utilitarianism developed between the late 18th century and the mid-19th century and is a legacy from both moral philosophy and classic economic theory. The moral philosophy component considers the satisfaction of an individual's desires or utility. Philosophically, maximization of each individual's satisfaction automatically leads to maximum satisfaction of the wants of all. Translated into more familiar terms, "the greatest good for the greatest number" is an underlying principle of utilitarianism.

Three basic assumptions about individuals and exchange relations are added from classic economic theory. First, individuals are purposive and motivated to maximize material benefits from exchanges with others in a free and competitive marketplace. Second, as agents in a free market, individuals have access to all the information needed to weigh alternatives and calculate costs for each alternative. Third, based on their own calculations, individuals are able to rationally choose the activities that will maximize their profits (Turner, 2003).

## MODERN SOCIAL EXCHANGE THEORIES

The influence of utilitarianism is evident in modern exchange theories to varying degrees. Utilitarian principles were reformulated for modern exchange theories in an attempt to explain human interactions in all social contexts, and without the limitations

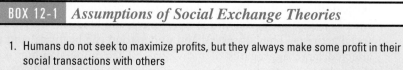

**BOX 12-1**  *Assumptions of Social Exchange Theories*

1. Humans do not seek to maximize profits, but they always make some profit in their social transactions with others
2. Humans are not perfectly rational, but they do engage in calculations of costs and benefits in social transactions
3. Humans do not have perfect information on all available alternatives, but they are usually aware of at least some alternatives, which form the basis for assessment of costs and benefits
4. Humans always act under constraints, but they still compete with one another in seeking to make a profit in their transactions
5. Humans always seek to make a profit in their transactions, but they are limited by the resources that they have when entering an exchange relation
6. Humans do engage in economic transactions in clearly defined marketplaces in all societies, but these transactions are only a special case of more general exchange relations occurring among individuals in virtually all social contexts
7. Humans do pursue material goals in exchanges, but they also mobilize and exchange nonmaterial resources, such as sentiments, services, and symbols

Source: Turner (1991).

imposed by a pure economic framework, hence the label "social" exchange theory. Assumptions of social exchange theories as outlined by Turner (2003) are listed in Box 12-1.

The *social exchange* perspective emerged in American sociology in the 1960s with the work of Homans (1961) and Blau (1964) and later with Nye (1979) and Emerson (1981), and in social psychology with Thibaut and Kelley (1959). Modern exchange theories emphasize the social and psychological motivation of individuals. There are two major divisions of social exchange theories: the individualistic or microlevel theories and the societal/collectivist or macrolevel theories.

Within the *individualistic social exchange* framework, the central focus is motivation; human beings are motivated by self-interest to act. Relationships are deemed successful and continue when each party feels that the nature of an exchange is fair and beneficial. Beneficial or rewarding relationships require commitment to sustain them. When *reciprocity* is absent or unrewarding within the relationship, or costs exceed rewards, individuals tend to withdraw from further exchanges. This premise applies to all social groups, including the family. Divorce is an example of withdrawing from an unsatisfactory exchange relationship.

In contrast to the individualistic or microlevel perspective are the macrolevel theories. This second broad division of social exchange theories is derived from a *collectivist* tradition and gives greater weight to society. Collectivism has its roots in the perspective of French anthropologist Levi-Strauss (1969), whose work emphasized the integration of exchanges from larger social structures. In this perspective, the focus is on reciprocity from an institutional level.

Three fundamental exchange principles relate to the concept of integration as proposed by Levi-Strauss (1969). First, individuals incur costs in all exchange relations, but costs are attributed to the customs, rules, laws, and values of society, as opposed to the individual motives found in economic or psychological explanations of exchange. Second, social norms and values regulate the distribution of all scarce and valued resources. Third, the norm of reciprocity governs all exchange relations (Turner, 2003). An example of costs associated with customs is the money dance conducted at

TABLE 12-1 *Central Concepts in Social Exchange Theories*

| Concept | Meaning |
| --- | --- |
| Agency | Individuals actively create or construct their social world, and as thinking, feeling, and acting beings, they are motivated to control or to condition the situations that affect their social lives to maximize their advantage. |
| Rationality | Individuals are acquisitive and success oriented, and motivated for immediate rewards. Therefore, to gain the most benefit, individuals calculate costs and the probabilities of receiving rewards or avoiding punishments in social interactions. |
| Structure | Social and cultural influences that constrain and shape an individual's behavior and conscious experiences are assumed to be located in the unconscious mind, in material relationships, in the symbolic relationships of myth or language, or in repetitive patterns of permanent interactions. |

Source: Waters (1994).

some wedding receptions in the United States. During the designated dance, currency is "pinned" on the bride and groom in exchange for a brief portion of the dance. This ritual signifies a socially sanctioned way for guests to give cash to the newlyweds and for the young couple to reciprocate.

*Rational choice* theory (Coleman, 1990; Hechter, 1987) is an example of an exchange theory. Rational choice theory attempts to explain the macrolevel behavioral processes of both small and large social systems. Rational choice theory has a systems focus, but the psychological needs and motives of individuals are removed.

Three major sociologic concepts, *agency*, *rationality*, and *structure*, are evident in the assumptions and propositions of contemporary social exchange theories (Table 12-1). The individualistic perspective emphasizes *agency* and considers that individuals actively shape their social lives, rather than being passive recipients. Individuals affect their own lives by adapting to, negotiating with, and changing social structures.

Inherent in the concept of *rationality* is the assumption that every individual has control over a supply of socially valued resources, either material or psychological, that serve as bartering tools. Individuals barter these resources in the social "marketplace" to maximize rewards by enhancing the valuables they control. Homans (1961) attempted to "soften" the more utilitarian or calculative perspective by emphasizing the influence of personal values on determining what individuals view as rewarding. The last concept, *structure*, is highly abstract and not directly observable. Social structure generally refers to the enduring and recurring patterns of behavior in groups and society.

Subsumed in these concepts (agency, rationality, and structure) are related issues of *inequality*, *power*, and *conflict*. A generation or so prior to its appearance in exchange theorizing, Karl Marx (1977) noted that inequality exists in hierarchical class structures where those who have control of resources with high economic value also have the power to exploit those with fewer such resources. Conflict, according to Marx, is inevitable with oppression, and resolution of conflict requires emancipatory actions. Factors associated with positions of privilege and power include gender, age, ethnicity, and socioeconomic status. Conflict theories are discussed in detail later in this chapter.

### Application to Nursing

Recent nursing studies that used social exchange theories as their conceptual framework were identified in the literature. For example, Mossop and Wilkinson (2006) drew upon social exchange theory to understand and address concerns of older clients in institutions to reciprocate the care and attention they received from student nurses. Reciprocity was found to be difficult for older adults to achieve as a result of diminishing resources. The social exchange perspective was also found to have potential to understand resource exchange in client–nurse interactions within the context of maternal–child home visits (Byrd, 2006). Finally, Appel, Giger, and Davidhizar (2005) incorporated concepts from rational choice theory into a conceptual model designed to reduce the health disparities in the cardiovascular health of low-income rural southern African-American women.

In another research study, Kane-Urrabazo (2006) incorporated concepts from social exchange theory in her exploration of the manager's role in shaping organizational culture. She concluded that certain managerial characteristics facilitate an effective workplace for both employees and the organization.

## RELATED THEORIES

There are many theories, principles, and concepts derived from, or related to, exchange theories. Exchange theories that are commonly used by nurses include systems theory and social networks.

### General Systems Theory

*General systems theory* (GST) is one type of exchange theory. GST or, more specifically, *open systems theory* (OST) (von Bertalanffy, 1968), is regarded as a universal grand theory because of its unique relevancy and applicability (Johnson & Webber, 2005).

The GST was initially introduced in the 1930s by von Bertalanffy. In GST, systems are composed of both structural and functional components that interact within a boundary that filters the type and rate of exchange with the environment. Living systems are open because there is an ongoing exchange of matter, energy, and information. The following elements are common to systems (Figure 12-1):

- Input—matter, energy, and information received from the environment
- Throughput—matter, energy, and information that is modified or transformed within the system
- Output—matter, energy, and information that is released from the system into the environment
- Feedback—information regarding environmental responses used by the system (may be positive, negative, or neutral) (Kenney, 1995)

Basic tenets of GST are that (1) a system is composed of subsystems, each with its own function; (2) systems contain energy and matter; (3) a system may be open or closed (open systems exchange energy and closed systems have clearly defined boundaries); and (4) open and closed systems reach stationary states (Mason & Attree, 1997).

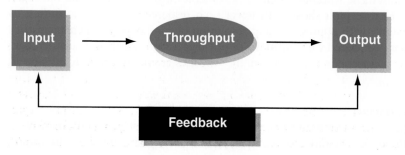

FIGURE 12-1 Elements of a system.

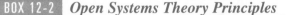

| BOX 12-2 | *Open Systems Theory Principles* |
| --- | --- |

1. A system is a unit that is greater than the sum of its parts (wholeness is a major premise of both GST and OST)
2. A system is comprised of subsystems that are themselves part of suprasystems (hierarchically "nested")
3. A system has boundaries (i.e., abstract entities such as rules, norms, and values) that permit exchange of information and resources both into (inputs) and out of (outputs) the system (boundaries can also hinder or block exchange processes)
4. Communication and feedback mechanisms between system parts are essential for system function
5. A change in one part leads to change in the whole system (*circular causality*)
6. A system goal or end point can be reached in different ways (*equifinality*)

For survival, a system must achieve a balance internally and externally (equilibrium). Equilibrium depends on the system's ability to regulate input and output to achieve a balanced relationship of the interactive parts. The system uses various adaptation mechanisms to maintain equilibrium. Adaptation may occur through accepting or rejecting the matter, energy, or information, or by accommodating the input and modifying the systems responses. Several OST principles that are purported to be applicable to all systems are shown in Box 12-2.

*Application to Nursing*

Systems theory has been frequently applied to nursing practice. Way and MacNeil (2007), for example, used systems theory as a framework for exploring a proposed baccalaureate nursing degree requirement and its potential impact on the nursing profession. Kurz and Hayes (2006) used GST as the foundation to measure the impact of an educational program on registered nurses' death anxiety, death attitudes, and knowledge. A systems theory framework helped illustrate the need for thorough assessment and implementation of systematic changes for appropriating staff (Upenieks, Akhavan, & Kotlerman, 2008). Finally, in clinical research, GST was used to examine the impact of alcohol dependence and depression on both the individual and their families and to guide implementation of focused advance practice nurse interventions (Fowler, 2006).

**Social Networks**

The study of *networks* can be a productive approach to understanding systems in nursing. In terms of the health and well-being of individuals, *social support networks*, as actual or potential resources, are especially relevant. Among members of social support networks, reciprocity and commitments are shaped by culturally mandated norms. This particularly relates to family networks (Logan & Spitze, 1996; Oliker, 1989; Stack, 1974).

The study of social networks should examine the underlying patterns of social relations (Turner, 2003). The units to be examined can range from individuals to positions, such as those found in health care organizations (e.g., nurses, physicians, pharmacists, administrators). In *network analysis* these units are referred to as *points*. Ties link points and represent the directional flow of resources. Figure 12-2 illustrates the exchange process in a simplistic diagram. In this figure, **A, B, C, D,** and **E** represent points, and arrows indicate ties. In the illustration B has reciprocal ties to all other points, but **A, C, D,** and **E** have ties to only three other points. In the social world,

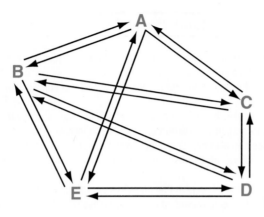

FIGURE 12-2 Example of resource flows in a noncomplex network.

resource exchanges can be instrumental, as in the exchange of information or materials, or *affective*, as shown by respect, approval, or an empathic ear.

Examples of techniques or tools for capturing and mapping network patterns include Moreno's (1953) *sociograms*, which plot the patterning of sentiments among group members; the echo-map used in family assessments to diagram exchange relations between families and their external environment; and the exchange theory and network analysis program developed by Emerson (1981). In contrast to more traditional exchange theories, Emerson's approach focuses on mapping the structure of exchange relations among *actors*, rather than the motivation of individuals. The idea of the analysis is to discover the events that may affect the relational unit (Turner, 2003).

### Application to Nursing

Resources, both affective and instrumental, flow through network exchange processes. Support from social networks is widely regarded as mediating the adverse effects of stressful events, as has been shown in numerous nursing studies. For example, social support was identified as one of the mediating variables for menopausal depression in Korean women (Choi, Lee, Lee, Kim, & Ham, 2004). Similarly, Sammarco and Konecny (2008) found that social support and uncertainty played a significant role in the quality of life for Latino breast cancer survivors. Another study looked at adherence to diet and fluid restrictions and the relationship of perceived social support for persons receiving hemodialysis (Kara, Caglar, & Kilic, 2007). In this work, social support was found to be a key factor in treatment adherence.

Several studies were identified examining the relationship between social support and pregnancy outcomes. These included Leahy-Warren's (2007) study of social support for first-time mothers, which suggested that nursing interventions need to acknowledge the women's own social network. Adolescents were the focus of a study by Meadows-Olivier and others (2007) that examined sources of stress and supportive resources of homeless teenage mothers, and a bioecological model was used to examine social support in postpartum adolescents (Logsdon, Hertwick, Ziegler, & Pinto-Foltz, 2008).

## Interactionist Frameworks

In the late 19th century, the focus of sociology shifted from macrostructures and processes (e.g., evolution, class conflict) to social interactional processes that link individuals to each other and to society. A diverse group of interactionist theories resulted from this shift. Two of these theories, symbolic interactionism and role theory, are discussed in the following sections.

## SYMBOLIC INTERACTIONISM

The early foundation for what was later to be called symbolic interactionism by Blumer (1969) was laid in the late 1800s. Three scholars from the philosophical tradition called *pragmatism* are credited with the seminal ideas from which symbolic interactionism sprang. From James' (1890) typology of selves came the concept of the "self." The concept of self was refined by Cooley (1902) a few years later to include the notion of "the looking glass self," or the self that comes from the process of symbolic communication with others in the "primary group." Dewey (1922) contributed his idea of "mind" as a process that emerges from, and is sustained through, interactions with others.

Mead (1934), the acknowledged father of symbolic interactionism, synthesized the concepts of self, mind, and society or social environment, which he perceived to be inseparable. Central to Mead's work is the notion that humans adapt to, and survive in, their environment by sharing common symbols, both verbal and nonverbal. A distinctive feature of this symbolic interaction is that humans can imagine themselves in other social roles, a concept termed *role-taking*, and internalize the attitudes, values, and norms of the "generalized other" or social group. Mead outlined stages of interactional learning by which he believed humans acquire social understanding. For Mead, the self is nonexistent at birth, and emerges as the result of social experience. Mead's basic assumptions are listed in Box 12-3.

"What humans define as real has real consequences" (Thomas & Thomas, 1928, p. 572) is a basic principle from social psychology. This principle is referred to as the *definition of the situation*, and links how individuals perceive their environment and how they respond or act in that environment. Mead stressed that this environmental perception and response is in actuality a problem-solving interaction. From these interactions comes the phenomenon Mead viewed as society, because it is through the processes of mind and self that society is both altered and maintained (Turner, 2003).

The focus for symbolic interactionism is on the connection between *symbols* (shared meanings) and *interactions*. Mead emphasized the process of role-taking as a basic mechanism by which interactions occur. Role-taking refers to the ability to not

---

**BOX 12-3** *Assumptions of Symbolic Interactionist Theories*

1. Human beings have the capacity to create and use symbols
2. Through the capacity to create and use symbols, humans have freed themselves from most of their instinctual and biologic programming
3. Human beings adapt and survive in the social world
4. Humans use words and language symbols to communicate, and they also use nonverbal gestures that have common meanings
5. Humans can effectively communicate because of their ability to read symbols produced by others and can take on the position or point of view of another person
6. Humans acquire a mind and self from interactions with others
7. Human interactions form the basis of society

Sources: Lindesmith and Strauss (1968); Turner (1991).

only put oneself in the role of another person, but also to anticipate how that person will think, feel, or respond (Mead, 1934; Stryker & Statham, 1985). Although they are sometimes used interchangeably, role-taking and empathy are not synonymous. Role-taking is a cognitive process, whereas empathy emphasizes the affective. The concept of role was extended to include the expectations attached to structural positions in society, and the concept of self became associated with the multiple roles played within these positions.

### Application to Nursing

Several qualitative research studies were found that used symbolic interaction as a conceptual framework to examine nursing per se. Deppoliti (2008), for example, used symbolic interaction to explore experiences that contributed to hospital nurses' construction of professional identity and Ware (2008) examined the socialization process of developing the self-concept of "professional nurse" in baccalaureate nursing students. Bankston (2005) incorporated symbolic interactionism into the conceptual framework for her study that examined predictors to collaborative practice behaviors used by registered nurses and physicians in acute care hospitals. Finally, Beel, Hawranik, McClement, and Daenincl (2006) used an interactionist framework to examine nurses' perceptions and experiences with palliative sedation.

In clinical research, Garcia and Saewyc (2007) used symbolic interaction to guide their focused ethnography on the health-related perceptions of recently immigrated Mexican adolescents. They used their research to encourage the design of culturally and developmentally appropriate mental health services.

## ROLE THEORY

The concept of "role" comes from the theater and conveys the notion that normative expectations and requirements, such as culturally defined behavioral rules, are attached to positions (status) in social organizations (e.g., family, corporation, society). Succinctly stated, an individual occupies a status, but plays a role (Lindesmith & Strauss, 1968).

Through the enactment of roles, static social positions are brought to life. Roles can be assumed to carry certain rights and privileges as well as certain duties and obligations. For example, a registered nurse has the right to be paid on time, and in turn has the obligation to report to work when scheduled and in a timely manner.

A status may include a number of roles, with each role appropriate to a specific social context. For instance, a woman who occupies the status of chief executive officer of a large company has multiple roles attached to that position. She may also have duties and obligations associated with other statuses such as daughter, sister, wife, mother, Red Cross volunteer, and so on. Role behavior, in any given situation, depends on the statuses occupied by interacting individuals. Staff nurses, for example, behave one way toward their clients, another way toward their coworkers, and yet another way toward their supervisors.

Social positions are *ascribed* based on such characteristics as class (e.g., poor, middle class, wealthy), gender, and racial or ethnic group membership, or are *achieved* through education, training, and so forth. There are societal constraints on all statuses. For instance, an African-American male nurse occupies several relevant statuses. He is a qualified professional, but there will undoubtedly be situations in which others will expect him to enact behaviors traditionally associated with his other ascribed status(es) (i.e., male, African-American, son, brother, father).

*Role strain*, or role stress, is a subjective experience produced by such conditions as *role ambiguity*, *role incongruity*, *role overload*, and *role conflict*. Ill-defined, vague, or unclear role expectations can result in role ambiguity (e.g., the staff nurse assigned to temporarily act as head nurse with no preparation). Role incongruity can occur when role expectations run counter to the individual's values and self-perception (e.g., a staff nurse who takes pride in her caring and supportive behaviors toward clients and coworkers is promoted to supervisor and must "trim the budget"). The nurse faced with an imbalance in ratio of demands (excessive) and time (inadequate) on an under-staffed acute intensive care unit may experience *role overload*. Occupying more than one status at a time increases the likelihood of an individual being unable to enact the roles associated with one status without violating those of another status (e.g., admin-istrative/supervisor–professional nurse/client advocate). The individual faced with such mutually exclusive or contradictory role expectations will likely experience *role conflict*.

The roles an individual plays have a profound effect on attitude and behavior as well as on self-perceptions. As society in general and health care systems in particular become increasingly more complex and resources shrink, role stress can be expected to continue and expand.

### Structural Role Theory

No one scholar is credited with *structural role theory*; contributions came from many sources. A descriptive analogy for understanding the overall assumptions of this ap-proach comes from a passage in William Shakespeare's *As You Like It*:

> *All the world's a stage*
> *and all the men and women merely players:*
> *They have their exits and their entrances;*
> *And one man in his time plays many parts.* (Act II, scene vii)

Human interaction is viewed as being similarly structured; individual actors adhere to societal norms or "scripts" attached to statuses or positions they occupy. Role di-rectives come from those with power, and actors adjust their responses or "perfor-mances" to others with whom they interact, as well as their reference group or "audience." Through self-concepts and role-playing, individuals develop their own unique interactional styles (Turner, 2003).

Structural role theorists de-emphasize the creative aspects of mind and self and place more emphasis on the impact of social structure on interaction. Structural role theorists posit that individuals spend a great deal of time in groups of one kind or an-other and are shaped or socialized by the groups to which they belong. An individual uses groups to help define personal beliefs, attitudes, and values; these are called *ref-erence groups*. The influence of reference groups continues even when that individual is away from the group members because the group's norms and values have been in-ternalized. The internalized norms and values are continually used as a measuring stick by which the behaviors of one's self and others are evaluated. An example of a reference group for student nurses would be professional nurses. Reference groups can be positive or negative; the former have individuals that are desirable to emulate, whereas the latter provide a model to avoid.

### Process Role Theory

Role theory focuses on the impact of behavior on self-conceptions and is viewed by some as being too structured and deterministic (Turner, 2003). *Process role theory* pro-poses a different perspective. There are three dominant characteristics of process role theory: (1) individuals negotiate their roles in most social contexts; (2) roles are gen-eral configurations about conduct; and (3) roles are not fixed and predetermined. In most social encounters (including highly structural situations) individuals actively make roles and negotiate with others their right to enact a given role (Turner, 1962).

*Application of Role Theory to Nursing*

A significant amount of research on role theory and related concepts among nurses has been performed. Junious and colleagues (2004), for example, examined job satisfaction among school nurses and determined that role strain contributed to low morale among the group. In other works, Sewell (2008) studied journaling as a mechanism to facilitate graduate nurses' role transition and Holt (2008) explored how advance practice nurses adapt and adjust to their roles in primary care settings.

Caregiver roles have been examined by a number of researchers. For example, the effects of caregiving on families of persons receiving cancer treatment was studied by Schumacher, Stewart, Archbold, Caparro, Mutale, and Agrawal (2008) and Wells, Cagle, Bradley, and Barnes (2008). Bern-Klug and Forbes-Thompson (2008) studied the self-imposed role expectations of family members of nursing home residents.

In other research, role theory has been used to examine role strain among client groups. For instance, the effectiveness of using role-exit theory for marital counseling following extended military deployment was studied and found effective (Gambardella, 2008). Schachman, Lee, and Lederman (2004) examined an intervention to reduce role strain among military wives. Then, in another work Koniak-Griffin, Logsdon, Hines-Martin, and Turner (2006) explored the numerous and diverse factors that impact the mothering role in contemporary society and provided guidelines for nursing interventions that permit individual and cultural differences.

## Conflict Theories

Society is generally regarded as a system, composed of interdependent and essentially harmonious parts that are linked together into a boundary-maintaining whole. Social integration results from the mixing of parts and consensus on societal goals and cultural values. With cooperation being the primary social process, change is gradual and adaptive, and society remains stable (Eitzen & Baca-Zinn, 1998).

But individuals' perceptions of the water glass as being either half-empty or half-full are similar to how society can be viewed. The same social phenomenon can be seen as maintaining system balance and integrity (a functionalistic perspective), or it can be seen as generating divisiveness and conflict.

The conflict perspective sees conflict as endemic to social organizations. This is due to the existence of structural constraints, which result in the unequal distribution of power. These imbalances of power may result in competitive interactions among and between groups. Social problems (e.g., gender, class, and racial/ethnic inequality; poverty, violence, and health disparities) are in actuality "societally induced conditions" (Eitzen & Baca-Zinn, 1998, p. 57).

How the causes, consequences, and interventions of social problems are addressed depends on the theoretical perspective of either conflict or order. The order perspective tends to "blame the victim" (Ryan, 1976) or labels the "deviant." Rehabilitating individuals is the remedy. From the conflict perspective, rehabilitation of individuals is like treating symptoms and ignoring the root cause(s). What needs to be fixed is society because society has failed to meet the needs of individuals and needs restructuring.

According to conflict theory, social problems are "found within the institutional framework of society . . . and are not the exclusive functions of individual pathologies" (Eitzen & Baca-Zinn, 1998 p. 58). Eitzen and Baca-Zinn (1998) propose a synthesis

---

**BOX 12-4** *Assumptions of the Order and Conflict Synthesis Model*

1. Processes of stability and change are properties of all societies. Human societies are paradoxical—they are always ordered and always changing.
2. Societies are organized, but the process of organization generates conflict. Conflict is generated by the unequal distribution of power in decision-making processes over scarce resources, in a system of social stratification.
3. Society is an imperfect social system. Parts of the system may have complementary and consensual as well as exclusive and incompatible interests and goals.
4. Societies are held together by complementary interests, by consensus on cultural values, and also by coercion.
5. Social change is common to all societies; it may be gradual or abrupt, reforming or revolutionary.

Source: Eitzen and Baca-Zinn (1998).

---

of the order and conflict models. Assumptions of their proposed synthesis model are summarized in Box 12-4.

Conflict theories share common ground in the elements analyzed in human societies: inequality, power/authority, domination/subjugation, interests, and conflict. Modern conflict theories have their roots in the writings of Karl Marx, the most famous conflict theorist, with later influences from Max Weber (1958) and Georg Simmel (1956). Marx argued that economic-based class conflict is the most basic and influential source of all social change. He viewed class conflict as inevitable because of the unequal allocation of goods and services in capitalist societies. Marx's model of conflict was shaped by Europe's transition from a feudal to a capitalistic society and he wrote that capitalism is an economic system that perpetuates inequality. Marx believed that the only means for emancipatory social change within a capitalist society was violent revolution, with the workers fighting against the capitalists. He argued that the ideology of any society is always the ideology of the ruling class or the powerful people, because those in power use ideology to ensure that the value system reigns (Eitzen & Baca-Zinn, 1998).

Weber (1958) rejected Marx's dichotomous model of the relationships between conflict and power. He believed that the potential for conflict decreases as societies move from traditional authoritarian relationships to relationships organized around rational/legal authority in industrial/bureaucratic societies.

Simmel (1956) shared Marx's and Weber's view that conflict was an "inevitable and ubiquitous feature" of society resulting from divergent interests, but believed that conflict also came from the innate aggressive instincts of humans. He perceived conflict to be necessary for adaptation and growth of humans and society. Without conflict there could be no adaptation and growth. It was from these conflict-driven processes that solidarity was promoted, both within and between human groups. Conflict was therefore functionally necessary.

Modern conflict theories have modified Marx's model. Dahrendorf (1958), a conflict theorist, regarded Marx's theory of class conflict and social change as too simplistic because other social groups (e.g., political groups) also experience conflict. Implicit in his perspective is the notion that conflict meets systems' functional need for change. Society is characterized by struggles between social classes and between powerful and less powerful groups because of the inequality embedded in hierarchical social structures. The potential for conflict is then inherent in the majority of human relationships because social organization means, among other things, the unequal distribution of power resulting in the "haves" and the "have-nots" (Eitzen & Baca-Zinn, 1998).

Coser (1956) was critical of the failure of Marx and Dahrendorf to acknowledge the integrative and adaptive functions of societies. In his view, conflict acts to alert social systems of problems. Through the process of addressing problems, a system adapts and structurally becomes better suited to remediate future problems. According to Coser, an inverse relationship exists between goals and level of conflict.

Three perspectives or types of conflict theory—feminism, critical social theory, and cultural bias—are used frequently by nurses in research, and are applicable in practice. They are described in the following sections.

## FEMINIST THEORY

Gender differences and subordination have traditionally been viewed as both natural and inevitable, but some believe that gender is socially constructed and tends to justify the subordination and exploitation of women. A core assumption in feminist theories is that women are oppressed. This perspective has been determined to be too simplistic, however, and beginning in the 1960s, new views of feminism were presented (Eitzen & Baca-Zinn, 1998).

A rather wide range of perspectives fall under the rubric of feminist theory. Feminist theory has been defined as "an analysis of women's subordination [within families and all other institutions] for the purpose of figuring out how to change it" (Eitzen & Baca-Zinn, 1998, p. 107). There are many issues, themes, and assumptions that are common in feminism. Osmond and Thorne (1993) discuss relevant themes in feminist theory; some of these are summarized in Box 12-5.

### Variations of Feminist Theory

There is considerable variation among feminist perspectives. A few of the most commonly encountered are described in this section.

*Liberal feminism* is concerned with the political life and well-being of women. Friedan (1963) is probably the most well-known liberal feminist. She argued against the entrapment of women by the *feminine mystique*, an ideology that claims women

---

**BOX 12-5** *Themes in Feminist Theories*

1. Women's experiences are central, normal, and valuable; experiences open new ways of knowing the world.
2. Gender is a basic organizing concept. The concept of "gender" involves two interrelated elements: (a) the social construction and exaggeration of differences between women and men (i.e., there is a fundamental basis of inequality, or social stratification, similar to social class and race), and (b) gender distinctions are used to legitimize and perpetuate power relations between women and men (i.e., compared with men, women are devalued and socially, economically, politically, and legally subordinated).
3. Gender distinctions occur in daily processes of constructing and reconstructing differences between women and men and devalue women. However, rather than passive victims, women participate in gendering processes as active agents, actors, and creators of culture.
4. Gender relations must be analyzed within specific sociocultural and historical contexts.
5. Monolithic, bounded notions (e.g., "the family") contribute to an ideology that contains class, cultural, and heterosexual biases, and supports the oppression of women.

Source: Osmond and Thorne (1993).

are separate, but special, by extolling the virtues of women's traditional roles of wife and mother. Especially noteworthy is Freidan's examination of differences in women's pathologies (e.g., married women compared to unmarried women are more susceptible to diseases/disorders).

*Socialist (Marxist) feminism* is exemplified by Millet's (1971) work describing the impact of patriarchy on the social structure, which she saw as a masculine system of political domination. She questioned the persistence of patriarchal beliefs and attitudes into an era where women are educated and free, yet continue to be subordinate and devalued. She determined that because patriarchal domination is socially constructed, women can take emancipatory actions and reconstruct gender relations.

Firestone's *The Dialectic of Sex* (1970) is perhaps the epitome of *radical feminism*. She refuted Marx's notion of economic class and argued instead that "sex class divisions" are at the root of women's oppression. "[T]o assure the elimination of sexual classes requires the revolt of the underclass (women) and the seizure of control of *reproduction*" (Waters, 1994, p. 267).

Brownmiller (1975), another radical feminist, argued that it is not women's biologic constraints, but sexual relationships that subordinate women. She focused on violence against women, and believed that rape is possible because human sexual behavior is unique. According to Brownmiller, rape is about power and control and therefore about domination and power over women.

A branch of radical feminism is *cultural feminism*, which focuses on women's differences. Cultural feminism condones separatism and suggests that rather than striving to be like men, women should work toward reorganizing society around a female-dominated community—"womanculture."

*Psychoanalytic feminism* takes the male-centered and sexist assumptions of Freudian theory and reworks them. Chodorow (1989) refuted the notions of the Oedipal complex and penis envy by connecting the role of mothering to the construction of gendered personalities. Gilligan (1982) addressed the "different voice" of moral reasoning. These two theorists, as well as others, have helped to bridge the gap to consider the internal psyches of girls and women (Osmond & Thorne, 1993).

### Application of Feminist Theory to Nursing

Feminist theory and philosophy have been frequently cited in the nursing literature. Beginning in the late 19th century, Florence Nightingale wrote on gender roles. Examples of Nightingale's feminist views included her efforts to obtain women's right to education, self-development, and occupations, and her criticism of the double sexual standard of the times (Chinn, 1999; Pfettscher, de Graff, Tomey, Mossman, & Slebodnik, 1998).

Nursing research studies have been conducted using feminist concepts and theories. For example, Rose and Glass (2008) studied the significance of emancipatory research to the subjective experiences of nurses and to the future of nursing practice. In a similar work, Giddings (2005) examined the challenges that nurses face in addressing institutionalized social injustices that lead to health disparities. Finally, Prakke, Wrubel, Moskowitz, Chesla, and Benner (2004) used a feminist perspective for their qualitative study that explored maternal caregivers' concerns, knowledge and needs in caring for their chronically ill children.

## CRITICAL SOCIAL THEORY

The early foundation for *critical social theory* can be found in Marx's argument that oppressive arrangements require revolutionary action. The concept of emancipatory alternatives has replaced Marx's revolutionary (and more violent) action in contemporary critical social theories. To identify and address oppressive social arrangements, individuals cannot simply accept that how they perceive the social world is indeed factual. Rather, they must question their assumptions to identify oppressive social arrangements. This is made possible through the unique capacity for self-reflection that humans possess.

Critical social theory uses societal awareness to expose social inequalities that keep people from reaching their full potential. It is derived from the belief that social meanings structure life through social domination. Proponents of critical social theory maintain that social exchanges that are not distorted by power imbalances will stimulate the evolution of a more just society. Furthermore, critical theory assumes that truth is socially determined (Butterfield, 2007).

Habermas (1991) is perhaps the best-known contemporary critical social theorist. In opposition to Marx's revolutionary action, Habermas argued that emancipation from domination is possible through "[rational] communicative [inter-] action." He supported employment of negotiation as integral to communicative action, realizing that negotiation must be conducted without the use of power or coercion by either of the interacting parties. With his emphasis on interaction through communication, Habermas discounted the importance of both material and structural constraints on changing social systems.

In the health care industry, health maintenance organizations provide an example of purposive and rational social structures that are not designed with "communicative action" between client and health care providers in mind. Authority relationships are maintained within these agencies, and negotiation is often not a possibility.

### Application to Nursing

Concepts from critical social theory have been described in recent nursing literature, typically within the context of working with disadvantaged groups. For example, Bateman (2005) used critical social theory to illuminate oppressive elements that impede mental health service access and to empower individuals for action for change.

Other nursing authors used critical social theory to discuss general aspects of the discipline of nursing. For example, guided by critical social theory, Sumner and Danielson (2008) examined the nurse–patient relationship in the current acute health care delivery system in three countries and concluded that nurses care about and are proud of the work they do but are tired and desire acknowledgement of their efforts. Verkaaik (2007) studied the relationship between nurse manager leadership attributes and nurse clinical autonomy in both *magnet* and *nonmagnet* hospitals. Results showed the relationship contributes to magnet status.

## CULTURAL DIVERSITY AND CULTURAL BIAS

An interest in cultural diversity and cultural bias is not a phenomenon peculiar to the social sciences or sociology in particular. Culture, as socially patterned human thought and behavior (Bodley, 2000), is an integral and highly influential component of the interface between humans and their social environment. The word *culture* comes from the Latin root *colere*, to inhabit, cultivate, or honor. In general it refers to human activity; different definitions of culture reflect different theories for understanding, or criteria for valuing, human activity. The interest in and the study of culture in the United States have been steadily pushing their way to the forefront since the mid-1980s (Alexander & Smith, 2001). It was also during this time that a shift occurred in U.S. population demographics and the corresponding increase in diverse ethnic groups became more pronounced, resulting in the concepts of culture and cultural diversity becoming an increasingly relevant topic.

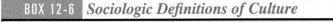

## BOX 12-6 *Sociologic Definitions of Culture*

- A way of life, a system of ideas, values, beliefs, knowledge, and customs passed on from generation to generation
- All the learned and shared products of a society
- The entire complex of ideas and material objects that people of a society (or group) have created and adopted for carrying out the necessary tasks of collective life

Source: Ferrante (1992).

There is little consensus among sociologists in this specialized area of study as to just what the concept of culture means. From a sociologic perspective culture can be broadly conceived as the symbolic/expressive dimension of social life. Examples of three different sociologic definitions are listed in Box 12-6 with an anthropological comparison in Table 12-2.

Despite the disagreement on definition, sociologists agree on the essential principles of culture. These principles are that (1) culture consists of tangible (material) and intangible (nonmaterial) components; (2) people inherit and learn a culture; (3) biological, environmental, and historical forces shape and change culture; and (4) culture is a tool that people use to evaluate other societies and to adapt to problems of living (Ferrante, 1992).

The word *bias* refers to an inclination for or against some phenomenon that inhibits impartial and objective judgment that can, in the extreme, constitute prejudice. *Cultural bias*, interpreting and judging phenomena in relation to one's own culture, is an ever-present danger and central to human societies. A multitude of historical and contemporary examples of cultural biases deal with the "isms": racism, sexism, classism, and ageism. An alternate perspective views cultural bias as a normative response to safeguard that which is known and familiar to the individual—ethnocentrism. Any normative belief about human beings can be reasonably isolated as a cultural belief and consequently lead to a biased perspective.

### Application to Nursing

Nursing research has shown that cultural beliefs, including those related to age, class, sex, and race/ethnicity, promote biases that may be contributing factors in health disparities.

### TABLE 12-2 *Anthropological Definitions of Culture*

| | |
|---|---|
| Topical | Culture consists of everything on a list of topics, or categories, such as social organization, religion, or economy |
| Historical | Culture is social heritage, or tradition, that is passed on to future generations |
| Behavioral | Culture is shared, learned human behavior, a way of life |
| Normative | Culture is ideals, values, or rules for living |
| Functional | Culture is the way humans solve problems of adapting to the environment or living together |
| Mental | Culture is a complex of ideas, or learned habits, that inhibit impulses and distinguish people from animals |
| Structural | Culture consists of patterned and interrelated ideas, symbols, or behaviors |
| Symbolic | Culture is based on arbitrarily assigned meanings that are shared by a society |

Source: Bodley (2000).

This includes gaps in access, questionable diagnostic practices, and limited provision of optimum interventions (Bernstein, 2007; Crowe, 2006; DeSocio, Elder, & Puckett, 2008; Guamero, 2007; Hampton, 2007). Other studies have shown that ethnocultural variations in symptoms can set the stage for diagnostic bias that can result in inappropriate interventions (Chang & Roberts, 2008) and their expression (Arnault, Sakamoto, & Moriwaki, 2005). Similarly steadfast adherence to the Western illness-based model can marginalize persons with disabilities (Hill, 2006).

In other nursing research, Wang and Chan (2005) looked at the impact of a culturally appropriate education program for Chinese Americans with type 2 diabetes and Whittemore (2007) conducted a similar study for Hispanic adults. Another study investigated critical care nurses' provision of culturally congruent care to Arab Muslims (Marrone, 2008). And finally, data from a phenomenological study of African-American registered nurses in southeastern Louisiana led the author to encourage the nursing profession to promptly address the problems of cultural diversity among its own practitioners (Wilson, 2007).

## Chaos Theory

A problem with explaining chaos theory is that the word *chaos* immediately brings to mind the common meaning of "a condition or place of great disorder or confusion" or of randomness—"having no specific pattern." When used in the scientific context, chaos, as will be explained, means something very different. A second problem lies in simplifying the somewhat exotic and strange terminology (Ward, 1995). Application poses an additional problem because much of the argument of the theory has been developed through complex mathematical formulae (Weigel & Murray, 2000). The last problem is that large data sets with long-time sequences are necessary for chaos to become evident (Shelley & Wagner, 1998). This section discusses concepts related to chaos theory, and their application in nursing and health care.

The modernist theories of Western science (e.g., GST, germ theory) focus on linearity, homeostasis, order, equilibrium, predictability, and control (e.g., causal models). These concepts form a sort of invisible template that constrains many scientists from examining the "noise" or variation in their data (e.g., outliers); thus, they are unable to "look outside the box." An emerging postmodern science of nonlinear dynamic systems, in particular chaos theory, takes science "outside that box."

Chaos theory has its origins in meteorology in the 1960s (Johnson & Webber, 2005) and is part of an emerging postmodern science. The interdisciplinary application of chaos theory has steadily gained momentum since the 1990s. Chaos theory is the study of unstable, aperiodic behavior in deterministic (nonrandom) nonlinear dynamical systems. *Dynamical* refers to the time varying behavior of a system and *aperiodic* is the nonrepetitive but continuous behavior that results from the effects of any small disturbance. Prediction of future states in such systems is impossible.

More simply stated, chaos theory is about finding the underlying order in the apparent disorder of natural and social systems, and understanding how change occurs in nonlinear dynamical systems over time (Hayles, 1999) (Box 12-7). According to Young (1992), chaos theory provides "insight and guidance into the delicate and shifting relationship between order and disorder in ways not permitted in modern science nor imagined in more traditional knowledge processes" (p. 446). Based on chaos theory, therefore, natural and social systems survive precisely because of their nonlinear behavior. Examples of dynamical instability in the real world include disease, political unrest, and families and communities in trouble. Chaos may also be found in

**BOX 12-7** *Principles of Chaos Theory*

- Systems, no matter their level of complexity, rely on an underlying order and seek stability and survive precisely because of their nonlinear behavior or *orderly disorder*
- Simple events can result in very complex behaviors or events

the physical body in heart rhythms, electrical brain activity, and chemical reactions (e.g., neurotransmitters).

## CONCEPTS FROM CHAOS THEORY

Sociology (and nursing), as well as other social science disciplines, have much to gain in the way of useful knowledge by adopting the concepts and logics of chaotic dynamics (Young, 1991). This section presents four of those concepts.

*Sensitive dependence on initial conditions,* the hallmark of chaotic systems, is where even small differences can cause dramatically divergent paths. Because equilibrium is never reached in a dynamical system, trajectories that start from "arbitrarily close" points will ultimately diverge exponentially (Mark, 1994). This sensitivity to initial conditions is commonly referred to as the "butterfly effect"—where hypothetically, a butterfly flapping its wings on one side of the world can cause a tornado the next month on the other side of the world. This concept was dramatized in the 2004 release of the movie "The Butterfly Effect," but it has been at least intuitively known for centuries, as written in the well-known proverb:

> For want of a nail, the shoe was lost;
> For want of a shoe, the horse was lost;
> For want of a horse, the rider was lost,
> For want of a rider, a message was lost;
> For want of a message, the battle was lost;
> For want of a battle, the kingdom was lost!

A small change—no nail—resulted in the huge concluding event of a lost kingdom.

This effect was illustrated by Heaton and Call (1995). They examined the relationship between age at time of marriage for a large sample of couples in two age groups: 23–26 and 27–29 years. The marriage survival rates were almost identical at 5 years, but divergent trajectories became increasingly evident at 10 and 15 years. At 20 years, the marital survival rates were significantly higher for the 27–29 year olds. The age difference between the two groups was small, yet those differences caused two groups of nonlinear dynamical systems to take divergent paths.

*A strange attractor* (strange because its appearance was unexpected) is similar to a magnet that exerts its pull on objects to return them to their original starting point. With this controlling action, an attractor provides a boundary "beyond which processes of differentiation and elaboration cannot go" (Shelley & Wagner, 1998, p. 365). For example, an attractor in relationships is "the behavioral pattern that underlies the period of stability" (p. 435). In a clinical example, Gottman (1991) identifies a sense of "we-ness" as an attractor in stable marriages. An attractor can be visualized (with appropriate software) by graphing the changing behavior of an attribute(s) of a system. Figure 12-3 is an example of a strange attractor showing chaotic motion from a simple three-dimensional model; note the butterfly resemblance.

3. Select one of the grand nursing theorists and review her work. Identify any concepts, principles, and theories drawn from the social sciences. Share findings with colleagues.

## INTERNET RESOURCES

http://sprott.physics.wisc.edu/cda.htm

Link to a program called "Chaos Data Analyzer"—a research and teaching tool designed to detect "seemingly random time series" within data.

http://www-chaos.umd.edu/

Link to University of Maryland's website describing nonlinear dynamics.

http://www.societyforchaostheory.org/

Society for Chaos Theory in Psychology and life sciences; provides basic information on the history and study of chaos theory.

## REFERENCES

Alexander, J. C., & Smith, P. (2001). The strong program in cultural sociology. In J. Turner (Ed.), *The handbook of sociological theory* (chap. 7). New York: Kluwer.

Appel, S., Giger, J., & Davidhizar, R. E. (2005). Opportunity cost: The impact of contextual risk factors on the cardiovascular health of low-income rural southern African-American women. *Journal of Cardiovascular Nursing, 20*(5), 315–324.

Arnault, D., Sakamoto, S., & Moriwaki, A. (2005). The association between negative self-descriptions and depressive symptomology: Does culture make a difference? *Archives of Psychiatric Nursing, 19*(2), 93–100.

Bankston, K. D. (2005). *Collective self-esteem and attitudes toward collaboration as predictors to collaborative practice behaviors used by registered nurses and physicians in acute care hospitals.* Abstract retrieved September 24, 2008, from http://www.ohiolink.edu/etd/.

Bateman, A. L. (2005). *Utilization of a critical social thinking perspective in an analysis of mental health service.* Paper presented at the Sigma Theta Tau International Conference. Abstract retrieved January 20, 2009, from http://www/nursinglibrary.org.

Beel, A., Hawranik, P., McClement, S., & Daenincl, P. (2006). Palliative sedation: Nurses' perceptions. *International Journal of Palliative Nursing, 12*(10), 510–518.

Bern-Klug, M., & Forbes-Thompson, S. (2008). Family members' responsibilities to nursing home residents "she is the only mother I got." *Journal of Gerontological Nursing, 34*(2), 43–52.

Bernstein, K. S. (2007). Mental health issues among urban Korean American immigrants. *Journal of Transcultural Nursing, 18*(2), 175–180.

Blau, P. (1964). *Exchange and power in social life.* New York: Wiley.

Blumer, H. (1969). *Symbolic interactionism.* Engle-wood Cliffs, NJ: Prentice-Hall.

Bodley, J. H. (2000). *Cultural anthropology: Tribes, states, and the global system* (3rd ed.). New York: McGraw-Hill.

Brownmiller, S. (1975). *Against our will.* New York: Simon & Schuster.

Butterfield, P. G. (2007). Thinking upstream: Conceptualizing health from a population perspective. In M. A. Nies & M. McEwen (Eds.), *Community health nursing: Promoting the health of populations* (4th ed., pp. 48–62). Philadelphia: Elsevier/ Saunders.

Byrd, M. (2006). Social exchange as a framework for client–nurse interaction during public health nursing maternal–child home visits. *Public Health Nursing, 23*(3), 271–276.

Chang, C., & Roberts, B. (2008). Cultural perspectives in feeding difficulty in Taiwanese elderly with dementia. *Journal of Nursing Scholarship, 40*(3), 235–240.

Chinn, P. L. (1999). Gender and nursing science. In E. C. Polifroni & M. Welch (Eds.), *Perspectives on philosophy of science in nursing: An historical and contemporary anthology* (pp. 462–466). Philadelphia: Lippincott Williams & Wilkins.

Chodorow, N. (1989). *Feminism and psychoanalytic theory.* New Haven, CT: Yale University Press.

Choi, M., Lee, D., Lee, K., Kim, H., & Ham, E. (2004). A structural model of menopausal depression in Korean women. *Archives of Psychiatric Nursing, 18*(6), 235–242.

Coleman, J. (1990). *Foundations of social theory.* Cambridge, MA: Belknap Press.

Cooley, C. H. (1902). *Human nature and the social order.* New York: Charles Scribner's Sons.

Coser, L. A. (1956). *The functions of social conflict.* London: Free Press of Glencoe.

Crowe, M. (2006). Psychiatric diagnosis: Some implications for mental health nursing care. *Journal of Advanced Nursing, 53*(1), 125–131.

Dahrendorf, R. (1958). Toward a theory of social conflict. *Journal of Conflict Resolution, 2*(2), 170–183.

Deppoliti, D. (2008). Exploring how new registered nurses construct professional identity in hospital settings. *Journal of Continuing Education in Nursing, 39*(6), 255–262.

DeSocio, J., Elder, L., & Puckett, S. (2008). Bridging cultures for Latino children: School nurse and advanced practice nurse partnership. *Journal of Child and Adolescent Psychiatric Nursing, 21*(3), 146–153.

Dewey, D. (1922). *Human nature and human conduct.* New York: Henry Holt.

Eitzen, D. S., & Baca-Zinn, M. (1998). *In conflict and order: Understanding society* (8th ed.). Boston: Allyn & Bacon.

Emerson, R. (1981). Social exchange theory. In M. Rosenberg & R. Turner (Eds.), *Social psychology* (pp. 30–65). New York: Basic Books.

Ferrante, J. (1992). *Sociology: A global perspective.* Belmont, CA: Wadsworth.

Firestone, S. (1970). *The dialectic of sex.* London: Paladin.

Fowler, T. (2006). Alcohol dependence and depression: Advance practice nurse interventions. *Journal of the American Academy of Nurse Practitioners, 18*(7), 303–308.

Friedan, B. (1963). *The feminine mystique.* London: Gollancz.

Gambardella, L. C. (2008). Role-exit theory and marital discord following extended military deployment. *Perspectives in Psychiatric Care, 44*(3), 169–174.

Garcia, C. M., & Saewyc, E. M. (2007). Perceptions of mental health among recently immigrated Mexican adolescents. *Issues in Mental Health Nursing, 28*(1), 37–54.

Giddings, L. S. (2005). Health disparities, social injustice, and the culture of nursing. *Nursing Research, 54*(5), 304–312.

Gilligan, D. (1982). *In a different voice: Psychological theory and women's development.* Cambridge, MA: Harvard University Press.

Gottman, J. M. (1991). Chaos and regulated change in families: A metaphor for the study of transitions. In P. A. Cowan & M. Hetherton (Eds.), *Family transitions* (pp. 247–272). Hillsdale, NJ: Lawrence Erlbaum.

Guamero, P. A. (2007). Family and community influences on the social and sexual lives of Latino gay men. *Journal of Transcultural Nursing, 18*(1), 12–18.

Habermas, J. (1991). The critical theory of Jurgen Habermas. In J. Turner (Ed.), *The structure of sociological theory* (pp. 254–281). Belmont, CA: Wadsworth.

Haigh, C. A. (2008). Using simplified chaos theory to manage nursing services. *Journal of Nursing Administration, 16*(3), 298–304.

Hamilton, P., West, B., Cherri, M., Mackey, J., & Fisher, P. (1994). Preliminary evidence of nonlinear dynamics in births to adolescents in Texas, 1964–1990. *Theoretic and Applied Chaos in Nursing, 1*(1). Retrieved May 1, 2009, from http://www.southernct.edu/chaos-nursing/volume1.htm.

Hampton, M. D. (2007). The role of treatment setting and high acuity in the over diagnosis of schizophrenia in African Americans. *Archives of Psychiatric Nursing, 21*(6), 327–335.

Hayles, N. K. (1999). From chaos to complexity: Moving through metaphor to practice. *Chaos and Complexity in Nursing, 4.* Retrieved July 23, 2004, from http://www.southernct.edu/chaos-nursing/chaos4.htm.

Heaton, T. B., & Call, V. R. A. (1995). Modeling family dynamics with event history techniques. *Journal of Marriage and the Family, 57*(4), 1078–1090.

Hechter, M. (1987). *Principles of group solidarity.* Berkeley, CA: University of California Press.

Hill, D. L. (2006). Sense of belonging as connectedness: American Indian worldview and mental health. *Archives of Psychiatric Nursing, 20*(5), 210–216.

Holt, I. G. S. (2008). Role transition in primary care settings. *Quality in Primary Care, 16*(2), 117–126.

Homans, G. (1961). *Social behavior.* London: Rutledge.

James, W. (1890). *The principles of psychology.* New York: Henry Holt.

Johnson, B. M., & Webber, P. B. (2005). *An introduction to theory and reasoning in nursing* (2nd ed.). Philadelphia: Lippincott Williams & Wilkins.

Junious, D. L., Johnson, R. J., Peters, R. J., Markham, C. M., Kelder, S. H, & Yacoubian, G. S. (2004). A study of school nurse job satisfaction. *Journal of School Nursing, 20*(2), 88–93.

Kane-Urrabazo, C. (2006). Management's role in shaping organizational culture. *Journal of Nursing Management, 14*(3), 188–194.

Kara, B., Caglar, K., & Kilic, S. (2007). Nonadherence with diet and fluid restrictions and perceived social support in patients receiving hemodialysis. *Journal of Nursing Scholarship, 39*(3), 243–248.

Kenney, J. W. (1995). Relevance of theory-based nursing practice. In P. J. Christensen & J. W. Kenney (Eds.), *Nursing process: Application of conceptual models* (4th ed., pp. 3–17). St. Louis: Mosby.

Kim, D. S. (2005). *An explanation of cancer patients' hope just after surgery under the idea of chaos theory.* Paper presented at the Sigma Theta Tau International Conference. Abstract retrieved January 14, 2009, from http://www.nursinglibrary.org.

Koniak-Griffin, D., Logsdon, M., Hines-Martin, V., & Turner, C. (2006). Contemporary mothering in a diverse society. *Journal of Obstetric, Gynecologic, and Neonatal Nursing, 35*(5), 671–678.

Kurz, J., & Hayes, E. (2006). End of life issues action: Impact of Education. *International Journal of Nursing Scholarship, 3*(1). Retrieved January 20, 2009, from http://bepress.com/ijnes/vol3/iss1/art18.

Leahy-Warren, P. (2007). Social support for first-time mothers: An Irish study. *The American Journal of Maternal Child Nursing, 32*(6), 368–374.

Levi-Strauss, C. (1969). *The elementary structures of kinship.* Boston: Beacon Press.

Lindesmith, A., & Strauss, A. (1968). *Social psychology.* New York: Holt, Rinehart & Winston.

Logan, J. R, & Spitze, G. (1996). *Family ties: Enduring relations between parents and their grown children.* Philadelphia: Temple University Press.

Logsdon, M., Hertwick, P., Ziegler, C., & Pinto-Foltz, M. (2008). Testing a bioecological model to examine social support in postpartum adolescents. *Journal of Nursing Scholarship, 40*(2), 116–123.

Lorenz, E. N. (1999). Lorenz: An auspicious salutation. *Chaos and Complexity in Nursing, 4*. Retrieved July 23, 2004, from http://www.southernct.edu/chaos-nursing/chaos4.htm.

Mark, B. A. (1994). Chaos theory and nursing systems research. *Theoretic and Applied Chaos in Nursing, 1*(1). Retrieved May 1, 2009, from http://www.southernct.edu/chaos-nursing/volume1.htm.

Marrone, S. R. (2008). Attitudes, subjective norms, and perceived behavioural control: Critical nurses' intentions to provide culturally congruent care to Arab Muslims. *Journal of Transcultural Nursing, 19*(1), 8–15.

Marx, K. (1977). *Capital: A critical analysis of political economy* (Vol. 1, B. Folkes, Trans.). New York: Vintage Books.

Mason, G., & Attree, M. (1997). The relationship between research and the nursing process in clinical practice. *Journal of Advanced Nursing, 26*(5), 1045–1049.

Mead, K. (1934). *Mind, self, and society* (Lecture notes). C. W. Morris (Ed.), Chicago: University of Chicago Press.

Meadows-Olivier, M., Sadler, L., Swartz, M., & Ryan-Krause, P. (2007). Sources of stress and support and maternal resources of homeless teenage mothers. *Journal of Child and Adolescent Psychiatric Nursing, 20*(2), 116–125.

Millet, K. (1971). *Sexual politics*. New York: Avon/Equinox.

Mills, C. W. (1959). *The sociological imagination*. New York: Oxford University Press.

Moreno, J. (1953). *Who shall survive?* New York: Beacon Press.

Mossop, M., & Wilkinson, T. (2006). Nursing education in gerontological clinical settings: What do elderly patients think of student-centered care? *Journal of Gerontologist Nursing, 32*(6), 49–55.

Nye, F. I. (1979). Choice, exchange, and the family. In W. R. Burr, R. Hill, F. I. Nye, & I. I. Reiss (Eds.), *Contemporary theories about the family* (pp. 1–41). New York: Free Press.

Oliker, S. J. (1989). *Best friends and marriage: Exchanges among women*. Berkeley, CA: University of California Press.

Osmond, M. W., & Thorne, B. (1993). Feminist theories: The social construction of gender in families and society. In P. G. Boss, W. J. Doherty, R. LaRossa, W. R. Schumm, & S. K. Steinmetz (Eds.), *Sourcebook of family theories and methods: A contextual approach* (pp. 591–623). New York: Plenum Press.

Pfettscher, S. A., de Graff, K. R., Tomey, A. M., Mossman, C. L., & Slebodnik, M. (1998). Florence Nightingale. In A. M. Tomey & M. R. Alligood (Eds.), *Nursing theorists and their work* (4th ed., pp. 69–85). St. Louis: Mosby.

Prakke, H., Wrubel, J., Moskowitz, J., Chesla, C., & Benner, P. (2004). *Maternal caregivers concerns, knowledge and needs in caring for their chronically ill children: An interpretive phenomenological study.* Abstract retrieved January 20, 2009, from http://www.nursinglibrary.org.

Prigogine, I., & Stengers, I. (1984). *Order out of chaos, Man's new dialogue with nature*. New York: Bantam.

Rose, J., & Glass, N. (2008, in press). The importance of emancipatory research to contemporary nursing practice. *Contemporary Nurse, 28*(1). Abstract retrieved October 2, 2008, from http://mra.e-contentmanagement.com/archives/vol/1/issue/1/article/2001/theimportance-of.

Ray, M. A. (1994). Complex caring dynamics: A unifying model of nursing inquiry. *Theoretic and Applied Chaos in Nursing, 3*. Retrieved September 12, 2004, from http://www.southernct.edu/chaos-nursing/volume1.htm.

Ryan, W. (1976). *Blaming the victim*. New York: Pantheon.

Sammarco, A., & Konecny, L. (2008). Quality of life, social support, and uncertainty among Latino breast cancer survivors. *Oncology Nursing Forum, 35*(5), 844–849.

Schachman, K. A., Lee, R. K., & Lederman, R. P. (2004). Baby boot camp: Facilitating maternal role adaptation among military wives. *Nursing Research, 53*(2), 107–112.

Schug, V., Forneris, S., & Kalb, K. (2007). *A recipe for leading change: Context, content, and conduct*. Paper presented at the Sigma Theta Tau International Conference. Abstract retrieved from http://www/nursinglibrary.org.

Schumacher, K., Stewart, B., Archbold, P., Caparro, M., Mutale, F., & Agrawal, S. (2008). Effects of caregiving demand, mutuality, and preparedness on family caregiver outcomes during cancer treatment. *Oncology Nursing Forum, 35*(1), 49–56.

Sewell, E. A. (2008). Journaling as a mechanism to facilitate nurses' role transition. *Nurses Staff Development, 24*(2), 49–52.

Shelley, R. K., & Wagner, D. (1998). Chaos in social theory: Explaining complex events with simple ideas. *Sociological Focus, 31*(4), 357–372.

Simmel, G. (1956). *Conflict and the web of group affiliations* (K. H. Wolff Trans.). Glencoe, IL: Free Press.

Stack, C. B. (1974). *All our kin*. New York: Basic Books.

Stryker, S., & Statham, A. (1985). Symbolic interaction and role theory. In G. Lindzey & E. Aronson (Eds.), *The handbook of social psychology* (3rd ed., pp. 311–378). New York: Random House.

Sumner, J., & Danielson, E. (2008). Critical social theory as a means of analysis of caring in nursing. *International Journal for Human Caring, 11*(1), 30–37.

Swindermann, T. D. (2005). The magnetic appeal of nurse informaticians: Caring attractor for emergence. Doctoral dissertation, Florida Atlantic University. Abstract retrieved from CINAHL database.

Thibaut, J. W., & Kelley, H. M. (1959). *The social psychology of groups*. New York: Wiley.

Thomas, W. I., & Thomas, D. S. (1928). *The child in America: Behavior problems and programs*. New York: Knopf.

Turner, J. H. (1991). *The structure of sociological theory*. Belmont, CA: Wadsworth Publishing.

Turner, J. H. (2003). *The structure of sociological theory* (7th ed.). Belmont, CA: Wadsworth Publishing.

Turner, R. H. (1962). Role taking: Processes versus conformity. In A. Rose (Ed.), *Human behavior and processes* (pp. 20–40). Boston: Houghton Mifflin.

Upenieks, W., Akhavan, J., & Kotlerman, J. (2008). Value-added care: A paradigm shift in patient care delivery. *Nursing Economics, 26*(5), 294–301.

Verkaaik, C. A. (2007). The relationship between nurse manager leadership attributes and nurse clinical autonomy: Magnet versus non-magnet hospitals. Doctoral dissertation, University of San Diego, California. Abstract retrieved from CINAHL database.

von Bertalanffy, L. (1968). *General system theory: Foundation, development, and applications.* New York: Braziller.

Wang, C., & Chan, S. (2005). Culturally tailored diabetes education program for Chinese Americans: A pilot study. *Nursing Research, 54*(5), 347–353.

Ward, M. (1995). Butterflies and bifurcations: Can chaos theory contribute to our understanding of family systems? *Journal of Marriage and the Family, 57*(3), 629–638.

Ware, S. M. (2008). Developing a self-concept of nurse in baccalaureate nursing students. *International Journal of Nursing Education Scholarship, 5*(1). Abstract retrieved January 24, 2009, from http://www.bepress.com/ijnes/vol5/iss1/art5/.

Waters, M. (1994). *Modern sociological theory.* Thousand Oaks, CA: Sage.

Way, M., & MacNeil, M. (2007). Baccalaureate entry to practice: A systems view. *The Journal of Continuing Education in Nursing, 38*(4), 164–169.

Weber, M. (1958). *The Protestant ethic and the spirit of capitalism.* New York: Charles Scribner's Sons.

Weigel, D., & Murray, C. (2000). The paradox of stability and change in relationships: What does chaos theory offer for the study of romantic relationships? *Journal of Social and Personal Relationships, 17*(3), 425–449.

Wells, J., Cagle, C., Bradley, P., & Barnes, D. (2008). Voices of Mexican American caregivers for family members with cancer. *Journal of Transcultural Nursing, 19*(3), 223–233.

Whittemore, R. (2007). Culturally competent interventions for Hispanic adults with type 2 diabetes. *Journal of Transcultural Nursing, 18*(2), 157–166.

Wilson, D. W. (2007). From their own voices. *Journal of Transcultural Nursing, 18*(2), 142–149.

Young, T. R. (1991). Chaos theory and symbolic interaction theory: Poetics for the postmodern sociologist. *Symbolic Interaction, 14*(3), 321–334.

Young, T. R. (1992). Chaos theory and human agency: Humanistic sociology in a postmodern era. *Humanity and Society, 16*(4), 441–460.

# 13

# Theories From the Behavioral Sciences

## M a r t h a   K u h n s   a n d   M e l a n i e   M c E w e n

*D*arlene Williams is in a master's degree program that will allow her to become a psychiatric clinical nurse specialist. In a course on the application of theory in nursing, one of her assignments is to write a paper describing how she has applied a theory in providing care for a client. Although Darlene has been working as a nurse in a psychiatric hospital for the past 10 years, she found this assignment difficult because thus far in the course the instructor had focused primarily on grand nursing theories. Darlene knew little about these theories because in her practice she uses a broad, eclectic approach, predominantly applying theories from the behavioral sciences.

Darlene discussed her dilemma with her professor and learned that she could use any theory or set of theories for the assignment; it was not necessary to rely strictly on nursing theories. The discussion with her professor enlightened Darlene about the necessity of applying nonnursing theories to nursing practice. With the realization of the importance of theories from other disciplines to nursing, Darlene's interest in the many psychologically based theories was piqued and she conducted a literature review.

The person that Darlene chose for her assignment was Alan, a 41-year-old white man, who was married and the father of two adolescents. Alan was admitted to the hospital with diagnoses of major depression, substance dependence with physiologic dependency, and hepatitis C. Assessments revealed that he had problems with his primary support group, problems related to the social environment, occupational problems, and problems related to interaction with the legal system.

Although this was Alan's first hospitalization, he had a long history of alcohol abuse. He also admitted to using cocaine on the weekends and to using heroin occasionally. His father was an alcoholic who died at the age of 44 with cirrhosis of the liver. Although not actively suicidal, Alan expressed passive death wishes. Alan is a well-known member of the community and owns a large software business, which is on the verge of bankruptcy. His motivation for entering treatment is that his wife threatened to divorce him unless he stops using alcohol and drugs.

*In reviewing Alan's care, Darlene planned to use a holistic approach, incorporating principles and concepts from various theories. The first theory that Darlene chose was Freud's psychoanalytic theory because of Alan's denial. This theory was relevant because Freud discussed how an individual uses defense mechanisms to decrease anxiety, and Darlene knew that a major defense mechanism of alcoholism is denial. Darlene also thought the cognitive-behavioral theories were appropriate because she believed that humans need to change cognition to change behavior. Because Darlene assumed that drinking and using drugs were means of coping, she planned to use Lazarus's coping theory to help Alan develop more effective coping strategies. Finally, Darlene planned to apply humanistic psychology because she believes that Alan, like all individuals, has the potential to change and social psychology theories address health beliefs and intent to change.*

---

As discussed in Chapter 1, nursing is a practice discipline, and practice disciplines are considered to be applied sciences rather than pure or basic sciences (Johnson, 1959). The object of both pure and applied sciences is the same (to achieve knowledge), but according to Folta (1968), the difference between the two is their emphasis. In pure science, the emphasis is on basic research, which focuses on the application of the scientific method to add abstract knowledge. In contrast, the emphasis in applied science is on research related to the application and testing of the abstract concepts (Folta, 1968). Thus, applied sciences use the scientific method to apply and test fundamental knowledge or principles in practice. Historically, nursing science has drawn much of its knowledge from the basic sciences and then applied that knowledge to the discipline of nursing.

In learning about theories used in nursing, it is important to remember that nursing has evolved over decades and that the knowledge base for the discipline is a compilation of phenomena from many different disciplines. In the case study, Darlene discovered the notion of "borrowed" versus "unique" theory. Johnson (1968) has defined borrowed theories as knowledge that has been identified in other disciplines and is used in nursing. According to Johnson, knowledge does not belong to any discipline but is shared across many disciplines; thus, nursing science draws on the knowledge of other disciplines to enhance the knowledge required for nursing practice.

One of the areas from which nurses draw theoretical understanding are the psychological sciences, sometimes referred to as the behavioral sciences. The contribution of the behavioral sciences to knowledge in nursing science and nursing practice cannot be denied. Even though the basic theories, concepts, and frameworks are derived from another discipline, they are applied in nursing practice. Additionally, they are frequently applied in nursing research as well as nursing education and administration.

There are many psychological theories, and it would be impossible to cover all of them in this chapter. Major theories were chosen to illustrate concepts that are used in nursing. For the purposes of this chapter, the psychological theories will be viewed in four categories: psychodynamic theories, behavioral and cognitive-behavioral theories, humanistic theories, and stress-adaptation theories. These theories look at an individual and how an individual responds to stimuli. In psychology there is also a special field known as social psychology, which examines how society or groups of individuals respond to various stimuli. This chapter will examine two theories of social psychology commonly used in nursing: the Health Belief Model and the Theory of Reasoned Action.

# Psychodynamic Theories

The late 1800s saw the creation of a new discipline, psychology/psychiatry, with a new body of knowledge. Before Sigmund Freud presented his radical works describing human thoughts and behaviors, people were considered to be either "good" or "bad," "normal" or "crazy." His work led to a major paradigm shift as scientists began to consider the thought processes of "man" and to speculate about human personality. From this paradigm shift came a number of psychological theories.

Freud's thinking was considered radical in the early 1900s. Even now in the early 21st century many people still consider his work radical, yet others believe it to be antiquated. Despite this, his basic ideas and concepts have been used and modified extensively in the development of numerous theories about human thought and behavior.

Psychodynamic theories attempt to explain the multidimensional nature of behavior and understand how an individual's personality and behavior interface. They also provide a systematic way of identifying and understanding behavior. This section describes three psychodynamic theories—the works of Freud, Erikson, and Sullivan. These three theories are also called "stage theories," meaning that they describe clearly defined stages at which new behaviors appear based on social and motivational influences. Table 13-1 compares the developmental stages of the three theories.

## PSYCHOANALYTIC THEORY: FREUD

According to Freudian theory, behavior is nearly always the product of an interaction among the three major systems of the personality: the id, ego, and superego. Even though each of these systems has its own functions, properties, and components, they interact so closely that it is difficult to distinguish their effects on behavior. Behavior is generally an interaction among these three systems; rarely does one system operate to the exclusion of the other two (Freud, 1960).

TABLE 13-1 *Stages of Development*

| Theorist | Developmental Emphasis | Stages |
|---|---|---|
| Sigmund Freud | Psychosexual | 1. Oral<br>2. Anal<br>3. Phallic<br>4. Latency<br>5. Genital |
| Erik E. Erikson | Psychosocial | 1. Trust versus mistrust<br>2. Autonomy versus shame and doubt<br>3. Intimacy versus guilt<br>4. Industry versus inferiority<br>5. Identity versus identity confusion<br>6. Intimacy versus isolation<br>7. Generativity versus stagnation<br>8. Integrity versus despair |
| Harry S. Sullivan | Interpersonal | 1. Infancy<br>2. Childhood<br>3. Juvenile<br>4. Preadolescence<br>5. Early adolescence<br>6. Late adolescence |

According to Freud, the id is the original system of the personality, and it is the matrix in which the ego and superego differentiate. The id is unable to tolerate an increase in energy, which is experienced as an uncomfortable state of tension. This increased tension can be perceived either internally or externally. The id discharges the tension to return the body to a state of equilibrium. This tension release is known as the pleasure principle (Freud, 1960).

The ego distinguishes between things in the mind and things in the external world. The ego is said to follow the reality principle with the aim of preventing tension until an appropriate object is found to satisfy the need. The ego has control over all cognitive and intellectual functions, and is considered to be the executive of the personality because it controls behavior. It does this by mediating the conflicting demands of the id, superego, and external environment (Freud, 1960).

The third system is the superego. The main functions of the superego are to (1) inhibit the impulses of the id; (2) encourage the ego to substitute moralistic goals for realistic goals; and (3) strive for perfection. The focus of the superego is on moral issues: "what is right" and "what is wrong" (Freud, 1960).

Freud based his theory on the scientific view of the late 19th century, which regarded the human body as an energy system. He proposed that because the body derives its energy from the work of the body (e.g., respiration, digestion), then memory and thinking are also defined by the work they perform. He labeled this concept psychic energy and stated that an instinct is an inborn state of somatic excitement. Furthermore, an instinct is a quantum of psychic energy or, as Freud said, "a measure of the demand made upon the mind for work" (1960, p. 168). All the instincts together yield the sum total of psychic energy (Freud, 1953).

The four characteristics of an instinct are source, aim, object, and impetus. Whereas source is the need, the aim is the removal of the tension. Object is what will satisfy the need and also includes all behaviors that occur to obtain the necessary object. The impetus of an instinct is the force or strength, which is determined by the intensity of the underlying need. Thus, psychic energy is displaced to the object to satisfy the instinctual need. Freud believed that instincts are the sole energy source for human behavior (Freud, 1953).

The environment plays two roles with regard to instinct. It either satisfies or threatens the development of the person. The individual responds with increased tension; an increase in tension is known as anxiety. The function of anxiety is to warn the person of impending danger. Anxiety motivates the person to do something; thus, a behavior is seen. As a result of increased tension or anxiety, an individual is forced to learn new methods of reducing the tension. According to Freud, these new methods are called ego defense mechanisms (Freud, 1956). "All defense mechanisms have two characteristics in common: (1) they deny, falsify, or distort reality and (2) they operate unconsciously so that the person is not aware of what is taking place" (Hall & Lindzey, 1978, pp. 91–92).

Freud was one of the first theorists to emphasize the developmental aspect of personality. He believed that the personality was developed within the first five years of life. Each of his stages of development, excepting latency, during which focus lies outside of one's own body, is defined as a mode of reaction to a particular zone of the body. Freud's stages were related to psychosexual development and included oral, anal, phallic, latency, and genital stages (Freud, 1953).

## Application to Nursing

Although nursing theories are not based on Freud's theory, many of his ideas and concepts are relevant to nursing practice. These concepts include anxiety, developmental stages, defense mechanisms, and the identity of self.

Freud's theory helps to explain the complex nature of a person and how a person's past influences his or her personality. The complex processes of the past, which are found in the unconscious mind, suggest an explanation for the diversity in a person's behaviors. Even though the emphasis in much of nursing is on the "here and now," understanding the person's relevant past experiences can help the nurse identify underlying themes and improve care.

The id, ego, and superego are the components of the self. When there is a disequilibrium among these concepts, the self becomes lost and must be reconstructed. Nurses can help clients who have undergone a loss of self to discover a more active sense of self, put the self into action, and use the enhanced self as a refuge. Furthermore, an understanding of the concepts of id, ego, and superego helps the nurse understand the needs of the client and helps the nurse respond more appropriately to the behaviors.

In Alan's situation from the opening case study, the domination of the id would lead to increased substance use because of the pleasure principles. When Alan sobered, the superego would cause him to have feelings of shame and guilt. Darlene can now help Alan choose acceptable ways of behaving, thus causing an equilibrium among the id, ego, and superego. This equilibrium would help to relieve Alan's feelings of anxiety.

A behavior is the way an individual responds to increased tension or anxiety, and, in this case, Alan responded to increased tension by abusing substances (e.g., alcohol, cocaine, heroin). Alan denied that he used substances inappropriately; he stated he used alcohol "socially," and the drugs were only done on weekends and therefore "no big deal." Alan also stated that he had no marital problems when, in fact, his wife was going to divorce him. Alan was demonstrating Freud's concept of defense mechanisms, specifically denial. Defense mechanisms are used to help reduce anxiety and tension. Denial describes a client's behavior and the main two definitions range from adaptive to maladaptive responses. In this case study, Alan uses denial as a maladaptive response. By using denial, Alan was able to decrease the feelings of rejection from his wife and the shame and guilt associated with abusing substances. Because Darlene recognized and understood the use of this maladaptive defense mechanism, she was able to develop a plan of care to help Alan develop more adaptive defense mechanisms to relieve anxiety.

Although denial is used in the case study to explain substance abuse, nurses encounter the use of denial with clients in almost all areas of nursing. Examples include those with amputations, cancer, hypertension, diabetes, and cardiac problems, just to mention a few. The use of denial is a way of protecting the self from a threat that could harm the person physically and decrease self-concept. When denial is used, the individual does not believe that he or she has a problem, and this can lead to noncompliant behavior. Noncompliance is one of the biggest challenges facing nursing today.

Recent nursing literature that reports on application of psychoanalytic theory covers a variety of issues. For example, Kozuki and Kennedy (2004) examined cultural aspects of psychotherapy, comparing Western practices with those of Japanese traditions. Thomas and Hynes (2007) used a psychoanalytic perspective to describe interaction and cohesion among therapeutic group members, and Franks (2004) employed psychoanalytic methods to discuss the uniqueness of the nurse–patient relationship within the rubric of evidence-based nursing. Other nursing authors have used psychoanalytical theory to examine such concepts as emotional boundaries in fertility nursing (Allan & Barber, 2005), acceptance and denial-related chronic illness (Telford, Kralik, & Koch, 2006), and transference and counter-transference in nursing practice (Jones, 2005).

## DEVELOPMENTAL (OR EGO DEVELOPMENTAL) THEORY: ERIKSON

Erikson's Psychosocial Developmental Theory emerged as an expansion of Freud's concept of ego. In Erikson's theory, specific stages of a person's life from birth to death are formed by social influences that interact with the physical/psychological, maturing organism. Erikson described this as a "mutual fit of individual and environment" (Erikson, 1975, p. 102). He is the only developmental theorist who extends development through adulthood; the other theorists stop with adolescence.

Erikson's theory lists eight stages of development: the first four stages occur in infancy and childhood, the fifth stage occurs in adolescence, and the last three stages occur during the adult years. In his work, Erikson emphasized the adolescent stage, that time in an individual's life when the person makes the transition from a child to an adult. This transitional period has the greatest influence on the adult personality. Erikson believed that each stage of development builds on the next, thus contributing to the formation of the total person. Also, even though Erikson gave a chronological timetable, it is not strict because he believed that each person has his or her own timetable for development (Erikson, 1963).

Erikson further developed the concept of ego to incorporate qualities that expanded the Freudian concept. He believed the ego is the most powerful of the three parts of the personality (id, ego, and superego) and described the ego as being robust and resilient. According to Erikson, the ego uses a combination of inner readiness and outer opportunities, with a sense of vigor and joy, to find creative solutions at each stage of development. This concentration of the potential strength of the ego empowers people to deal effectively with their problems (Erikson, 1968).

### Application to Nursing

Developmental theory is often a foundational element in nursing theories, and it is important in nursing practice (Wadensten & Carlsson, 2003). For example, an essential part of the assessment process is to determine age appropriateness or arrested development. Although developmental issues are generally thought to be associated with only pediatrics, this is not the case. By assessing the developmental stage of the adult and elderly person, data can be collected about interpersonal skills and behaviors because behavioral manifestations are clues to issues that need to be addressed in client care. Furthermore, individual responsibility and the capacity to improve one's functioning are issues to be addressed by nurses.

Erikson's theory identified the degree of mastery with regard to a person's chronological age. This mastery is known as ego strength. Bjorklund (2000) believed that promoting assessment from the perspective of ego strengths, instead of ego deficits, is a valuable skill for nurses who then can use the data for assessment and treatment outcomes. Early and GlenMaye (2000) also proposed that nurses work with clients from an ego strength perspective, particularly when including the family in the plan of care. Besides using ego strengths for assessment and interventions, the nurse can also use them to empower the client to take control of his or her life and to deal effectively with problems (Ryles, 1999).

Identifying and assessing Alan's ego strengths helped Darlene locate where Alan falls on the developmental continuum, thus providing data to develop therapeutic goals. When Darlene graduates and becomes a clinical nurse specialist, she can conduct family therapy, and Erikson's theory would be helpful in working with Alan's children, especially from the perspective of ego strength.

Developmental theory is not only used in psychiatric nursing, but in other specialty areas of nursing and is integral to holistic nursing practice (Reed, 1998). Nursing researchers and scholars commonly employ developmental theory in research studies or in describing practice guidelines for various groups. For example, Mamhidir and colleagues (2007) used developmental theory to examine the effect of manipulation of meal routines to improve weight gain among Alzheimer's patients. Other nurses have used developmental theory to improve nursing care among children.

For example, Taylor (2008) promoted using developmental theories to care for children during surgery, and Deering (2000) incorporated developmental theory in describing how school-aged children deal with disasters. In other examples, Harrison (2003) wrote about developmental issues related to aging among women with disabilities and Handley and Ward-Smith (2005) described issues faced by young and middle-aged adults who are addicted to alcohol. These examples demonstrate that developmental theory is used throughout the life continuum (i.e., children, adults, elderly) and is used in pediatric, psychiatric, geriatric, and medical-surgical nursing. Further examination of these research studies suggests that both ego strengths and ego deficits are being studied by nurses.

## INTERPERSONAL THEORY: SULLIVAN

Harry Stack Sullivan based his developmental theory on the premise that an individual does not, and cannot, exist apart from his or her relations with other people. He stated that from the first day of life, a baby is dependent on interpersonal situations, and that this dependence continues throughout the person's life. Even if the person becomes a recluse and withdraws from society, the person carries the memories of interpersonal relationships, which continue to influence behavior and thinking. Sullivan stated that it is a "relatively enduring pattern of recurrent interpersonal relationships which characterize a human life" (Sullivan, 1953, p. 111).

To explain this phenomenon, the term *dynamism* must be understood. Dynamism, as defined by Sullivan, is "the relatively enduring pattern of energy transformation which recurrently characterizes the organism in its duration as a living organism" (Sullivan, 1953, p. 105). The individual's dynamisms characterize interpersonal relations. Although all people have the same dynamisms, the mode of expression varies with the situation and life experience of the individual. Although most dynamisms satisfy the basic needs of the individual, an important dynamism develops as a result of anxiety; this is known as the dynamism of self or the self-system (Sullivan, 1953). Anxiety is a product of interpersonal relationships. Anxiety may produce a threat to the security of the self, thus causing the person to use various types of protective and behavioral control measures. This, in turn, reduces anxiety, but may interfere with being able to live constructively with others (Sullivan, 1953).

Sullivan also described the concept of personification, which is the image that a person has of himself or herself. Personification is a combination of feelings, attitudes, and conceptions that grow out of experiences with need satisfaction and anxiety. If interpersonal experiences are rewarding, it is known as the "good me" personification. On the other hand, if interpersonal experiences are anxiety arousing, it is known as the "bad me" personification. A synonym for personification is self-concept; thus, the "good me" personification is a high self-concept and the "bad me" personification is a low self-concept (Sullivan, 1953).

Sullivan viewed the individual as an energy or tension system. The goal of the tension system is to reduce anxiety. According to Sullivan, the two main sources of anxiety are the tensions that arise from the needs of the organism and tensions that result from anxiety (Sullivan, 1953).

Sullivan believed that "tensions can be regarded as needs for particular energy transformations that will dissipate the tension of awareness with an accompanying change of 'mental' state, a change of awareness" (Sullivan, 1953, p. 85). Anxiety is the experience of tension that results from real or imagined threats to one's security. High levels of anxiety produce a reduction in the efficacy of satisfying needs, disturbance of interpersonal relationships, and confusion in thinking. Thus, Sullivan hypothesized that an individual learns to behave in a certain way related to the resolution or exacerbation of tension (Sullivan, 1953).

Sullivan took his theory further and described the sequence of interpersonal events to which a person is exposed from infancy to adulthood and ways in which these situations contribute to the development of that individual. Besides the six stages of interpersonal development, Sullivan also developed a three-fold classification system of cognitions: prototaxic, parataxic, and syntaxic. Although Sullivan formally rejected the importance of instinct with regard to development, he acknowledged the importance of heredity. Furthermore, he did not believe that personality is set at an early age, but that it may change at any given time because new interpersonal situations arise and the human organism is malleable (Sullivan, 1953).

From Sullivan's theory, a new paradigm developed; this was the conception of participant–observer. Prior to this conception, the therapist observed only what was occurring. Now the therapist becomes an active part of the treatment. Another concept developed from Sullivan's interpersonal theory was that the environment plays an important role in treatment, thus creating the concept of a therapeutic milieu (Sullivan, 1953).

### Application to Nursing

Peplau (1952, 1963) based her nursing theory, Interpersonal Relations in Nursing, on Sullivan's theory, Interpersonal Theory of Psychiatry. Orlando (1961) based her nursing theory on Peplau's theory and Sullivan's theory. Thus it is clear that Sullivan's theory has been important to nursing.

From Sullivan's concept of degree of anxiety, Peplau developed the four levels of anxiety (mild, moderate, severe, and panic levels) that are the standards nurses use in assessing anxiety. Peplau believed that nurses play an important role in helping clients reduce their anxiety and in converting it into constructive action. Peplau also believed that the nurse's role is to help the client decrease insecurity and improve functioning through interpersonal relationships. These interpersonal relationships can be seen as microcosms of the way the person functions in his or her relationships (Thompson, 1986). This is very similar to Sullivan's concepts of the development of interpersonal relationships.

To educate the client and assist the person in gaining personal insight, Peplau (1963) elaborated on Sullivan's concept of participant–observer. According to her, nurses cannot be isolated from the therapeutic milieu if they want to be effective. Peplau's belief was that the nurse must interact with the client as a human being, with respect, empathy, and acceptance.

A major focus of Orlando's theory is client participation, which correlates with both Sullivan's and Peplau's concept of participant–observer. The formation, development, use, and termination of the nurse–client relationship is a phenomenon that is studied in nursing because it is a vital component of care and helps to determine the efficacy of treatment outcomes (Erci, Sezgin, & Kacmaz, 2008; Potter, Vitale-Nolen, & Dawson, 2005; Potter, Williams, & Costanzo, 2004; Sheldon & Ellington, 2008).

Another important concept of Sullivan's theory is the therapeutic milieu (i.e., a therapeutic environment). Almost all facilities today support the concept of a therapeutic environment that aids in facilitating all interactions. The therapeutic milieu is an important component of nursing practice, especially in the psychiatric setting. This concept was studied by Echternacht (2001) in relation to group therapy, and O'Neill, Moore, and Ryan (2008) when examining psychosocial interventions used by mental health nurse practitioners.

Sullivan also acknowledged the importance of heredity in development. Even though the heredity concept is a biologic perspective, psychologists, such as Sullivan, acknowledge the importance of heredity in personality development. In the case study, Darlene thought consideration of hereditable influences was important in working with Alan because Alan's father was an alcoholic.

# Behavioral and Cognitive-Behavioral Theories

The psychodynamic theories grew from the beliefs that (1) personality is based on how the person develops, (2) development stops at a certain age, and (3) behaviors associated with development cannot be changed. In other words, a person's destiny is set at an early age. Finding these theories problematic, the behavioral theorists postulated that personality consists of learned behaviors. More explicitly, personality is synonymous with behavior, and if the behavior is changed, the personality is changed.

Initially, behavioral studies focused on human actions without much attention to the internal thinking processes. When the complexity of behaviors could not be accounted for by strictly behavioral explanations, a new component was added: a component of cognitions or thought processes. The cognitive approach is an outgrowth of behavioral and psychodynamic theories and attempts to link thought processes with behaviors. Cognitive-behavioral theory, then, focuses on thinking and behaving rather than on feelings.

One of the best known behavioral theorists is B. F. Skinner. Additional cognitive-behavioral theories discussed in this section are those proposed by Beck and Ellis.

## OPERANT CONDITIONING: SKINNER

Like Freud, Skinner believed that all behavior is determined, but the two have different theories regarding the origin of the behavior. Although Skinner followed the ideologies of Pavlov and Watson (two early behaviorists), he expanded the notion of stimulus–response behavioral approaches of learning to include the concept of reinforcement. The Pavlovian theory, basically a biologic theory, states that a stimulus elicits a response. Skinner took this theoretical principle further and applied it to the psychological sciences. He held that it is possible to predict and control the behaviors of others through a contingency of human reinforcers, and he expanded on Pavlovian thinking by adding motivation and reinforcement to the principles of learning (Skinner, 1969).

*Operant conditioning* was the term coined by Skinner to label his theory. Operant conditioning refers to the manipulation of selected reinforcers to elicit and strengthen desired behavioral reinforcers. According to Skinner, an individual performs a behavior (discharges an operant) and receives a consequence (reinforcer) as a result of performing the behavior. The consequence is either positive or negative, and the consequence will most likely determine if the behavior will be repeated. Thus, although negative consequences have a deterrent effect on the behavior, positive consequences generally result in repetition of the behavior. Absence of reinforcement generally decreases the behavior. Skinner's premise was that reinforcement ultimately determines the existence of behavior (Skinner, 1969).

Skinner defined a reinforcer as anything that increases the occurrence of a behavior. It is important to note that the value of the reinforcer depends on its meaning to a particular individual, and the same reinforcer may have different effects on different people. According to Skinner, there are two types of reinforcers: primary and secondary. Primary reinforcers are important to survival (e.g., food, water, and sex) and secondary reinforcers are conditioned reinforcers (e.g., money, material goods, and praise) (Skinner, 1969).

Behaviors are generally multidimensional, and complex behaviors need to be broken down into smaller steps. This allows for the shaping of behavior, which consists of progressively reinforcing the smaller steps needed to achieve a certain behavior (Skinner, 1987).

## COGNITIVE THEORY: BECK

Aaron Beck based his cognitive theory on the work he did with depressed persons. He posited that biased cognitions are faulty, and he labeled these thoughts as *cognitive distortions*. Cognitive distortions are habitual errors in thinking that Beck stated are verbal or pictorial events that are formed in the conscious mind. When cognitions are distorted, an individual incorrectly interprets life events, jumps to inaccurate conclusions, and judges himself or herself too harshly. These distorted cognitions create a false basis for beliefs, particularly regarding the self, and influence one's basic attitude about the self. Thought distortions are the catalysts for how an individual perceives events in his or her life; they may keep the individual from reaching a desired goal. The process of changing cognitive distortions is called cognitive restructuring (Beck, 1976).

Although cognitive distortions are in the conscious mind, Beck believed that they are influenced by an automatic thinking schema that originates in the unconscious mind. The automatic thinking schemata are themes that have developed in childhood and have been reinforced throughout life. The automatic thinking schemata influence cognitions and can cause them to be faulty. Beck stated that an individual expresses illness through thoughts and attitudes. In other words, thoughts influence emotions, and behavior is controlled by thoughts. If thoughts are distorted, then illness occurs. To treat the illness the cognitive distortions must be changed (Beck, 1976).

## RATIONAL EMOTIVE THEORY: ELLIS

Another cognitive theorist was Albert Ellis, who described Rational Emotive Theory, which focuses on thinking and behavior rather than on feelings. The underlying premise is that an individual has the cognitive ability to think, decide, analyze, and do, and that he or she thinks either rationally or irrationally. The repetition of irrational thoughts reinforces dysfunctional beliefs, which, in turn, produce dysfunctional behaviors. These dysfunctional beliefs lead to self-defeating behaviors and the person experiences self-blame. Ellis stated that the individual learns these self-defeating behaviors and that the individual is capable of understanding their limitations. Ellis further posited that if behaviors are learned, they can be unlearned. A person can change beliefs by changing thoughts and thinking rationally. If this occurs, then the behavior is changed (Ellis, 1973).

### Application of Behavioral and Cognitive-Behavioral Theories to Nursing

The behavioral approach is a concrete method of monitoring or managing behavior. Nurses often use it with children or adolescents and people with chronic illness because it is often successful in changing targeted behaviors.

By combining behavioral theory with cognitive theory, the nurse can help alter behaviors by encouraging the individual to change irrational beliefs through problem-solving. An individual who is ill may express feelings of worthlessness, anger, and self-blame. The nurse using a cognitive-behavioral approach can point out specific positive qualities of the individual. This helps reduce self-blame and the person gradually begins to feel better about himself or herself because the belief system is changing. In essence, the nurse has changed behavior by presenting positive (secondary) reinforcement to the person, thus helping to change self-cognitions. This, in turn, changes the individual's belief system.

A cognitive-behavioral approach also helps the nurse point out the use of maladaptive defense mechanisms (e.g., projection). Projection is "attributing one's own thoughts or impulses onto another person. Through this process, the individual can attribute: intolerable wishes, emotional feelings or motivation onto another person" (Stuart & Sundeen, 1995, p. 990). People sometimes blame others for their problems. This is particularly true for those who are addicted to drugs and alcohol (like Alan); addicts frequently do not take responsibility for their substance use, misuse, and abuse. Using a cognitive approach, specifically Ellis, the nurse teaches the person to take responsibility for his or her own behaviors. While Ellis is used more with substance abuse because of the confrontational approach, Beck is used more with depressed persons because it focuses on an empathic approach. In the case study, Alan has a dual diagnosis of depression and substance abuse, and Darlene would most likely use a cognitive-behavioral approach in planning his nursing care.

In nursing, cognitive-behavioral strategies have been used to manage urinary incontinence (Palmer, 2004), and reduce symptoms in patients with advanced cancer (Sherwood et al., 2005). Cognitive-behavioral approaches have also been used to treat posttraumatic stress disorder (Childs-Clarke, 2003), manage generalized anxiety disorder (Antai-Otong, 2003), assist those coping with traumatic provider interactions (Sorenson, 2003), and treat individuals with dual diagnoses (Romana, 2003).

## Humanistic Theories

Humanistic theories developed in response to the psychoanalytic thought that a person's destiny was determined early in life. Proponents of humanistic psychology believed that psychoanalytic theories explicitly exclude human potential. In other words, there was no hope for a person. Humanistic theories emphasize a person's capacity for self-actualization; thus, they present a relatively hopeful and optimistic perspective about humans. Humanists believe that the person contains within himself or herself the potential for healthy and creative growth. The theories of Maslow and Rogers are discussed in the following sections on humanistic theories.

### HUMAN NEEDS THEORY: MASLOW

Abraham Maslow, known as the father of humanistic psychology, believed that psychology takes a pessimistic, negative, and limited conception of humans. He charged the discipline to examine human strengths and to stress human virtue instead of human frailties, and he proposed that human science should explore individuals who realize their full potential. Furthermore, he believed that the inner core of the person is the self, which is a unique individual who possesses both characteristics similar to others and characteristics uniquely distinct to the person (Maslow, 1963).

Motivation is the key to Maslow's theory because he assumed that instead of being passive, an individual is an active participant who strives for self-actualization. Maslow's theory is basically a hierarchy of dynamic processes that are critical for development and growth of the total person. There are six incremental stages of Maslow's theory: physiologic needs, safety needs, love and belonging needs, self-esteem needs, self-actualizing needs, and self-transcendent needs. The goal of Maslow's theory is to attain the sixth level or stage: self-transcendent needs (Maslow, 1963).

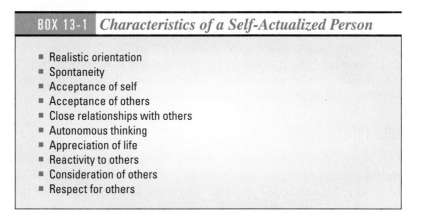

**BOX 13-1** *Characteristics of a Self-Actualized Person*

- Realistic orientation
- Spontaneity
- Acceptance of self
- Acceptance of others
- Close relationships with others
- Autonomous thinking
- Appreciation of life
- Reactivity to others
- Consideration of others
- Respect for others

In Maslow's scheme, needs are divided into "D" motives and "B" motives. "D" motives are deficiency needs. This means that these needs are basic and have the greatest strength because they are essential to human survival. "D" motive needs must be satisfied for a person to turn his or her attention to the satisfaction of the higher-level needs. These higher-level needs are called "B" motive needs and include self-esteem and self-actualization. Such needs are reflective of growth potential (Maslow, 1963).

Until basic deficiency needs are met, the individual does not pursue personal growth needs to develop his or her fullest potential as a human being. Maslow postulated an optimistic assessment by focusing on the individual's strengths instead of personal deficits. According to Maslow (1963), when a person strives for personal growth, it leads the person to her or his fullest potential. In other words, it is the person at her or his best. This means that the person develops a problem-solving approach to life, identifies with humankind, and transcends the environment. The person is able to look realistically at life and make rational decisions; this brings about inner peace. When a person accomplishes this, Maslow referred to the person as being self-actualized. Box 13-1 lists characteristics of a self-actualized person. This philosophical perspective helps a person get in touch with who he or she is and what he or she can become (Maslow, 1963).

### Application to Nursing
Maslow's theory can be applied to nursing practice in three ways:

1. It allows the nurse to emphasize the person's strengths instead of focusing on the individual's deficits.
2. It focuses on human potential, thus giving the person hope.
3. It provides a blueprint for prioritizing client care according to a hierarchy of needs.

By focusing on a person's strengths, the nurse empowers the individual. In the case study, when Darlene began planning Alan's care, she followed Maslow's hierarchy by giving priority to his "D" needs (i.e., physical and safety needs that help the individual feel safe and secure). She helped him withdraw safely from the addictive substances and treated active symptoms of hepatitis C. She knew that his physical needs must be met before she could address the "B" needs (i.e., his potential for personal growth, self-esteem, and self-actualization).

Considerable nursing research has been done in humanistic psychology, largely using Maslow's theory. This research has focused on examining health-promotion interventions for people with spinal cord injury (Sarhan & Cummings, 2008), enhancing quality of life for clients diagnosed with dementia (Hendry & Douglas, 2003), increasing physical activity among adults (Yap, Hemmings, & Davis, 2009), and improving holistic nursing care among elders in nursing homes (Weaver, 2005). Additionally, van Maanen (2006) used Maslow's theory to study the meaning and significance of health among British and American elders.

## PERSON-CENTERED THEORY: ROGERS

Carl Rogers developed a person-centered model of psychotherapy that emphasizes the uniqueness of the individual. He believed that every individual has the potential to develop his or her talents to the maximum potential; he called this the actualizing tendency. Furthermore, each individual possesses everything that is needed for self-understanding and for changing attitude and behavior (Rogers, 1959).

Two constructs are fundamental to Rogers' theory: organism and the self. Organism is the locus of all experience. Experience includes the awareness of everything potentially available that is going on within the organism at any given time. This totality of experience constitutes the phenomenal field, which has several components. The first component is that an individual's frame of reference can only be known by that person. The second component is that a person's behavior depends on the phenomenal field and is not dependent on stimulating conditions. The third component of a phenomenal field is that it is made up of conscious and unconscious experiences (Rogers, 1959).

A portion of the phenomenal field gradually differentiates; this is known as the self or self-concept. Self or self-concept denotes the "organized, consistent conceptual gestalt composed of perceptions of the characteristics of 'I' or 'me' and the perceptions of the relationship of the 'I' or 'me' to others and to various aspects of life with the values attached to these perceptions" (Rogers, 1959, p. 200). In addition to the self, there is an ideal self, which is what the person would like to be (Rogers, 1959).

The basic significance of the structural concepts organism and self is directly related to congruence and incongruence. These terms represent the acceptance or nonacceptance of the organism with the self. Congruence is when the self accepts the organismic experience without threat or anxiety; thus, the person is able to think realistically. Incongruence between self and organism makes an individual feel threatened and anxious, thus causing defensiveness and constricted and rigid thinking. This results in behavioral problems (Rogers, 1959).

According to Rogers, "behavior is basically the goal-oriented attempt of the organism to satisfy its needs as experienced" (Rogers, 1951, p. 491). Behaviors occur for the organism to maintain and enhance itself. Rogers believed that an individual has two learned needs, positive-regard and self-regard. Rogers stated, "If an individual should experience only unconditional positive regard, then no conditions of worth would develop, self-regard would be unconditional, the needs for positive regard and self-regard would never be at variance with organismic evaluation, and the individual would continue to be psychologically adjusted, and would be fully functioning" (Rogers, 1959, p. 224). This is not the case when an individual receives both positive and negative evaluations by others, causing an individual to learn to differentiate between actions and feelings that are worthy or unworthy.

Organism and self are subject to strong influences from the environment, especially from the social environment. Rogers did not provide a timetable of significant changes through which an individual passes; instead, he focused on ways in which evaluation of an individual by others tends to influence the experience of the organism and the experience of the self (Rogers, 1951).

### Application to Nursing

The major contribution that Rogers added to nursing practice is the understanding that each client is a unique individual, who is basically good, with an inherent potential for self-actualization. He introduced the concept of a person-centered approach, which is easily adapted to nursing. Not only does this approach view the individual as unique, but there is equal collaboration between the nurse and the client in the individual's care.

Darlene followed Rogers' philosophy that each individual is unique. Even though Alan had characteristics that were similar to others, he was an individual who had characteristics that were unique to him. Darlene collaborated with Alan to develop his plan of care. This is important in all areas of nursing because clients need to feel they are special and unique and that they have a say in their care. Their input into their treatment will motivate them to accomplish their goals; thus, treatment outcomes will be enhanced.

Rogers also identified the conditions that are needed for an effective nurse–client relationship: unconditional positive regard, empathic understanding, and genuineness. An effective nurse–client relationship will help to facilitate change in the person and produce a positive outcome to treatment.

# Stress Theories

Although the previous theories have dealt with the development of personality and mental illness, the stress theories deal with normal human functioning. Stress, adaptation, and coping are all natural parts of life. Stress is inevitable in everyone's life, and people must deal with stress by adapting through coping. The stress theories provide nursing with a framework to understand the effects that stress has on the individual and how the individual responds to stressful situations or life events. Although the ability to successfully adapt to stress leads to the equilibrium of the individual, the inability to adapt successfully leads to disequilibrium. The disequilibrium may result in physiologic or psychological disorders. The important thing to remember with stress theories is that stress is different for everyone. The following sections discuss Selye's general adaptation syndrome in relation to Peplau's levels of anxiety and Lazarus' Stress Coping Adaptation Theory.

## GENERAL ADAPTATION SYNDROME: SELYE

Hans Selye pioneered research into stress and proposed the general adaptation syndrome (GAS). Because Selye defined stress as wear and tear on the body, the GAS explains the physiologic responses to stress. An explanation of the GAS is presented in Chapter 14, but it will be discussed here briefly because Selye's GAS is also discussed in psychological literature.

The GAS has three stages: alarm, resistance, and exhaustion. The first stage is the alarm reaction. This stage mobilizes the body's defense forces and activates the fight or flight syndrome, which puts the body in a state of disequilibrium. The second stage is resistance and focuses on the body's physiologic responses to regain homeostasis. The final stage is exhaustion. In this stage the body has exhausted all its resources and a diseased state can occur (Selye, 1956).

Selye concentrated on the physiologic changes in the body and did not elaborate on the psychological changes. Kneisl and Ames (1986) correlated the three levels of

TABLE 13-2 *Selye's and Peplau's Anxiety States*

| Selye's Stages of the General Adaptation Syndrome | Peplau's Levels of Anxiety | Characteristics of Levels of Anxiety |
|---|---|---|
| Alarm alert | Level 1 (mild) Level 2 (moderate) | Increased alertness Increased awareness Increased efforts to reduce anxiety Narrowing of perceptual field Problem-solving is present Coping is increased |
| Resistance | Level 2 (moderate) Level 3 (severe) | Feels threatened Feels overloaded Problem-solving difficulties Selective inattention Depressed Irritable Psychosomatic symptoms |
| Exhaustion | Level 3 (severe) Level 4 (panic) | Feels helpless Feelings of awe, dread, terror Loss of control Personality disorganization Loss of rational thoughts Decreased ability to relate rationally to others Out of touch with reality Dissociation Disease process (physical and emotional) |

the GAS with Peplau's levels of anxiety. Table 13-2 compares the stages of Selye's syndrome with Peplau's levels of anxiety. In the alarm stage, there is an increased level of alertness and anxiety is found at levels 1 (mild) and 2 (moderate). The individual focuses on the immediate task, which is to reduce the stressor. If the threat is eliminated, the person has adapted successfully. If the threat is not effectively resolved, the individual advances to the next stage (Kneisl & Ames, 1986).

In the resistance stage, the individual experiences levels 2 (moderate) or 3 (severe) of anxiety. This is the stage the individual increases the use of coping mechanisms to adapt to the stressor. Psychosomatic symptoms may appear in this stage. If the individual is unable to adapt to the stressor, the individual becomes overwhelmed with the stressor and advances to the next stage (Kneisl & Ames, 1986).

The stage of exhaustion results when the stressor is not or cannot be neutralized. This occurs because the stress may have lasted too long, the person is totally overwhelmed by the stressor, or the individual's normal coping mechanisms have been exhausted. At this stage the individual experiences anxiety at levels 3 (severe) or 4 (panic) of Peplau's levels of anxiety. The person becomes dysfunctional and a multitude of psychopathologic symptoms can occur: disorganized thinking, disorganized personality, delusions, hallucinations, stupor, or violence (Kneisl & Ames, 1986).

## STRESS, COPING, ADAPTATION THEORY: LAZARUS

Lazarus' theory deals with how a person copes with stressful situations. Whereas Selye's focus is on the body's physiologic responses, Lazarus focused on the person's psychological responses. He viewed these responses as a process and stated that a process-oriented approach is directed toward what an individual actually thinks and does within the context of a specific encounter, and includes how these thoughts and actions change as the encounter unfolds. "Coping, when considered as a process, is characterized by dynamics and changes that are functions of continuous appraisals and reappraisals of the shifting person environmental relationship" (Folkman & Lazarus, 1988, p. 3).

The two major factors that are precedents to stress are the person–environment relationship and appraisals. The person–environment relationship includes such factors as personality, values, beliefs, commitments, social networks, social supports, demands and constraints, social cultural factors, and life events. The three cognitive appraisals are primary, secondary, and reappraisal. Primary appraisal refers to the judgment that an individual makes about a particular event or stressor. Secondary appraisal is the evaluation of how an individual responds to an event. Reappraisal is simply appraisal after new or additional information has been received (Lazarus & Folkman, 1984).

Lazarus posited that stress is much more complicated than just stimulus and response. He focused on the idea that coping is not due to anxiety itself, but how the person perceives the threat. Lazarus identified this perception as an appraisal and explained that a person's evaluation of a stressor or events is classified as a cognitive appraisal. He defined stress as "a particular relationship between the person and the environment that is appraised by the person as taxing or exceeding his/her resources" (Lazarus & Folkman, 1984, p. 18).

To manage the demands and emotions generated by the appraised stress, coping occurs. Coping is the process by which a person manages the appraisal. The two types are problem-focused and emotion-focused coping. Problem-focused coping actually changes the person–environment relationship, and emotion-focused coping changes the meaning of the situation. Once the person has successfully coped with a situation, reappraisal occurs. Reappraisal allows for feedback about the outcome and allows for adjustment to new information (Lazarus & Folkman, 1984).

Successful coping results in adaptation. Adaptation is "the capacity of a person to survive and flourish" (Lazarus & Folkman, 1984, p. 182). Adaptation affects three important areas: health, psychological well-being, and social functioning. These three areas are interdependent, and when one area is affected, all three areas are affected. For example, if a person develops an illness, it can cause problems in work performance, which in turn elicits a negative self-concept.

### Application of Stress Theories to Nursing

Stress and adaptation are the basis of Roy's Adaptation Model (Roy & Andrews, 1991) and Neuman's System Model (Neuman, 1989). Roy and Andrews (1991) stated that the goal of nursing is the promotion of adaptive responses through the mode of coping. Neuman's theory deals with a person's responses to stress (Neuman, 1989).

The application of stress theories to nursing is important. Indeed, they provide a framework for nurses to assess the effects of stress, both physical and psychological, on the individual and the coping processes that the individual uses. When assessing a client's stressors, it is important for the nurse to also consider the meaning of the stressor to the individual and the resources and support that the person has in coping with the stressors. The nurse can help with problem-solving or cognitive restructuring to facilitate effective coping and adaptation. This can also lead to the development of new coping strategies for the individual.

Stress theories are very important in nursing practice, and nurses using them as research frameworks have done considerable research. For example, Puskar and colleagues (2008) examined how stress and coping influenced weight perception and depressive symptoms among adolescents in a rural community. The coping behaviors of caregivers of children undergoing liver transplantation were researched by LoBiondo-Wood, Williams, and McGhee (2004), and Akintola (2008) studied coping behaviors of volunteers providing care for patients with AIDS in South Africa. Finally, experimental studies using Lazarus' theory included an examination of the efficacy of therapeutic play interventions in preparing children for surgery (Li & Lopez, 2008) and the efficacy of education and telephone counseling interventions to enhance emotional, physical, and social adjustment in patients with breast cancer and their partners (Budin et al., 2008).

## Social Psychology

Health professionals use many different models for understanding behavior change because it is a complex process. Further, behavior change is often difficult to achieve and sustain. When health professionals attempt to encourage healthy behaviors, they are competing against powerful influences. These powerful influences involve social, psychological, and environmental conditioning. In order for change to occur, the benefits of behavior must be desired and perceived to be beneficial to the person. Although education is an important factor in facilitating change, information is frequently not enough. The benefits of behavior change must be compelling. When implementing change, a multilevel, interactive perspective clearly shows the advantages of incorporating behavioral and environmental components. Social psychology helps to predict health behavior, and is widely used in health promoting activities.

Two models that address this issue are the Health Belief Model (HBM) and the Theory of Reasoned Action/Theory of Planned Behavior. The HBM addresses a person's perceptions of the threat of a health problem and the accompanying appraisal of a recommended behavior for preventing or managing the problem, which is manifested as a behavior. The Theory of Reasoned Action assumes that people are rational and make decisions based on the information available to them. The important determinant of a person's behavior is intent. Both of these theories will be discussed in more detail in the following sections.

## HEALTH BELIEF MODEL

The HBM was one of the first models that adapted theories from the behavioral sciences to predict health behaviors. This was done by focusing on the attitudes and beliefs of individuals. The HBM was originally developed in the 1950s by a group of social psychologists working for the U.S. Public Health Service who wanted to improve the public's use of preventive services (Rosenstock, 1974). Their assumption was that people fear disease and that health actions were motivated in relation to the degree of the fear and the benefits obtained. The HBM explained health behavior in terms of several constructs: perceived susceptibility of the health problem, perceived severity, perceived benefits, perceived barriers, and cues to action (Rosenstock, 1990).

Perceived susceptibility refers to one's opinion of chances of getting a condition, whereas perceived severity is one's opinion of how serious a condition and its sequelae are. One's opinion of the efficacy of the advised action to reduce risk or seriousness of impact is known as perceived benefits. Perceived barriers are one's opinion of the tangible and psychological cost of the advised action (Rosenstock, 1974).

**Individual Perceptions**  **Modifying Factors**  **Likelihood of Action**

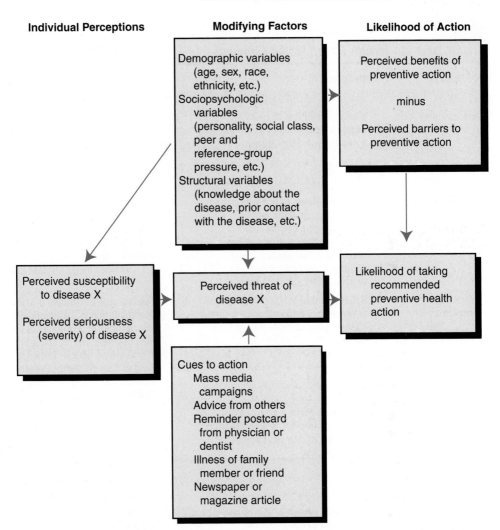

FIGURE 13-1 The Health Belief Model. (From Becker, M. H., Haefner, D. P., Kasl, S. V., et al. (1977). Selected psychosocial models and correlates of individual health-related behaviors. *Medical Care*, 15, 27–46, with permission.)

These four concepts were proposed as accounting for people's readiness to action. Thus, another concept was identified as "cues to action." These cues to action would activate the readiness to act and stimulate overt behaviors (Rosenstock, 1990) (Figure 13-1).

In 1988, Rosenstock added another concept to the HBM, which he identified as self-efficacy. Self-efficacy is one's confidence in the ability to successfully perform an action. This concept was used to help the HBM better fit the challenges of changing habitual, unhealthy behaviors such as smoking, overeating, and being sedentary (Rosenstock, 1990). Table 13-3 summarizes the major concepts of the HBM.

## THEORY OF REASONED ACTION (THEORY OF PLANNED BEHAVIOR)

The Theory of Reasoned Action (TRA) was initially developed in the late 1960s by social psychologists Icek Ajzen and Martin Fishbein (Fishbein & Ajzen, 1975). The TRA explains the relationship among beliefs, attitudes, intentions, and behavior.

TABLE 13-3 *Health Belief Model Concepts*

| Concept | Definition | Examples |
|---------|-----------|----------|
| Perceived susceptibility | Subjective risk of contracting a condition; belief or opinion regarding chances of acquiring a health problem or threat | Does a teenage girl believe she will get pregnant during a single sexual encounter? Does an elderly man believe he will get the flu this winter? Does a middle-aged woman with a strong family history of breast cancer believe that she is vulnerable? |
| Perceived severity | Concern related to the seriousness of a health condition and understanding of potential difficulties the condition might cause; belief or perception of seriousness or consequences of a health threat or condition | A teenage girl believes that pregnancy would change her life dramatically. An elderly man understands that pneumonia is a potential complication of the flu. A middle-aged woman knows her grandmother died of breast cancer. |
| Perceived benefits | Beliefs related to the effectiveness of preventive actions; opinion that changing behavior(s) may reduce the treat | The teenage girl knows that using contraception will dramatically reduce the chances of a pregnancy. The elderly man believes that flu shots are effective in preventing illness. The middle-aged woman recognizes that yearly mammograms are effective in reducing deaths from breast cancer. |
| Perceived barriers | Perception of the obstacles to changing behavior; opinion related to tangible and/or psychological costs of action | The teenage girl may be embarrassed about going to a clinic to obtain contraceptives. The elderly man may not have transportation to take him to the clinic to receive a flu shot. The middle-aged woman's insurance does not cover the cost of mammograms. |
| Cues to action | A stimulus (external or internal) that triggers health-related behaviors; something that makes the individual aware of a health threat | The teenage girl attends a school-sponsored program on problems encountered by teenage mothers. The elderly man sees a posted flyer that a mobile van will be nearby the following week to provide free flu shots. The middle-aged woman learns from a public service radio ad that low-cost mammography is available at a nearby hospital. |
| Self-efficacy | Belief that one has the ability to change one's behaviors; recognition that personal health practices and choices can positively influence health | The teenage girl decides to postpone intercourse. The elderly man attends the shot clinic provided by the mobile van. The middle-aged woman makes an appointment for a mammogram. |

It assumes that people are rational and make decisions based on the information available to them. The goal of the TRA, therefore, is to understand and predict behaviors that are largely under the individual's control (Poss, 2001). The TRA was later modified to the Theory of Planned Behavior (TPB) (Montano & Kasprzyk, 2002).

According to the TPB, the most important determinant of a person's behavior(s) is intention. Intention is the cognitive representation of the individual's readiness to perform a behavior and is determined by (1) attitude toward the behavior; (2) subjective norms; and (3) perceived behavioral control.

Attitude, or behavioral beliefs, refers to the individual's positive or negative evaluation of performing the behavior; it is concerned with his/her beliefs about the consequences of performing the behavior. Attitude has been viewed as a combination of feelings, beliefs, intentions, and perceptions. Combined with knowledge, these factors analyze the acceptability of performing a behavior in relation to a bipolar scale of positive/negative or yes/no. The determinant of attitude component is called "salient belief." A person's attitude toward a behavior can be predicted by multiplying the evaluation of each of the behavior's consequences by the strength of the belief. Beliefs are formed about an issue/object by associating it with all kinds of characteristics, qualities, and attributes. This leads to the development of an attitude (Ajzen & Fishbein, 1980).

Subjective norm, or normative beliefs, is seen as the social pressure upon a person to perform or not perform a behavior. In deciding whether to perform an action or behavior, an individual may consider what his/her parents, friends, or others will think about the behavior, as well as how important it is to comply with the wishes of others. It involves both one's beliefs about the opinions of others and the person's motivation to conform to the wishes of those others. Thus, people often behave as they believe others expect them to behave.

Control beliefs, or perceived behavioral control, refer to the perceived power of factors that may facilitate or impede the behavior. In general, the more favorable the attitude and subjective norm, the greater the perceived control and the stronger would be the person's intention to perform the behavior. According to the TPB, behavioral intention is the most immediate determinant of any social behavior, but only under conditions where the behavior in question is under volitional control.

The TPB proposes that an individual's intention is determined, in turn by his/her attitude and subjective norm regarding the performance of the behavior. Furthermore, attitude to the behavior is accounted for by beliefs about the outcomes of the behavior and evaluations of those outcomes. Subjective norm is determined by perceived pressure from specified significant others to carry out the behavior and motivation to comply with the wishes of significant others. Figure 13-2 depicts the components of the Theory of Planned Behavior.

## Application of Social Psychology Theories to Nursing

The application of social psychology theories in nursing typically relates to the area of health promotion. Nurses can propose strategies and develop programs to make people aware of health problems. They can then implement these programs using the social theories to change unhealthy behaviors to healthy behaviors. That is the reason that nurses must advocate health promotion for patients using a multidimensional approach: organizational change efforts, policy development, economic supports, and environmental change. In today's society, disseminating the message is much easier. It can be delivered through printed educational material, electronic mass media, or directly in one-to-one counseling (Glanz, Rimer, & Lewis, 2008). Social psychology theories are useful in promoting healthy behaviors, and nurses should be challenged to use them to make people aware of health problems and to propose positive behavioral change.

In the case study, Darlene might use a social psychology theory, such as the Theory of Planned Behavior, to examine factors that might influence Alan's intention to change his behavior. For example: What is Alan's attitude toward stopping drinking? What is his understanding of his family's attitudes and beliefs related to his alcohol use?

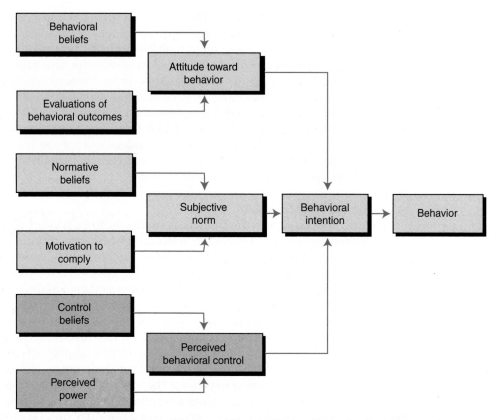

FIGURE 13-2 Theory of Reasoned Action and Theory of Planned Behavior. (From Ajzen, I., & Fishbein, M. (1980). *Understanding attitudes and predicting social behavior.* Englewood Cliffs, NJ: Prentice-Hall. Reproduced by permission of Pearson Education, Inc.) The lighter-shaded upper section shows the Theory of Reasoned Action; the entire figure shows the Theory of Planned Behavior.

What does he perceive as his level of control over his behavior? Examining each of these areas can help Darlene predict Alan's intention to change and ultimately, his behavior relative to alcohol use and abuse.

As mentioned, the HBM was developed to help explain health-related behaviors. Besides being a guide to help identify leverage points for change, it can also be a useful framework for designing change strategies. Indeed, its use in nursing research and practice has been notable. During the last decade, more than 130 articles have been published in the nursing literature employing or testing the HBM.

For example, Wood (2008) used the HBM to examine motivation to exercise to reduce risk for breast cancer; and Hall and colleagues (2007) used the HBM to examine the effectiveness of a culturally sensitive education program on the beliefs of Hispanic women related to breast cancer. In other studies, Raftopoulos (2008) used constructs from the HBM to predict acceptance of the flu vaccine among nurses; and Chan, Kwong, Zang, and Wan (2007) used it to determine the efficacy of an educational program to prevent osteoporosis. Numerous other works describing application of the HBM (e.g., Li, Stotts, & Froelicher, 2007; Michaels, McEwen, & McArthur, 2008; Morton, 2008; Schroeter & Peck, 2008; Weld, Padden, Ramsey, & Bibb, 2008) can be found in the nursing literature.

The Theory of Reasoned Action/Theory of Planned Behavior, likewise, has been used frequently in nursing studies. Review of the literature indicated more than 300 citations in recent nursing journals. Research examining the prediction of exercise intent and behaviors, for example, was conducted by several groups (Conn, Tripp-Reimer, & Maas, 2003; Downs & Hausenblas, 2004; Prosser, Thomas, & Darling-Fisher, 2007). Other researchers have used the Theory of Reasoned Action to look at health-promotion behaviors in diverse areas including intention to stop smoking and prevent initiation of tobacco use (Tingen, Waller, Smith, Baker, Reyes, & Trieber, 2006), to donate bone marrow among African-Americans (Glasgow & Bello, 2007), to undergo repeat mammography screening (Lopez-McKee, McNeill, Bader, & Morales, 2008), and to predict sexual intercourse and condom use (Villarruel, Jemmott, Jemmott, & Ronis, 2004).

## Summary

This chapter has presented five families of theories that attempt to explain human behavior. Although each theory emphasizes a different concept or viewpoint, no one theory best explains the complexity of human behavior. The psychodynamic theories attempt to explain an individual's behavior in terms related to the development of the self that is formed by adulthood. The behavioral theorists believe that behavior is learned by reinforcement; whereas the cognitive theorists believe that the reinforcements are related to an individual's thought patterns. Humanistic theories propose that individuals have within themselves the capacity to change. This potential for healthy and creative growth occurs throughout the individual's life span; thus, the behavior of an individual is a dynamic process. The stress-adaptation theories are associated with behaviors identified with the way a person adapts to stress through individual coping mechanisms. Finally, the social psychology theories look at how a person changes and ways to incorporate change through the promotion of health. Table 13-4 offers a brief comparison of these theories.

The case study helped to illustrate the complexity of humans and that using a single theory will not fully explain all of the variables that are associated with behavior and its impact on health. Therefore, most nurses adopt an eclectic approach to theory utilization in providing care. This means that the nurse chooses concepts from various theories that best explain the behaviors of the person. Due to the interrelatedness of the concepts in the theories (e.g., the self, anxiety, hope, development, cognitions, reinforcements, empowerment, health promotion), concepts from multiple theories can be used. The concepts from the various theories chosen for the individual will depend on the patient's particular behavior, needs, or problems. By knowing how behavior is formed, the nurse can better plan effective care to change behaviors to improve health.

## LEARNING ACTIVITIES

1. Consider the case of a school nurse who is working with a 14-year-old student suspected of being addicted to alcohol. Discuss with classmates what concepts from the various theories described could be used in planning nursing interventions. Using the theories from social psychology, how could the nurse set up a health-promotion campaign for teenage drug and alcohol program?

2. Consider the following case: A 30-year-old woman arrives in the emergency department. She is diagnosed with a drug overdose. Assessment data reveal the

TABLE 13-4 *Comparison of Behavioral Theories*

| Theory | Theorist | Emphasis | Key Concepts |
|---|---|---|---|
| Psychodynamic | Freud | The study of unconscious mental processes of the psychodynamics of behavior | Personality structure: id, ego, superego; libido, pleasure principle, reality principle, instincts, stages of psychosexual development |
| | Erikson | Psychosocial factors that influence development | Id, ego, superego; conscious, preconscious, unconscious; developmental tasks; eight stages of biopsychosocial development |
| | Sullivan | Interpersonal experiences that influence development | Self-system, anxiety, security operations, personifications, modes of experience; stages of interpersonal growth and development |
| Cognitive-behavioral | Skinner | Analysis of human behavior observed in the current situation | Operant conditioning; positive and negative reinforcement |
| | Beck | Cognitive distortions | Arbitrary inference, overgeneralization, selective abstraction, magnification and minimization, underlying assumptions, entitlement, perfection, automatic thoughts |
| | Ellis | The values and assumptions that govern much of people's lives | ABC theory of rational emotive theory |
| Humanistic | Maslow | Fulfilling human potential | Hierarchy of needs, self-actualization |
| | Rogers | Person-centered | Organism and the self; congruence and incongruence; positive-regard and self-regard |
| Stress-adaptation | Selye | Analysis of stress at the physiologic and biochemical levels of functioning | Stressor, general adaptation syndrome, alarm reaction, stages of resistance, stages of exhaustion |
| | Lazarus | Cognitive model of stress | Appraisal, coping, outcome |
| Social psychology | Rosenstock | Perceived threat and net benefits | Perceived susceptibility, perceived severity, perceived benefits, perceived barriers, cues of action, self-efficacy |
| | Ajzen and Fishbein | People make rational decisions based on the information they have | Intent, attitude, subjective norms |

following information: she has three children (18 months, 4 years old, and 14 years old); she is in the process of her second divorce; she took 25 Valium tablets (2 mg/tablet), which her doctor had given her for stress; she is unemployed; and she did not graduate from high school. Which theory(ies) should be used to direct her care? What concepts from other theories could be used to enhance her care?

3. Consider the following case: A 65-year-old woman is being admitted for a mastectomy due to cancer. She expresses fear and depression during the nursing assessment. What concepts from the various theories could be used in planning

her care? How might her care be changed if the woman were 25 years old or 45 years old? How have the social psychology theories been used in promoting breast cancer awareness?

4. Consider the following case: A 52-year-old man is admitted to the hospital for hypertension for the third time in the past year. Each time he stopped taking his medications because he was "feeling good." What concepts from the various theories could be used to change his behavior? How could the nurse set up a health-promotion program for managing hypertension in the hospital? In the community?

## REFERENCES

Ajzen, I., & Fishbein, M. (1980). *Understanding attitudes and predicting social behavior.* Englewood Cliffs, NJ: Prentice-Hall.

Akintola, O. (2008). Defying all odds: Coping with the challenges of volunteer caregiving for patients with AIDS in South Africa. *Journal of Advanced Nursing, 63*(4), 357–365.

Allan, H., & Barber, D. (2005). Emotional boundary work in advance fertility nursing roles. *Nursing Ethics, 12*(4), 391–399.

Antai-Otong, D. (2003). Current treatment of generalized anxiety disorder. *Journal of Psychosocial Nursing and Mental Health Services, 41*(12), 20–29.

Beck, A. T. (1976). *Cognitive therapies and the emotional disorders.* New York: International University Press.

Bjorklund, P. (2000). Assessing ego strengths: Spinning straw into goals. *Perspectives in Psychiatric Care, 36*(1), 14–23.

Budin, W. C., Hosking, C. N., Haber, J., Sherman, D. W., Maislin, G., Cater, J. R., Cartwright-Alcarese, F., Kowalski, M. O., McSherry, C. B., Fuerbach, R., & Shukla, S. (2008). Breast cancer: Education, counselling, and adjustment among patients and partners: A randomized clinical trial. *Nursing Research, 57*(3), 199–213.

Chan, M. F., Kwong, W. S., Zang, Y., & Wan, P. Y. (2007). Evaluation of an osteoporosis prevention education programme for young adults. *Journal of Advanced Nursing, 57*(3), 270–285.

Childs-Clarke, A. (2003). Nursing care following trauma: A cognitive behavioral approach. *Mental Health Practice, 7*(3), 34–40.

Conn, V. S., Tripp-Reimer, T., & Maas, M. L. (2003). Older women and exercise: Theory of Planned Behavior beliefs. *Public Health Nursing, 20*(2), 153–163.

Deering, C. G. (2000). A cognitive developmental approach to understanding how children cope with disasters. *Journal of Child and Adolescent Psychiatric Nursing, 13*(1), 7–16.

Downs, D. S., & Hausenblas, H. A. (2004). Women's exercise beliefs and behaviors during their pregnancy and postpartum. *Journal of Midwifery and Women's Health, 49*(2), 138–144.

Early, T. J., & GlenMaye, L. F. (2000). Valuing families: Social work practice with families from a strengths perspective. *Social Work, 45*(2), 118–130.

Echternacht, M. R. (2001). Fluid group: Concept and clinical application in the therapeutic milieu. *Journal of the American Psychiatric Nurses Association, 7*(1), 39–44.

Ellis, A. (1973). *A humanistic psychotherapy: The rational-emotive approach.* New York: Julian Press.

Erci, B., Sezgin, S., & Kacmaz, Z. (2008). The impact of therapeutic relationship on preoperative and postoperative patient anxiety. *Australian Journal of Advanced Nursing, 26*(1), 59–66.

Erikson, E. H. (1963). *Childhood and society.* New York: Norton.

Erikson, E. H. (1968). *Identity: Youth and crisis.* New York: Norton.

Erikson, E. H. (1975). *Life history and the historical movement.* New York: Norton.

Fishbein, M., & Ajzen, I. (1975). *Belief, attitude, intention and behavior: An introduction to theory and research.* Reading, MA: Addison-Wesley.

Folkman, S., & Lazarus, R. S. (1988). *Manual for the ways of coping questionnaire.* Palo Alto, CA: Consulting Psychologist Press.

Folta, J. R. (1968). Perspectives of an applied science. *Nursing Research, 17*(6), 502–507.

Franks, V. (2004). Evidence-based uncertainty in mental health nursing. *Journal of Psychiatric and Mental Health Nursing, 11*(1), 99–105.

Freud, S. (1953). Three essays on sexuality. In *Standard edition of the complete psychological works of Sigmund Freud* (Vol. 7). London: Hogarth (First German edition, 1905).

Freud, S. (1956). Inhibitions, symptoms and anxiety. In *Standard edition of the complete psychological works of Sigmund Freud* (Vol. 20). London: Hogarth (First German edition, 1926).

Freud, S. (1960). *The ego and the id.* (J. Strachey, Trans.). New York: Norton.

Glanz, K., Rimer, B. K., & Lewis, F. M. (2008). *Health behavior and health education: Theory, research and practice* (4th ed.). San Francisco, CA: Jossey-Bass.

Glasgow, M. E. S., & Bello, G. (2007). Bone marrow donation: Factors influencing intentions in African Americans. *Oncology Nursing Forum, 34*(2), 369–377.

Hall, C. P., Hall, J. D., Pfriemer, J. T, Wimberley, P. D., & Jones, C. H. (2007). Effects of a culturally sensitive education program on the breast cancer knowledge and beliefs of Hispanic women. *Oncology Nursing Forum, 34*(6), 1195–1202.

Hall, C. S., & Lindzey, G. (1978). *Theories of personality.* New York: Wiley.

Handley, S. M., & Ward-Smith, P. (2005). Alcohol misuse, abuse and addiction in young and middle adulthood. *Annual Review of Nursing Research, 23*(1), 213–244.

Harrison, T. (2003). Women aging with childhood onset disability. *Journal of Holistic Nursing, 21*(3), 242–259.

Hendry, K. C., & Douglas, D. H. (2003). Promoting quality of life for clients diagnosed with dementia. *Journal of the American Psychiatric Nurses Association, 9*(3), 96–102.

Johnson, D. E. (1959). The nature of nursing science. *Nursing Outlook, 7*(5), 291–294.

Johnson, D. E. (1968). Theory in nursing: Borrowed and unique. *Nursing Research, 17*(3), 206–209.

Jones, A. C. (2005). Transference, counter-transference and repetition: Some implications for nursing practice. *Journal of Clinical Nursing, 14*(10), 1177–1184.

Kneisl, C. R., & Ames, S. W. (1986). *Adult health nursing: A biopsychosocial approach.* Menlo Park, CA: Addison-Wesley.

Kozuki, Y., & Kennedy, M. G. (2004). Cultural incommensurability in psychodynamic psychotherapy in Western and Japanese traditions. *Journal of Nursing Scholarship, 36*(1), 30–38.

Lazarus, R. S., & Folkman, S. (1984). *Stress appraisal and coping.* New York: Springer.

Li, H. C., & Lopez, V. (2008). Effectiveness and appropriateness of therapeutic play intervention in preparing children for surgery: A randomized controlled trial study. *Journal for Specialists in Pediatric Nursing, 13*(2), 63–69.

Li, W. W., Stotts, N. A., & Froelicher, E. S. (2007). Compliance with antihypertensive medication in Chinese immigrants: Cultural specific issues and theoretical application. *Research and Theory for Nursing Practice, 21*(4), 236–254.

LoBiondo-Wood, G., Williams, L., & McGhee, C. (2004). Liver transplantation in children: Maternal and family stress, coping and adaptation. *Journal for Specialists in Pediatric Nursing, 9*(2), 59–66.

Lopez-McKee, G., McNeill, J. A., Bader, J., & Morales, P. (2008). Comparison of factors affecting repeat mammography screening of low-income Mexican American women. *Oncology Nursing Forum, 35*(6), 941–947.

Mamhidir, A. G., Karlsson, I., Norberg, A., & Kihlgren, M. (2007). Weight increase in patients with dementia and alteration in meal routines and meal environment after integrity promotion care. *Journal of Clinical Nursing, 16*(9), 987–996.

Maslow, A. H. (1963). *Towards a psychology of being* (2nd ed.). Princeton, NJ: Van Nostrand.

Michaels, C., McEwen, M. M., & McArthur, D. B. (2008). Saying "no" to professional recommendations: Client values, beliefs and evidence-based practice. *Journal of the American Academy of Nurse Practitioners, 20*(12), 585–589.

Montano, D. E., & Kasprzyk, D. (2002). The theory of reasoned action and the theory of planned behavior.

In K. Glanz, B. K. Rimer, & F. M. Lewis (Eds.), *Health behavior and health education: Theory, research and practice* (3rd ed., pp. 67–98). San Francisco: Jossey-Bass.

Morton, J. L. (2008). "I Feel Good!" A weekly wellness radio broadcast for elementary school children. *The Journal of School Nursing, 24*(2), 83–87.

Neuman, B. (1989). *The Neuman systems model* (2nd ed.). East Norwalk, CT: Appleton & Lange.

O'Neill, M., Moore, K., & Ryan, A. (2008). Exploring the role and perspectives of mental health nurse practitioners following psychosocial interventions training. *Journal of Psychiatric and Mental Health Nursing, 15*(7), 582–587.

Orlando, I. (1961). *The dynamic nurse–patient relationship.* New York: Putnam.

Palmer, M. H. (2004). Use of health behaviour change theories to guide urinary incontinence research. *Nursing Research, 53*(6S), S49–S55.

Peplau, H. E. (1952). *Interpersonal relations in nursing.* New York: Putnam.

Peplau, H. E. (1963). A working definition of anxiety. In S. F. Burd & M. A. Marshall (Eds.), *Some clinical approaches of psychiatric nursing* (pp. 323–327). Toronto: Macmillan.

Poss, J. E. (2001). Developing a new model for cross-cultural research: Synthesizing the Health Belief Model and the Theory of Reasoned Action. *Advances in Nursing Science, 23*(4), 1–15.

Potter, M. L., Vitale-Nolen, R., & Dawson, A. M. (2005). Implementation of safety agreements in an acute psychiatric facility. *American Psychiatric Nurses Association Journal, 11*(3), 144–155.

Potter, M. L., Williams, R. B., & Costanzo, R. (2004). Using nursing theory and a structured psycho educational curriculum with inpatient groups. *Journal of the American Psychiatric Nurses Association, 10*(3), 122–128.

Prosser, R. A., Thomas, A. C., & Darling-Fisher, C. S. (2007). Physical activity intervention in an academic setting. *American Association of Occupational Health Nurses Journal, 55*(11), 448–452.

Puskar, K., Bernardo, L. M., Fertman, C., Ren, D., & Stark, K. H. (2008). The relationship between weight perception, gender and depressive symptoms among rural adolescents. *Online Journal of Rural Nursing and Health Care, 8*(1), 13–23.

Raftopoulos, V. (2008). Attitudes of nurses in Greece towards influenza vaccination. *Nursing Standard, 23*(4), 35–42.

Reed, P. G. (1998). A holistic view of nursing concepts and theories in practice. *Journal of Holistic Nursing, 16*(4), 415–419.

Rogers, C. R. (1951). *Client-centered therapy: Its current practice, implications, and theory.* Boston: Houghton Mifflin.

Rogers, C. R. (1959). A theory of therapy, personality, and interpersonal relationships as developed in the client-centered framework. In S. Koch (Ed.), *Psychology: A study of science* (Vol. 3, pp. 184–256). New York: McGraw-Hill.

Romana, M. D. (2003). Cognitive-behavioral therapy: Treating individuals with dual diagnoses. *Journal of Psychosocial Nursing and Mental Health Services, 41*(12), 30–35.

Rosenstock, I. M. (1974). The health belief model and preventive health behavior. *Health Education Monographs, 2*, 354–436.

Rosenstock, I. M. (1990). The Health Belief Model: Explaining health behavior through expectancies. In K. Glanz, F. M. Lewis, & B. K. Rimer (Eds.), *Health behavior and health education: Theory, research and practice* (pp. 39–62). San Francisco: Jossey-Bass.

Roy, C., & Andrews, H. A. (1991). *The Roy Adaptation Model: The definitive statement*. East Norwalk, CT: Appleton & Lange.

Ryles, S. M. (1999). A concept of empowerment: Its relationship to mental health nursing. *Journal of Advanced Nursing, 29*(3), 600–607.

Sarhan, F., & Cummings, P. (2008). Health promotion for people with spinal cord injury: Improving quality of life. *British Journal of Neuroscience Nursing, 4*(8), 374–381.

Schroetter, S. H., & Peck, S. D. (2008). Women's risk of heart disease: Promoting awareness and prevention—a primary care approach. *MEDSURG Nursing, 17*(2), 107–113.

Selye, H. (1956). *The stress of life*. St. Louis: McGraw-Hill.

Sheldon, L. K., & Ellington, L. (2008). Application of a model of social information processing to nursing theory: How nurses respond to patients. *Journal of Advanced Nursing, 64*(4), 388–398.

Sherwood, P., Given, B. A., Given, C. W., Champion, V. L., Doorenbos, A. Z., Azzouz, F., Kazachik, S., Wagler-Ziner, K., & Monahan, P. O. (2005). A cognitive behavioural intervention for symptom management in patients with advanced cancer. *Oncology Nursing Forum, 32*(6), 1190–1198.

Skinner, B. F. (1969). *Contingency of reinforcement: A theoretical analysis*. New York: Appleton-Century-Crofts.

Skinner, B. F. (1987). Whatever happened to psychology as the science of behavior? *American Psychologist, 42*, 780–786.

Sorenson, D. S. (2003). Healing traumatizing provider interactions among women through short-term group therapy. *Archives of Psychiatric Nursing, 17*(6), 259–269.

Stuart, G. W., & Sundeen, S. J. (1995). *Principles and practice of psychiatric nursing* (5th ed.). St. Louis: Mosby.

Sullivan, H. S. (1953). *The interpersonal theory of psychiatry*. New York: Norton.

Taylor, E. (2008). Providing developmentally based care for preschoolers. *Association of periOperative Registered Nurses Journal, 88*(2), 267–275.

Telford, K., Kralik, D., & Koch, T. (2006). Acceptance and denial: Implications for people adapting to chronic illness: Literature review. *Journal of Advanced Nursing, 55*(4), 457–464.

Thomas, M., & Hynes, C. (2007). The darker side of groups. *Journal of Nursing Management, 15*(3), 375–385.

Thompson, L. (1986). Peplau's theory: An application to short term therapy. *Journal of Psychosocial Nursing and Mental Health Services, 24*(8), 26.

Tingen, M. S., Waller, J. L., Smith, T. M., Baker, R. R., Reyes, J., & Trieber, F. A. (2006). Tobacco prevention in children and cessation in family members. *Journal of the American Academy of Nurse Practitioners, 18*(1), 169–179.

Van Maanen, H. M. T. (2006). Being old does not always mean being sick: Perspectives on conditions of health as perceived by British and American elderly. *Journal of Advanced Nursing, 53*(1), 54–64.

Villarruel, A. M., Jemmott, J. B., Jemmott, L. S., & Ronis, D. L. (2004). Predictors of sexual intercourse and condom use intentions among Spanish-dominant Latino youth: A test of the planned behavior theory. *Nursing Research, 53*(3), 172–183.

Wadensten, B., & Carlsson, M. (2003). Nursing theory views on how to support the process of ageing. *Journal of Advanced Nursing, 42*(2), 118–124.

Weaver, D. (2005). Addressing residents' social, emotional and identity needs. *Nursing and Residential Care, 7*(9), 389–393.

Weld, K. K., Padden, D., Ramsey, G., & Bibb, S. C. G. (2008). A framework for guiding health literacy research in populations with universal access to healthcare. *Advances in Nursing Science, 31*(4), 308–318.

Wood, M. E. (2008). Theoretical framework to study exercise motivation for breast cancer risk reduction. *Oncology Nursing Forum, 35*(1), 89–95.

Yap, T. L., Hemmings, A., & Davis, L. S. (2009). The systematic development of a tailored E-mail intervention for health behaviour change toward increasing intentional physical activity. *Western Journal of Nursing Research, 31*(3), 330–346.

# 14

# Theories From the Biomedical Sciences

## Melanie McEwen

*M*aria Leon is in her final year of a graduate program preparing to become a certified registered nurse anesthetist (CRNA). During the course of her graduate education, Maria observed that most people reported a burning sensation as propofol (a drug used to induce general anesthesia) was administered intravenously (IV). In conducting a review of the literature and discussing her observations with other CRNAs, Maria found several techniques used to minimize the injection pain. Based on this information, Maria decided that she would like to conduct a research study to examine the effectiveness of using lidocaine to reduce the injection pain of propofol. This project would fulfill the capstone requirement for her master's degree.

A literature review of pain management led Maria to the gate control theory, which posits that there is a gating mechanism in the spinal cord. When pain impulses are transmitted from the periphery of the body by nerve fibers, the impulses travel to the dorsal horns of the spinal cord, specifically to the area of the cord called the substantia gelatinosa. According to the theory, when the gate is open, pain impulses ascend to the brain; when the gate is partially open, only some of the pain impulses can pass through. Pain medication has an effect on the gate, and if pain medication is administered before the onset of pain, it will help keep the gate closed, allowing fewer pain impulses to pass through.

In planning her research project, Maria used the gate control theory to guide the design and structure of the study. For the study, she decided to compare two techniques for pain prevention. One technique involved mixing 20 mL of a 1% propofol solution with 5 mL of a 2% lidocaine solution and injecting 1 mL of the mixture immediately before administration of the propofol. The second technique involved the placement of a tourniquet inflated to 50 mm Hg on the arm in which the IV access device was placed. Then 5 mL of 2% lidocaine would be injected and the tourniquet would be removed 1 minute later; propofol would then be injected. A time frame of 20 seconds would allow the clients to report pain in the arm before the propofol took effect. Maria also planned to have a control group that did not have either of the pain prevention interventions.

*If the theory was correct, Maria hypothesized that both experimental groups would have less pain from the injection because the gate that allowed pain sensations would not open, or would only partially open. She did not know which of the two experimental procedures would be more effective in preventing pain, but was enthusiastic about conducting the study and adding to the body of knowledge on pain prevention in anesthesia.*

Theories from the biomedical sciences (e.g., biology, medicine, public health, physiology, pharmacology) have had a tremendous impact on nursing practice since Nightingale's time. Indeed, many of these theories are so integral to nursing practice that they are overlooked or taken for granted. For example, at the beginning of the 21st century, the germ theory seems almost too elemental to mention, because even kindergarten children are taught the basic concept of germs and how to prevent infection. But nurses should recognize the relatively recent discovery of this revolutionary theory (late 1800s) and understand that a significant amount of nursing care is based on it. Other theories, concepts, and principles are similarly ingrained within nursing practice.

Biomedical theories have been the basis for research efforts of physiologists, physicians, and laboratory-based scientists for many years. Nurses have also been involved in research of this type and are increasingly directing studies that have a physiologic or biologic basis. As with any study, the underlying theories or conceptual frameworks may be broad (e.g., germ theory) or very narrow (e.g., gate control theory).

This chapter presents some of the most commonly used theories and principles from the biomedical sciences to illustrate how they are being used in studies conducted by nurses and applied in nursing practice. The number of these theories is staggering; thus, space allows for discussion of only a few. Although there is some overlap, the theories will be grouped into two large categories: theories of disease causation (e.g., germ theory, natural history of disease) and theories related to physiology (e.g., stress and adaptation, cancer causation, pain).

## Theories and Models of Disease Causation

On a day-to-day, moment-to-moment basis, nurses in practice use any one of a number of concepts, principles, and theories from biology and public health. These theories are often related to disease causation and progression. This includes pathogenesis and infection, as well as multiple epidemiologic concepts and principles (e.g., risk factor, exposure, prevention). This section provides a review of a few of these principles, theories, and models and shows how they are used in nursing practice and nursing research.

### EVOLUTION OF THEORIES OF DISEASE CAUSATION

Disease refers to any condition that disturbs the normal functioning of an organism, whether it affects one organ or several systems. The term has also been defined as the failure of an organism to respond or adapt to its environment. The concept has changed dramatically over the course of time, however, and ideas about the cause of disease have been influenced by the prevailing culture and scientific thought.

In ancient times, disease was frequently viewed as a divine intervention or punishment. Early human beings attributed diseases to the influence of demons or spirits, and magic was a large of treatment and prevention. As time passed, other interventions or treatments, such as the use of plant extracts, became more common.

As humans formed into societies and distinct cultural groups, two trends, or approaches, to medicine evolved. Sorcerers and priests embraced a magico-religious approach, whereas early physicians and scientists developed an empirico-rational approach. The empirico-rational approach was based on experience and observation and was practiced at first by priests but was adapted by nonclerical physicians. Modern medicine arose primarily from the empirico-rational approach, as the human body and its functions became better known and as science led medical practice away from superstition and focus on the spiritual realm to include scientific processes and reasoning.

In the 17th century, William Harvey, an English physician and anatomist, demonstrated the dynamics of blood circulation (Kalisch & Kalisch, 2004). Detailed studies of the organs, diseases, and processes, such as physiology and respiration, quickly followed, conducted by eminent physicians and scientists of the time. Medical debates focused on minute features of the body and how to treat particular diseases. Philosophies and theories developed that were largely reductionistic and deductive, focusing on cause and effect; the medical model quickly evolved.

In the latter part of the 19th century, scientists began to unravel the basic causes of infectious disease. Modern medicine began with the advent of Pasteur's germ theory, which posited that a specific microorganism was capable of causing an infectious disease (Black & Hawks, 2009). The focus on single agent or single organism cause for disease persisted for a number of decades and resulted in multiple successes in both treating and preventing communicable diseases. Today, however, the predominant general model of disease causation is multicausal, involving invasive agents, immune responses, genetics, environment, and behavior.

A number of theories and models describe disease causation and the properties that relate to disease processes and prevention. Some of the most frequently encountered models in nursing practice and research are discussed in the following sections.

## GERM THEORY AND PRINCIPLES OF INFECTION

Louis Pasteur first proposed the germ theory in 1858. He theorized that a specific organism (i.e., a germ) was capable of causing an infectious disease (Kalisch & Kalisch, 2004). Today, this seems like a simple theory, but it is one that was critical to the development of modern medical care. Its impact has been phenomenal and has helped to radically reduce the number of deaths from infection.

At the beginning of the 21st century, this theory, or theories of infection, are most often applied to prevent infection (e.g., practicing strict handwashing, cleansing a scrape and applying antibiotic ointment, or prophylactically treating a surgery client with antibiotics) or to describe the process that seeks to identify, understand, and manage infectious diseases. This process initiates the search for the causative agent of an infection and method(s) of transmission. Once this has been accomplished, the focus can shift to the development of ways to prevent and treat the disease.

One of the most recent and dramatic examples of this process was the outbreak of acquired immunodeficiency syndrome (AIDS). The syndrome was first identified by the Centers for Disease Control and Prevention in September of 1982, but months passed before it was determined that the causative agent was a retrovirus, later termed the human immunodeficiency virus (HIV) (Ungvarski & Flaskerud, 1999). Early in the process, even before the virus was isolated, methods of transmission (e.g., sexual, transplacental, via blood products) were recognized and interventions for prevention proposed. Research on treatment has produced somewhat successful results in recent years and is ongoing.

Another, even more current, example involves bovine spongiform encephalopathy (BSE), or mad cow disease, and its relationship with Creutzfeldt–Jakob disease (CJD). It has been hypothesized that the causative agent of BSE is a *prion*, which is not truly a germ, but a protein that is transmitted through ingestion of contaminated meat; the principles of infection, however, are similar (Sheff, 2005). Much additional work will be necessary to support this theory and to enhance preventive efforts. Ultimately, it is hoped that effective treatments for CJD will be found.

### Application to Nursing

Research studies use the germ theory to identify the causes or agents of infection. For an infection to occur, the host must be susceptible to the invasive organism. This susceptibility may be termed *risk*. For example, a person who has experienced severe burns is at higher risk of infection because one of the first lines of defense, the skin, is damaged. Many nursing articles that present practice guidelines and nursing research studies have focused on prevention and management of infection as well as identifying factors that place an individual at risk for developing infections. These studies and guidelines use principles from the germ theory, although this is rarely acknowledged.

Examples from recent literature that detail aspects of nursing practice related to prevention of infection include guidelines for choosing sterile or nonsterile gloves (Flores, 2008), techniques of hair removal prior to surgery (Waddington, 2008), and guidelines for prevention of infections related to urinary catheters, central lines and ventilator-associated pneumonia in intensive care units (Kanouff, DeHaven, & Kaplan, 2008). Bubacz (2007) and Alex and Letizia (2007) presented guidelines for prevention of community-acquired methicillin-resistant *Staphylococcus aureus* (MRSA) in worksites and schools, respectively. With respect to the previous discussion of CJD, strategies to prevent prion infection were presented by Lovasik (2004), Rentz (2008), and Sheff (2005).

## THE EPIDEMIOLOGIC TRIANGLE

The classic epidemiologic model, particularly useful in the depiction of communicable disease, is the epidemiologic triangle (Figure 14-1). This model is often used to illustrate the interrelationships among the three essential components of host, agent, and environment with regard to disease causation. A change in any of the three components can result in the disease process. For example, exposure at school (environment) of a child who has not been immunized (host) to the measles virus (agent) will probably result in a case of measles.

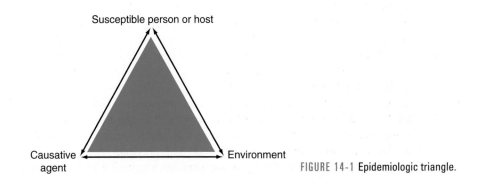

FIGURE 14-1 Epidemiologic triangle.

Within the epidemiologic triangle, prevention of disease lies in averting exposure to the agent, enhancing the physical attributes of the host to resist the disease, and minimizing any environmental factors that might contribute to disease development. Host, agent, and environmental factors that affect health can also influence progression of the disease process. Host factors include age, gender, race/ethnicity, marital status, economic status, state of immunity, and lifestyle factors (e.g., diet, exercise patterns, hygiene, occupation, sexual health). Agent factors include presence or absence of biologic organisms (e.g., bacteria, fungi, viruses), exposure to physical factors (e.g., radiation, extremes of temperature, noise), and exposure to chemical agents (e.g., poisons, allergens, gases). Last, environmental factors include such things as physical elements or properties (e.g., climate, seasons, geology), biological entities (e.g., animals, insects, food, drugs), or social/economic considerations (e.g., family, public policy, occupation, culture) (McEwen & Pullis, 2009).

## THE WEB OF CAUSATION

To explain disease and disability caused by multiple factors, MacMahon and Pugh (1970) developed the concept of "chain of causation," later termed the "web of causation." Prior to that time, it had been observed that chronic diseases (i.e., coronary artery disease and most types of cancer) are not attributable to one or two factors or causative agents. Rather, they result from the interaction of multiple factors. An example of the application of the web of causation to the development of coronary heart disease is presented in Figure 14-2.

The web of causation can also be applied to many health-related threats and conditions. The problem of teenage pregnancy, for example, is attributable to a complex interaction among a number of causative and contributing factors including lack of knowledge about sexuality and pregnancy prevention, lack of easily accessible contraception, peer pressure, low self-esteem, social patterns in which teen mothers are more likely to be children of teen mothers, use of alcohol or other drugs, and so on. Family violence, cocaine use, and gang membership are examples of other threats to health and well-being that can be more accurately explained through a model of multiple causations.

Recognition that many health problems have multiple causes leads to the recognition that there are rarely simple solutions to these health problems. When trying to manage teen pregnancy, for example, the solution is not as simple as addressing a knowledge deficit regarding sexuality and contraception. Many (if not most) teens are well informed about contraception and the mechanics of how one gets pregnant, and they still fail to take preventive measures. To prevent heart disease in an individual at risk, interventions include health education addressing a number of areas including smoking cessation, weight loss, cholesterol reduction, and exercise. Likewise, to prevent teen pregnancy, interventions should include health teaching on improving self-esteem, participating in role-playing exercises on how to say "no," encouraging orientation toward the future, enhancing parental supervision, and providing recreational alternatives (sports and other after-school activities), as well as giving information on sexuality, the mechanics of reproduction, and methods of contraception.

### Application to Nursing

Nurses have developed interventions and proposed strategies to address complex health problems with multifactorial etiologies. For example, from a large-scale study, Nonnemacher and others (2008) outlined risk factors for development of pressure ulcers among hospitalized individuals. These included: previous occurrence of pressure ulcers, limited mobility, skin problems, insufficient nutrition, and friction/shearing movement.

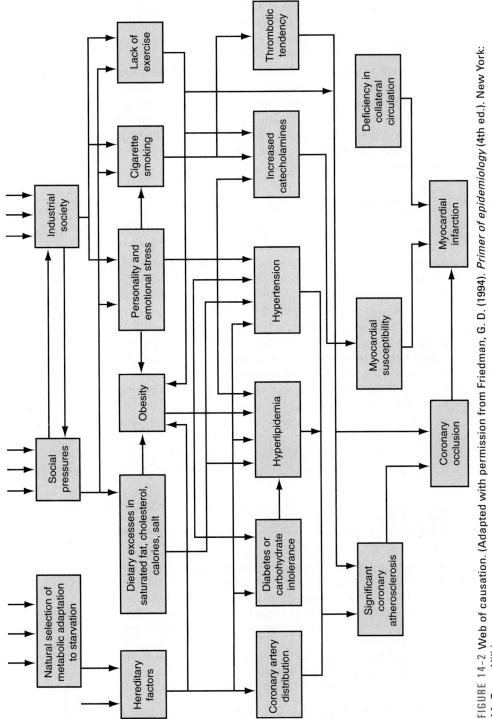

FIGURE 14-2 Web of causation. (Adapted with permission from Friedman, G. D. (1994). *Primer of epidemiology* (4th ed.). New York: McGraw-Hill.)

In another study, DiNapoli (2003) described the multiple risk factors as well as protective factors that may contribute to violent behavior in girls. These factors include social influences, such as media exposure, behaviors of peers relative to use of alcohol, cigarettes, and other substances, parental communication, GPA, race/ethnicity, and personal health. Other variables that can affect violence in girls include being friends with "bad kids," friends who fight, use of illegal drugs, pregnancy, history of psychological counseling, and having attempted suicide.

In other works, Siegel (2007) used the web of causation as the theoretical framework in her examination of the predictors of overweight in children in 6th, 7th, and 8th grades, and Van Dyke (2005) used the web of causation to explain the complex interrelationships explaining domestic violence. Finally, Selby-Harrington and Tesh (2000) developed a web of causation for infant mortality combining race/ethnicity, maternal age, parity, marital status, socioeconomic and educational status, and prenatal care.

## NATURAL HISTORY OF DISEASE

The natural history of a disease refers to the progress of a disease process in an individual over time. In their classic model, Leavell and Clark (1965) described two periods in the natural history of disease, prepathogenesis and pathogenesis. In this model, the prepathogenesis stage occurs prior to interaction of the disease agent and human host when the individual is susceptible. For example, an adult male smokes, a teenage girl considers becoming sexually active, or a preschooler attends a party also attended by a sick child. After exposure or interaction, the period of prepathogenesis proceeds to early pathogenesis (i.e., alterations in lung tissue, pregnancy, chickenpox) and on through the disease course to resolution—either death, disability, or recovery (i.e., lung cancer, teen motherhood, immunity to chicken pox).

In addition to the description of the natural history of disease progression, Leavell and Clark (1965) also outlined three levels of prevention—primary prevention, secondary prevention, and tertiary prevention—that correlate with the stages of disease progression (Box 14-1). Each of the three levels of prevention is applied at the appropriate stage of pathogenesis in an attempt to halt progression (Figure 14-3). Thus, at the primary prevention stage, interventions focus on general health promotion

---

**BOX 14-1**    *Levels of Prevention*

- *Primary prevention:* Activities that are directed at preventing a problem before it occurs. This includes altering susceptibility or reducing exposure for susceptible individuals in the period of prepathogenesis. Primary prevention consists of two categories: *general health promotion* (e.g., good nutrition, adequate shelter, rest, exercise) and *specific protection* (e.g., immunization, water purification).
- *Secondary prevention:* Early detection of and prompt intervention for a disease or health threat during the period of early pathogenesis. Screening for disease and prompt referral and treatment are secondary prevention.
- *Tertiary prevention:* Consists of limitation of disability and rehabilitation during the period of advanced disease and convalescence, where the disease has occurred and resulted in a degree of damage.

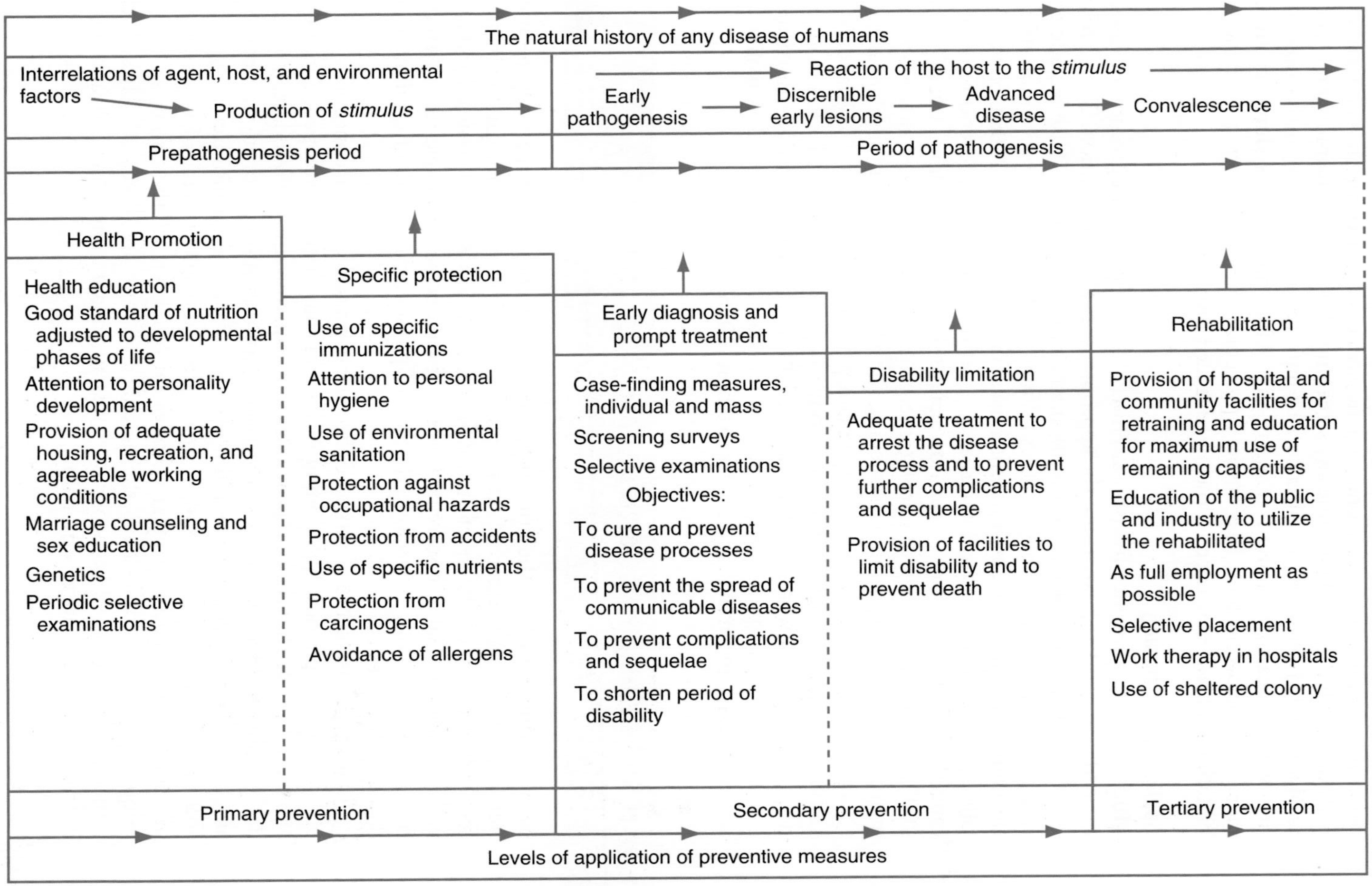

The natural history of any disease of humans

Interrelations of agent, host, and environmental factors → Production of *stimulus*

Reaction of the host to the *stimulus*

Prepathogenesis period → Period of pathogenesis

Early pathogenesis → Discernible early lesions → Advanced disease → Convalescence

**Health Promotion**

Health education
Good standard of nutrition adjusted to developmental phases of life
Attention to personality development
Provision of adequate housing, recreation, and agreeable working conditions
Marriage counseling and sex education
Genetics
Periodic selective examinations

**Specific protection**

Use of specific immunizations
Attention to personal hygiene
Use of environmental sanitation
Protection against occupational hazards
Protection from accidents
Use of specific nutrients
Protection from carcinogens
Avoidance of allergens

**Early diagnosis and prompt treatment**

Case-finding measures, individual and mass
Screening surveys
Selective examinations

Objectives:
To cure and prevent disease processes
To prevent the spread of communicable diseases
To prevent complications and sequelae
To shorten period of disability

**Disability limitation**

Adequate treatment to arrest the disease process and to prevent further complications and sequelae
Provision of facilities to limit disability and to prevent death

**Rehabilitation**

Provision of hospital and community facilities for retraining and education for maximum use of remaining capacities
Education of the public and industry to utilize the rehabilitated
As full employment as possible
Selective placement
Work therapy in hospitals
Use of sheltered colony

Primary prevention | Secondary prevention | Tertiary prevention

Levels of application of preventive measures

FIGURE 14-3 Natural history of disease. (Adapted with permission from Leavell, H. R., & Clark, E. G. (1965). *Preventive medicine for the doctor in his community: An epidemiologic approach* (p. 18). New York: McGraw-Hill.)

activities (e.g., encouraging a healthful diet and promoting regular exercise) and efforts to prevent specific health problems (e.g., vaccination, encouraging use of seatbelts and car seats, promoting oral hygiene). Secondary prevention is concerned with early detection and would include any screening activity (e.g., mammography, cholesterol screening) and subsequent efforts to limit disease progression for those identified with a health condition (e.g., taking statin medications, lumpectomy with radiation/chemotherapy). Last, tertiary prevention involves efforts to enhance rehabilitation and convalescence following advanced disease.

### Application to Nursing

Much of nursing practice focuses on efforts to prevent the progression of disease at the earliest period or phase using the appropriate levels of prevention. There are many examples of applying primary prevention strategies in practice. These include efforts to prevent skin cancer among athletes (Wiggs, 2007), primary prevention of cancer through modification of environmental risks (Giarelli & Jacobs, 2005), prevention of falls among elders (Bucher, Szczerba, & Curtin, 2007), and prevention of cervical cancer through promoting vaccination against the human papilloma virus (Ehrhardt, 2007). Excellent examples of nursing interventions targeted to secondary prevention include a program to promote screening for alcohol use and misuse among elders (Naegle, 2008), lead screening for pregnant women and children (Cleveland, Minter, Cobb, Scott, & German, 2008), and counseling and testing for BRCA gene mutations among at risk women (Zimmerman, 2002). Tertiary prevention efforts include information to help nurses work to prevent reoccurrences and secondary malignancies among long-term survivors of cancer (Mahon, 2005).

## Theories and Principles Related to Physiology and Physical Functioning

Many theories based on the normal physiologic functioning of the body are used in nursing practice and research. Although much of normal physiologic functioning is regarded as fact (e.g., the heart pumps blood, the lungs exchange oxygen and carbon dioxide), a great deal of research still is being conducted to uncover the mysteries of the body's physiology. Therefore, theories of physiologic functioning still need to be developed and tested.

Over the past century scores of theories, principles, and concepts related to physiology and physical functioning of humans have been developed. Among others, these include theories and principles of aging, immunity, wound healing, cancer development, inflammation and infection, hormone action, nutrition, metabolism, and body systems (renal system, pulmonary gas exchange, cardiovascular physiology, and nervous system functioning). Space does not allow detailed explanation or presentation of multiple, similar theories on one topic. Rather, some of the most frequently cited examples from the nursing literature are discussed. These include principles or theories of homeostasis, stress and adaptation, immunity and immune function, genetics, cancer, and pain.

## HOMEOSTASIS

Claude Bernard, a physiologist in the 20th century, first conceived the idea of homeostasis. He hypothesized that an organism must have the capacity to maintain its internal environment to live. A 20th century physician, Walter Canon, developed the concept of feedback mechanisms to further explain Bernard's principles of regulation. He coined the term *homeostasis* referring to the dynamic equilibrium and flexible on-going processes that maintain certain biological factors within a range (Lipsitz, 2000). The principles of homeostasis state that all healthy cells, tissues, and organs maintain static conditions in their internal environment.

Dr. Eugene Yates introduced the related concept of "homeodynamics" to show that there is continuous change in physiologic processes (e.g., heart rate, blood pressure, nerve activity, hormonal secretion), based on changes within or external to the organism. Thus, to survive, the body system depends on a dynamic interplay of multiple regulatory mechanisms (Lipsitz, 2000). Homeostasis or homeodynamics includes physiologic principles often described in terms of organ-based systems (e.g., cardiovascular, respiratory, endocrine, immune, and neurologic systems). However, in reality, the body systems are integrated and are continually adapting to environmental changes.

### Application to Nursing

There are a number of illustrations of how principles of homeostasis are applied in nursing practice. For example, Hankins (2006) explained the physiologic process of homeostasis in the human body, focusing on the role of albumin in fluid and electrolyte balance; and Place and Phillips (2005) provided a detailed discussion of the importance of maintaining homeostasis and blood glucose levels in patients in the intensive care unit. In articles focusing on infants in children, Davis, Parker, and Montgomery (2004) used the principles of homeostasis to describe the physiology and function of sleep in healthy infants and young children, and Koo and Warren (2003) presented the benefits in maintaining calcium homeostasis to promote bone health in infants.

In research, the concept of homeostasis served as a theoretical framework in a study to determine the effect of soothing music on neonatal behavioral states in the hospital newborn nursery. In this study, it was hypothesized that because the newborn nursery is noisy, the sounds might interfere with the neonate's efforts to achieve physiologic and behavioral homeostasis. This study showed a significant difference in the number of high arousal states when infants were exposed to normal newborn nursery conditions and when soothing music was played. The researchers determined that music may assist newborns reach a state of homeostasis in a newborn nursery (Kaminski & Hall, 1996).

## STRESS AND ADAPTATION: GENERAL ADAPTATION SYNDROME

In addition to the principles of homeostasis, Walter Canon also developed the concept of fight or flight to explain the body's reaction to emergencies. This fight or flight response prepares the body for muscular activity (i.e., running, self-defense) when reacting to a perceived or actual threat. The fight or flight response is a series of chemical reactions that are initiated by the adrenal medulla, which produces epinephrine (adrenaline) and norepinephrine. This reaction increases the heart rate, respiratory rate, blood pressure, and blood glucose levels. Blood is shunted to the muscles of the legs, heart, and lungs from the intestines; this prepares the body for quick response to danger (Black & Matassarin-Jacobs, 1997).

In the 1960s and 1970s, Hans Selye built on Canon's work by developing a framework to describe how the body responds to stress. Selye derived his theories of stress from the observations he made while caring for people who were ill. The clinical manifestations he noted were loss of appetite, weight loss, feeling and looking ill, and generalized muscle aching and pains. Selye called this response the general adaptation syndrome (GAS) because it involved generalized changes that affect the body.

Selye believed that changes in organs occur in three stages. Stage 1, the alarm phase, begins with the fight or flight response. In this stage, the adrenal glands enlarge and release hormones including adrenocorticotropic hormone (ACTH). This increases blood glucose and depresses the immune system. If the stress continues, the body begins to experience detrimental changes (e.g., shrinkage of the thymus, spleen, lymph nodes, and other lymphatic structures). Other physical manifestations, such as gastric and duodenal ulcers, can also develop.

Stage 2 (resistance) occurs when the body starts to react and return to homeostasis. If the stressor ends, the body should be able to return to normal. Stage 3 (exhaustion) occurs when the stressor persists and the body cannot continue to produce hormones as in Stage 1, or when damage has occurred to other organs (Table 14-1) (Selye, 1976).

Selye thought that the body's response to stress is nonspecific; that is, the body reacts as a whole organism. Also, it is not just bad things that cause stress, but good things as well. Health conditions thought to be related to stress include cancer, hypertension, heart disease, cerebrovascular accident, peripheral vascular disease, asthma, tuberculosis, emphysema, irritable bowel syndrome, sexual dysfunction, obesity, anorexia, bulimia, connective tissue disease, ulcerative colitis, Crohn's disease, infections, and allergic and hypersensitivity diseases.

Selye's syndrome theory has been the basis of many studies. Holmes and Rahe (1967) conducted one classic study. They proposed that a large number of life changes cause stress, which in turn may cause disease. The researchers asked individuals of various socioeconomic and cultural groups to rank a number of life changes according to the amount of energy needed to adapt to change. These events were ranked and a certain number of life change units (LCUs) were assigned to each one. This scale was named the Social Readjustment Rating Scale (SRRS). The total number of LCUs experienced by a person accumulates over time, and theoretically indicates the amount of stress a person has experienced. A significant accumulation of stress increases the likelihood of an incidence of major illness.

TABLE 14-1 *Selye's Stages of Stress*

| Stage | Characteristics | Physical Responses |
|---|---|---|
| Alarm | Begins with alarm; body prepares for survival (fight or flight); physiologic changes are coordinated by the central nervous system (CNS) and the sympathetic nervous system (SNS), which stimulates the adrenal medulla to secrete norepinephrine and epinephrine; the adrenal cortex is stimulated by the pituitary gland's release of ACTH. | CNS involuntary responses include secretion of specific hormones and metabolism and fluid regulation. SNS responses include increased heart rate, contraction of the spleen, release of glucose, increase in respiratory rate, decrease in clotting time, dilation of pupils, increased perspiration, and piloerection (hairs standing on end). |
| Resistance | The body recognizes a continued threat and physiologic forces adapt to maintain increased resistance to stressors; begins with a decrease in ACTH, and the body concentrates on organs that are most involved in the specific stress responses. | Adaptation implies return or improvement in physical health. Ineffective resistance leads to a state of maladaptation in which there is deterioration in the level of physical functioning. Chronic resistance eventually causes damage to the involved systems. |
| Exhaustion | The body enters exhaustion when all energy for adaptation has been used; ACTH secretion increases and the organ or organ systems show evidence of deterioration. | Symptoms include hypertrophy of the adrenal glands, ulceration in the gastrointestinal tract, and atrophy of the thymus gland. |

### Application to Nursing

In research studies, several nurses have used the SRRS. One study (Samuels-Dennis, 2007) used the SRRS as one measure to examine the relationships among employment status, stress, and depressive symptoms in single mothers. Another study (Welsh, 2006) used the SSRS to study the correlation between stress and depression in medical-surgical hospital nurses.

In a discussion relative to nursing practice, Motzer and Hertig (2004) described potential gender differences in the response to stress using Selye's model as a framework. Trethewey (2004) used the GAS and Pender's Health Promotion Model to outline a detailed plan of care for advanced practice nurses to assist them in managing patients diagnosed with systemic lupus erythematosus. In a similar work, Mulvihill (2005) used Selye's model to review the long-term impact of childhood trauma on the victim's psychological health.

## THEORIES OF IMMUNITY AND IMMUNE FUNCTION

The immune system comprises a complex, coordinated group of systems that produces physiologic responses to injury or infection. The purpose of the immune system is to neutralize, eliminate, or destroy microorganisms that invade the body. Extensive interactions affect the manufacture of products that alter the structure and function of cells.

Immunity involves specific recognition of what is designated as an antigen, memory for particular antigens, and responsiveness on reexposure. The immune system is related to other systems involved in inflammation and healing. Each system is involved in the response of inflammation and has two characteristics: (1) recognition of a stimulating structure by specific receptors and (2) response by one or more effector elements that aims to alter or eliminate the stimulating structure.

The immune system contains a large variety of cells, called leukocytes, that protect the body against foreign invasion. The five classes of leukocytes are neutrophils, eosinophils, basophils, monocytes, and lymphocytes; each has a specific function in the immune response. The granulocytes (neutrophils, eosinophils, and basophils) are short-lived phagocytic cells. They search out bacteria or cell debris and destroy them through phagocytosis (Workman, 2008).

Monocytes mature into macrophages in tissues and defend against tumor cells. They secrete monokines (i.e., interleukin-1) that assist in immune and inflammatory responses. Lymphocytes originate from stem cells in the bone marrow and mature into either B or T cells. The T cells differentiate in the thymus gland, and the B cells mature in the bone marrow. Both T and B lymphocytes continually recirculate between blood, lymph, and lymph nodes. The surface of B lymphocytes is coated with immunoglobulin, and when the appropriately matched antigen is detected by a B cell, the surface immunoglobulin will bind with it. The T lymphocytes play a role in cell-mediated immunity. There are a variety of T cell subsets; some are regulatory T cells, which include helper T cells and suppressor T cells (Black & Hawkes, 2009).

The complement system consists of some 24 interacting molecules found in serum and on cells. The complement system participates in inflammation by coordinating elements of the inflammatory response to microorganisms and tissue injury through generation of peptides that initiate effects such as leukocyte activation, chemotaxis, and mast cell degranulation. The system facilitates phagocytic function by coating the target particle with biologically active peptides and fragments of molecules activating the system. A series of proenzymes and other molecules initiate an attack on the cell membranes of microorganisms (Winchester, 2000).

Antibody-mediated immunity involves antigen–antibody actions to neutralize, eliminate, or destroy foreign proteins. Antibodies for these actions are produced by B lymphocytes. The B lymphocytes become sensitized to a specific foreign protein (antigen) and synthesize an antibody directed specifically against that protein. The antibody (rather than the actual B lymphocyte) participates in action to neutralize, eliminate, or destroy that antigen. Cell-mediated immunity involves many leukocytic actions, reactions, and interactions. Lymphocyte stem cells and lymphoid tissues regulate activities and inflammation by producing and releasing cytokines. T lymphocytes can be natural killer cells or helper cells (T4 or Th cells) (Workman, 2008).

### Application to Nursing

Principles of immune function can be used as a theoretical framework for research. A number of recent nursing research studies can be identified that look at factors related to immune status. For example, a study by Hughes and colleagues (2008) concluded that as an adjunct intervention, massage therapy helps reduce side effects of treatment and may boost immune function in children with cancer. Two other studies (Dowling, Hockenberry, & Gregory, 2003; MacDonald, 2004) noted the positive effect of humor on immune function.

The interrelatedness of the nervous, endocrine, and immune systems were described in two recent works on psychoimmunology. In one report, Ruiz and Avant (2005) examined the literature and found that maternal prenatal stress may prove to be detrimental to the immune system of both mother and developing infant. Another work (Starckweather, Witek-Janusek, & Mathews, 2005) presented an overview of the interaction of cytokines and hormones at the cellular level, and discussed how they might affect immune functioning; their review was intended to serve as a framework for conducting nursing research.

## GENETIC PRINCIPLES AND THEORIES

Although genetic principles and theories date back to Gregor Mendel's work in the 1860s, advances in molecular biology have only recently begun to transform health care delivery. The Human Genome Project is an organized effort initiated in 1990 and completed in 2001 to create a biologically and medically useful database of the genome structure and sequence in humans. (The term human genome refers to the entire complement of genetic material contained on the 46 chromosomes.) It is anticipated that information gained from the Human Genome Project will increase understanding of inherited conditions, both single gene and complex diseases as well as responses to treatment (Beery, 2008; Biesecker, Biesecker, & Collins, 2000; Lea & Tinley, 1998).

A gene is the fundamental and functional unit of heredity. It is composed of a double strand of DNA, and each of the strands has thousands to millions of bases. The order of the bases codes information that directs the manufacture of a specific protein (Lea & Tinley, 1998). A gene mutation is an alteration in DNA coding that results in a change in the protein product. Mutations in some genes cause clinical disease because of the absence of the normal protein. Sickle cell anemia, for example, results when one base is substituted with another.

Gene discoveries have provided information on genetic disorders that cause symptoms in a large proportion of persons who have abnormal genotypes. Successes include the isolation of genes for cystic fibrosis, neurofibromatosis, muscular dystrophy, Huntington's disease, and some types of breast cancer (Biesecker et al., 2000). Many other diseases have a genetic susceptibility component that results from the interaction of multiple genes with environmental factors. Because these diseases involve many genes and many possible mutations, an enormous number of combinations of genotypes are possible. Determining the molecular pathophysiology of human disease will provide opportunities for diagnosis, prevention, and treatment.

### Application to Nursing

Genetics will greatly affect the way health care is practiced in the future, and nurses will need to incorporate genetic technology and discovery into practice and research at the individual, family, and community levels. Nurses familiar with genetics and who are able to "think genetically" can ask appropriate questions of patients to assess genetic risk factors, communicate with patients and their families about inherited risks, make referrals to genetic counselors, reinforce counseling, and administer gene therapy or genetically specific drugs (Kirk, Lea, & Skirton, 2008; Lashley, 2000). Table 14-2

TABLE 14-2 *A Nursing Model for Genetics in Health Care*

|  | Nursing Science | Genetic Education | Ecogenetic Nursing |
|---|---|---|---|
| Individual | Caring behavior and support role | Predictive genetic testing | Educating patients on genetic testing |
|  | Care across the life span | Gene discoveries for diseases | Assisting patients to determine need for testing |
|  | Patient counseling | Genes in pedigrees | Genetic consulting |
|  | Medication | Pharmacogenetics | Educating about individualized medication therapy |
| Family | Pedigrees | Genetic role in disease | Interpreting and sharing genetic risk and health promotion |
|  | Health promotion | Molecular pathology | Individualizing genetic testing and health promotion |
|  | Multidisciplinary practice | Genetic specialist on the health care team | Referring to and interfacing with genetic specialists |
|  | Informed consent | Genetic research concerns | Explaining risks and benefits of genetic study |
|  | Teaching and counseling families | Genetic risks | Assessing and counseling families—reproductive risks and prenatal diagnosis |
| Community | Community assessment | Population-based screening | Community readiness for genetic screening and intervention |
|  | Design and implement screening programs and follow-up service | Genetic testing | Availability and voluntary access to genetic information, testing, and assurance of follow-up services |
| Population | Clinical trials | New technology | Coordinating genetically focused research |
|  | Nursing research | Genetic research | Collaborative research: focusing on ecogenetics, ethics, and psychosocial issues |
|  | Patient advocacy | Ethical issues surrounding genetic tests | Ensuring that patients remain the priority of clinical treatment and research |

suggests a nursing model for application of genetics in health care illustrating how and where genetics education can be added to basic nursing science. The result is preparation of the nurses for "ecogenetic nursing."

A practicing nurse must be sensitive to issues of ethics and confidentiality related to genetic testing and genetic information. Indeed, genetics is one area of health care where technology precedes the ethical framework for dealing with issues and creates problems previously unknown; nurses must be prepared to deal with these problems (Beery, 2008; Kirk, Lea, & Skirton, 2008). Nurses knowledgeable in genetics can ensure that patients and families make informed and voluntary decisions about genetic information. Nurses can also serve as patient advocates as they obtain informed consent to participate in genetic clinical trials or to undergo genetic tests.

Nurses knowledgeable in genetics can have an important role in counseling patients at risk for complex diseases. Because complex diseases occur much more frequently than single-gene disorders, and because the number of diseases found to have genetic determinates is increasing rapidly, there will not be enough genetic counselors to serve all who are at risk (Beery, 2008; Johnson & Brensinger, 2000). Nurses must use their knowledge of genetics to identify and differentiate genetic risks in patients with complex disorders and refer these patients to a genetic counselor whenever appropriate (Fessele, 2008; Kirk et al., 2008).

Nurses are becoming more involved with managing genetic information because it is often collected and recorded when the nurse takes a family history and obtains certain blood tests (e.g., screening for breast cancer, sickle cell trait). Genetic testing and counseling combines the provision of genetic information with psychosocial counseling. It is nondirective, voluntary, and personal, and should precede testing to allow informed decision making. Counseling should include an explanation of risk factors, exploration of the person's perception of the condition, and discussion of childbearing options. Potential outcomes of decisions are examined to facilitate decision making, and follow-up counseling is recommended (Biesecker et al., 2000; Fessele, 2008; Monsen et al., 2000). Goals of genetic counseling are to help clients and family members comprehend the medical genetic information, appreciate the genetic contribution to health and illness, understand health options and alternatives, and make informed health choices (i.e., whether to pursue further testing, evaluation, and treatment). Genetic counseling frequently includes referral and follow-up for family members to gain more information and possible treatment.

Nurses have also studied specific genetically based illnesses. For example, Frazier, Johnson, and Sparks (2005) reported on a review of research on the genetic basis for developing cardiovascular disease (CVD). They determined that understanding genes and genetic pathways can improve clinical practice and development of strategies to prevent CVD and reduce related mortality. Recognizing the impact of inherited mutations on the *BRCA1* and *BRCA2* genes and the associated increased risk of breast cancer, Nogueira and Appling (2000) described risk factors and risk factor analysis and provided strategies for prevention and early detection of breast cancer. In a similar work, Houshmand, Campbell, Briggs, Mc-Fadden, and Al-Tweigeri (2000) described three options for women with tests positive for *BRCA1* and *BRCA2* genes. These were "watch and wait," prophylactic mastectomy, and chemoprevention.

Nurses are involved in researching other aspects of how genetics influences health. For example, Frazier, Turner, Schwartz, Chapman, and Boerwinkle (2004) pointed out genetic difference affecting the blood pressure lowering effects of diuretics.

# CANCER THEORIES

The altered behavior of cancer cells is thought to result from several factors, including exposure to chronic irritants, chemicals, radiation, infectious agents, and genetic aberrations. Cancer cells are similar to normal cells in their basic biology and biochemistry, but regulation of their proliferation and differentiation is defective. Cells taken from malignant tumors typically differ from normal tissue cells in several ways. They are less sensitive to differentiation-inducing factors and they can divide indefinitely. Also, key regulatory factors (i.e., oncogenes, tumor suppressor genes, and cyclins) are altered in cancer cells (Wicha, 2000).

Cancer presents as a complex series of diseases involving multiple steps. It is thought to begin with an event that leaves a cell premalignant; this is followed by a number of promotional steps that increase the potential for an initiated cell to become malignant. The strong age correlation (i.e., incidence increases with age) supports the concept that most cancers result from the cumulative impact of multiple exposures over the lifetime (Blattner, 2000).

One theory of cancer development suggests that cancer arises as a series of genetic errors (Cavence & White, 1995). In this theory, there are three stages of cancer development: (1) initiation (referred to as the original genetic error), (2) promotion (genetic changes that continue and favor uncontrolled growth and metastasis), and (3) progression or latency (uncontrolled growth and full-blown malignant activity) (Figure 14-4).

This theory of cancer development states that cancer begins with one change in a normal cell. That change may alter cell production or cell function. This initiated cell may undergo additional malignant changes, especially if the environment supports the malignant activity. The cancer process can be stopped during the initiation stage, and even in the promotion stage, if the cellular environment is enabled to repair or control the carcinogenic genetic alteration (Foltz & Mahon, 2000).

Between 30% and 40% of all cancer deaths are preventable by modifying lifestyle factors, such as tobacco and alcohol use and diet. For example, it is thought that combined exposure to alcohol and smoking accounts for approximately 75% of all oral and pharyngeal cancers. Alcohol alone contributes to about 3% of all instances of colon, colorectal, esophageal, pancreatic, prostate, and breast cancers (Blattner, 2000). Table 14-3 lists some of the lifestyle, therapeutic, environmental, and host factors that appear to affect the development of cancer.

Theories dealing with cancer have been tested in a multitude of studies, with a goal of identifying the cause(s) of cancer, improving care, and ultimately finding cures. Studies that provided a basis for a relationship between lifestyle and cancer prevention have been conducted. For example, a growing body of evidence suggests that food choices may have a protective effect on carcinogenesis (Fuchs et al., 1999).

### Application to Nursing

Several works were found that addressed aspects of cancer prevention. For example, Loud, Peters, Fraser, and Jenkins (2002) focused on the use of genetic information to prevent, diagnose, and treat cancer. Zimmerman (2002) also focused on use of genetics to test patients at risk for genetic markers (*BRCA1* gene mutation) and described how to use that information in cancer prevention.

Ingram and Visovsky (2007) discussed efforts to promote exercise as an intervention to modify physiologic risk factors in cancer survivors. They noted that there is growing evidence that exercise contributes to improvements in body weight and

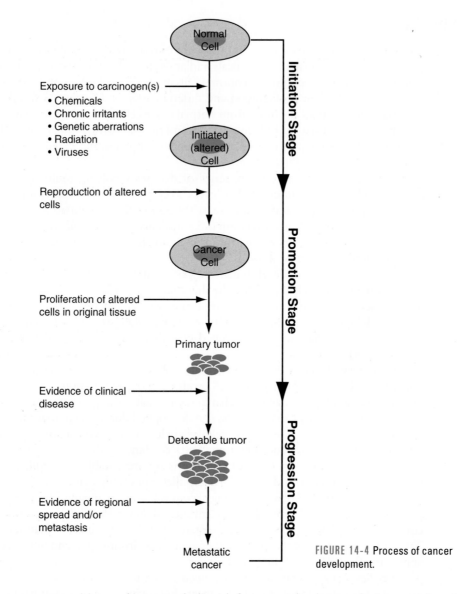

FIGURE 14-4 Process of cancer development.

composition, reduces metabolic risk factors, and enhances the immune function leading to overall survival in patients who have experienced cancer.

## PAIN MANAGEMENT

Pain is a phenomenon that has received a great deal of attention in health care. Early pain theories emphasized the specific pathways of pain transmission. Later theories attempted to uncover the complexity of central processing of pain in specific areas of the brain. The specificity theory of pain, for example, was proposed in the early 1800s. The theory was based on the recognition that free nerve endings exist in the periphery of the body and suggested that there are highly specific structures and pathways responsible for pain transmission. These nerve endings act as pain receptors that are capable of accepting sensory input and transmitting this information along specific nerve fibers. This theory set the stage for further studies on pain and pain management (Keene, McMenamin, & Polomano, 2002).

TABLE 14-3 *Factors That Contribute to Cancer Development*

| Factor | Examples | Type of Cancer |
|---|---|---|
| Lifestyle factors | Use of tobacco and alcohol, diet | Lung, oral, and pharyngeal cancers (smoking and alcohol); colon and rectal cancer (alcohol, diet) |
| Therapeutic factors | Medically prescribed drugs (hormones, anticancer drugs, immunosuppressive agents) | Vaginal and cervical cancer (*in utero* exposure to diethylstilbestrol [DES]), endometrial cancer (synthetic estrogens), breast cancer (possible link to use of synthetic estrogens), leukemia (some anticancer drugs), non-Hodgkin's lymphoma (drug-induced immunosuppression) |
| Environmental factors | Ionizing radiation, ultraviolet radiation, occupation, pollution, some infectious agents | Skin cancers (ultraviolet radiation), leukemias and thyroid cancer (ionizing radiation), lung cancer (some occupations and pollutants), cervical cancer (some subtypes of human papilloma virus), hepatocellular carcinoma (hepatitis B and C viruses) |
| Host factors | Inherent sensitivities to carcinogenesis | Colon and rectal cancers (familial adenomatous polyposis), site-specific breast cancers, cancer of the ovary, retinoblastoma |

Source: Blattner (2000).

A biochemical theory of pain perception was proposed in the 1970s following iden-tification of endorphins and opioid receptors. This theory postulates that morphine-like substances attach to pain receptors to modulate or decrease pain. Endorphin, which is synthesized in the pituitary and basal hypothalamus, is released into the bloodstream from the pituitary gland and mediates pain at the spinal cord level through circulating spinal fluid. Opioid receptors modulate pain by binding endogenous opioid peptides. When acute pain is elicited, endogenous opioids are released and are associated with the stress response to modulate or decrease pain. If pain-relieving medications are ad-ministered, they will attach to specified sites and result in pain relief. Pain can be con-trolled with drugs that bind to receptors (Summers, 2000).

### Gate Control Theory

The gate control theory (GCT) was proposed in 1965 to explain the relationship between pain and emotion. Melzack and Wall (1982) concluded that pain is not just a physiologic response, but that psychological variables (i.e., behavioral and emotional responses) influence the perception of pain. According to the GCT, a gating mechanism occurs in the spinal cord. Pain impulses are transmitted from the periphery of the body by nerve fibers (A delta and C fibers). The impulses travel to the dorsal horns of the spinal cord, specifically to the area of the cord called the *substantia gelatinosa*. The cells of the *substantia gelatinosa* can inhibit or facilitate pain impulses that are conducted by the transmission cells. If the activity of the trans-mission cells is inhibited, the gate is closed and impulses are less likely to be con-ducted to the brain. When the gate is opened, pain impulses ascend to the brain. Similar gating mechanisms exist in the descending nerve fibers from the thalamus and cerebral cortex. A person's thoughts and emotions can influence whether pain impulses reach the level of conscious awareness (Helms & Barone, 2008; Keene et al., 2002).

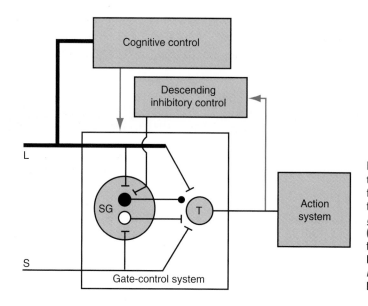

FIGURE 14-5 Gate control theory. *L*, large-diameter fibers; *S*, small-diameter fibers; *SG*, *substantia gelatinosa*; *T*, transmission. (Adapted with permission from Watt-Watson, J. H., & Donovan, M. I. (1992). *Pain management* (p. 20). St. Louis: Mosby.)

The gate control model (Figure 14-5) differentiates the excitatory (*white circle*) and inhibitory (*black circle*) links from the *substantia gelatinosa* to the transmission cells as well as descending inhibitory control from brainstem systems. The round knob at the end of the inhibitor link implies that its action may be presynaptic, postsynaptic, or both. All connections are excitatory, except the inhibitory link from *substantia gelatinosa* to the transmission cell (Melzack & Wall, 1982).

As mentioned in the case study, it is believed that pain medication has an effect on the gating mechanism. If pain medication is administered before the onset of pain (i.e., before the gate is opened), it will help keep the gate closed longer and fewer pain impulses will be allowed to pass through. The greater the degree of pain, the greater the number of pain impulses passing through the gate. If fewer pain impulses are allowed through the gate, the person will experience less pain. If the gate is allowed to open completely, a higher dosage of pain medication is required to close the gate. Therefore, in theory, prevention and management of pain are linked to keeping the gate closed.

### Application to Nursing

The GCT has also been the model for several reports related to pain management. Findlay (2004), for example, presented the GCT as an example of evidence-based practice in a work explaining application of the theory to the practice of neonatal nursing. In other examples, Hickman, Bell, and Preston (2005) used GCT to support the use of acupressure to help relieve postoperative nausea and vomiting; and Muldoon (2006) used it to promote the intervention of skin cooling to help relieve pain related to chronic wound healing. Oliver and Ryan (2004) used GCT to discuss therapeutic options that help relieve pain related to osteoarthritis and rheumatoid arthritis.

In nursing research, Friesner, Curry, and Moddeman (2006) used GCT as the framework in a research study to compare two strategies for removal of chest tubes. They determined that encouraging slow, deep-breathing relaxation helps manage pain during chest tube removal. In another experimental study, Hatfield (2008) showed that administration of an oral sucrose solution prior to immunization is effective in helping relieve pain in infants receiving routine vaccinations. Finally, Jacobson (2006) used the GCT to compare the effect of three different cognitive-behavioral interventions (music, kaleidoscope, and guided imagery) on pain perception during insertion of intravenous catheters. She found no statistically significant differences in pain reported among the three different intervention groups nor in comparison with a control group.

## Summary

Nurses continually use concepts and principles from multiple biomedical theories in practice and in research. Indeed, these concepts, principles, and theories are so integral to nursing that they are difficult to differentiate and set aside for detailed inspection.

The biomedical theories used by nurses include theories of disease and disease causation, as well as theories related to physiology and physical functioning. Nurses, particularly advanced practice nurses such as Maria from the case study, should study these theories. They should understand their relevance to nursing practice and recognize how they are used and supported in nursing research.

Because of length constraints, only a few concepts and theories were described in this chapter. But it is hoped that these discussions will lead the reader to recognize the importance of understanding theory and to apply theory to guide practice and research. Ultimately, this will improve the care of clients.

## LEARNING ACTIVITIES

1. Search current nursing journals for research studies that use epidemiologic, biologic, or physiologic theories as a framework. What theories are being tested?

2. Review the original work of one of the grand nursing theorists. Identify the epidemiologic, biologic, or physiologic concepts that are components of the theory.

3. With colleagues, discuss what theories or types of theories are used in routine nursing practice. How are different theories used in various specialty areas (e.g., pediatric oncology, geriatrics, transplantation) or settings (e.g., labor and delivery, critical care unit, clinics)? What theories are used across all settings and specialty areas?

4. Outline a potential research study using one of the theories or models presented in this chapter as a framework as depicted in the opening case study. Show how the model or theory can be used to generate testable hypotheses.

## REFERENCES

Alex, A., & Letizia, M. (2007). Community-acquired methicillin-resistant *Staphylococcus aureus*: Considerations for school nurses. *Journal of School Nursing, 23*(4), 210–213.

Beery, T. (2008). Genetics for advanced nursing practice. *The Nurse Practitioner, 33*(11), 10–18.

Biesecker, L. G., Biesecker, B. B., & Collins, F. S. (2000). The genome project and molecular diagnosis. In H. D. Humes (Ed.), *Kelley's textbook of internal medicine* (4th ed., pp. 9–11). Philadelphia: Lippincott Williams & Wilkins.

Black, J. M., & Hawks, J. H. (2009). *Medical surgical nursing: Clinical management for positive outcomes* (8th ed.). Philadelphia: Elsevier.

Black, J. M., & Matassarin-Jacobs, E. (1997). *Nursing clinical management for continuity of care* (5th ed.). Philadelphia: Saunders.

Blattner, W. A. (2000). Etiology of malignant disease. In H. D. Humes (Ed.), *Kelley's textbook of internal medicine* (4th ed., pp. 141–147). Philadelphia: Lippincott Williams & Wilkins.

## TRAIT THEORIES OF LEADERSHIP

The Great Man Theory approach to defining leadership evolved into trait theories in the 1930s and 1940s. The trait theories assert that leaders possess certain characteristics (i.e., physical or personality traits and talents) that nonleaders do not. Attributes, such as shyness, laziness, and aggressiveness, are considered the antithesis of characteristics a leader should possess. An example of a physical attribute associated with leadership is height (i.e., a tall person may be able to look down on others and, therefore, may cut an imposing figure of authority). The converse may be true as well. Some individuals believe if someone is born shorter than most people, the individual may have to be more assertive or aggressive and those behaviors may result in the development of a strong leader. Personality traits or characteristics associated with leaders include intelligence, self-confidence, charisma, initiative, self-awareness, self-control, the ability to communicate effectively with individuals and in groups, goal-orientation, self-directedness, the ability to assume consequences for actions and decisions, and the ability to tolerate stress. In lesser leadership positions, technical competence is important because it would be difficult to establish rapport with group members if the leader did not understand the technical details of the work (DuBrin, 2005). For example, a nurse whose clinical area of expertise is maternal–child health would probably have a difficult time assuming the position of Director of Critical Care Services because of the level of technical expertise required in critical care nursing.

Research studies designed to test trait theories of leadership have been inconsistent. The trait theories are limited by focusing only on leadership characteristics to the exclusion of the environment, the situation, and other possible confounding variables. Additionally, they focus on the attributes the leader brings to a particular situation rather than focusing on what specific actions the leader takes to address the situation.

Research attempts to identify traits consistently associated with leadership over time have been successful. Six traits have been identified that seem to best delineate the differences between leaders and nonleaders. These leader traits are the desire to lead, honesty and integrity, self-confidence, drive, intelligence, and job-relevant knowledge (Drafke, 2009).

## EMOTIONAL INTELLIGENCE

An interest in the inner or personal qualities of leaders has recently reemerged, particularly with respect to ethical qualities and charisma. This interest has been fueled by the demand for leaders with vision and charisma. Personality traits and characteristics have an important influence on leader effectiveness. The traits and characteristics that are most relevant tend to vary with the situation at hand. A foundational trait for leadership effectiveness that does not vary from situation to situation is self-awareness (DuBrin, 2005).

Self-awareness is one of the four key factors in emotional intelligence (EI). According to Goleman, Boyatzis, and McKee (2001), EI is a major contributor to leader effectiveness. The concept of EI refers to managing one's self and one's relationships effectively. EI includes the abilities of self-confidence, empathy, and visionary leadership. Passion for the work and for the people who do the work is particularly important to a leader with a high degree of EI. It is difficult, if not impossible, to inspire or motivate others if the leader is not passionate about the major work activities. The leader with high EI is able to sense and articulate a group's shared, yet possibly unexpressed, feelings, and is able to develop a mission that inspires others to achieve a common goal (DuBrin, 2005). EI includes understanding one's own feelings, sensitivity, and empathy for others, and the regulation of emotions.

Goleman et al. (2001) define four key competencies of EI:

- Self-awareness—the ability to understand and modulate one's own emotions. Goleman contends this is the most essential of the four major competencies. A self-aware individual knows his or her own strengths and weaknesses and has a high level of self-esteem. The self-aware leader seeks feedback continually to determine how well his or her actions and decisions are received by others.
- Self-management/self-control—the ability to control one's emotions; control over mood and temper. The leader who is self-controlled acts with honesty and integrity in a consistent and dependable manner.
- Social awareness—the leader has empathy for others including subordinates; is intuitive about organizational "political" forces. The socially aware leader shows genuine care for others in the organization.
- Social skills/relationship skills—the ability to communicate clearly and convincingly. The leader who has social and relationship skills disarms conflicts; builds strong personal and professional bonds; uses social skills to spread enthusiasm and to solve disagreements and problems; uses kindness and humor often; and constantly expands network of contacts and supporters within and outside of the organization (DuBrin, 2005; Hellriegel et al., 2005).

Goleman discovered that the most effective leaders are alike in one essential way—they all possess a high degree of EI. Without a high degree of EI, a leader will never become a great leader (DuBrin, 2005).

## BEHAVIORAL THEORIES OF LEADERSHIP

Movement away from trait theories to explain and define leadership began as early as the 1940s. Leadership research from the 1940s through the mid-1960s focused instead on behavioral styles that leaders demonstrated (i.e., specific behaviors of leaders that make some more effective than others) (Hitt, Black, & Porter, 2009). This set of theories is referred to as the behavioral or functional theory of leadership. The major difference between trait theories and behavioral theories is that trait theories are concerned with the leader's individual characteristics, whereas behavioral theories seek to explain specific actions taken by the leader (Wagner & Hollenbeck, 2005).

Lewin and Lippett conducted some of the first studies of leadership behavior at the University of Iowa in the late 1930s. The researchers, using an after-school study group of 20 boys, aged 11, explored autocratic, democratic, and laissez-faire leadership behaviors or styles. The results of this study revealed that when the boys had a democratic leader, groups were more cohesive, the boys were more motivated, and originality of work was higher. With a democratic leader, the boys produced less work, but the work was of a higher quality than the work produced when the group leader used an authoritarian or laissez-faire leadership style. Nineteen of the 20 boys preferred the democratic style of group leadership over the other two styles (Lewin & Lippitt, 1938).

Other studies of autocratic versus democratic leadership styles concluded that democratic leadership styles produced higher performance results in some studies, whereas in other studies, performance was higher in groups with an authoritarian leader. However, what was consistent among study groups was that the level of satisfaction of group members was higher with the democratic style of leadership than with other styles.

Tannenbaum and Schmidt (1973) further explored satisfaction with leader style and developed a model known as the continuum of leader behavior. This model provides for a range of leadership behaviors from leader centered (autocratic) to employee centered (laissez-faire). In determining which leader behavior the manager should implement, the authors proposed that the manager evaluate the following three variables: characteristics of the manager (i.e., experience with a certain leadership style), characteristics of the employees (i.e., level of experience with the process/job), and characteristics of the situation (i.e., offering a new product or service for the first time). Tannenbaum and Schmidt recommended an employee-centered approach or style because this approach most often led to increased employee satisfaction, motivation, and high performance and quality of the work product.

### Leader–Member Exchange Theory

Leader–Member Exchange (LMX) Theory was developed by George Graen and James Cashman. The central focus of LMX theory is the relationship and interaction between the supervisor (leader) and the subordinate (group member). The exchange between the superior and the subordinate is the unique, underlying premise of LMX. Interest in LMX has increased in recent years, leading to many field studies to test the propositions of the theory.

The theory recognizes that superiors develop unique working relationships with each subordinate or group member. According to LMX theory, leaders categorize subordinates into one of two groups: the in-group (high-quality relationship with the leader) or the out-group (low-quality relationship). Often the leader's first impression of the subordinate's competence heavily influences the leader's assignment of the subordinate to the in- or the out-group. The theory proposes that leaders do not interact with subordinates equally because supervisors have limited time and resources (Graen & Cashman, 1975).

Members of the in-group often have attitudes and values similar to the leader and interact frequently with the leader. They have a special exchange or relationship with the leader. In-group members perform their jobs in accordance with the expectations of their employment contracts. In addition, they can be counted on by the leader to volunteer for extra work and to take on additional tasks and responsibilities. As a result, in-group members are given additional rewards (increased job latitude, extra attention from the leader, and inside information that is not available to all employees), responsibility, and trust by the supervisor in exchange for their loyalty and performance. Research on LMX in field studies reveals that members of the in-group enjoy higher degrees of autonomy, job satisfaction, and trust from the supervisor as compared to members of the out-group.

Out-group members have less in common with the leader and are detached from the leader. There is limited reciprocal trust and support in the leader–subordinate relationship. Members of the out-group receive few rewards from supervisors and are more likely to quit because of job dissatisfaction.

Supervisors who aspire to be the most effective leaders create a special exchange relationship with all of their subordinates (Graen & Uhl-Bien, 1995; Wang, Law, Hackett, Wang, & Chen, 2005). The intent is not necessarily to treat all employees the same. Those subordinates who by virtue of their position in the organization have greater responsibility or administrative authority will have a deeper level of exchange with the superior. However, it is possible and highly desirable that the leader engender relationships of mutual trust, respect, and support with all followers.

LMX theory postulates that the quality of the subordinate's relationship with the supervisor has a large impact on job behavior and performance and the quality of that relationship has important job consequences (Bolino, 2007). Therefore, it is imperative that subordinates be evaluated based on their competencies rather than on the leader's favoritism (Graen & Uhl-Bien, 1995).

# MOTIVATIONAL THEORIES OF LEADERSHIP

The motivational theories expanded on the behavioral theories of leadership by focusing on factors that enhance worker/employee satisfaction and motivation and identifying factors that have a negative impact on those factors. Many of the motivational theories were based on the work of Maslow's Hierarchy of Needs Theory (1968). Maslow's work included the concepts of five basic needs (i.e., physiologic, safety, love, esteem, and self-actualization), which he described as being the driving forces or motivators of human behavior. Lower-level physiologic needs, including food and rest, must be satisfied before an individual can work on accomplishing higher-level needs such as self-esteem and self-actualization. Even though his theory was derived as a motivational theory, Maslow's early works were not originally applied to motivation in the workplace.

### Theory X and Theory Y

Douglas McGregor first published his work on Theory X and Theory Y in an article in 1957. McGregor was influenced by the works of Maslow, Herzberg, Argyris, and Likert. McGregor believed the structure of bureaucratic organizations, as well as prevailing management philosophy and policies, resulted in a situation in which power resided exclusively with management. In this structure, the role of management was to direct workers under the assumption that all workers were unmotivated, unambitious, lazy, and preferred to be led. These assumptions were labeled by McGregor as Theory X. McGregor's theory was that workers who had no input in the performance of the job lacked interest in the job and satisfaction with the work, resulting in resistance to change.

McGregor proposed a different set of assumptions and practices for meeting organizational goals in a more effective, humanistic manner; he designated this Theory Y. Management's priorities in Theory Y are to develop worker potential, remove obstacles, create opportunities for worker growth, and provide guidance, rather than control direction, for the worker. Theory Y encourages worker responsibility and participation in decision making. McGregor believed this style of participatory management would result in greater productivity, creativity, and worker satisfaction.

Because McGregor failed to operationalize concepts in his theories, there have been few direct tests of his theories. When the theories were tested, conflicting results were obtained (Caplan, 1971; Gray, 1978; Green, 1981; Kay, 1973; Malone, 1975; Morse & Lorsch, 1970). Most recently, Kopelman, Prottas, and Davis (2008) attempted to test the substantive validity of McGregor's theory by measuring the focal construct of the central concept utilizing an investigator-developed Theory X/Y attitude measure. The researchers viewed this as a critical first step in testing the many assumptions of the theory. The new measure is content valid and has adequate reliability. Finally, although a few contemporary companies are using Theory X management, many companies subscribe to the tenets of Theory Y (Daft & Marcic, 2009).

### Motivation–Hygiene Theory (Herzberg's Two-Factor Theory)

Motivation–hygiene, or two-factor theory, was established by psychologist Frederick Herzberg in 1959. Herzberg sought to describe the differences between factors that are true motivators for individuals (i.e., recognition for a job well done, opportunities for promotion or advancement, challenging and rewarding work), and hygiene or maintenance factors. Examples of hygiene or maintenance factors include salary, quality of supervision, interpersonal relationships with coworkers, and good working conditions (Herzberg, 1966).

According to Herzberg (1966), hygiene factors, although they keep workers from becoming dissatisfied, do not act as real motivators. Hygiene factors are most often extrinsic and usually cannot be changed by employee behaviors; hygiene factors do not motivate employees. Motivators are most often intrinsic factors and are correlated with increased job satisfaction. Thus, when managers want to motivate employees, motivators should be emphasized.

## CONTINGENCY THEORIES OF LEADERSHIP: LEADERSHIP AND MANAGEMENT BY SITUATION

As research into leadership became increasingly complex, it was recognized that leader characteristics, traits, and behaviors were not sufficient to explain the concept. The focus of research then shifted to include components of the situation or the environment into the equation as well. In other words, various external factors, such as conditions in the situation and the nature of the task to be accomplished, help to determine the leadership style that would be most effective in a particular situation.

### The Fiedler Contingency Theory of Leadership

One of the earlier efforts to address contingencies in leadership situations was the Fiedler Contingency Theory of Leadership (Fiedler, 1967). Fiedler, Chemers, and Mahar (1976) state:

> This theory holds that the effectiveness of a group or organization depends on two interacting or 'contingent' factors. The first is the personality of the leaders to determine their leadership style. The second factor is the amount of control and influence which the situation provides leaders over the group's behavior, the task, and the outcome. This factor is called situational control. (p. 3)

Fiedler (1967) developed the Least Preferred Coworker (LPC) Scale to determine and classify leadership styles. The instrument, an 18-item semantic differential scale, uses contrasting adjectives (e.g., friendly/unfriendly, open/guarded, and insincere/sincere) to direct the leader to describe an LPC. From the leader's responses on the scale, an LPC score is obtained. A leader with a high LPC score describes an LPC in a generally favorable manner. Fiedler believed this leader tends to be relationship oriented and considerate about the feelings of coworkers. Conversely, a leader with a low LPC score would be described by Fiedler as task oriented. Leaders who fall in the midrange of scores are a mix of the two types of leaders and should determine for themselves to which group they ultimately belong. Fiedler's assumption is that a leader's style is innately either relationship or task oriented and that style cannot be changed as the situation changes (Fiedler et al., 1976).

Once the leader's style has been determined by the LPC score, the next step is to match or fit the leader with the situation. Fiedler used the term "situational control" to describe three major group classifications or variables that may be used to evaluate an individual situation (Box 15-1).

Leader–member relations can be classified as good or poor, task structure as high or low, and position power as strong or weak. According to Fiedler, the better the leader–member relations, the higher the task structure; the stronger the position power, the more control or influence the leader has. For example, a nurse who is in an autonomous position as the vice president of patient care services (strong position power), who is highly respected (good leader–member relations) by a group of nurse practitioners (high task structure), and employed by the hospital, is influential to the nurse practitioner group.

---

> ### BOX 15-1  *Group Classifications*
>
> - *Leader–member relations:* Confidence in the leader and support of the group is effective in influencing the group's performance. (This is the most important factor in determining the leader's control and influence over the group.)
> - *Task structure:* Structure of the task is on a continuum from a well-defined, step-by-step procedure, to a vague and undefined one.
> - *Position power:* Authority is vested in the leader's position by the organization.

---

In Fiedler's studies of greater than 1,200 groups since the 1950s, the low LPC leader (task oriented) has been found to be most effective in very favorable situations (position power is strong and leader–member relations are good) and in very unfavorable situations (position power is weak and leader–member relations are weak). Also, the low LPC leader is most effective when tasks are clear and highly structured. The high LPC leader (relationship oriented) is most effective in moderately favorable situations when position power is weak, task structure is low, and leader–member relations are good (Hitt et al., 2009).

Numerous studies have been undertaken to test the validity of the contingency model's assumptions (Chemers, Harp, Rhodewalt, & Wysocki, 1985; Fiedler, 1969; Minor, 1980). These comprehensive studies, including a meta-analysis of 125 tests of the contingency model, provide strong support for the model's validity.

### Path–Goal Theory

Robert House (1971, 1996) developed the Path–Goal Theory as an extension of the earlier work of Georgopoulos, Mahoney, and Jones (1957) and from research related to the expectancy theories of motivation (Vroom, 1964). Situational factors that are examined in this theory include the nature and scope of the task to be accomplished, the employee's perceptions and expectations of the task, and the role of the leader in the work process. Expectations of the leader in this theory are to assist followers in determining and attaining goals and to provide the necessary direction and support to ensure that employee goals are compatible with those of the organization. The role of the leader is also to provide motivation and some type of reward (i.e., recognition for the employee once the task has been completed or the goal has been reached) (Podsakoff, Bommer, Podsakoff, & Mackenzie, 2005). The leader is responsible for helping the employee determine and clarify the path the worker is to take to reach the goal. An important aspect of the leader's role is to identify and remove obstacles from the path of the worker to enable him or her to successfully attain the goal.

House (1971) identified four leadership behaviors to test the assumptions of his theory. The *directive* leader provides specific guidance and direction to workers on how the task is to be accomplished; the *supportive* leader is concerned with the accomplishment of the task as well as the needs of the worker; the *participative* leader involves workers in making decisions about how the task or goal should be accomplished; and the *achievement-oriented* leader sets challenging goals and has high expectations that employees will perform at the highest level. House assumes leaders are flexible and are able to use any of the leadership behaviors described above as the situation warrants.

The Path–Goal Theory also proposes two sets or classes of situational or contingency variables that influence the relationship between the leadership behavior and

motivation, and commitment to actualize the vision. Leaders must be able to express the vision in ways other than verbally. That is, the vision should be expressed in the leader's behavior. Extending the vision entails making the vision meaningful to followers in different contexts and different situations (i.e., the vision should be shared by management and staff as well as across departments and levels of the organization).

# Organizational/Management Theories

Frederick Taylor, a mechanical engineer in steel plants in Pennsylvania, is recognized as the father of scientific management (Williams, 2009). In 1911, Taylor published *The Principles of Scientific Management*, which revolutionized the way work was accomplished in organizations in the United States. This change led to the use of the scientific method to help determine the "one best way" for a job to be done. Taylor's work is credited with beginning modern management theory.

## SCIENTIFIC MANAGEMENT

Taylor's work evolved because of what he perceived as inefficiencies on the job by workers and management, which he believed led to only one-third of the possible output. These inefficiencies included workers applying differing techniques to get the same job done, employees working at a deliberately slow pace, management not matching worker expertise and talents to the job, and management making decisions based on hunches and intuition. Taylor (1911) devised four principles of management (Box 15-2).

As a result of implementation of Taylor's principles and ideas, profits and productivity in American organizations rose dramatically. His methods gave U.S. companies a competitive advantage over foreign companies—an advantage that lasted for approximately 50 years.

## THEORY OF BUREAUCRACY/ORGANIZATIONAL THEORY

Max Weber, a political theorist and sociologist in prewar Germany, was attempting to address social and political concerns when he developed his definition of bureaucracy (Williams, 2009). Weber considered a bureaucracy to be an ideal form for an

---

**BOX 15-2** *Taylor's Principles of Management*

- Using scientific methods (i.e., time and motion studies), work can be organized to produce maximum efficiency and productivity while capitalizing on the expertise of the individual worker.
- Workers with specific attributes and qualifications should be hired and then trained and matched to the job that would make the best use of their capabilities.
- Workers should be rewarded monetarily if production exceeds established goals rather than being paid an hourly wage; workers should know where and how they fit into the organization and should be informed of the organization's mission and how they can help to accomplish the mission.
- Managers and workers should work cooperatively; however, the role of management is to plan and supervise, and the role of the worker is to get the work done.

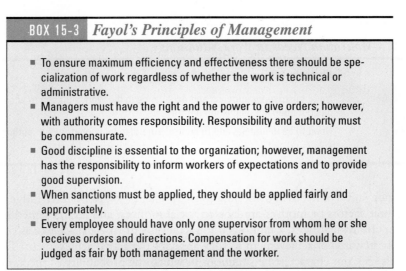

**BOX 15-3** *Fayol's Principles of Management*

- To ensure maximum efficiency and effectiveness there should be specialization of work regardless of whether the work is technical or administrative.
- Managers must have the right and the power to give orders; however, with authority comes responsibility. Responsibility and authority must be commensurate.
- Good discipline is essential to the organization; however, management has the responsibility to inform workers of expectations and to provide good supervision.
- When sanctions must be applied, they should be applied fairly and appropriately.
- Every employee should have only one supervisor from whom he or she receives orders and directions. Compensation for work should be judged as fair by both management and the worker.

organization in which there is a clearly defined hierarchy and division of labor operating in a system of detailed rules and regulations. Weber's theory emphasized the concepts of authority, command, power, domination, and discipline. For example, in a bureaucracy, the authority for decision making depends on the individual's position in the organization (i.e., the higher the individual is ranked in the organization, the greater the level of authority of that individual) (Weber, 1970). Many of Weber's principles are still used in large health care organizations today.

## CLASSIC MANAGEMENT THEORY

Henri Fayol, a French mining engineer and industrialist, successfully brought the Commentry-Fourchambault Mining Company from the brink of bankruptcy in 1888 and made it into a thriving, successful company. He accomplished this by using 14 principles of administration and management (DuBrin, 2009). These principles address areas, such as division or specialization of work, authority, employee discipline, unity of direction or supervision, remuneration of workers, chain of command, equity, initiative, and esprit de corps (Fayol, 1949). Examples of Fayol's principles of management are included in Box 15-3. Many, if not most, of Fayol's principles are used in organizations today.

# Motivational Theories

The ability to motivate others is a characteristic shared by leaders. Motivational theories are derived predominantly from the work of psychologist Abraham Maslow and his theory. McGregor's and Herzberg's theories were presented as evolving from Maslow's theory. The following sections discuss contemporary theories of motivation including Achievement–Motivation or Three Needs Theory, Expectancy Theory, and Equity Theory.

## ACHIEVEMENT–MOTIVATION THEORY

The Achievement–Motivation Theory was developed by Atkinson, McClelland, and Veroff. It focuses on aspects of personality characteristics and proposes three forms of

TABLE 15-1 *Motivation Needs in Work Situations*

| Need | Characteristics |
|---|---|
| Achievement (n-Ach) | Need to strive for success and excellence in the work situation to accomplish what has not been accomplished before |
| Power (n-Pow) | Need to be influential and to control others; to be in charge or in authority |
| Affiliation (n-Aff) | Need to be liked, accepted, and respected by others |

motivation or needs in work situations (Drafke, 2009; Robbins & Judge, 2009). These three factors or motives are labeled social motives, and are presented in Table 15-1.

Individuals with a high need for achievement (n-Ach) are not as concerned with the rewards of achievement as they are with the actual achievement. These individuals seek out characteristic situations in which the probability of success is neither too high nor too low, in which success can be achieved through one's own efforts, and in which personal credit can be received for a good or successful outcome. For example, if the probability of success is too high, an n-Ach individual will find motive satisfaction low—he or she perceives that there is not a sufficient challenge. High n-Ach individuals are often attracted to entrepreneurial activities such as developing their own businesses (Rue & Byars, 1977).

Research indicates that a high need to achieve is not necessarily synonymous with being a good manager. Other research has revealed that the needs for affiliation and power are closely related to managerial success. That is, the best managers appear to be those individuals who have a high need for power and a low need for affiliation (Robbins & Judge, 2009).

## EXPECTANCY THEORY

Victor Vroom developed Expectancy Theory in the 1960s. Major concepts of this theory include the effects of ability and motivation on performance; they can be expressed as a mathematical statement:

$$\text{Performance} = \text{Ability} \times \text{Motivation}$$

Vroom (1960) concluded that managers should attempt to develop and motivate employees simultaneously. However, he recognized that the successful motivation of employees depends on the employee's aptitude and ability as well.

In a later work, Vroom (1964) added the concepts of expectancy, instrumentality, and valence to motivation. This premise can also be expressed as a mathematical statement:

$$\text{Motivation} = \text{Expectancy} \times \text{Instrumentality} \times \text{Valence}$$

*Expectancy* is defined as the association between the action and the outcome of the action. Action will lead to the achievement of a goal. *Instrumentality* describes the type of outcome derived because of an action; it is the perception that achievement of a goal will lead to a reward. *Valence* is the value placed on the desirability of the outcome by the employee (Vroom, 1964).

In short, the Expectancy Theory states that an individual will act (performance) in a certain manner because there is an expectation (motivation) that the act will result in an outcome. Employee performance is also based on the attractiveness of that outcome (reward) to the individual. Note that the attractiveness of the outcome or reward is what the *employee* perceives it to be, not what the manager perceives. An individual's own perceptions of performance and reward will determine the employee's level of effort. Therefore, it behooves managers to make certain employees understand and see the connection between performance and rewards and to determine what rewards are valued (and expected) by workers.

## EQUITY THEORY

J. Stacy Adams, a research psychologist, developed Equity Theory in 1963. This theory is based on the concepts of cognitive dissonance and distributive justice. It attempts to describe the relationship in which an individual gives something (input) and in exchange receives something (outcome) (Adams, 1965).

In a work situation, an individual expects that if he or she works hard at a job (input) he or she will receive compensation or recognition (outcome) based on what he or she has put in. The individual then compares this input–outcome ratio with relevant others in the same job situation (inside or outside of the organization). If the worker perceives the input–outcome ratio of the relevant others is equal to his or her own, then a state of equity exists. If the ratios are not equal (i.e., if the workers perceive themselves to be over- or under-rewarded), a state of inequity exits and the employee will attempt to correct the inequity (Robbins & Judge, 2009). The corrections may take several forms and include lower or higher inputs or outputs and increased absenteeism. The presence of inequity results in employee dissatisfaction.

## Concepts of Power, Empowerment, and Change

In society and in organizations the words power and authority are often used synonymously and sometimes interchangeably. However, the two concepts are not synonymous.

## POWER

*Power* is the larger concept from which authority is derived. Power can be defined as influence wielded by an individual or group of individuals to change behaviors and attitudes and to sway decisions. Power implies a dependency relationship. In other words, the more dependent an individual is on another, the more power is generated by the individual in possession of the desired attribute (e.g., wealth, information, prestige, etc.). Power can have positive or negative connotations. For example, among disenfranchised groups, power may have a negative connotation, as in abusing power or by engendering feelings of powerlessness.

*Authority*, on the other hand, is a formal right based on the manager's position in the organization. Authority is a source of legitimate power; however, some individuals (and organizations) are more proficient than others in using and delegating authority. Authority can be under- and over-used. Usually the higher one is (by virtue of vertical position) in an organization, the greater one's authority.

French and Raven (1959) conducted early research related to the concept of power. They classified five bases or sources of power: reward, coercive, legitimate, referent, and expert power (Table 15-2). Coercive, reward, and legitimate power are considered formal bases of power; referent and expert power are personal bases of

TABLE 15-2 *Sources of Power*

| Type of Power | Characteristics | Examples |
|---|---|---|
| Reward | The transfer of positive reinforcers from the leader to the follower | Praise, compensation, and other rewards the follower values |
| Coercive | The use of negative sanctions to achieve results desired by the leader | Unfavorable work assignments; unappealing work schedules |
| Legitimate | Power derived by virtue of the position or title held within the organization | Vice president of patient care services; chief nursing officer; charge nurse; team leader |
| Referent | Power that some individuals possess by virtue of their association with a more powerful individual or entity | Being on the faculty of a well-known university; working for a renowned nurse |
| Expert | Power derived through an individual's knowledge, experience, and expertise or skill in a certain discipline or area of specialization | A clinical nurse specialist consulting in the case of a pregnant oncology patient; a nursing professor chairing a curriculum change committee |

power. Two other bases of power, *informational power* and *charismatic power*, have subsequently been identified in the literature (Heineken & McCloskey, 1985). Informational power is the power held by an individual who has the information necessary for others to accomplish a task or goal. Charismatic power can be distinguished from referent power as a type of personal power rather than reflected power. Charismatic power is the power that attracts one individual to another.

Power bases can be used individually or in combination. The effect of the power bases is additive; that is, the more power bases an individual uses, the greater or broader the power that individual will exert or exercise. Research indicates that personal sources of power are most effective (Carson, Carson, & Roe, 1993).

# EMPOWERMENT

In many organizations, including some health care organizations, power has shifted from residing exclusively with management to the worker or a group or workers, often in a team configuration. *Empowerment*, in organizational terminology, is the transfer or delegation of responsibility and authority from managers to employees; empowerment is the sharing of power. Empowerment also involves the sharing of vision, mission, knowledge, expertise, decision making, and resources necessary for employees to reach organizational goals. The concept of empowerment can be operationalized as a continuum with employees in some organizations having virtually no say in how the work is to be accomplished, to the other end of the continuum where employees have complete control over work processes (Daft & Marcic, 2009).

Empowerment is consistent with the contemporary views of leadership (i.e., transformational, visionary, etc.). In today's competitive economic environment, organizations that have been successful from an economic and quality standpoint are those that have empowered employees to "get the job done." This usually involves removing bureaucratic barriers to success such as forcing workers to wait days or weeks for management approval of new work methods or for allocation of necessary resources to accomplish a task or goal. To exploit competitive marketplace advantages, decisions and changes are made rapidly and at a lower level in the organizational structure than in traditional companies. Empowered employees are often more creative and responsive to the needs of the customer or consumer.

# CHANGE

Today, nursing and, in a broader view, health care, are arenas that seem to be in a constant state of flux or change. For most individuals, change elicits feelings of uncertainty, anxiety, and upheaval. Kurt Lewin, a German psychologist, proposed a method of planned change, which is controlled change or change by design. Theorists who have expanded the work of Lewin include Havelock, whose theories on change include six phases; Kilmann, who postulated five stages of organizational planned change; Kotter, who describes a process that includes eight stages for leading change; and Smith, who identified seven levels of change (Tomey, 2009).

## Planned Change Theory

Lewin described a method in his field theory that provides a basis for considering the process of *planned* change (Lewin, 1951). Planned change occurs by design, as opposed to change that is spontaneous or that occurs by happenstance or by accident. When Lewin's process is used correctly and in its entirety by a group or a system, effective change is implemented.

Central to Lewin's theories on planned change are the concepts of field and force. A *field* can be viewed as a system; therefore, when change occurs in one part or aspect of the system, the whole system must be examined to determine the effect of that change. *Force* is defined as a directed entity that has the characteristics of direction, focus, and strength. Lewin states that change is a move from the status quo that results in a disruption in the balance of forces or disequilibrium between opposing forces (Lewin, 1951).

According to Lewin (1951), there are two forces involved in change, *driving forces* and *restraining forces*. As the name implies, a driving force encourages or facilitates movement to a new direction, goal, or outcome. A restraining force has the opposite effect; restraining forces block or impede progress toward the goal. In planned change, driving forces should be identified and accentuated. If possible, restraining forces should also be identified and minimized to achieve the desired outcome or change. Lewin describes effective change as the return to equilibrium as a result of balancing opposing forces. If driving forces and restraining forces can be identified, it may be possible to predict if and when change would be successful. Lewin (1951) identifies three phases that must occur if planned change is to be successful: unfreezing the status quo, moving to a new state, and refreezing the change to make it permanent. In the unfreezing stage, individuals involved must be informed of the need for change and should agree that change is needed. Change, particularly in the work environment, often leads to feelings of uneasiness, uncertainty, and loss of control. Change, just for the sake of change, is viewed by most individuals as stressful and unnecessary.

Driving forces should exceed restraining forces during movement, the second phase of the planned change process. The initiator of the change, the change agent, should recognize that change takes time, should be accomplished gradually, and should be thoughtfully and comprehensively planned before implementation.

During the refreezing phase, stabilization occurs. If stabilization is successful, the change is assimilated into the system. Change disrupts the comfort of the status quo; it leads to disequilibrium. Therefore, resistance to change should always be anticipated and expected.

Kotter (1995) expanded Lewin's theory by devising a more detailed eight-step approach for implementing change that correlates to the unfreezing, movement, and refreezing phases in Lewin's model. Kotter analyzed common mistakes made when managers attempt to initiate a change. Based on these mistakes, Kotter's Eight Step Plan for Implementing Change was devised. The eight steps include:

1. Create a sense of urgency for the change
2. Form coalitions to have enough power to lead the change
3. Create a new vision to direct the change; strategies must be developed to achieve the new vision
4. Communicate the new vision purposefully and effectively throughout the organization
5. Remove barriers to change, empower others to act on the new vision, encourage an atmosphere of creativity and risk-taking
6. Plan rewards for short-term "wins" when the organization begins to move toward the new vision
7. Continually assess the effects of the change and make adjustments as necessary in new programs
8. Reinforce the changes by linking new behaviors to organizational success (Robbins & Judge, 2009)

Uncertain and dynamic environments often characterize the environments of organizations today. In this environment, stability and predictability rarely exist. Disruptions in the status quo are the norm. Organizations today face constant change, often bordering on chaos. Leaders in today's environments of continual change must be prepared to efficiently and effectively adapt to change and must be able to manage all aspects of change—from both external and internal forces.

## Problem-Solving and Decision-Making Processes

Decision making is typically viewed as but one component of problem solving. Decision making can occur without taking the time to complete a comprehensive analysis, a step that is usually required in problem solving. Also, a decision can be made without identifying the real problem. Factors that play a role in an individual's process or method of decision making include the individual's values, life experiences, preferences, and inherent ways of thinking.

Early attempts to arrive at a scientific or rational method of decision making were described in the Rational Decision-Making Model. More recently, research conducted by Vroom and Yetton (1973), and Vroom and Jago (1988) related to decision making has resulted in quantitative decision technology. This method can help managers select a decision-making style based on input and mathematical computation of effects of leader and situational variables.

### THE RATIONAL DECISION-MAKING MODEL

The primary assumption of the Rational Decision-Making Model, which has ties to the classic theories of economic behavior, is that of economic rationality. Economic rationality contends that people always attempt to maximize their individual economic outcomes when weighing decisions. Individuals or managers evaluate potential outcomes of their decisions based on current or prospective monetary worth. In a business decision-making situation, a manager weighs the alternative outcomes of a decision based in terms of profit-and-loss potential. The alternative selected as part of the decision-making process is the alternative that reaps the highest expected worth. *Expected worth* equals the sum of the expected values of the associated costs and benefits of the outcomes resulting from that alternative (Wagner & Hollenbeck, 2005).

Other assumptions of the model include the following:

- The problem is easy to discern and is without ambiguity.
- There is one well-defined goal to be achieved.
- All possible alternatives and consequences to action are known to the decision maker.
- There are no time or cost constraints.
- The final choice that is made will have the maximum economic payoff.

However, the assumptions of rationality often do not hold true. For example, in today's health care environment how often does the manager have the luxury of no time or cost constraints?

Simon (1965), an economist and psychologist, concluded that most managers did not make decisions based on objective rationality. Simon proposed that there are bounds or limits to the ability of humans to make rational decisions at all times. *Bounded rationality*, a term devised by Simon, means that humans are unable to make entirely rational decisions because of the limits of human mental abilities and because of the influence of external factors on decision making. As a result, most people who make decisions do not have the time or capability to wait for the best possible solution to every problem. Decisions are made using incomplete knowledge and without attempting to determine all possible consequences. The final decision is good enough or "satisficing." Most people stop the search for alternatives when they find a satisficing alternative.

There are several influences on the decision-making process, which contribute to bounded rationality. These include intuition, personality and cognitive intelligence, EI, quality and accessibility of information, political considerations, degree of certainty, crisis and conflict, the values of the decision maker, procrastination, and decision-making styles (DuBrin, 2009).

## GROUP DECISION MAKING

In organizations, groups or teams of people typically make decisions rather than individuals. Group decision making is often used when the decision is complex, such as when a new process or product is being developed. Advantages of group decision making include: the decision made may be of higher quality because of the collective wisdom of the group members, major errors may be avoided because of the ability of the group members to evaluate each member's thinking, and commitment or "buy-in" of the group may be increased because of members role in the outcome of the decision (DuBrin, 2009).

There are several disadvantages to group decision making. It often takes longer to reach a decision using a group. In addition, decision making in groups may lead to compromises that really do not solve the problem. Because of the often increased time involved for group decision making, group decision making should be reserved for problems that are multifaceted, complex, and important enough to warrant the efforts of the group (DuBrin, 2009).

An example of a group decision-making process is the nominal group technique (NGT). Use of this technique allows a manager to explore potential alternatives to a problem and the reaction to implementation of specific alternatives. NGT follows a very structured format that begins by identifying the problem and ends with developing an action plan to implement a chosen solution. Once the plan is implemented, the group reconvenes to discuss progress and to evaluate outcomes (DuBrin, 2009).

## ORGANIZATIONAL QUANTITATIVE DECISION-MAKING TECHNIQUES

Many organizations today, particularly health care organizations, rely on data-based decision making. That is, leaders and managers in those organizations rely on results of facts and quantitative measures to make decisions although intuition and judgment still influence the decision-making process.

Examples of quantitative approaches used in decision making include the utilization of the following: Paretto diagrams for problem identification; Gantt charts and milestone charts to monitor the progress of scheduled projects; break-even analyses (a method to determine profitability of new ventures or programs); decision trees; graphic illustrations of all possible alternatives to solve a particular problem; and sophisticated inventory-control techniques (DuBrin, 2009).

## Conflict Management

Conflict can be positive or negative and functional or dysfunctional, although most people tend to shy away from situations in which there may be conflict. Negative conflict can be detrimental if allowed to continue for long periods without intervention from management. In general, a conflict situation has the following characteristics:

- At least two parties are involved.
- Strong emotions and behavior, directed toward defeating or suppressing the opponent, are apparent.
- Mutually exclusive needs or values exist or are perceived to exist.
- Opposing parties attempt to gain power over each other (Katz & Lawyer, 1985).

## CONFLICT MODE MODEL

When a conflict occurs, Thomas (1976) recommended that the first course of action is to discern the other party's intent in causing the conflict before determining how to respond. Response is guided by two behaviors or dimensions: cooperativeness and assertiveness. Cooperativeness is used if one is more focused on satisfying the other person's concerns. Assertiveness is used if one is more focused on satisfying one's own concerns (Thomas, 1976).

Thomas and Kilmann (1974) defined five conflict-handling modes or strategies: competing, accommodating, avoiding, collaborating, and compromising. *Competing* or *forcing* is used when the issue is important, needs speedy resolution, and "buy-in" from individuals other than the manager is unnecessary. When the issue in conflict is of relative unimportance to the manager or when the manager "gives in" to the other party involved in the conflict, *accommodation* is used. *Avoidance* should be used when emotions are still high and when the conflict is trivial; confrontation should be postponed until a more opportune time arrives. *Collaboration* is the opposite of avoidance and is used when the issue is too important to each side to be compromised; all parties want a win-win solution. *Compromise* is used for complex issues when conflicting parties are similar in power. Compromise can also be used to craft a temporary solution (Daft & Marcic, 2009).

Integrating the five conflict-handling modes with the two dimensions of cooperativeness and assertiveness results in the following conflict resolution options for managers: competing (assertive, but uncooperative), collaborating (assertive and cooperative), avoiding (unassertive and uncooperative), accommodating (unassertive, but cooperative), and compromising (midrange on both assertiveness and cooperation). Each option has its inherent strengths and weaknesses and no one option is ideal for every situation.

## Quality Control and Quality Improvement

One of the integral values of American society that has evolved in the last several decades is access to health care at reasonable cost in terms of resources. With increasing demands on health service organizations for improved quality and lower costs, the entire health care system has been forced to evaluate modes of operation and traditional quality assurance (QA) programs. As a result, many health care organizations have incorporated concepts of quality improvement (QI).

QI is the commitment and approach used to scrupulously examine and continuously improve every process in every part of an organization. The ultimate intent of this methodology is meeting and exceeding customer expectations. QI empowers individuals and teams within systems to look at the way service is delivered to customers, to identify root causes of problems in the system, and then to creatively adopt solutions to the problems. Many health care organizations can accurately claim substantial improvements in both service effectiveness and efficiency as a result of this commitment and approach to quality.

In the field of QI, just as in the field of QA, there exists a complex, ever-changing vocabulary. Even the term QI is not consistently used as the primary label for quality-related concepts. Other labels (and their abbreviations) frequently noted in the literature include continuous quality improvement (CQI), total quality management (TQM), total quality systems (TQS), quality systems improvement (QSI), and total quality (TQ), and among others.

### QUALITY IMPROVEMENT VERSUS QUALITY ASSURANCE

What is the relationship of QI to QA in health care? Several limitations to traditional QA approaches have been identified. These limitations include the static approach of QA, the focus of QA as too narrow to meet modern health care needs, the focus of QA on physician practice, and under emphasis on nonphysician providers and on systems processes, which have a strong impact on provision of quality care. Other limitations of traditional QA programs that have been identified include: QA is department or individually focused; QA has little emphasis on error-free work; and QA places too much emphasis on external accreditation standards.

### QUALITY IMPROVEMENT FRAMEWORKS

For more than four decades, two Americans, W. Edwards Deming and J. M. Juran, were the primary champions of the quality movement throughout the world (Port, 1991). Deming was the developer of statistical quality control, whereas Juran was the innovator of total quality control. Both are credited with playing major roles as statistical and managerial consultants to Japanese industry in Japan's successful revitalization after the devastation of World War II. (Port, 1991).

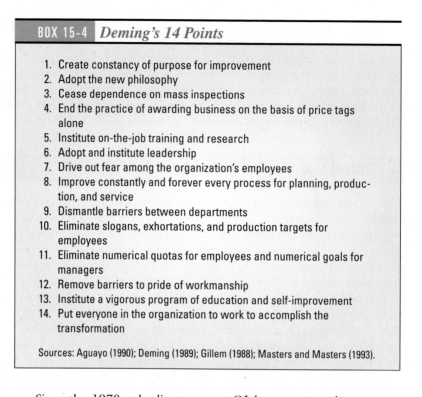

**BOX 15-4**  *Deming's 14 Points*

1. Create constancy of purpose for improvement
2. Adopt the new philosophy
3. Cease dependence on mass inspections
4. End the practice of awarding business on the basis of price tags alone
5. Institute on-the-job training and research
6. Adopt and institute leadership
7. Drive out fear among the organization's employees
8. Improve constantly and forever every process for planning, production, and service
9. Dismantle barriers between departments
10. Eliminate slogans, exhortations, and production targets for employees
11. Eliminate numerical quotas for employees and numerical goals for managers
12. Remove barriers to pride of workmanship
13. Institute a vigorous program of education and self-improvement
14. Put everyone in the organization to work to accomplish the transformation

Sources: Aguayo (1990); Deming (1989); Gillem (1988); Masters and Masters (1993).

Since the 1970s, the literature on QI has grown and many experts have contributed their ideas on QI. In the United States, the quality theories of Deming, Juran, and Crosby predominate. Deming's (1989) major thesis is that the cause of inefficiency and low quality can generally be traced back to system inadequacies rather than individual worker inadequacy. It is management's responsibility to improve the system with the involvement of all employees. This management theory focuses on improving quality, productivity, and competitive position in the marketplace and is referred to in the literature as Deming's 14 points (Box 15-4).

Deming's goal was to gear an organization's workforce to pursue specific organization-wide goals that were aimed at satisfying customer requirements for quality, price, and service. Juran (1988) defined quality as "fitness for use." To satisfy customers, a product or service must have two components—features that a customer wants and as free from deficiencies as possible. According to Juran, one or the other of these two components alone does not constitute high quality. Juran offered three processes whereby managers can maintain and improve quality. These are commonly referred to as Juran's trilogy (Table 15-3; Juran, 1988).

Crosby (1979) emphasized the importance of systems knowledge and improvement, the disadvantages of reliance on inspections, and the need for statistical quality control. Crosby termed his major concepts the "four absolutes":

1. The definition of quality is conformance requirements.
2. The system of quality is prevention and on not relying solely on "after-the-fact" methods to improve quality.
3. The performance standard is zero defects.
4. The measurement of quality is the price of nonconformance, which involves all costs in doing things wrong. In service companies, the cost of nonconformance is 35% of operating costs, whereas the cost of conformance is a far lower figure (Crosby, 1979).

TABLE 15-3 *Juran's Trilogy: Processes Used to Maintain and Improve Quality*

| Process | Activities |
|---|---|
| Quality planning | Building quality into the processes and the product |
| Quality control | Evaluating actual performance, comparing that performance to predetermined goals, and taking action on the differences |
| Quality improvement (breakthrough) | Encouraging attainment of previously unprecedented levels of performance by the organization |

Although experts on QI differ somewhat on their approaches, their theories share several characteristics (Daft & Marcic, 2009). These include:

- QI is driven by the leaders of the organization.
- Customer-mindedness permeates the organization.
- A transition is made from inspection-based management to process improvement.
- Formal process-improvement methods and statistical tools are used.
- All employees are involved in the exploration and refinement of work processes.

## ORGANIZATIONAL LEADERSHIP ROLE AND QUALITY IMPROVEMENT

Organizational leadership has a profound impact on the successful implementation of QI. All of the experts agree that the organization's leaders must be committed to QI if an organization-wide program is to succeed. They also agree the move to QI is not a move that can be accomplished in a short time. QI is not a "quick fix," but requires 2–5 years at a minimum for complete implementation (Varkey, Reller, & Resar, 2007).

The QI organization calls for changes that include a shift from individual responsibility to group or collective responsibility, a shift from administrative authority for problem solving to participative problem solving, a replacement of rigid procedures with flexibility and spontaneity, and a problem focus yielding to emphasis on continuous improvement and entrepreneurial thinking (Williams, 2009). Contemporary approaches to the measurement of quality in health care organizations today include the plan-do-study-act (PDSA) process, six-sigma, and lean strategies. Some institutions use principles from different QI methodologies on the same QI project. An example is the use of the "lean-sigma" approach, which is a combination of the lean and six-sigma approaches (Varkey et al., 2007).

# Evidence-Based Practice

In recent years, terms such as evidence-based medicine (EBM), evidence-based practice (EBP), evidence-based nursing, evidence-based health care, and best practices guidelines (BPGs) have emerged and assumed a significant position in health care literature. These terms are probably best understood as decision-making frameworks that assist health care providers with making complex decisions utilizing research and other forms of evidence on a routine basis when formulating those decisions (Melnyk & Fineout-Overholt, 2005). Evidence-based decision frameworks are used to describe methods adopted by practitioners and others in an effort to increase the quality of health care, to decrease variability of care, and to decrease the costs related to providing health care.

Utilization of EBP and BPGs increases the quality of care by attempting to bridge the gap between the discovery of knowledge in health care and the time that knowledge is applied in practice. The Institute of Medicine (IOM) suggests that time-lag may be as long as 20 years (IOM, 2001). The use of EBP and BPGs should decrease inappropriate variability in practice patterns, which often leads to increased costs. For example, a woman diagnosed with Stage II breast cancer in Provo, Utah, should receive the same level of care as a woman who is diagnosed with the same stage of breast cancer in Tampa, Florida, if health care practitioners subscribe to and utilize the latest evidence-based or practice guidelines for the treatment and management of Stage II breast cancer.

Evidence-based medicine utilizes a defined method in four major steps:

1. Eliciting, describing, defining, and refining a structured question about a target population, outcome, and typically, an intervention
2. Systematic and comprehensive review of the literature in an attempt to answer the question
3. Evaluation of the data and data sources retrieved for methodologic rigor (i.e., data obtained as a result of randomized clinical trials as compared to data from anecdotal reports)
4. Analysis of the data uncovered to answer the question (Donald, 2002)

The limitations of EBP include the absence of organizational support and structure to properly utilize this decision-making framework; insufficient skills to frame the question, retrieve the data or analyze the data; and gaps in the literature that make it impossible to sufficiently answer the question. In addition, some clinicians argue that EBP decreases or threatens clinical autonomy in decision making.

The role of the advanced practice nurse in EBP is continuing to expand. APNs are often relied upon to be the clinical leader of EBP. This leadership role includes continually researching and acquiring the most updated versions of BPGs or clinical guidelines; interpreting the guidelines for other staff and for patients and families; successfully implementing the recommendations of the guidelines; and conducting research to determine the effectiveness of the guidelines from clinical, quality, and cost perspectives after implementation. Chapter 17 contains additional information on EBP.

## Summary

This chapter provides a basis for the advanced practice nurse to achieve understanding and appreciation for the utility of leadership and management theories in contemporary nursing practice. By virtue of their roles, advance practice nurses are viewed as leaders and, as such, often have quite visible positions in organizations and the community.

Allison, the CNS in the opening case study, is in a position in which she needs to define her role. To be an effective leader, she must develop a leadership style that considers her personal strengths and weaknesses and fits the needs and personality of the unit. She will also need to use a number of management concepts and principles, particularly related to motivation and change. She must also be prepared to implement QI strategies that will affect the unit to improve client care.

Assimilation of strategies to improve leadership, motivation, change, decision making, and other concepts discussed in this chapter into the practice repertoire of the advanced practitioner in nursing is crucial to the viability and sustainability of the role.

## LEARNING ACTIVITIES

1. Analyze the leadership style of your current supervisor. Does the supervisor's leadership behavior vary from situation to situation? Would the supervisor be classified as a transformational, transactional, charismatic, visionary, or other leader? Why?

2. Assess the organization in which you work today. Are Fayol's and Taylor's principles of management evident in this organization? Give examples.

3. Think back to the last time a major change occurred in your work environment. Was the change a planned change? What were the driving forces and restraining forces? Who was the change agent? Did the change occur as planned?

4. Investigate the integration of evidence-based practices (EBP) in your community and in your specialty area. Have health care providers in your area made a commitment to the integration of EBP? If not, why? If so, to what extent and in what specialty areas?

## REFERENCES

Adams, J. S. (1965). Inequity in social exchanges. In L. Berkowitz (Ed.), *Advances in experimental psychology* (pp. 267–300). New York: Academic Press.

Aguayo, R. (1990). *Dr. Deming: The American who taught the Japanese about quality*. New York: Fireside.

Avolio, B. J., Zhu, W., Koh, W., & Puja, B. (2004). Transformational leadership and organizational commitment: Mediating role of psychological empowerment and moderating role of structural distance. *Journal of Organizational Behavior, 25*, 951–968.

Bass, B. M., Avolio, B. J., Jung, D. I., & Berson, Y. (2003). Predicting unit performance by assessing transformational and transactional leadership. *Journal of Applied Psychology, 88*(2), 207–218.

Bennis, W. (1984). The four competencies of leadership. *Training and Development Journal, 38*(8), 15–19.

Bolino, M. C. (2007). What about us? Relative deprivation among out-group members in Leader-Member Exchange relationships. *Academy of Management Proceedings*, 1–5.

Bono, J. E., & Judge, T. A. (2003). Self concordance at work: Toward understanding the motivational effects of transformational leaders. *Academy of Management Journal, 46*(5), 554–571.

Burns, J. M. (1978). *Leadership*. New York: Harper & Row.

Caplan, E. (1971). *Management accounting and behavioral science*. Reading, MA: Addison-Wesley.

Carson, P. P., Carson, K. D., & Roe, C. W. (1993). Social power bases: A meta-analytic examination of interrelationships and outcomes. *Journal of Applied Psychology, 23*, 1150–1169.

Chemers, M., Harp, R., Rhodewalt, F., & Wysocki, J. (1985). A person–environment analysis of job stress: A contingency model explanation. *Journal of Personality and Social Psychology, 49*(3), 628–635.

Conger, J. A., & Kanungo, R. N. (1988). Behavioral dimensions of leadership. In J. A. Conger & R. N. Kanungo (Eds.), *Charismatic leadership*. San Francisco: Jossey-Bass.

Crosby, P. B. (1979). *Quality is free*. New York: McGraw-Hill.

Daft, R. L., & Marcic, D. (2009). *Understanding management* (6th ed.). Mason, OH: South-Western Cengage Learning.

Deming, W. F. (1989). *Out of the crisis*. Cambridge, MA: Massachusetts Institute of Technology Press.

Donald, A. (2002). How to practice evidence-based medicine. *Medscape General Medicine, 5*(1). Available at: http:www.medscape.com/viewpublication/122_index.

Drafke, M. (2009). *The human side of organizations* (10th ed.). Upper Saddle River, New Jersey: Pearson Prentice-Hall.

DuBrin, A. J. (2005). *Fundamentals of organizational behavior* (3rd ed.). Mason, OH: Thomson South-Western.

DuBrin, A. J. (2009). *Essentials of management* (8th ed.). Mason, OH: South-Western Cengage Learning.

Fayol, H. (1949). *General and industrial management*. London: Pitman & Sons.

Fiedler, F. (1967). *A theory of leadership effectiveness*. New York: McGraw-Hill.

Fiedler, F. (1969). Style or circumstances: The leadership enigma. *Psychology Today, 2*(10), 38–43.

Fiedler, F., Chemers, M., & Mahar, L. (1976). *Improving leadership effectiveness: The leader match concept*. New York: Wiley.

French, J., & Raven, B. (1959). The bases of social power. In D. Cartwright (Ed.), *Studies in social power*. Ann Arbor, MI: University of Michigan.

Georgopoulos, B., Mahoney, G., & Jones, N. (1957). A path-goal approach to productivity. *Journal of Applied Psychology, 53*, 345–353.

Gillem, T. (1988). Deming's 14 points and hospital quality: Responding to the consumer's demand for the best value health care. *Journal of Nursing Quality Assurance, 2*(3), 70–78.

Goleman, D., Boyatzis, R., & McKee, A. (2001). Primal leadership: The hidden driver of great performance. *Harvard Business Review, 79*(11), 42–51.

Graen, G., & Cashman, J. F. (1975). A role-making model of leadership in formal organizations: A developmental approach. In Hunt, J. G., & Larson, L. L. (Eds.), *Leadership frontiers* (pp. 143–165). Kent, OH: Kent State University Press.

Graen, G., & Uhl-Bien, M. (1995). Relationship-based approach to leadership: Development of the leader-member exchange (LMX) theory of leadership over 25 years: Applying a multi-level, multi-domain perspective. Special issue: Leadership: The multiple-level approaches (Level 1). *Leadership Quarterly, 6,* 219–247.

Gray, E. R. (1978). The non-linear systems experiment: A requiem. *Business Horizons, 21,* 31–36.

Green, J. P. (1981). People management: New directions for the 1980s. *Administrative Management, 42,* 22–26.

Heineken, J., & McCloskey, J. (1985). Teaching power concepts. *Journal of Nursing Education, 24*(1), 40–42.

Hellriegel, D., Jackson, S. E., & Slocum, J. W. (2005). *Management: A competency-based approach* (10th ed.). Mason, OH: Thomson South-Western.

Hersey, P., & Blanchard, K. (1977). *Management of organizational behavior: Utilizing human resources.* Englewood Cliffs, NJ: Prentice-Hall.

Herzberg, F. (1966). *Work and the nature of man.* Cleveland: World.

Hitt, M. A., Black, J. S., & Porter, L. W. (2009). *Management* (2nd ed.). Upper Saddle River, NJ: Pearson Prentice-Hall.

House, R. (1971). A path-goal theory of leader effectiveness. *Administrative Science Quarterly, 16,* 321–338.

House, R. J. (1977). A 1976 theory of charismatic leadership. In J. G. Hunt & L. L. Larson (Eds.), *Leadership: The cutting edge.* Carbondale, IL: Southern Illinois University Press.

House, R. J. (1996). Path-goal theory of leadership: Lessons, legacy, and a reformulated theory. *Leadership Quarterly, 7*(3), 323–352.

Institute of Medicine (IOM) (2001). *Crossing the quality chasm: A new health care system for the 21st century.* Washington, DC: National Academy Press.

Jens, R., & Heinitz, K. (2007). Transformational and charismatic leadership: Assessing the convergent, divergent, and criterion validity of the Multifactor Leadership Questionnaire and the Conger and Kanungo Scales. *Leadership Quarterly, 18,* 121–133.

Judge, T. A., & Piccolo, R. F. (2004). Transformational and transactional leadership: A meta-analytic test of their relative validity. *Journal of Applied Psychology, 89*(5), 755–768.

Jung, D. D., & Sosik, J. J. (2006). Who are the spellbinders? Identifying personal attributes of charismatic leaders. *Journal of Leadership and Organizational Studies, 12*(4), 12–26.

Juran, J. M. (1988). *Quality control handbook.* New York: McGraw-Hill.

Katz, N. H., & Lawyer, J. W. (1985). *Communication and conflict resolution skills.* Dubuque, IA: Kendall/Hunt.

Kay, A. (1973). Where being nice to workers didn't work. *Business Week, 1,* 98–100.

Kopelman, R. E., Prottas, D. J., & Davis, A. L. (2008). Douglas McGregor's Theory X and Y: Toward a construct-valid measure. *Journal of Management Issues, 20*(2), 255–271.

Kotter, J. P. (1995, Mar/Apr). Leading changes: Why transformation efforts fail. *Harvard Business Review,* pp. 59–67.

Lewin, K. (1951). *Field theory in social science.* New York: Harper & Row.

Lewin, K., & Lippitt, R. (1938). An experimental approach to the study of autocracy and democracy: A preliminary note. *Sociometry, 1,* 292–300.

Malone, E. (1975). The non-linear systems experiment in participative management. *Journal of Business, 48,* 52–64.

Maslow, A. (1968). *Toward a psychology of being.* New York: Van Nostrand Reinhold.

Masters, M. L., & Masters, R. J. (1993). Building TQM into nursing management. *Nursing Economics, 11*(5), 274–291.

Melnyk, B. M., & Fineout-Overholt, E. (2005). *Evidence-based practice in nursing and healthcare.* Philadelphia: Lippincott Williams & Wilkins.

Minor, J. (1980). *Theories of organizational behavior.* Hinsdale, IL: Dryden.

Morse, J., & Lorsch, J. (1970). Beyond theory Y. *Harvard Business Review, 48*(3), 61–68.

Peters, T. (1987). *Thriving on chaos.* New York: Alfred A. Knopf.

Podsakoff, P. M., Bommer, W. H., Podsakoff, N. P., & Mackenzie, S. B. (2005). Relationships between leader reward and punishment behaviour and subordinate attitudes, perceptions, and behaviours: A meta-analytic review of existing and new research. *Organizational Behavior and Human Decision Processes, 99,* 113–142.

Port, O. (1991, October 25). Dueling pioneers. *Business Week,* p. 17.

Robbins, S. P., & Coulter, M. (2005). *Management* (8th ed.). Upper Saddle River, NJ: Prentice-Hall.

Robbins, S. P., & Judge, T. A. (2009). *Organizational behavior* (13th ed.). Upper Saddle River, NJ: Pearson Prentice-Hall.

Rue, L. W., & Byars, L. (1977). *Management—Theory and application.* Homewood, IL: Richard D. Irwin.

Schaubroeck, J., Lam, S. K., & Cha, S. E. (2007). Embracing transformational leadership: Team values and the impact of the leader behavior on team performance. *Journal of Applied Psychology, 92*(4), 1020–1030.

Schriesheim, C. A., Castro, S. L., Zhou, X. T., & DeChurch, L. A. (2006). An investigation of path-goal and transformational leadership theory predictions at the individual level of analysis. *Leadership Quarterly, 17,* 21–38.

Simon, H. A. (1965). *The shape of automation for man and management*. New York: Harper Textbooks.

Tannenbaum, R., & Schmidt, W. H. (1973). How to choose a leadership pattern. *Harvard Business Review, 5*, 162–180.

Taylor, F. W. (1911). *The principles of scientific management*. New York: Harper.

Thomas, K. W. (1976). *Handbook of industrial and organizational psychology*. Chicago: Rand-McNally.

Thomas, K. W., & Kilmann, R. H. (1974). *The Thomas-Kilmann conflict mode instrument*. Tuxedo Park, NY: Xicom.

Tomey, A. M. (2009). *Guide to nursing management and leadership* (8th ed.). St. Louis: Mosby Elsevier.

Varkey, P., Reller, M. K., & Resar, R. K. (2007). Basics of quality improvement in health care. *Mayo Clinic Proceedings, 82*(6), 735–739.

Vecchio, R. P., Justin, J. E., & Pearce, C. L. (2008). The utility of transactional and transformational leadership for predicting performance and satisfaction within a path-goal theory framework. *Journal of Occupational and Organizational Psychology, 81*, 71–82.

Vroom, V. H. (1960). *Some personality determinants of the effects of participation*. Englewood Cliffs, NJ: Prentice-Hall.

Vroom, V. H. (1964). *Work and motivation*. New York: Wiley.

Vroom, V. H., & Jago, A. G. (1988). *The new leadership: Managing participation in organizations*. Englewood Cliffs, NJ: Prentice-Hall.

Vroom, V. H. & Jago, A. G. (2007). The role of situations in leadership. *The American Psychologist,* 17–24.

Vroom, V. H., & Yetton, P. W. (1973). *Leadership and decision-making*. Pittsburgh: University of Pittsburgh Press.

Wagner, J. A., & Hollenbeck, J. R. (2005). *Organizational behavior* (5th ed.). Mason, OH: Thomson South-Western.

Walumbwa, F. O., Avolio, B. J., & Zhu, W. (2008). How transformational leadership weaves its influence on individual job performance: The role of identification and efficacy beliefs. *Personnel Psychology, 61*, 793–825.

Wang, H., Law, K. S., Hackett, R. D., Wang, D., & Chen Z. X. (2005). Leader–member exchange as a mediator of the relationship between transformational leadership and followers' performance and organizational citizenship behavior. *Academy of Management Journal, 48*(3), 430–432.

Washington, R. R. (2007). Empirical relationships between theories of servant, transformational, and transactional leadership. *Academy of Management Proceedings,* 1–6.

Weber, M. (1970). Bureaucracy. In W. Sexton (Ed.), *Organization theories* (pp. 39–43). Columbus, OH: Charles E. Merrill.

Williams, C. R. (2009). *Management* (5th ed.). Mason, OH: South-Western Cengage Learning.

# 16

# Learning Theories

## Evelyn Wills and Melanie McEwen

*B*arbara Davis is a family nurse practitioner working in a community clinic. Recently, she cared for Frank Young, a 65-year-old African-American who came to the clinic at his wife's insistence because of recurring, severe headaches. Mr. Young reported that his headaches started about 6 months ago; he attributed them to stress caused by his recent retirement.

Mr. Young's physical findings indicated that he was about 50 lbs overweight and that his blood pressure while sitting was 204/110. His lower legs and feet were slightly edematous, and laboratory tests revealed a total cholesterol reading of 290 mg/dL. All other laboratory blood and urine results were normal.

Barbara explained to Mr. Young that he has high blood pressure and asked to discuss the problem with both him and his wife. She led the Youngs to a room in which they sat in comfortable chairs around a small table. Barbara began the discussion by asking if the couple had any experience with hypertension (HTN). She explained the relationship among HTN, race, age, gender, and weight and described its prevalence among various groups. She showed the Youngs a short video that used nonmedical terms to describe HTN, visually illustrated the physiologic changes that cause HTN, and then explained some of the possible complications. After the video, Barbara questioned the Youngs to evaluate their level of understanding. A 15-minute discussion followed in which Barbara described management strategies. She gave Mr. Young two prescriptions and explained what they were for and how to take them. Following the explanation, she had him repeat the information to her. They also discussed the importance of limiting sodium intake, and Barbara gave the Youngs a booklet that highlighted the sodium content in various foods.

At the end of the appointment, they reviewed the ways to lower Mr. Young's blood pressure and made a follow-up appointment for the following week. Barbara encouraged Mrs. Young to accompany her husband to the follow-up meeting and set up an appointment with the clinic's dietitian to go over ways the Youngs could reduce the amount of fat and salt in their diet.

One of the most important roles of the advanced practice nurse (APN) is teaching. Teaching performed by the APN is usually more informal than formal. That is, the APN teaches clients and their families, or students and colleagues, more often on a one-to-one basis as the need arises than in a formal, planned teaching session in a classroom setting. But teaching includes more than just providing clients with information. Because someone has been "told" something does not mean that learning has occurred. Many factors are involved for learning to be successful, and providing information is only one of them.

This chapter provides the APN with tools to facilitate learning for patients, families, and staff. Basic theories of learning can serve as a framework for the APN in all teaching endeavors. Theories provide a way to organize thinking for what will be communicated to other people. They may offer a mechanism whereby the instructor can look at a situation in a different way when current methods are not working, or they may provide a map for charting completely unfamiliar territory. In any event, application of theories helps ensure that learning is optimized, and facilitating learning is an essential objective of the APN.

## What Is Learning?

Learning can be defined as a change in behavior, or a change in mental or emotional functioning (Bastable, 2008, p. 12). Learning occurs as individuals interact with their environment, incorporating new information into what they already know (Braungart & Braungart, 2008; Vandeveer, 2009). Further, if learning is to be permanent, it must be treated as a process that occurs over time rather than an isolated event. Time and repeated contacts are required for an individual to acquire new knowledge that is meaningful and significant (Forrest, 2004).

Learning can be grouped into three categories: psychomotor learning (the acquisition and performance of skills); affective learning (a change in feelings, values, or beliefs); and cognitive learning (acquiring information). Examples of psychomotor learning would include a nursing student mastering certain patient care procedures (e.g., inserting an IV or changing a sterile dressing) and a patient learning to self-inject insulin. Illustrations of affective learning include an alcoholic acquiring strategies to overcome addiction and a nurse developing cultural sensitivity when caring for immigrants. Cognitive learning generally involves the addition of new information, as when a new mother learns how to care for her infant or a novice nurse learns to recognize the signs and symptoms of congestive heart failure. Although not always recognized, psychomotor learning tends to be more easily accomplished and measured than affective and cognitive learning (Rankin & Stallings, 2005). Nurses must understand all three types of learning and know how to facilitate each in patients and their families as well as among other nurses and ancillary staff.

The process of assimilating new knowledge into our daily lives makes all humans constant learners, because learning is necessary for survival. Although all animals can learn, humans are capable of using their knowledge to be creative, predict the future, explain the past, or deal with the present. Indeed, learning is such an important human experience that it has created the desire or curiosity to discover how people learn. This search to understand how people learn has led to the development and formalization of learning theories.

## What Is Teaching?

It must be recognized that while teaching and learning are interrelated, learning occurs as a separate and individual process apart from teaching. Teaching refers to the intentional act of communicating information and is often defined as the facilitation of learning (Bastable, 2008). To accomplish this, teachers must be aware of the learning styles and learning needs of the individual, and how capable that individual is of responding to the demands of instruction (Forrest, 2004).

It is a common assumption that teaching is helping one to gain knowledge. While that is certainly an important component of teaching, knowledge is seldom enough to elicit a change in behavior or thinking. Knowing what should be done and acting on that knowledge are two different things (Saarmann, Daugherty, & Riegel, 2000). For example, a patient with chronic renal failure may *know* that salt and potassium are to be avoided in the diet, but learning has not occurred until that knowledge has been incorporated as a change in behavior.

Anyone who teaches, including a mother or father teaching a child how to put away toys, or a woman teaching a friend to crochet, has some belief regarding how learning occurs. Unfortunately, sometimes the knowledge the teacher possesses about learning is simplistic: "I told you; therefore, you should know." An individual's beliefs about learning can influence that person's behavior regarding what should happen to make learning occur. By understanding basic theories of learning, the APN will be better prepared to help the learner make the transition from gaining knowledge to learning. This chapter presents some of the many theories of learning and describes how they are used to solve problems encountered in the teaching–learning process. These theories may be used by nurses in practice, as well as for designing, implementing, and evaluating research projects.

## Categorization of Learning Theories

Some nurses might question why it is important to understand the process of learning and to know about some of theories of learning. Learning theories describe the processes used to bring about changes in the ways individuals understand information and changes in the ways they perform a task or skill. Further learning theories can help provide a focus for creating an environment and conditions in which teaching can occur more effectively (Vandeveer, 2009). Kurt Lewin is credited with the adage: "There is nothing so practical as a good theory." A good theory enables you to make choices confidently and consistently and to explain or defend why you made the choice you did. Thus, although nursing theory provides the framework for professional assessment of the client's condition or needs and the specific language the nurse uses when making a diagnosis or charting, learning theories explain *how* this information is assimilated and suggests effective ways to present it to the client as an intervention. Learning theory, then, combined with nursing theory, gives APNs guidance as they interact with clients.

There are many different types of learning theories and only a few of the most commonly used in nursing are described in the following sections. The main categories as categorized by Bigge and Shermis (1999) are the behavioral learning theories and the cognitive learning theories. Behavioral learning theories include the works of Pavlov, Skinner, and others. Cognitive learning theories include cognitive-field theories, information-processing theories, interaction theories, and developmental theories (social cognitive/social learning theory), psychodynamic theory (humanistic learning theory), and adult learning theory. Some of the major theories for each group will be discussed briefly, with examples of application from the nursing literature.

# Behavioral Learning Theories

Behavioral theories were among the first to be widely recognized and used in education. Indeed, they were so pervasive in the American educational system in the 1950s and 1960s that many people still associate the term "learning theories" with behavioral theories. Behavioral learning theories served the growing American educational system well during the 20th century. They provided the rapidly expanding system with an organized, systematic approach.

*Behaviorism* focuses on what is directly observable in learners. It is largely based on the works of Ivan Pavlov and Edward Thorndike, who researched how both humans and animals learned, and their work became the basis for behavioral psychology (Hergenhahn & Olson, 2004; Olson & Hergenhahn, 2009; Vandeveer, 2009). In behavioral theories, behavior (response) is viewed as the result of stimulus conditions. The behavioral learning theories that evolved from this perspective are sometimes referred to as the stimulus–response (S–R) model of learning. Some of the major behaviorist theorists include Thorndike (connectionism), Pavlov (classical conditioning), Skinner (operant conditioning), Watson (behaviorism), and Hull (reinforcement). Table 16-1 summarizes the assertions of each of these theorists.

Edward L. Thorndike (1874–1949) was one of the first theorists to attempt scientific studies to understand the learning process. He perceived that learners are empty organisms who respond to stimuli in a random manner. He provided the original S–R framework for behavioral psychology. For Thorndike, learning was the result of associations formed between stimuli and responses (S–R), and the S–R connections were formed through trial and error. Such associations or habits become strengthened or weakened by the nature and frequency of the S–R pairings. The hallmark of connectionism was that learning could be adequately explained without referring to any observable internal states (Thorndike, 1932).

In a well-known study, Pavlov (1849–1936) taught his dog to salivate when a tuning fork was hit by rewarding him with meat powder placed into his mouth. Soon the dog would salivate when the tuning fork was hit even though no meat powder was provided. This involuntary reaction is known as *conditioning*. Pavlov's work is labeled

TABLE 16-1 *Comparison of Behavioral Learning Theories*

| Theorist | Theory Distinctions |
|---|---|
| Thorndike | Original stimulus–response framework; learners respond randomly to stimuli; learning is trial and error |
| Pavlov | Classical conditioning; responses are involuntary and based on experience |
| Skinner | Operant conditioning; learning produces a desirable behavior because it is reinforced or strengthened |
| Hull | Stimulus–response framework (based on Thorndike); includes reinforcement as a characteristic of learning |
| Watson | Behaviorism (based on Pavlov); classical conditioning and "extinguishing" behaviors |

as classical conditioning to differentiate it from other types of S–R associations that deal with voluntary behavior (Braungart & Braungart, 2008). Classical conditioning is what one sees in a child's response to the sight of a needle. The conditioned stimulus (the sight of the needle) is able to evoke the response (crying) formerly reserved for the unconditional stimulus (actual pain from an injection). Response to the sight of a needle is learned behavior based on experience.

To B. F. Skinner (1904–1990), the purpose of psychology is to predict and control the behavior of individuals. He defined learning as a change in probability of response and coined the term *operant conditioning*. An *operant* is a set of behaviors that constitutes an individual doing something. Operant conditioning is the learning process whereby a desirable behavior is made more likely to occur in the future or to occur more frequently because it is reinforced or strengthened (Olson & Hergenhahn, 2009; Ormrod, 2004). When the desired response occurs, whether accidental or planned, a reward that is meaningful to the learner is provided so recurrence of the desired response is increased. In the previously discussed classical conditioning, the person in question receives reinforcement no matter what he or she does, whereas in an operant conditioning situation the individual's behavior causes the reward to happen.

John B. Watson (1878–1958) was the first American psychologist to incorporate Pavlov's work into his own. While Watson's research methods would be called into question under today's standards, he did demonstrate classical conditioning in an experiment where he subjected a young boy named Albert to a white rat. At first, the boy was not afraid of the rat. However, Watson created a loud noise whenever the boy touched the rat. Eventually, the boy associated touching the rat with the noxious stimulus, and became afraid of the rat and other small animals. Watson then demonstrated the idea of "extinguishing" the conditioned behavior by offering the rat to the boy without the loud noise (Lefrancois, 2000; Ormrod, 2004). Watson's work has been used to explain and treat fears, phobias, and prejudices that people develop in response to situations and events. Watson is generally credited with originating the term behaviorism (Olson & Hergenhahn, 2009).

Clark L. Hull (1884–1952) based his studies on Thorndike's work, but included *reinforcement* as a major characteristic of learning. Reinforcement is a complex concept that is widely used in education today. Reinforcement is a consequence of an action that makes that action more likely to be repeated. Reinforcement may be internal/external, positive/negative, self-administered, social, or impersonal (Roberts, 1975). Reinforcement can be seen in many ways, from a simple smile (or frown) to aversion therapy (e.g., the quit smoking clinics that have individuals smoke one cigarette after another until they become sick). Problems can arise because the behavior the teacher intends to reinforce may not be the actual behavior that is reinforced.

Behaviorists are concerned with the observable and measurable aspects of human behavior. Basically, behaviorists believe that behavior can be controlled (and thus learning has occurred) through rewarding desirable behavior and ignoring or punishing behavior that is undesirable. Reinforcing or strengthening the behavior increases the chance of its recurrence in the future. These theorists are concerned with behavior modification and make much use of the concepts of reflexes, reactions, objective measurement, quantitative data, sequence of behavior, and reinforcement schedules (Ormrod, 2004; Ozmon & Craver, 2003). Box 16-1 summarizes characteristics of behavioral learning theories.

Teachers who subscribe to this viewpoint are considered designers and controllers of students' behavior. The teacher is responsible for what students should learn and for evaluating how, when, and if they have learned. Teachers are expected to be content experts, transmit prescribed content, control the way learners receive and use the content,

| BOX 16-1 | *Characteristics of Behavioral Learning Theories* |

- Focus on behavior modification, reflexes, reaction, and reinforcement
- Concerned with observable and measurable aspects of human behavior
- Posit that behavior can be controlled through rewarding desirable behavior and ignoring or punishing undesirable behavior

and then test to determine if they have received it (Knowles, 1981). Learning objectives (also called behavioral objectives, instructional objectives, or performance criteria) are broken down into a large number of very small tasks and reinforced one by one. The tasks are organized so that understanding develops progressively. This premise has led to the development of programmed texts and computer-assisted instruction. Tests are used in a classroom situation to measure the amount of knowledge a student has gained.

Use of behavioral theory encourages the development of clear behavioral outcomes and methods for evaluating those desired behaviors. It works well for many of the psychomotor skills that must be accomplished for both nurses and patients. Behavioral theory, however, is not without detractors. Because the learner assumes a relatively passive role, there is a possibility that old behaviors will be resumed once the learner is removed from the highly structured and controlled environments created by behaviorally based teaching methods. In other words, without the affective and cognitive components of learning, there has not been a change in feelings or thinking for the learner. Once they are returned to the original environment that fostered and rewarded the undesirable behavior, chances are high that the original behavior will return. Many question whether behavioral techniques alone are capable of producing permanent changes in behavior.

## APPLICATION TO NURSING

Behaviorist principles are widely used by nurses, nursing educators, and staff developers. For example, learning contracts with clients are an outgrowth of this perspective. Likewise, nurses often use reinforcement when they comment on how well clients are following their treatment regimens and when they correctly repeat instructions. Also, much of nursing education is directed toward having students meet behavioral objectives, which is a hallmark of behavioral theories (see Chapter 20).

## Cognitive Learning Theories

In contrast to behavioral theories, which generally ignore the thoughts, feelings, and cognitive processes of the learner, cognitive learning theories emphasize the mental processes and activities that go on within the learner (Vandeveer, 2009). Cognitive theorists do not view reward as a condition for learning, although they do not negate the role of reinforcement. The learner's own goals, thoughts, expectations, motivations, and abilities in the processing of information are seen as the foundations for learning.

Cognitive learning theory began to gain popular momentum in the 1960s when the recognition of the limitations of behavioral theories led to the development of more complete theories to frame and explain how people learn, and how permanent changes in behavior are accomplished. One of the most important theorists in cognitive science, Jean Piaget, however, developed major components of his theory in the 1920s.

Cognitive theories focus on the operations of the mind and on how thoughts influence an individual's actions in relation to the environment (Vandeveer, 2009). Several major subcategories of cognitive learning theories have evolved over time. Those described in the following sections include gestalt (cognitive-field) theories, information-processing theories, cognitive development theories, social learning theories, psychodynamic theory, and adult learning theory. Representative examples useful for nurses are presented in the following sections.

## COGNITIVE-FIELD (GESTALT) THEORIES

A break with behaviorism occurred when the concept of "insight" learning was introduced into the gestalt theories. "Gestalt" is a German word that refers to the configuration or patterned organization of cognitive elements (Braungart & Braungart, 2008). The gestalt view of learning focuses on organization of a person's perceptual field to organize and make sense of multiple parts. The scientific view underlying gestalt principles is field theory. Field theory espouses that a "field" is a dynamic, interrelated system in which any part can affect all other parts, and that the whole is more than the sum of the parts (Olson & Hergenhahn, 2009). Gestalt theory and field theory have become so closely associated that they are commonly referred to as cognitive-field theory.

The cognitive-field psychologists consider learning to be closely related to perception. They define learning in terms of reorganization of the learner's perceptual or psychological world—his or her field. The field includes a simultaneous and mutual interaction among all the forces or stimuli affecting the person—the internal environment as well as the external environment. Experience is the interaction of a person and his or her perceived environment, whereas behavior is the result of the interplay of these forces. Consequently, perception and experiences of reality are uniquely individual, based on a person's total life experiences. Nothing exists in and of itself, but only in relationship to something else. Learning, then, is the process of discovering and understanding the relationships among people, things, and ideas in the field. Learning is viewed as an active, goal-oriented process that is accomplished when information is processed and the "aha" moment is experienced. Transfer of information from the teacher to the student does not constitute learning. In order for learning to be accomplished, students must assume responsibility for learning and discover and assign their own meaning in order to understand and truly learn content. Through the learning process the learner gains new insights or changes old ones. The purpose of learning is to think more effectively in a wide variety of situations, and thus be able to solve problems.

Because cognitive-field theorists are concerned with the progressive development of the total person, they perceive self-actualization as the driving force that motivates all human behavior. Motivation involves the forces operating in a particular situation that cause the person to want to do something (as opposed to the behavioral theorists who think of motivation as a drive that reduces a perceived need). Growth and development are important in motivation and necessary for self-actualization to occur. As an individual matures, the forces operating to induce one to do something change.

Kurt Lewin (1890–1947), one of the major gestalt theorists, believed that humans have a basic need to bring order to a situation and that motivation to learn is stimulated by the ambiguity perceived in the situation. By involving students in the learning process the instructor helps learners see the need to learn. Through the use of verbal explanations, showing pictures, drawing diagrams, and other teaching activities, the instructor helps the individual understand significant relationships so that the learner can

| BOX 16-2 | *Characteristics of Cognitive-Field Learning Theories* |
|---|---|

- Learning is related to perception
- Perceptions of reality and experiences are uniquely individual and based on life experiences
- Thoughts influence actions
- Motivation is key to learning
- Self-actualization is the main motivating force

organize the experience into a functional pattern. By arranging a sequence of problems that flow hierarchically in level of difficulty and providing appropriate resources for the learner to use to solve the problems, the instructor creates a motivating environment for learning (Knowles, Holton, & Swanson, 2005).

Cognitive-field theorists believe people can learn information cognitively without changing their behavior and that motivation is the key. Motivation is an extremely difficult concept to implement. In the health care field one often hears reports that an individual is noncompliant, when in actuality the person is not motivated (for whatever reason) to do what the health care professionals perceive as the correct thing to do. Indeed, it often takes months and even years to find the right combination of factors that motivate an individual. As a child, Mr. Young, from the opening case study, would probably rebel against changing his eating habits, but he may be more likely to be motivated to do so as an adult because he understands the relationship between his diet and his headaches. Box 16-2 depicts characteristics of cognitive-field theories.

### Application to Nursing

Barbara, the nurse in the case study, used cognitive-field theory when she had the Youngs move into a room more conducive to learning. By controlling the external stimuli affecting the situation, she allowed the brain to focus more on the information she was presenting. By using visual models as well as her verbal explanation, she involved more senses in the learning process and thereby more of the whole person. Mr. Young's pain served as a good motivator, increasing his desire for relief and his willingness to participate in the learning process to prevent future episodes.

In reviewing recent nursing literature, cognitive-field theory and/or gestalt theory was used several times. Carter and Rukholm (2008) analyzed nurses' writing activities and teacher interactions and searched for evidence of critical thinking in an online setting. They found nurses' critical thinking and writing competence grew over time in the online activity. Leigh (2007) studied the incorporation of high-fidelity patient simulators and nursing students' feelings of self-efficacy and confidence in performing nursing care in an intensive care situation. She found that the feelings of confidence in the ability to think critically under stress were increased in the students.

## INFORMATION-PROCESSING MODELS

Information-processing theories emerged in the 1970s. They arose from the field of artificial intelligence as researchers attempted to create computer systems to simulate human cognitive skills (Byrnes, 2001; Vandeveer & Norton, 2005). Learning theorists using these models are concerned with the process of acquiring information, remembering it, and using it for problem solving. These theories propose an elaborate set of internal processes to account for how learning and retention occur (Ormrod, 2004).

In information-processing theories, human memory is thought to be composed of three stores: sensory store, short-term store, and long-term store. Information from the environment passes sequentially through the stores. The sensory store (also known as the sensory memory, iconic memory, or echoic memory) holds incoming information long enough that preliminary cognitive processing can begin. Information stored in the sensory memory is stored basically in the form in which it was sensed—visual input is stored visually, auditory input in an auditory form. Although the sensory store has unlimited capacity, information is stored very briefly.

The short-term memory is the most active component of the memory systems. Thinking occurs within the short-term memory and determines which information will be attended to within the sensory memory. The short-term memory holds information while it is being processed from both the sensory memory and the long-term memory. Interpretation of newly received environment input is interpreted in the short-term memory.

The long-term memory is the most complicated of the memory systems and the one that has received the most research. Long-term memory is thought to have an unlimited capacity, but the experts disagree regarding how long the information remains in storage. Some experts believe it is there forever, but others believe the information is lost through a variety of forgetting processes. Information is rarely stored in the long-term memory in the form in which it is received. What is stored is the "gist" of what was seen or heard rather than word-for-word sentences or precise mental images. Individuals organize the information that is stored in the long-term memory so related pieces of information are associated together (Ormrod, 2004).

In information-processing models, learning consists of strategies to transfer information from short-term storage to long-term storage. Information in the short-term memory (also known as the working memory) is lost within 5–20 seconds if action is not taken to reinforce it (Byrnes, 2001). For example, repeating the individual's name when introduced to a new person increases the ability to recall it at a later time. It is important for an instructor using this theory to present information in an organized manner, to overlap the information with previously learned knowledge, and to show the learner how the material is organized and how it relates to what was previously learned (Ormrod, 2004). External stimuli are thought to support several different types of ongoing internal processes involved in learning, remembering, and performing. Techniques such as visual imagery facilitate learning and the recall of information.

Along with remembering is the question of why people forget. Three theories have been proposed to explain this phenomenon: decay and interference theories, and the loss of retrieval cues. Decay theory proposes that information weakens over time, if it is not practiced or used. This is similar to the "use it or lose it" theory of muscle strength. Interference theory postulates that something interferes between the information already in storage and the new information being learned. If the new information being learned interferes with previously stored information, it is called retroactive interference; if old information interferes with the learning of new information, it is called proactive interference (Ormrod, 2004). Loss of retrieval cues involves the weakening of associations among the retrieval cues and records (Byrnes, 2001). For example, a nurse frequently sees a colleague from another unit in the cafeteria. The nurse knows this person's name and recognizes him or her. When the nurse meets this same person in the grocery store in street clothes, however, the nurse knows she knows the person, but may not recall from where or the name. Because the person is out of context, the associations are not readily available for recall.

### Application to Nursing

Nurses in practice and research have used information-processing theories. In the opening case study, by asking the Youngs to repeat some actions they could take to assist in lowering Mr. Young's blood pressure, Barbara was helping the information to be stored in their long-term memory. In examples from the nursing literature, O'Neill, Dluhy, and Chin (2005) used an information-processing theory as a framework for creating a computerized clinical decision-making model to assist novice nurses in making clinical judgments. In another work, Higgins (1999) used information-processing theories as a framework to study nurses' perception of collaborative nurse–physician decision making and its impact on client outcomes. The study concluded that the nurses' perception of collaboration did not predict client outcomes and that decision–task complexity did not have an impact on collaboration and client outcome prediction.

## COGNITIVE DEVELOPMENT OR INTERACTION THEORIES

Cognitive development theories assume that behavior, mental processes, and the environment are interrelated. Also termed interaction theories, they are concerned with the progressive development and changes in thinking, reasoning, and perception of individual learners. A major assumption of cognitive theories is that learning occurs as a sequential process. Learning takes place over time, as when a child explores and interacts with the environment.

The experiential learning model exemplifies the interaction theories, which postulate that individuals learn from their immediate experiences and that learning happens in all human settings (Kolb, 1984). Learning is how individuals adapt and cope with the environment (the world) in which they live. Because each person's experience is unique, individuals develop a preferred style for learning. Whereas behavioral objectives state what the student will learn, experiential learning focuses on the conditions of learning. The instructor's role is to create an environment for learning and the experiences that support student understanding of the whole rather than its separate parts (Rogers & Freiberg, 1994). This is achieved through activities such as group process, problem-solving activities, and simulation exercises. Some of the theories noted for this perspective are Piaget's cognitive development theory, Gagne's conditions of learning, Perry's theory of intellectual and ethical development, and Bandura's social learning theories. Box 16-3 summarizes characteristics of cognitive development/interaction theories.

### Piaget

Jean Piaget (1896–1980) is probably the best known of the cognitive development theorists. He believed that cognitive development occurs in stages and that the stages occur in a fixed order and are universal to persons everywhere. He identified the following stages: sensorimotor, preoperational, concrete operational, and formal operational.

---

**BOX 16-3** *Characteristics of Cognitive Development/Interaction Learning Theories*

- Behavior, mental processes, and the environment are interrelated
- Individuals learn from their experiences
- Learning is how individuals adapt to and cope with their environment
- Focus is on conditions that promote learning

According to Piaget, for learning to occur, an individual must be able to assimilate new information into existing cognitive structures or schemes; that is, the new experience must overlap with previous knowledge. Behavior becomes more intelligent as coordination between the reactions to objects becomes progressively more interrelated and complex. Cognitive development begins in the sensorimotor stage (which is evident from birth until about 2 years of age) with the baby's use of the senses and movement to explore its world. In the preoperational stage (from about 2 years old until about age 6 or 7), action patterns evolve into the symbolic but illogical thinking of the preschooler. In this stage, language ability grows rapidly (Berk, 2003; Bigge & Shermis, 1999). In the concrete operational stage, cognition is transformed into the more organized reasoning of the school-aged child (age 6–7 until about 11 or 12). Abstract reasoning begins with the formal operational stage of the adolescent where youth are able to construct ideals and reason realistically about the future (Berk, 2003; Ormrod, 2004).

In Piaget's work, it is the schemes, or psychological structures, that change with age. Individuals build new schemes by adapting their experiences into previous knowledge. Assimilation and accommodation processes make up the adaptive process (Berk, 2003).

Many adults, however, have not developed complete formal operational thinking and need concrete examples before being presented with abstract ideas. Thus, it is important for the teacher to present information in a manner appropriate for the stage of development. The APN has no formal means of testing an individual's cognitive development stage, but must rely on the individual's verbal interaction during the assessment process. In the case study, Barbara could do this by using a familiar example of a clogged sink to explain what was occurring inside the blood vessels.

### Application to Nursing

A significant number of nursing articles can be found that use Piaget's theory either as a conceptual framework for a research study or to interpret or describe findings or actions. For example, Dickey, Kiefner, and Beidler (2002) used Piaget's writings on development in a discussion on children's and adolescent's ability to assent, consent, or dissent to participation in medical research. Another study used Piaget's theory as the conceptual framework in a cross-cultural examination of children's fears of medical experiences (Mahat, Scoloveno, & Cannella, 2004), and a third used Piaget's work to describe the processes children use to cope with disasters (Deering, 2000). Finally, LaFleur and Raway (1999) presented a nursing study using Piaget's theory which compared the perception of pain intensity between school-aged children and adolescents. Subjects ranked the word descriptors "pain," "hurt," and "ache." Findings indicated that children and adolescents associate similar levels of intensity with each of the words, but associate different experiences with each.

### Gagne

Robert M. Gagne (1916–2002) believed that much of individual's learning (from sensorimotor to highly complex intellectual skills) requires different conditions for learning to be successful. He classified learning outcomes into five different categories: intellectual skills, verbal information, cognitive strategies, motor skills, and attitudes. Each category has subcategories and involves both internal and external conditions that contribute to, or interfere with, the learning process (Gagne, 1985). Gagne believed that there are eight different types of learning that proceed sequentially in a hierarchical order (Box 16-4).

For Gagne (1985), teaching means arranging the conditions that are external to the learner. When trying to get a client or patient to understand a concept (such as HTN in

| BOX 16-4 | *Gagne's Types of Learning* |
|---|---|

1. *Signal learning:* An involuntary response occurs to a specific stimulus (based on Pavlov's conditioned response).
2. *Stimulus–response:* A voluntary response occurs to a specific stimulus (similar to Skinner's operant conditioning).
3. Chaining: Two or more stimulus–response (S–R) associations occur and a sequence of behaviors is learned.
4. Verbal association: The chaining of verbal S–R connections.
5. Discrimination learning: The learner responds to one stimulus but not a similar one.
6. Concept learning: The learner organizes different stimuli into a class and then responds to any member of that class in the same way.
7. Principle or rule learning: A chain of two or more concepts.
8. Problem solving: The combination of two or more principles or rules to form higher-order thinking patterns.

Source: Gagne (1985).

the case study), it is important not only to provide a definition of the concept but also to give many positive examples to illustrate the concept, while at the same time giving negative examples to illustrate what the concept is not. The APN can test clients' understanding of a concept by asking them to think of their own examples and applications.

*Application to Nursing*

Gagne's principles have been used in some nursing studies. Shawler (2008) describes a strategy that uses standardized patients (actors instructed to simulate a set of symptoms) to teach graduate nursing students about complex mental disorders. In a survey of nurse anesthetists, respondents were asked to report the frequency of their experience of one of 24 selected untoward pathophysiologic conditions in their practice. The respondents overwhelmingly believed that experiential learning was required to prepare anesthetists to manage untoward events (Fallacaro & Crosby, 2000).

In another example, Ward and McCormack (2000) described how they created a learning culture as a subelement of the overall work environment. The intention was to shift the emphasis away from classroom-based education to learning at and from work, so as to remove the theory–practice gap and create a means of integrating learning with practice.

**Perry**

William G. Perry is a cognitive theorist who did most of his work on university-age students. His work had been criticized by psychologists and educators because his initial study sample consisted mainly of young male Harvard University students from privileged backgrounds (Perry, 1999). However, since 1970 his work has been replicated numerous times, and has been found to be valid and reliable. As a result, it has become influential in higher education (Vandeveer & Norton, 2005).

Perry's theory of intellectual and ethical development is similar to Piaget's regarding how individuals learn. Like Piaget, Perry's theory posits that learners move along a developmental continuum, both logically and psychologically (Perry, 1999). Also like Piaget, Perry believes that a certain amount of disequilibrium is necessary for accommodation to occur. However, rather than first being concerned with problem solving and application of logic, Perry's model is more concerned with how learners move from a dualistic (black versus white, right versus wrong) view of the world to a more relativistic view. Accepting the relativistic view requires the learner to adopt the notion that knowledge is not absolute, and that there is no absolute criteria or authority for deciding right or wrong. Also, like other learning models, Perry concludes that different learners require different learning environments (Kurfiss, 1996).

Perry's theory describes nine positions of intellectual development. The more advanced the position, the more the person is likely to utilize formal reasoning. Perry's nine positions are grouped into three periods of development. The first period, which is composed of positions 1, 2, and 3, is "dualism." The dualist considers knowledge to be absolute and his/her belief systems are unquestioned and unanswered. Authorities are considered to have all the right answers, and to question authority is unthinkable. Position 1 is termed "basic duality" and is composed of a child's basic set of understanding of issues of truth, morality, and values.

Perry's (1999) positions 2 and 3 of the first period (dualism) are termed "multiplicity prelegitimate" and "multiplicity subordinate," respectively. In these periods, much of the knowledge base is still considered absolute, but people begin to recognize that there are some gray areas. The learner can accept multiple perspectives, but rather than evaluate and apply reason to different viewpoints, the learner will simply seek to please the teacher and "go with the flow." Ironically, as the student actively seeks "what the teacher wants," the learner begins to acquire the fundamental mechanisms of independent thought (Kurfiss, 1996).

Relativism, the second period in intellectual development (positions 4, 5, and 6), requires recognition that all knowledge is not absolute truth. In this period, students progressively develop strategies for dealing with ambiguities and begin to consider the context when making decisions about questions of knowledge. Learners view authorities and experts as fellow learners, albeit more experienced at processing and making sense of the information in a given field. As the person moves from the end of this stage to the next period, there is a realization that one is responsible for defining oneself, and that the condition of one's existence is influenced by his or her own life choices.

The final period is termed "Commitments" (positions 7, 8, and 9) (Perry, 1999). Here the learner becomes skilled in rational processes and can commit to a system of values, beliefs, and opinions that is used to define the self. Decisions are made through conscious consideration of alternatives based on accumulated learning and experiences. There is willingness to accept alternate viewpoints and decisions made by others (Kurfiss, 1996).

### Application to Nursing

A few citations discussing use of Perry's work in the nursing literature were identified. For example, Rapps, Riegel, and Glaser (2001) used Perry's theory of cognitive development as the basis for developing a predictive model to enhance critical thinking in registered nurses. They examined the hierarchical levels of cognitive development (dualism, relativism, and commitment) and determined that critical thinking skills were significant only in the dualistic level. Aquilino (1997) used Perry's theory to examine the processes used by nursing students to obtain clinical knowledge. Using Perry's work to interpret her study, she determined that her findings supported the notion that college students fall in the multiplicity or early relativism phase of cognitive development. Finally, McGovern (1995) also used Perry's work to examine the relationship among cognitive development, moral development, and critical thinking in sophomore nursing students and determined that Perry's work benefited interpretation of the findings.

### Bandura

Albert Bandura's (1977a) Social Learning Theory was based on the concept of reciprocal determinism and concerned with the social influences that affect learning (e.g., groups, culture, and ethnicity). In this theory, environment, cognitive factors, and behavior interact with one another so each variable affects the other two. For example, people learn from the continual bombardment of environmental stimuli without being aware that they are doing so.

Bandura's theory focuses on how people learn from one another and encompasses such concepts as observational learning, imitation, and modeling (Bandura, 1977a). Many behaviors that people exhibit have been acquired through observation and modeling of others. Individuals can imitate behaviors of someone they admire. For example, teenagers often imitate the behavior of their latest movie or rock star idol, or a nursing student may imitate the behaviors of a registered nurse who exemplifies the student's concept of professionalism.

Learning by watching or listening to others (vicarious learning) can occur without imitating the behaviors observed. In this instance, people can verbally describe the behavior, but may not demonstrate it until later, when there is a need to do so. The concept of vicarious learning is used frequently by schools of nursing. Because not all students can care for clients with the same condition, nursing schools have students share their clinical experiences in postconferences. Students learn from each other's experiences, but may not have an opportunity to implement the learning until after they graduate.

In recent years, Bandura has focused more on the underpinnings of constructivism and social cognition. He has stressed that the learner is actively involved with the environment through personal selection, intentionality, and self-regulation of the learning process based on his own "filter" of the world. People may actively select their own role models and regulate their own attitudes and actions regarding learning. An important finding of Bandura's research for health care professionals is that self-efficacy promotes learning and productive human function. This implies that nurses should promote patients' independence and confidence rather than simply accepting and endorsing dependent behaviors in order to facilitate learning and health promotion.

*Application to Nursing*

Numerous recent nursing articles cite using Bandura's theory. Indeed, according to a review of published research reports, Montgomery (2002) found that Bandura's social cognitive theory, the health belief model, and the health promotion model were the most significant theories for nursing research related to adolescent health promotion. Bandura's theory has also been used by nurses to develop successful interventions. For example, Dougherty, Pyper, and Frasz (2004) described a nursing intervention based on Bandura's theory that was designed to improve physical functioning and psychological adjustment among patients who had received an implantable cardioverter defibrillator. Liaw (2003) described a study of a "developmentally supportive care training program" (p. 82) that used videotaped and personalized instruction to teach supportive care for preterm infants. The program was reportedly based on Bandura's cognitive learning theory and the study determined that the program was effective in teaching the nurses to provide quality care and improve the outcomes of these babies. Finally, Tsay (2003) described a Bandura-based intervention designed to promote adherence to a prescribed diet and fluid regimen for persons with endstage renal disease.

## PSYCHODYNAMIC LEARNING THEORY

While not technically a group of distinct learning theories, psychodynamic theory, which was based on the work of Sigmund Freud, does have implications for learning and behavior change (Braungart & Braungart, 2008). Some of the most important contributions to learning theory have come from the discipline of psychotherapy because psychotherapists are concerned with the reeducation of their clients. Freud contributed concepts such as the unconscious, subconscious, repression, and defense mechanism, which are used by learning theorists (Knowles et al., 2005). Freud believed emotions interfered with cognition and that human motivation comes from deep internal drives, many of which arise from the unconscious (Roberts, 1975). Individuals may or may not be conscious of their own motivations and why they think, feel, and act the way they do.

According to psychodynamic theorists, motivation for behavior can come from several sources. The most basic source of motivation comes from the primal instincts and desires we are born with. This is referred to as the *id*. According to Freud, the basic function of the *id* is to seek pleasure and avoid pain. On the other hand, motivation is also based on the function of the *superego*, which is an individual's conscience based on internalized values and societal standards. These primitive drives and highly developed conscience are mediated by the *ego*, which allows individuals to weigh decisions and make the best choices.

This psychodynamic view gives the APN perspective on teaching related to a patient's ego development. Patients with healthy ego development are able to make choices about their own care and maintain sometimes difficult courses of action to achieve outcomes. On the other hand, patients with poor ego development may choose the immediately gratifying course of action. When viewed from a learning theorist perspective, knowledge may not have a profound effect on the behaviors of patients who have poor ego development. For example, simply knowing about appropriate food choices for a diabetic patient may not be enough to incorporate healthy food choices into their behavior.

While psychodynamic theory provides a framework for understanding the behavior of others, it is largely speculative and abstract in nature. Health care professionals are cautioned that while these theories may provide some insight into the behavior of a person, they should not be used to dismiss a person's behavior or as a basis for decisions about whether or not to provide teaching.

## HUMANISTIC LEARNING THEORY

Whereas Freudian scholars saw emotions as negative influences, humanistic educators recognize that emotions can have a positive influence on the learning process. Humanistic psychologists, often referred to as "third force" psychologists, are concerned with human potential and are interested in helping individuals develop that potential. As individuals or groups achieve new abilities, the human potential improves; consequently, the individual is always "becoming." Human relations skills are one of the major human abilities that concerns humanistic educators. Humanistic educators want learners to have warm interpersonal relationships, to trust others and themselves, and to be aware of others' feelings. The teacher's role is to design experiences that help improve the learners' abilities to perceive, feel, wonder, sense, create, fantasize, imagine, and experience (Roberts, 1975).

By redefining the role of the educator and focusing on the needs and feelings of the learner, humanistic theory has given health professionals a useful tool for client-centered teaching and care. Humanistic theory is the foundation for many successful wellness programs, self-help groups, and palliative care (Braungart & Braungart, 2008).

### Rogers
Carl Rogers (1902–1987), one of the leaders of the humanistic perspective, transferred his principles about "client-centered" therapy to "student-centered" teaching.

For Rogers (1983), the learner is in the process of becoming, the goal of education is to develop a "fully functioning person," and the teacher's role is to facilitate the process. He believed learning is a natural process, entirely controlled internally by the learner, in which the individual's whole being interacts with the environment, as the learner perceives it. The learner has both the freedom to learn and to be self-directed (as opposed to teacher directed). By providing problems real and meaningful to the learner, intrinsic motivation is stimulated to solve the problem. Rogers perceived the only truly educated person to be the one who learns how to learn, knows how to adapt to changing circumstances, and is continually seeking knowledge.

### Application to Nursing

Nurses often use these principles in practice. For example, Vacek (2009) used concept mapping with students to promote critical thinking in a baccalaureate nursing program. The findings were that students using concept mapping experienced enhanced learning and critical thinking. Wong et al. (2008) adopted a problem-based learning approach in a clinical simulation. They found that the students learned in a stable, safe environment and could experience the full range of learning issues (p. 513) without endangering themselves or their patients. They found that this learning environment also has staff development value.

## DEVELOPMENTAL PSYCHOLOGY

In addition to Piaget, other developmental psychologists have contributed to a growing understanding of learning as it is affected by characteristics such as physical capabilities, mental abilities, interests, attitudes, values, creativity, and lifestyle. Noted developmental psychologists include Abraham Maslow (1908–1970), who wrote on needs hierarchy of motivation; Erik Erikson (1902–1994), who explored personality development; and Robert Havighurst (1900–1991), who described developmental tasks or life problems that lead to readiness to learn. Other developmental psychologists have also contributed to the understanding of the impact of maturation on learning. At one time, learning was thought to cease when an individual reached the mid-twenties in age. Thanks to developmental psychologists, it is now recognized that learning may occur throughout the life span.

### Constructivism

Constructivism is one of the newer developmental learning theories and is based on Piaget's work. Constructivists believe that knowledge has no existence outside the person's mind and that learners always interpret what is presented to them using preexisting knowledge, history, and typical ways of perceiving and acting (Byrnes, 2001). The basic operating processes in learning are assimilation, accommodation, and constructivism.

*Assimilation* is a process whereby an individual interacts with an object or event in a way that is consistent with what is already known. *Accommodation* is a process whereby an individual modifies the existing knowledge to account for a new event. Learning occurs when the individual incorporates an experience into his or her existing knowledge base. By attempting to make sense of the new experience, the learner *constructs* new knowledge (Ormrod, 2004). Therefore, the learner constructs new knowledge rather than acquiring new knowledge. The purpose of instruction is to support this construction, rather than to communicate information (Duffy & Cunningham, 1997).

One of the significant contributions of the developmental psychologists to learning is the recognition that there is a hierarchical basis in thinking from lower forms to higher forms with age and experience. Therefore, learners need a certain amount of education, experience, or practice before being capable of highest-order thinking. If the nurse presents new information before the first information has been received and translated, the collision of the information causes the information to "jam" in the client's brain, resulting in confusion. Nurses working with older people must recognize this phenomenon and incorporate it into their practice.

It is important for APNs to realize that geriatric clients are capable of learning. It simply may take a longer period of time to do so because of the increased time it takes for information to travel through the nervous system and be interpreted. For example, a 65-year-old person who has had a stroke can relearn to use muscles just as a 45-year-old person can, but the elder client will take several weeks or months longer to do so. Even a healthy 65-year-old individual may not mentally process information as rapidly as a 45-year-old person.

## ADULT LEARNING

Malcolm Knowles (1913–1997), although not the first educator to study adult learning, is credited with popularizing the notion of andragogy in North America. *Andragogy* is concerned with a unified theory of adult learning, as opposed to *pedagogy*, which focuses on youth learning. He views pedagogy as a content model and andragogy as a process model. For Knowles (Knowles et al., 2005) the single most important thing in helping adults to learn is to create a climate of physical comfort, mutual trust and respect, openness, and acceptance of differences. By responding to the needs of the learner, and providing the learning resources required for learning, teachers facilitate learning. To be effective, presenters (teachers) need to "tell it like it is" and stress "how I do it" rather than telling the learner what to do. Through self-direction, learners are responsible for their own learning. Knowles (Knowles et al., 2005) identified six assumptions regarding andragogy (Box 16-5).

Knowles (Knowles et al., 2005) believed that adults need to know why they need to learn something. As a result, the teacher can help learners understand how the knowledge is important to their future or the quality of their lives. Second, Knowles recognized the importance of self-concept in the adult learner. He taught that as people mature, their self-concept moves from one of being dependent toward one of being self-directed. Adult learners want others to see them as being capable of self-direction and resent having someone else's will imposed on them. A self-directing teacher avoids "talking down" to the learner, provides information that enhances the adults' ability to solve problems, and encourages independence.

---

### BOX 16-5   *Knowles' Assumptions of Adult Learners*

1. *Need to know:* Adults need to know why they need to learn something.
2. *Self-concept:* As people mature their self-concept moves from one of being dependent toward one of being self-directed.
3. *Experience:* As people mature they accumulate a large amount of experience that can serve as a rich resource for learning.
4. *Readiness to learn:* Real-life problems or situations create a readiness to learn in the adult.
5. *Orientation to learning:* As a person matures his or her time perspective changes from one of postponed application of knowledge to immediacy of application.
6. *Motivation:* Adults are primarily motivated by a desire to solve immediate and practical problems. As a person matures, motivation to learn is stimulated by internal stimuli rather than external stimuli.

A third assumption revolves around experience. Knowles (Knowles et al., 2005) explained that as people mature they accumulate a large amount of experience that can serve as a rich resource for learning. Adults learn better when their own experiences are incorporated into the learning process. New experiences contribute to the learner's self-identity. Ignoring or devaluing this experience is perceived as rejecting them as a person.

The fourth assumption involves readiness to learn. Real-life problems or situations create a readiness to learn in the adult. Adults are problem-oriented learners, as opposed to subject-oriented learners; they want information that will help them solve a specific problem rather than an inclusive discussion of the subject. As a person matures, readiness to learn becomes increasingly oriented to the developmental tasks of social roles. Organizing learning activities around these life experiences facilitates the learning process. Readiness to learn can be created by exposing the individual to superior models, simulation exercises, and other techniques.

Similarly, the fifth assumption centers on orientation to learning. As a person matures, his or her time perspective changes from one of postponed application of knowledge to immediacy of application. Accordingly, the orientation toward self-learning shifts from one of subject centeredness to one of problem centeredness (Knowles et al., 2005).

Finally, motivation is the cornerstone of the adult learning theories. According to Knowles (Knowles et al., 2005), adults are primarily motivated by a desire to solve immediate and practical problems. As a person matures, motivation to learn is stimulated by internal stimuli rather than external stimuli. The learner is self-directed, determines what is to be learned and how it is to be learned, and assumes the primary responsibility for learning. For example, some motivational force is exerted from external sources such as a desire for a better paying job, but a stronger force arises from internal sources such as job satisfaction.

Theorists subscribing to developmental approaches to learning generally agree that there is a natural progression in thinking from the lower forms to higher forms with age and experience. Therefore, people need to have a certain amount of education, experience, or practice before they can perform higher-order thinking (Byrnes, 2001). For example, the man with newly diagnosed diabetes, with little formal education and who has not known another diabetic person, will have difficulty comprehending the implications of diabetes on his lifestyle.

### Application to Nursing

There are numerous examples of the use of Knowles' theory in the nursing literature. Hammer and Craig (2008) employed a qualitative process to study nurses returning to clinical practice after a period of inactivity. They found that the more the nurses learned that was useful directly in clinical practice, the more easily they returned to the nursing role. Adult learning theory was the basis for a program in New Zealand to support midwives in clinical practice (Lennox, Skinner, & Foureur, 2008). They used mentorship, preceptorship, and clinical supervision in the training project. Doyle, Gallagher, Bell, and Roynane (2008) used adult education principles in a train-the-trainer project to educate nurses engaged in services to the elderly in Ireland.

## Summary of Learning Theories

As the previous discussions have illustrated, numerous learning theories have been posited over the past century. Table 16-2 summarizes the cognitive-focused theories described. Many other diverse areas of study have developed from both the behavioral and cognitive fields of learning theories. Examples are multiple intelligence (Gardner, 1999), whole

TABLE 16-2 *Summary of Cognitive Learning Theories*

| Group of Theories | Key Principles | Examples of Theorists |
|---|---|---|
| Cognitive-field (Gestalt) theories | Learning relates to perception; motivation is key; behavior is related to perception and experience. | Lewin |
| Information-processing theories | Memory is composed of sensory memory, short-term memory, and long-term memory; learning consists of strategies to transfer information from short-term memory to long-term memory. | Anderson Bahrick |
| Cognitive development (interaction) theories | Individuals learn from their experiences; learning is how individuals adapt and cope with their environment. | Gagne Piaget Bandura Perry |
| Psychodynamic theory; humanism | Reeducation of clients is important; focus is on human potential; emphasis is on collaboration in the learning process; recognizes that emotions can positively affect learning. | Freud Rogers |
| Developmental psychology | Learning is affected by many variables, including physical and mental ability, attitudes, interests, and values; learning interprets information based on previous knowledge and experiences; learning continues throughout life. | Maslow Erikson Piaget Havighurst |
| Andragogy (adult learning theory) | The process of learning rather than content is the focus; physical comfort, mutual trust and respect, openness, and acceptance are important concepts. | Knowles |

brain learning (Maxfield, 1990), learning styles (Kolb, 1976), assimilation (Ausubel, 1978), proficiency (Knox, 1980), transformational learning (Brookfield, 1991; Mezirow, 1981), memory (Atkinson & Shiffrin, 1968), self-directed learning (Tough, 1967), self-efficacy (Bandura, 1977b), and problem-solving (Newell & Simon, 1972).

# Learning Styles

It is widely recognized that most individuals have a preferred style of learning. Learning style is a characteristic that allows individuals to interact with instructional circumstances in such a way that learning is produced. Learning style preference relates to the likes and dislikes a person has for certain sensory modes, learning conditions, and learning strategies. Most people have probably not thought about how they learn, and if questioned would give an answer based on what they assume, rather than what is correct.

By carefully listening to verbal comments of a patient, the APN can obtain clues about the preferred learning style. For example, if the individual says something such as "I hear what you're saying," the preferred learning style is most likely auditory. This individual learns best by hearing a discussion, presentation, audiocassette, and so forth. If, however, the response is "I see what you mean," the learning style is probably visual, and the person responds better to pictures, movies, demonstrations, and so forth. Tactual and kinesthetic learners make statements such as "I feel this is very important." These learners will learn best if able to manipulate or physically maneuver material with their hands. The availability of paper and pencils for taking notes, highlighter pens for marking important information, and picture puzzles will assist these types of learners (Morse, Oberer, Dobbins, & Mitchell, 1998).

In addition to age, gender also influences one's learning style. Men tend to be more visual, tactile, and kinesthetic than women. They are also more peer oriented and nonconforming and need the freedom to move around in an informal setting (Dunn & Dunn, 1992, 1993; Dunn & Griggs, 1995). In contrast, during learning situations women tend to be more auditory, conforming, and authority oriented than men, and are more able to sit passively (Pizzo, Dunn, & Dunn, 1990).

An important factor influencing learning is whether the individual tends to learn better analytically or globally. Analytic learners learn facts, step by step in a logical progression building toward a whole. Global learners, by contrast, want to understand the whole before learning about the parts. Analytic learners will listen to all the facts as long as they believe they are heading toward a goal. Global learners need to know what they need to learn and why they need to learn it.

Different environments and different teaching strategies are required for global and analytic learners. Global learners learn better with intermittent periods of concentration and relaxation in a place with soft lighting, music, or other sound while sitting informally eating lots of snacks. Short stories, anecdotes, humor, and illustrations can be used to capture the attention of global learners (Morse et al., 1998). Conversely, the analytic learner needs a quiet, well-lit formal setting with few or no interruptions and few or no snacks (Dunn & Griggs, 1998).

## Principles of Learning

A common approach for teaching either individuals or groups is the use of learning principles. Principles of learning have been derived from multiple theories and are items that people can agree on no matter to which learning theory they subscribe. Whereas learning theories provide explanation about the underlying mechanisms involved in the learning process, principles identify specific elements that are important for learning and describe the particular effects of these variables on learning. The following are some other learning principles that may assist APNs as they attempt to provide health information to their clients.

- Learning is facilitated if information is provided from simple to complex, concrete to abstract, and known to unknown. This generally accepted learning principle recognizes the hierarchy in learning.
- Learning is facilitated if the information is personal and individualized. Learning occurs inside individuals and is activated by learners themselves. The client is more likely to remember what is taught if actively involved in the learning process.
- Learning is facilitated if it is relevant to the learner's needs and problems. What is relevant and meaningful is decided by the learner and must be discovered by him or her. Information that is meaningful is more easily stored and retrieved than information learned by rote memorization. What the APN perceives as important to the health of the client may not be what the client perceives as important.
- Learning is facilitated if the individual is attentive. Attention is essential for learning. Attention is the process through which information moves into the short-term memory. Any internal (e.g., fear) or external factor (e.g., noise) that distracts the client can interfere with the learning process.

## REFERENCES

Aquilino, M. L. (1997). Cognitive development, clinical knowledge, and clinical experience related to diagnostic ability. *Nursing Diagnosis, 8,* 110–120.

Atkinson, R. C., & Shiffrin, R. M. (1968). Human memory: A proposed system and its control processes. In K. W. Spence & J. T. Spence (Eds.), *The psychology of learning and motivation: Advances in research and theory* (Vol. 2, pp. 89–195). New York: Academic Press.

Ausubel, D. P. (1978). *Educational psychology: A cognitive view* (2nd ed.). New York: Holt, Rinehart & Winston.

Bandura, A. (1977a). *Social learning theory.* Englewood Cliffs, NJ: Prentice-Hall.

Bandura, A. (1977b). Self-efficacy: Toward a unifying theory of behavioral change. *Psychological Review, 84,* 191–215.

Bastable, S. B. (2008). Overview of education in health care. In S. B. Bastable (Ed.), *Nurse as educator: Principles of teaching and learning for nursing practice* (3rd ed., pp. 3–23). Boston: Jones & Bartlett.

Berk, L. E. (2003). *Child development* (6th ed.). Boston: Allyn & Bacon.

Bigge, M. L., & Shermis, S. S. (1999). *Learning theories for teachers* (6th ed.). New York: Addison Wesley Longman.

Braungart, M. M., & Braungart, R. G. (2008). Applying learning theories to health care practice. In S. B. Bastable (Ed.), *Nurse as educator: Principles of teaching and learning for nursing practice* (3rd ed., pp. 51–89). Boston: Jones & Bartlett.

Brookfield, S. D. (1991). *Developing critical thinkers.* San Francisco: Jossey-Bass.

Bruccoliere, T. (2000). How to make patient teaching stick. *RN, 63*(2), 34–38.

Byrnes, J. P. (2001). *Cognitive development and learning in instructional contexts* (2nd ed.). Boston: Allyn & Bacon.

Carter, L. M., & Rukholm, E. (2008). A study of critical thinking, teacher–student interaction and discipline-specific writing in an online educational setting for registered nurses. *Journal of Continuing Education in Nursing, 39*(3), 133–138.

Deering, C. G. (2000). A cognitive developmental approach to understanding how children cope with disasters. *Journal of Child and Adolescent Psychiatric Nursing, 13*(1), 7–16.

DeYoung, S. (2003). *Teaching strategies for nurse educators.* Upper Saddle River, NJ: Prentice-Hall.

Dickey, S. B., Kiefner, J., & Beidler, S. M. (2002). Consent and confidentiality issues among school-age children and adolescents. *Journal of School Nursing, 18*(3), 179–185.

Dougherty, C. M., Pyper, G. P., & Frasz, H. A. (2004). Description of a nursing intervention program after an implantable cardioverter defibrillator. *Heart & Lung, 33*(3), 183–190.

Doyle, S., Gallagher, J., Bell, M., & Roynane, S. (2008). Establishing a "train the trainer" education model for clinical skills development. *Nursing Older People, 20*(5), 34–37.

Duffy, T. M., & Cunningham, D. J. (1997). Constructivism: Implications for the design and delivery of instruction. In D. H. Jonassen (Eds.), *Handbook of research for educational communications and technology* (pp. 170–198). New York: Macmillan.

Dunn, R., & Dunn, K. (1992). *Teaching elementary students through their individual learning styles: Practical approaches for grades* 3–6. Boston: Allyn & Bacon.

Dunn, R., & Dunn, K. (1993). *Teaching secondary students through their individual learning styles: Practical approaches for grades* 7–12. Boston: Allyn & Bacon.

Dunn, R., & Griggs, S. A. (1995). *Multiculturalism and learning styles: Teaching and counseling adolescents.* Westport, CT: Greenwood Press.

Dunn, R., & Griggs, S. A. (1998). Learning styles: Link between teaching and learning. In R. Dunn & S. A. Griggs (Eds.), *Learning styles and the nursing profession* (pp. 11–23). New York: National League for Nursing Press.

Fallacaro, M. D., & Crosby, F. E. (2000). Untoward pathophysiological events: Simulation as an experiential learning option to prepare anesthesia providers. *Clinical Forum for Nurse Anesthetists, 11*(3), 138–143.

Fitzgerald, K. (2008). Instructional methods and settings. In S. B. Bastable (Ed.), *Nurse as educator: Principles of teaching and learning for nursing practice* (3rd ed., pp. 429–471). Boston: Jones & Bartlett.

Forrest, S. (2004). Learning and teaching: The reciprocal link. *Journal of Continuing Education in Nursing, 35*(2), 74–79.

Gagne, R. M. (1985). *The conditions of learning* (4th ed.). New York: Holt, Rinehart & Winston.

Gardner, H. (1999). *Intelligence reframed: Multiple intelligences for the 21st century.* New York: Basic Books.

Hammer, V. R., & Craig, G. P. (2008). The experiences of inactive nurses returned to nursing after completing a refresher course. *The Journal of Continuing Education in Nursing, 39*(8), 358–367.

Hergenhahn, B. R., & Olson, M. H. (2004). *An introduction to theories of learning* (7th ed.). Upper Saddle River, NJ: Prentice-Hall.

Higgins, L. W. (1999). Nurses' perceptions of collaborative nurse–physician transfer decision making as a predictor of patient outcomes in a medical intensive care unit. *Journal of Advanced Nursing, 29*(6), 1434–1443.

Knowles, M. (1981). *From teacher to facilitator of learning.* Follett Publishing Co., Educational Materials Catalog. (Reprinted in Knowles, M., Holton, E. F., & Swanson, R. A. (2005). *The adult learner: The definitive classic in adult education and human resource development* (6th ed., pp. 251–254). Burlington, MA: Elsevier).

Knowles, M., Holton, E. F., & Swanson, R. A. (2005). *The adult learner: The definitive classic in adult education and human resource development* (6th ed.). Burlington, MA: Elsevier.

Knox, A. B. (1980). Proficiency theory of adult learning. *Contemporary Educational Psychology, 5,* 378–404.

Kolb, D. A. (1976). *The learning style inventory.* Boston: McBer.

Kolb, D. A. (1984). *Experiential learning.* Englewood Cliffs, NJ: Prentice-Hall.

Kurfiss, J. G. (1996). *Critical thinking: Theory research, practice and possibilities: ASHE-ERIC/Higher education research report.* Washington, DC: George Washington University, Graduate School of Education and Human Development.

LaFleur, C. J., & Raway, B. (1999). School-age child and adolescent perception of the pain intensity associated with three word descriptors. *Pediatric Nursing, 25,* 45–50.

Lefrancois, G. R. (2000). *Theories of human learning* (4th ed.). Belmont, CA: Wadsworth/Thomson Learning.

Leigh, G. T. (2007). High Fidelity Patient Simulation and Nursing Students' self efficacy: A review of the literature. *International Journal of Nursing Education Scholarship, 5*(1), 1–17.

Lennox, S., Skinner, J., & Foureur, M. (2008). Mentorship, preceptorship and clinical supervision: Three key processes for supporting midwives. *New Zealand College of Midwives Journal, 39*(10), 7–12.

Liaw, J. (2003). Use of a training program to enhance NICU nurses' cognitive abilities for assessing preterm infant behaviors and offering supportive intervention. *Journal of Nursing Research, 11*(2), 82–92.

Mahat, G., Scoloveno, M. A., & Cannella, B. (2004). Comparison of children's fears of medical experiences across two cultures. *Journal of Pediatric Health Care, 18*(3), 302–307.

Maxfield, D. G. (1990). Learning with the whole mind. In R. M. Smith and associates (Eds.), *Learning to learn across the life span* (pp. 98–122). San Francisco: Jossey-Bass.

McGovern, M. W. (1995). The effect of developmental instruction strategies on the cognitive development of sophomore nursing students' relationship of cognitive development scores to measures of critical thinking and moral development. Philadelphia: Temple University, unpublished dissertation.

Mezirow, J. (1981). A critical theory of adult learning and education. *Adult Education, 32,* 3–27.

Montgomery, K. S. (2002). Health promotion with adolescents: Examining theoretical perspectives to guide research. *Research and Theory in Nursing Practice, 16*(2), 119–134.

Morse, J. S., Oberer, J., Dobbins, J. A., & Mitchell, D. (1998). Understanding learning styles: Implications for in-service educators. In R. Dunn & S. A. Griggs (Eds.), *Learning styles and the nursing profession* (pp. 27–40). New York: National League for Nursing Press.

Newell, A., & Simon, H. A. (1972). *Human problem solving.* Englewood Cliffs, NJ: Prentice-Hall.

Olson, M. W., & Hergenhahn, B. R. (2009). *An introduction to theories of learning.* Upper Saddle River, NJ: Pearson Prentice-Hall.

O'Neill, E. S., Dluhy, N. M., & Chin, E. (2005). Modeling novice clinical reasoning for computerized decision support system. *Journal of Advanced Nursing, 49*(1), 68–77.

Ormrod, J. E. (2004). *Human learning: Principles, theories and educational applications* (4th ed.). Englewood Cliffs, NJ: Prentice-Hall.

Ozmon, H., & Craver, S. (2003). *Philosophical foundations of education* (7th ed.). Upper Saddle River, NJ: Prentice-Hall.

Perry, W. G. (1999). *Forms of ethical and intellectual development in the college years: A scheme.* San Francisco, CA: Jossey-Bass.

Pizzo, J., Dunn, R., & Dunn, K. (1990). A sound approach to reading: Responding to students' learning styles. *Journal of Reading, Writing, and Learning Disabilities International, 6,* 249–260.

Rankin, S. H., & Stallings, K. D. (2005). *Patient education in health and illness* (5th ed.). Philadelphia: Lippincott Williams & Wilkins.

Rapps, J., Riegel, B., & Glaser, D. (2001). Testing a predictive model of what makes a critical thinker. *Western Journal of Nursing Research, 23*(6), 610–626.

Roberts, T. B. (1975). Freudian, (pp. 3–9); behavioral psychology (pp. 131–139); humanistic psychology (pp. 289–292); transpersonal psychology (pp. 395–401). In T. B. Roberts (Ed.), *Four psychologies applied to education: Freudian, behavioral, humanistic, transpersonal.* New York: Schenkman.

Rogers, C. R. (1983). *Freedom to learn for the 80's.* Columbus, OH: Merrill.

Rogers, C. R., & Freiberg, H. J. (1994). *Freedom to learn* (3rd ed.). New York: Macmillan College Publishing.

Saarmann, L., Daugherty, J., & Riegel, B. (2000). Patient teaching to promote behavioral change. *Nursing Outlook, 48*(6), 281–287.

Shawler, C. (2008). Standardized patients: A creative teaching strategy for psychiatric-mental health nurse practitioner students. *Journal of Nursing Education, 47*(11), 528–531.

Swartz-Kulstad, J. L., & Martin, W. E. (1999). Impact of culture and context on psychosocial adaptation: The cultural and contextual guide process. *Journal of Counseling and Development, 77,* 281–293.

Thorndike, E. L. (1932). *The fundamentals of learning.* New York: Teachers College Press.

Tough, A. (1967). *Learning without a teacher.* Toronto: Ontario Institute for Studies in Education.

Tracy, J. T., & Mayer, D. K. (2000). Perspectives on cancer patient education. *Seminars in Oncology Nursing, 16*(1), 47–56.

Tsay, S. (2003). Self-efficacy training for patients with end-stage renal disease. *Journal of Advanced Nursing, 43*(4), 370–375.

Vacek, J. E. (2009). Using a conceptual approach with concept mapping to promote critical thinking. *Journal of Nursing Education, 48*(1), 45–48.

Vandeveer, M. (2009). From teaching to learning: Theoretical foundations. In D. M. Billings & J. A. Halstead (Eds.), *Teaching in nursing: A guide for faculty.* St. Louis: Elsevier Saunders.

Vandeveer, M., & Norton, B. (2005). From teaching to learning: Theoretical foundations. In D. M. Billings & J. A. Halstead (Eds.), *Teaching in nursing: A guide for faculty.* St. Louis: Elsevier Saunders.

Ward, C., & McCormack, B. (2000). Creating an adult learning culture through practice development. *Nurse Education Today, 20,* 259–266.

Wong, F. K. Y., Cheung, S., Chung, L., Chan, K., Chan, A., To, T., & Wong, M. (2008). Framework for adopting a problem-based learning approach in a simulated clinical setting. *Journal of Nursing Education, 47*(11), 508–514.

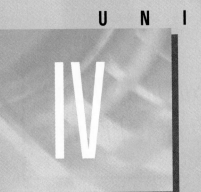

**IV**

*Application of Theory in Nursing*

# 17

# Application of Theory in Nursing Practice

## Melanie McEwen

*E*  *mily Chan is a clinical nurse specialist who coordinates a liver transplant program at a large medical center. In her position she serves as the case manager for a number of individuals. Emily was assigned to work with Sarah Bishop, a 45-year-old high school teacher who had recently received a new liver after contracting hepatitis C from a blood transfusion more than a decade ago. Sarah is married and has two teenage children.*

*The management of liver transplant clients is highly complex; it is essential to consider multiple facets of care over an extended period of time. In designing a plan of care for Sarah, Emily conducted a lengthy assessment. She was pleased to discover that Sarah was well educated and knew a great deal about her illness. Sarah asked many informed questions and was anxious to learn all she could from Emily. During the time that Emily worked with Sarah, she used a number of principles and theories in care delivery. She explained physiologic principles related to chronic liver disease and liver failure to Sarah, and she combined that information with pharmacologic principles related to the large number of medications required to prevent rejection. Complications of the disease, as well as side effects from the medications, were examined at length. For the educative processes, Emily used several different learning principles and theories and incorporated a variety of teaching techniques, including one-on-one time, printed materials, interactive computer programs, and videos.*

*To address the many psychosocial issues that Sarah and her family would face, Emily combined principles and concepts from different theories to plan interventions. She incorporated role theory, family theory, developmental theory, and others to help Sarah and her family understand how the illness might affect Sarah's roles as wife, mother, daughter, sister, and teacher. She encouraged family support and advocated for counseling for all family members. She also referred Sarah to a support group. Emily also guided Sarah in addressing the spiritual issues involved in living with a chronic, life-threatening illness. Among other concepts, she discussed hope, meaning, and transcendence.*

*Finally, a significant aspect of Sarah's care involved management of her finances. Emily carefully described the process of reimbursement and explained what services were covered. Incorporation of principles and concepts from management and economics was necessary for Emily to adequately understand and explain the financial aspects of Sarah's care.*

---

Theory is considered to be both a process and a product. As a process, theory has numerous activities and includes four interacting, sequential phases (analyzing concepts, constructing relationships, testing relationships, and validating relationships) that are implemented in practice. As a product, theory provides a set of concepts and relationships that may be combined to describe, explain, predict, and prescribe phenomena of interest; this information is then used to guide nursing practice (Kenney, 1995, 2006). In a practice discipline such as nursing, theory, and practice are inseparable. Indeed, development and application of theory affiliated with research-based practice has been seen as fundamental to the development of the profession and autonomous nursing practice.

Theory provides the basis of understanding the reality of nursing; it enables the nurse to understand why an event happens. To illustrate how theory is applied in practice, Dale (1994) used the example of a nurse who knows theories and principles of the anatomy of soft tissues and the related physiologic concept of pressure. This knowledge allows the nurse to recognize how a pressure sore can develop. Armed with this knowledge, the nurse can take steps to prevent it.

To improve the practice of nursing, nurses need to search the literature, critically appraise research findings, and synthesize empirical and contextually relevant theoretical information to be applied in practice. Further, nurses must continually question their practice and seek to find better alternatives (Rosswurm & Larrabee, 1999). Nurses cannot afford to think of theory and research as intellectual pursuits separate from clinical performance; rather, nurses should be aware that theory and research provide the basis for practice (Doane & Varcoe, 2005; Marrs & Lowry, 2006; Parker, 2006).

This chapter examines several issues related to the application of theory in nursing practice. First, the relationship between theory and practice and the concept of theory-based nursing practice are described. This is followed by a discussion of the perceived theory–practice gap that has persisted in nursing. Practice theories are then presented, followed by a discussion of the concept of evidence-based practice (EBP). The chapter concludes with examples illustrating how theory is used and applied in nursing practice.

## Relationship Between Theory and Practice

In the discipline of nursing, there should be a reciprocal relationship between theory and practice. Practice is the basis for nursing theory development, and nursing theory must be validated in practice. Theory is rooted in practice and refined by research, and it should be reapplied in practice. Box 17-1 shows several of the many ways in which theories influence nursing practice.

Theory provides nurses with a perspective with which to view client situations and a way to organize data in daily care. Theory allows nurses to focus on important information while setting aside less important, or irrelevant, data. Theory may assist in directing analysis and interpretation of the relationships among data and in predicting outcomes necessary to plan care. Further, a theoretical perspective allows the nurse to plan and implement care purposefully and proactively, and when nurses practice purposefully and systematically, they are more efficient, have better control

| BOX 17-1 | *Ways in Which Theory Influences Nursing Practice* |

- Identifies recipients/clients of nursing care
- Describes settings and situations in which practice should occur
- Defines which data to collect and how to classify the data
- Outlines actual and potential problems to be considered
- Aids in understanding, analyzing, and interpreting health situations
- Guides formulation of nursing diagnoses
- Describes, explains, and sometimes predicts client's responses
- Clarifies objectives and establishes expected outcomes
- Specifies actions or interventions to be provided
- Sets standards for practice
- Differentiates nursing practice from practice of other health disciplines
- Promotes responsibility and accountability for nursing care
- Identifies areas for research

Sources: Fawcett (1992); Kenney (2006); Young et al. (2001).

over the outcome of care, and are better able to communicate that care with others (Cody, 2003; Young, Taylor, & Renpenning, 2001; Ziegler, 2005). Thus, nurses need to use theoretical perspectives to help understand which data are important, how data are related, what can be predicted by relationships, and what interventions are needed to deal with special relationships.

For example, a nurse working in a postpartum unit should be aware of the theoretical basis for the development of postpartum depression. That nurse should know risk factors for postpartum depression, its signs and symptoms, and various management strategies. Further, if the nurse suspects postpartum depression in a teenage mother, she or he must know what additional data need to be gathered to address the complex issues created by this mother's special needs and circumstances. The additional information should be analyzed and interpreted based on an understanding of the specific problems and complications posed by teen pregnancy, and an appropriate plan of care for that young woman can be developed and goals and outcomes predicted.

Similarly, a nurse working in a pediatric clinic should understand the theoretical principles of immunity and disease prevention when explaining the importance of immunization to a new mother. If the mother expresses concerns about a potential complication of the vaccine, the nurse should gather additional information from the mother to understand her specific concerns. On learning that the mother had read recent reports that the measles/mumps/rubella vaccine might cause autism, the nurse must be able to articulate the rationale behind immunization and to direct the mother to sources of information about vaccine safety and potential complications, including the most recent and relevant research data. This information will allow the mother to make an informed decision about the care of her infant.

## Theory-Based Nursing Practice

Theory-based nursing practice is the "application of various models, theories, and principles from nursing science and the biological, behavioral, medical and sociocultural disciplines to clinical nursing practice" (Kenney, 2006, p. 295). Nursing practice is complex, and theory informs the practitioner to do what is right and just (good practice).

In nursing, practice without theory becomes rote performance of activities based on tradition, common sense, and following orders (Billings & Kowalski, 2006; Marrs & Lowry, 2006; Perry, 2004).

Theory can offer the practitioner a basis for making informed decisions that are based on deliberation and practical judgment. With increasing clinical experience, nurses are able to combine theoretical and clinical knowledge with critical thinking skills to make better clinical decisions and thereby improve practice. Nursing, like all practice disciplines, uses a special combination of theory and practice in which theory guides practice and the practice grounds theory. Nurses rely heavily on theoretical understanding, and practice will be improved not just by experience, but by an understanding of theory. As Cody (2003) pointed out, "one learns to practice nursing by studying nursing theories, and one learns to practice nursing very well by studying nursing theories very intensely" (p. 226).

Dreyfus and Dreyfus (1996) believe that as nurses gain knowledge, skills, and expertise, theory and practice intertwine in a mutually supportive process; however, only if both theory and research are encouraged and appreciated can full expertise in nursing practice be realized. Theory is needed to explain the ends and means of nursing practice, and the nurse who uses theory-based practice will be able to describe, explain, predict, and control nursing events and initiate preventive actions (Kikuchi, 2004). Theory-based practice, therefore, is purposeful and controlled; it includes preventive action and can be explained by the nurse.

It is sometimes difficult to decide where, when, and how to apply theory in nursing practice. This may be particularly true for nursing students and novice nurses. The application of theory in practice requires an understanding of concepts and principles associated with the needs of a particular client, group of clients, or community, and recognition of when and how to use these concepts and principles when planning and implementing nursing care. Chinn and Kramer (2008) suggested criteria for determining when theory should be applied in practice. These are shown in Table 17-1.

## The Theory—Practice Gap

Despite the decades-long study of theory in nursing and the development and evolution of nursing theory, the notion that there is a "gap" between theory and practice is a common perception among nurses (Billings & Kowalski, 2006; Gallagher, 2004). Indeed, according to Liaschendo and Fisher (1999), nurses in clinical practice rarely use the language of nursing theory, nursing diagnosis, or the nursing process unless mandated to do so by accrediting bodies or institutional practice policies.

Several reasons for this have been suggested. For example, theory development has historically been regarded as the domain of nurse educators rather than the concern of practitioners. Nursing theory and practice have been viewed as two separate nursing activities, with theorists seen as those who write and teach about the ideal, separated from those who implement care in reality.

Although most scholars believe that theory and practice are, or at least should be, reciprocal, Rolfe (1998) points out that the relationship between theory and practice appears to be unidirectional and hierarchical. Indeed, theory is seen as above or superior to practice and is positioned to direct practice; rarely does practice appear to affect theory. This has caused mistrust by practitioners who believe academic knowledge has little relevance in practice situations. Indeed, practitioners often complain that theory distorts practice, if it has any relevance to practice at all (Billings & Kowalski, 2006; Wilson, 2008).

**TABLE 17-1** *Guidelines for Application of Theory in Nursing Practice*

| Question | Process for Determining Application to Practice | Example |
|---|---|---|
| Are theory goals and practice goals congruent? | Examine the goal of the theory and compare it with the outcomes or goals of nursing practice (standards of practice, personal views of nursing). | A rehabilitation nurse developing a plan of care for a spinal cord injury must choose between a theory of coping and a theory of adaptation. |
| Is the context of the theory congruent with the practice situation? | Examine the theory to determine context for application and compare it with the context of the situation at hand. | A hospice nurse is concerned that a new agency policy on pain management is based on a theory for postsurgical pain relief. |
| Is there similarity between theory variables and practice variables? | Compare the theoretic variables (concepts) and the variables recognized to directly influence the practice situation to determine if all essential concepts are addressed in the theory. | A nurse working with AIDS clients believes a learning theory might not consider the health status of the learner (the learner is assumed to be healthy) on the outcome(s) of client education. |
| Are explanations of the theory sufficient to be used as a basis for nursing action? | Use expert judgment about nursing actions that are implied or explicit within the theory to determine sufficiency; examine correlation between theoretic and practice variables. | A theory of therapeutic touch might be intriguing to an oncology nurse, but sufficient study should be conducted to determine when and how to apply the intervention in an oncology unit. |
| Does research evidence support the theory? | Conduct a review of the literature for research support of the theory; critically examine study findings for validity and applicability to practice. | Before considering implementing expensive measures that might prevent nosocomial infection, the nurse manager of a surgical ICU conducts a literature review to learn how effective the measures have been in similar settings. |
| How can the theory influence nursing practice and the nursing unit? | Consider ways in which an approach will affect nursing practice and a nursing unit; plan changes including observation and recording of factors relevant to the theory's application. | A theory that partially explains medication errors is being incorporated into new policies and procedures on a general medical unit, and the unit supervisor wants to be sure that the procedures include data collection for outcomes evaluation. |

Source: Adapted from Chinn and Kramer (2008).

Language also contributes to the gap in theory and practice. Further, in the "ideal" world of nursing theory, nursing practice is discussed as being performed as it ought to be rather than as how it is. Further, many nurses believe that theory is irrelevant to practice because of the obscurity of academic language and focus on circumscribed, ideal situations (Doane & Varcoe, 2005).

Finally, Allmark (1995) observed that practice often develops without theory, and knowing theory is not a guarantee of good practice. Furthermore, many practices resist explanation. Practice changes and develops in the light of theory, but much of the knowledge of practice is different from theory.

A different view has been taken by some. Larsen, Adamsen, Bjerregaard, and Madsen (2002) conducted a study of nursing literature and determined that there is no inherent gap between theory and practice. They noted that although theorists and practitioners are situated in different environments, they share common and implicit understandings related to knowledge development and implementation of that knowledge in practice. Also, Nicoten and Andrews (2003) noted that theoretical principals are applied daily in practice, although nurses do not always recognize their use of theory.

## CLOSING THE THEORY–PRACTICE GAP

Despite repeated calls to merge theory, practice, and research, the interaction remains fragmented or unrecognized. To promote nursing's ability to meet its obligations to society, there needs to be an ongoing, reciprocal relationship among nursing theory, nursing science, and nursing practice. This will help close the perceived gap between theory and practice.

Several factors that interfere in the reciprocal interrelationship of theory, practice, and research in nursing need to be addressed. These factors include educational issues, interaction between nursing researchers/scholars and practicing nurses, and problems or issues central to contemporary nursing practice.

Lack of exposure to theoretical principles during the basic educational program is a major impediment to closing the theory–practice gap. Because more than half of nurses in the United States have been educated in associate degree or diploma schools of nursing, they are frequently not exposed to either theory or research, as is common among baccalaureate program. This lack of focus on theory has been recognized, and in recent years, there has been momentum in nursing education to enhance emphasis on research and knowledge development (Jerlock & Severinsson, 2003; Johnson & Webber, 2005).

It is equally important to stress theoretical concepts and principles following completion of formal education because nurses are required to continually assimilate and synthesize a sizable amount of information into their practice. The continued professional growth of practicing nurses is important and, fortunately, many practicing nurses read scholarly journals, research-based literature, and practice-based journals. It is imperative that all nurses in clinical practice also be encouraged to expand their knowledge through ongoing exposure to new theoretical concepts and nursing research in continuing educational offerings or formal educational programs.

A second issue relates to the disparity between the world of nursing theorists and scholars and the world of practicing nurses. Unfortunately, many nurse theorists and nurse researchers have limited clinical involvement, and time constraints restrict their ability to develop relationships with clinically based nurses. Conversely, the majority of nurses in practice have little or no direct contact with nurse theorists or nurse researchers. To address this problem, those who propose theory and conduct research have recognized the need to be directly involved in clinical practice. Further, many understand the importance of studying problems encountered in practice and using language and terminology that can be easily understood by clinical nurses who are working to implement these changes.

The final issue in closing the practice–theory gap relates to changes in health care delivery and the need to address current practices from a theoretical perspective. Nurses face many challenges posed by changes in the health care delivery system. For example, the decrease in length of stay has dramatically reduced the time available for preoperative and postoperative teaching and discharge planning. Likewise, reimbursement mechanisms have dramatically influenced the availability of home health care and largely determined when and how nurses care for clients and what services are provided. These changes, although somewhat successful in curbing the inflation of health care costs, have also had a negative impact on nursing care.

The demands of the changing health care system along with other anticipated problems must be addressed from a practice, theory, and research perspective. These problems include chronic illnesses (e.g., heart disease, cancer), aging of the population, and the increase in the number of persons from a variety of racial and cultural backgrounds. These factors have contributed to the growing need to integrate multiple concepts, principles, and theories into designing, planning, and implementing effective nursing care. Thus, as nursing continues to evolve to meet the challenges described, clinical practice will need to be more heavily based on theory and research and less reliant on routine, common sense, and tradition (Billings & Kowalski, 2006; Perry, 2004).

# Practice Theories in Nursing

Earlier chapters described different types and levels of theory used in nursing. In addition to borrowed or shared theories, this book has described grand nursing theories and middle range nursing theories. This section provides information about the theories often termed *practice theories*, which are narrow, circumscribed theories proposed for a specific type of practice. It is important to stress that they are not the only theories applied in nursing practice.

## DEFINITION AND CHARACTERISTICS OF PRACTICE THEORIES

Practice theories are nursing theories used in the actual delivery of nursing care to clients. Several characteristics are common to practice theories. First, they are used to carry out nursing interventions and often include or lead to the performance of psychomotor procedures (e.g., dressing changes, venipuncture, medication administration) or are related to communication (e.g., education, counseling). Second, practice theories may be derived from grand or middle range theories, from clinical practice, and/or from research, and may describe, explain, or prescribe specific nursing practices. Third, practice theories combine a set of principles or directives for practice and often have a role in testing theories. Finally, practice theories may benefit nursing practice and the development of nursing knowledge by allowing for an in-depth analysis of a particular nursing intervention or practice.

The term *situation-specific theory* is sometimes used to describe practice theory (Chinn & Kramer, 2008; Im, 2005; Meleis, 2007). Practice theories are clinically specific and reflect a particular context that may include directions or blueprints for action. Further, in comparison to grand or middle range theories, practice theories have a lower level of abstraction, are context specific, and are easily applied in nursing research and practice.

Practice theories often emerge from grounded theory research or from synthesizing and integrating research findings and applying this knowledge to a specific situation or population. Typically, the intent is to develop a framework or blueprint to understand that particular situation or group of clients. Many nursing scholars support developing theories that reflect nursing practice thus ensuring that nursing practice is a source for theory development. Table 17-2 lists some areas that have been proposed for the development of practice theories for nursing.

## EXAMPLES OF PRACTICE THEORIES FROM NURSING LITERATURE

The nursing literature contains few examples of practice theories or situation-specific theories per se. In searching for illustrations, most theories that could be termed "practice theories" are those that were developed through grounded theory research

TABLE 17-2 *Types of Practice Theories Needed in the Discipline of Nursing*

| Type of Practice Theory | Examples |
| --- | --- |
| Theories providing explanations about client problems | Theories of healing, airway patency, fatigue, and speech |
| Theories describing therapeutics for client problems | Theories of suctioning, wound care, rest, and learning |
| Theories providing the nurse with ideas about how to approach clients | Theories of caring, empowerment, and communication |
| Theories providing explanations or ideas about how the nurse makes or should make decisions | Theories of clinical inference and clinical decision making |
| Theories providing explanations about what happens in the actual delivery of nursing care | Theories describing outcomes of client care |

Source: Kim (1994).

or those developed through application of a grand theory or a borrowed theory to a specific aggregate or in a very defined set of circumstances. A few were identified that were reported to have resulted from quantitative research studies and literary synthesis. Also, as mentioned in Chapter 10, some of the theories that are termed by the author or others as "middle range" may be more appropriately labeled practice theories.

Examples of practice-level theories developed from qualitative, grounded theory studies include a work by Suh (2008) who examined breast cancer screening practice among immigrant Korean women in the United States. A situation-specific theory focusing on that subcultural group was proposed explaining the sociocultural context of adherence to health promotion practices. Also using grounded theory, Runquist (2007) developed a situation-specific theory titled "persevering through postpartum fatigue" to help practitioners understand the phenomenon and to assist in developing nursing interventions to reduce its consequences.

In another work, Kidner and Flanders-Stepans (2004) examined the experiences of pregnant women who developed the serious complication of the HELLP (hemolysis, elevated liver enzymes, and low platelets) syndrome. The result of the study was the Model of the Maternal Experience of HELLP Syndrome, which described the experience as a circular process in which the mothers experienced traumatic and very emotional events during delivery. Common themes that were expressed and incorporated into the model were premonition, physical changes or symptoms, betrayal, "whirlwind," and loss. Common emotions were fear of death, frustration, anger, and guilt. They also reported overwhelming feelings of lack of control and "not knowing."

An example of a practice theory based on a grand theory is a work presented by Hannon-Engel (2008) which applied concepts and linkages from Roy's Adaptation Model to develop a theoretical framework to help practitioners manage patients with bulimia nervosa. Similarly, Mefford (2004) developed a practice theory of health promotion for preterm infants based on Levine's Conservation Model. In this theory, nursing interventions are directed toward adaptation of both the family and the infant through conservation of energy, structural integrity, personal integrity, and social integrity. Wholeness (health) of the infant and family is reflected by physiologic stability and growth, minimal structural injury, neurodevelopmental competence, and stability of the family system. Additional examples of practice or situation-specific theories and information about each are presented in Table 17-3.

TABLE 17-3 *Examples of Practice Theories and Models*

| Practice Theory or Model | Target Population | Development Process | Goal and Activities or Actions Prescribed |
|---|---|---|---|
| Symptom-focused diabetes care (Skelly, Leeman, Carlson, Soward, & Burns, 2008) | African-American women | Review of the literature and intervention protocols | Guides community-based, culturally sensitive diabetes interventions |
| Theory of breast-feeding (Nelson, 2006) | Maternal/infant dyad | Review of the literature; guidelines and recommendations | Promotes "salutary breastfeeding," which strives to promote congruity and minimize conflict to balance the positive benefits of breast-feeding for both the infant and mother |
| Progressively lowered stress threshold model (McCloskey, 2004) | Persons with dementia | Developed from clinical care for persons with Alzheimer's through application of theories of confusion, client-centered therapy, anxiety, stress, and coping | Directs care for patients with Alzheimer's and other dementias: minimize stressors and agitation by modifying or controlling factors that increase stress |
| Cancer patients pain experience (Im, 2006) | Caucasian cancer patients | Integrative approach to theory development (Im, 2005; Im & Meleis, 1999) | Describes the transitions of cancer patients' pain experience (e.g., types, patterns, properties), and their personal conditions and patterns of response, and shows how nursing therapeutics can respond |
| Theory of health promotion for preterm infants (Mefford, 2004) | Preterm infants in NICU | Application of Levine's Model; quantitative study involving 235 infants | Seeks to improve health outcomes of preterm infants through applying conservation principles; guides neonatal nursing practice |
| Taking care of oneself in a high-risk environment (Rew, 2004) | Vulnerable individuals in high-risk environments (homeless youth) | Grounded theory study of 15 homeless adolescents; incorporation of concepts of Orem's theory | Describes the socialization process experienced by homeless youth; suggests the need for nurses to support health, growth, and development among this group |
| Migration transition model (Clingerman, 2007) | Mexican and Mexican-American female migrant farmworkers | Qualitative research study of female farmworkers | Presents the transition processes experienced by this cohort and describes their patterns of response; presents potential nursing actions or therapeutics |
| Model of maternal experience of HELLP syndrome (Kidner & Flanders-Stepans, 2004) | New mothers who survived HELLP syndrome | Grounded theory study of nine women | Describes the emotional experiences of this population; suggests interventions for health providers to support and educate women who experience this condition |
| Maintaining hope in transition (Davidson, Dracup, Phillips, Padilla, & Daly, 2007) | People with heart failure | Application of Transition Theory to patients with heart failure | Use hope to focus on positive future orientation and emphasize the individual's ability to cope with and adjust to heart failure |

# Evidence-Based Practice

Over the past several years, the concept of EBP has appeared with increasing frequency in the nursing literature. EBP is similar to research-based practice and has been called an approach to problem solving in clinical practice that conscientiously uses the current "best" evidence in the care of patients (LoBiondo-Wood & Haber, 2006). It involves identifying a clinical problem, searching the literature, critically evaluating the research evidence, and determining appropriate interventions. Some nursing scholars believe that EBP will help fill the gap between research, theory, and practice (Billings & Kowalski, 2006). Because it is closely tied to the subject of research and theory, several issues relating to EBP are described in the following sections.

## OVERVIEW OF EVIDENCE-BASED PRACTICE

The concept of EBP originated in medicine in the late 1980s. EBP was built on the premise that health professionals should not center practice on tradition and belief, but on sound information grounded in research findings and scientific development (Melnyk & Fineout-Overholt, 2005; Upton, 1999). Until recently, the concept of EBP was more common in Canadian and English nursing literature than in U.S. nursing literature. The term, however, is becoming increasingly common; this is attributed in part to the guideline initiatives of the Agency for Health Care Quality (DiCenso, Guyatt, & Ciliska, 2005; Hudson, Duke, Haas, & Varnell, 2008). Several nursing scholars (DiCenso et al., 2005; Ingersoll, 2000; Melnyk & Fineout-Overholt, 2005; Rycroft-Malone, 2004; Titler, 2006) have pointed out that EBP and research are not synonymous. They are both scholarly processes, but focus on different phases of knowledge development—application versus discovery. EBP refers to the integration of individual clinical expertise with the best available external clinical evidence from systematic research. EBP is based on clinical research studies, particularly studies using clinical trials, meta-analysis, and studies of client outcomes, and it is more likely to be applied in practice settings that value the use of new knowledge and in settings that provide resources to access that knowledge.

## DEFINITION AND CHARACTERISTICS OF EVIDENCE-BASED PRACTICE

In medicine, EBP has been defined as the conscientious, explicit, and judicious use of the current best evidence in making decisions about the care of individual patients. It is an approach to health care practice in which the clinician is aware of the evidence that relates to clinical practice and the strength of that evidence (Jennings & Loan, 2001; Tod, Palfreyman, & Burke, 2004).

To distinguish nursing from medicine regarding EBP, a number of definitions have been presented in the literature. Sigma Theta Tau (2005, para 4) defined evidence-based nursing as "an integration of the best evidence available, nursing expertise, and the values and preferences of the individuals, families and communities who are served." Similarly, DiCenso and colleagues (2005) defined EBP as "the integration of best research evidence with clinical expertise and patient values to facilitate clinical decision making" (p. 4). Both of these use similar terms (e.g., best evidence, expertise, patient values). Ingersoll (2000) used slightly different terms when she suggested that evidence-based nursing practice "is the conscientious, explicit, and judicious use of theory-derived, research-based information in making decisions about care delivery to individuals or groups of patients and in consideration of individual needs and preferences" (p. 152).

In nursing, EBP generally includes careful review of research findings according to guidelines that nurse scholars have used to measure the merit of a study or group of studies. Evidence-based nursing de-emphasizes ritual, isolated, and unsystematic clinical experiences, ungrounded opinions, and tradition as a basis for practice, and stresses the use of research findings. Other measures or factors, including nursing expertise, health resources, patient/family preferences, quality improvement, and the consensus of recognized experts, are also incorporated as appropriate (DiCenso et al., 2005).

EBP has several critical features. First, it is a problem-based approach and considers the context of the practitioner's current experience (Melnyk, 2004). In addition, EBP brings together the best available evidence and current practice by combining research with tacit knowledge and theory. Finally, EBP facilitates the application of research findings by incorporating first- and second-hand knowledge into practice (French, 1999).

## CONCERNS RELATED TO EVIDENCE-BASED PRACTICE IN NURSING

Despite growing acceptance of the concept of EBP in nursing, some criticisms and concerns have been voiced in the nursing literature. For example, there is the concern that EBP is more focused on the science of nursing than on the art of nursing. It is believed that strict concentration on empirically based knowledge will lead to the failure to capture the uniqueness of nursing and the importance of holistic care in contemporary practice (Fawcett, Watson, Neuman, Walker, & Fitzpatrick, 2001; Hudson et al., 2008; Upton, 1999).

Another concern is that strict reliance on EBP will place nurses in the role of medical extender or medical technician, where nursing will be reduced to a technical practice. This concern was voiced as equating EBP with "cookbook care" and a disregard for individualized patient care (Melnyk & Fineout-Overholt, 2005). Indeed, although evidence may provide direction for development of procedures, techniques, and protocols for nursing, it has been established that these are not the only knowledge that informs the nursing practice and that consideration of individual needs and values is essential (Hudson et al., 2008; Mitchell, 1999).

Third, because research involving humans is complex, findings may be open to interpretation, and therefore should not be the sole basis for practice. Research must be considered within the context of the practice prescribed by theory, and it must integrate the values and beliefs of nursing philosophy (Fawcett et al., 2001; McKenna & Slevin, 2008; Mitchell, 1999).

A fourth concern relates to promoting a link with evidence-based medicine and its emphasis on positivist thinking and the dominance of randomized clinical trials as the major evidence. This concern is related to the absence of consideration of evidence gathered through qualitative research and theory development (Fawcett et al., 2001; Jennings & Loan, 2001).

A fifth concern relates to the potential for linking health care reimbursement exclusively to interventions that can be substantiated by a documented body of evidence (Ingersoll, 2000). This leads to a number of ethical questions and issues that should be considered.

Finally, it is argued that not all practice in the health professions can or should be based on science. In many cases, researchers have yet to accumulate a sufficient body of knowledge. In other cases, a different frame of reference provides a different rationale for action (McKenna & Slevin, 2008). In these instances, strict reliance on EBP may result in numerous voids when developing a plan of care.

Concerns such as these have been addressed by DiCenso and colleagues (2005), who assert that a fundamental principle of EBP is that research evidence alone is not sufficient to plan care. Other ethical and pragmatic factors, such as benefits and risks, associated costs, and patient's wishes, should be considered. Further, they note that "best research evidence" can be quantitative or qualitative and does not necessarily rely on randomized control studies. These notions are also supported by Rycroft-Malone (2004), who maintains that well-conceived and well-conducted qualitative and quantitative research evidence, clinical experience, and patient experiences, combined with local or organizational influences, are necessary to facilitate EBP.

## PROMOTION OF EVIDENCE-BASED PRACTICE IN NURSING

Tod and others (2004) contend that, because it is relatively new, the concept of EBP in nursing is still somewhat unsophisticated because many nursing practices are based on experience, tradition, intuition, common sense, and untested theories. It is argued that the need to move to EBP is growing, whereas the actual implementation has lagged somewhat due to the continued lack of implementation of nursing research findings in practice (Sams, Penn, & Facteau, 2004). There is concern that nurses in clinical environments rarely take advantage of knowledge and theory derived from research findings; Melnyk and Fineout-Overholt (2005) have outlined barriers to implementation of research and EBP in nursing (Box 17-2).

There is significant support for increasing emphasis on EBP in nursing. Indeed, practitioners, researchers, and scholars should welcome it. A systematic process of EBP may assist nurses in reducing the gap between theory and practice. However, it should be recognized as only one component of nursing knowledge and, thereby, only one component of nursing practice. Rosswurm and Larrabee (1999) developed a six-phase model to promote EBP, as summarized in Table 17-4.

---

**BOX 17-2** *Barriers to Evidence-Based Practice in Nursing*

- Lack of knowledge regarding EBP strategies
- Misperceptions or negative views about research and evidence-based care
- Lack of belief that EBP will result in more positive outcomes than traditional care
- Voluminous amounts of information in professional journals
- Lack of time and resources to search for and appraise evidence
- Overwhelming patient loads
- Organizational constraints (e.g., lack of administrative support)
- Demands from patients for a certain type of treatment
- Peer pressure to continue with practices that are steeped in tradition
- Inadequate content and skills regarding EBP in educational programs

Source: Melnyk and Fineout-Overholt (2005).

TABLE 17-4 *Evidence-Based Practice Model*

| Step | Examples of Activities |
|---|---|
| 1. Assess need for change in practice. | Involve stakeholders in process of change; collect internal data about current practices; compare internal data with external data; identify problem(s). |
| 2. Link problem interventions and outcomes. | Use standardized classification systems and standardized language; identify potential interventions and activities; select outcome indicators. |
| 3. Synthesize best evidence. | Search research literature related to major variables; critique and weigh evidence; synthesize best evidence; assess feasibility, benefits, and risks. |
| 4. Design practice change. | Define proposed change; identify needed resources; plan implementation processes; define outcomes. |
| 5. Implement and evaluate change in practice. | Perform pilot study demonstration; evaluate process and outcomes; decide to adapt, adopt, or reject practice change. |
| 6. Integrate and maintain change in practice. | Communicate recommended change to stakeholders; present staff in-service education program on change in practice; integrate into standards of practice; monitor process and outcomes. |

Source: Rosswurm and Larrabee (1999).

## Application of Theory in Nursing Practice

A lack of understanding of theory leads to a failure to recognize the use of theory on a day-to-day, even minute-to-minute, basis in the practice of nursing. For example, the practice of washing hands prior to client contact is based directly on the principles of germ theory and the epidemiologic concepts of disease transmission and disease prevention. Barnum (1998) used the term *implied theory* to refer to those theories used by practicing nurses during routine client care. Examples of application of theory can be taken from several sources within practice-based nursing literature. With few exceptions, as in real practice, the theoretical principles are implicit rather than explicit.

This section illustrates the application of a variety of theories, principles, and concepts in nursing journals and the nursing intervention classification system. The intent of this exercise is to show where and how nurses use theoretical principles in practice. For the most part, these theories are implied and extrapolated rather than explicitly stated in the works in question. Some readers may argue whether the theories/principles/concepts are addressed at all in the examples. Furthermore, the theories/principles/concepts discussed will most likely not be the only ones suggested in the work; indeed, there are probably countless others.

### THEORY IN NURSING TAXONOMY: EXAMPLES FROM THE NURSING INTERVENTION CLASSIFICATION SYSTEM

To illustrate the use of theory in nursing taxonomies, two interventions from the Nursing Intervention Classification (NIC) system are discussed. The NIC is a comprehensive list of 514 nursing interventions grouped into 30 classes and 7 domains. Nurses in all specialties and in all types of settings perform these interventions. The NIC includes physiologic, behavioral, safety, family, and community interventions, and there are interventions for illness treatment, illness prevention, and health promotion (Bulechek, Butcher, & Dochterman, 2008).

The intervention of intermittent urinary catheterization is used to highlight the incorporation of theories and principles from biology, physiology, and medicine into nursing. In a second discussion, theories related to behavioral interventions (i.e., learning theories and psychosocial theories and principles) are examined in the intervention of patient contracting.

### Intermittent Urinary Catheterization

Intermittent urinary catheterization refers to the "regular periodic use of a catheter to empty the bladder" (Bulechek et al., 2008, p. 779). The procedure may be performed by the nurse, another caregiver, or the client, and may be done in the home or in an institutional setting. The purposes are to eliminate residual urine in the bladder, reduce urinary infections, prevent incontinent episodes, regain bladder tone, achieve dilatation of the urethra, increase client control of urinary elimination, and facilitate self-care.

The authors presented incidence data to support the need and rationale for the intervention and explained how the problem of urinary incontinence is underreported. The data presented comparing rates and percentages were an example of the use of epidemiologic principles. Discussion of complications and side effects, including urinary tract infection and fistulas resulting from indwelling catheters, related to principles of anatomy and physiology as well as disease processes. Description of costs of alternative strategies implied the use of economic principles. Mention of reluctance to report incontinence suggested incorporation of psychosocial theories, and encouraging self-care related to several nursing theories, such as those of Orem and Erickson, Tomlin, and Swain.

The activities that comprise the intervention of intermittent urinary catheterization largely focus on prevention and identification of infection and teaching needs related to the psychomotor skills used by nurses and others providing care. Table 17-5 lists a few of the activities for the intervention and suggests a broad theoretical basis for each.

**TABLE 17-5** *Intermittent Urinary Catheterization: Theoretical Basis for Activities*

| Activity | Possible Theory Base |
|---|---|
| Perform comprehensive urinary assessment, focusing on causes of incontinence. | Physiology, certain disease processes |
| Teach client/family purpose, supplies, methods, and rationale of intermittent catheterization. | Teaching/learning principles and theories |
| Teach client/family clean intermittent catheterization technique. | Germ theory (principles of asepsis) |
| Use clean or sterile technique for catheterization. | Germ theory (principles of asepsis) |
| Maintain client on prophylactic antibacterial therapy for 2–3 weeks at initiation as appropriate. | Pharmacology, health promotion/prevention strategies |
| Establish a catheterization schedule based on individual needs. | Developmental theory, role theory, needs theory |
| Teach client/family signs and symptoms of urinary tract infection. | Principles of disease processes |

Source: Bulechek et al. (2008).

TABLE 17-6 *Patient Contracting: Theoretical Basis for Selected Activities*

| Activity | Possible Theory Base |
| --- | --- |
| Encourage the client to identify own strengths and abilities. | Role theory, developmental theory, needs theory |
| Assist client in identifying the health practice he or she wishes to change. | Self-determinism |
| Assist the client in identifying present circumstances that may interfere with achievement of goals. | Role theory, developmental theory, health beliefs, motivation theory |
| Encourage the client to identify appropriate, meaningful reinforces/rewards. | Motivation theory |

Source: Bulechek et al. (2008).

### Patient Contracting

One of the many behaviorally focused NIC interventions is patient contracting. Patient contracting is defined as "negotiating an agreement with an individual which reinforces a specific behavior change" (Bulechek et al., 2008, p. 541). The patient contracting intervention uses a seven-step process, which includes (1) behavioral analysis; (2) goal setting; (3) determination of responsibilities of all parties; (4) use of positive reinforcement; (5) use of potential consequences or sanctions for nonfulfillment of responsibilities; (6) determination of specific dates for initiation, negotiation, and termination; and (7) use of a signed, written contract.

The major theoretical basis of the intervention is principles from behavior modification and operant conditioning. The intervention also uses concepts and principles from other theories. These concepts include motivation, compliance/noncompliance, and risk factor management. In addition, patient contracting is based on the premise that all individuals have the right to self-determination to make their own choices and to be active in their own health care, and that health care providers must offer treatments that empower patients to identify their own priorities, strengths, weaknesses, and goals. These are ethical principles, which are fundamental to professional nursing practice.

Bulechek and colleagues (2008) developed a long list of activities that might be used in patient contracting. Table 17-6 lists a few of these activities and identifies a possible theoretical basis for each.

## EXAMPLES OF THEORY FROM NURSING LITERATURE

The general nursing literature is replete with examples of how theories are applied in routine nursing practice. This section presents several examples of practice—application of borrowed or "implied" theories as described earlier, as well as application of middle range and grand theories.

### Application of "Borrowed" and "Implied" Theories in Nursing Practice

Examples of application of borrowed theories in practice are easily identified in the literature. For example, Cleveland and others (2008) provided an explanation of the bases for current recommendations for screening and strategies for managing lead exposure in pregnant women and children. This discussion included epidemiologic information describing risk factors and demographic data accounting for the disparities of distribution of high lead levels. Additionally, environmental concepts and theories of lead contamination and related prevention strategies were examined.

Finally, the pathophysiology of lead absorption was explained, and this discussion included an overview of potential treatment for high lead levels (celation therapy) and the related biomedical and pharmacological aspects of the therapy.

Manning (2004) described the educator role within the advanced practice specialty of gastrointestinal nursing. This work focused on how the role of advanced practice nurse as educator requires knowledge and ability to apply concepts from a number of theories. She described how change theory, learning theory, motivation theory, communication, aging processes theory, and cultural diversity were incorporated into planning and implementing educational experiences.

In a final example of application of borrowed theories in nursing practice, Morton (2008) reported on the development and implementation of a health education program for school children. She used the Health Belief Model (HBM) as a guide to develop a series of weekly broadcasts over the participating schools' public announcement systems. Topics included head lice awareness, sleep, seat belt safety, and dental care. The intent of the education program was to provide health information that would enhance children's understanding of their individual risk for health threats and the perceived benefits of health promoting behaviors. In addition to HBM constructs, this program also illustrated application of other theories, models, and concepts including learning theories, biomedical concepts (principles of infection), and epidemiology (prevention).

### Application of Grand and Middle Range Theories in Nursing Practice

Articles showing how grand and middle range nursing theories have been applied in nursing practice can readily be found in the nursing literature. Martinez (2005) used Orem's self-care deficit theory to develop a plan of care for an elderly woman who needed an ileostomy. The author described how she used Orem's theory to assess her patient's self-care agency and therapeutic self-care demands and determined that her self-care demands exceeded her self-care agency. The goal was to increase her self-care agency to adequately and effectively meet her self-care demands.

In another work, Kavanaugh and colleagues (2006) used Swanson's middle range theory of caring to assist nurses in the process of recruiting and retaining vulnerable participants for research studies. The authors described how the theory could be used with different vulnerble groups to help alleviate potential for coercion and reduce the difficulty in recruiting potential study participants. Aspects of the theory were explained; these included the constructs of "maintaining belief," "knowing," "being with," "doing for," and "enabling." Numerous examples of how each construct was addressed during the implementation stages were provided, and included conveying hope, maintaining realistic optimism, and finding meaning (maintaining belief), being with, conveying availability and enduring with (being with), and informing and supporting (enabling).

The middle range comfort theory was used to direct nursing practice in a postanesthesia care unit (PACU) (Wilson & Kolcaba, 2004). These nurses described how comfort theory was able to direct more holistic care through employment of "comfort care interventions." These interventions were grouped as standard comfort interventions (i.e., vital signs, patient assessment, medication administration); coaching interventions (i.e., emotional support, education, listening); and "comfort food for the soul" (therapeutic touch, music therapy, personal connections). The writers concluded that these measures enhanced comfort in PACU patients.

How the Synergy Model has been used in guiding nursing practice can easily be found in the literature. For example, Smith (2006) described how the Synergy Model could be used to plan and provide spiritual nursing care in critical care settings. Then, in another work, Reilly and Humbrecht (2007) explained how the Synergy Model could be used to develop nursing interventions for remote telemetry monitoring.

## Summary

Many nursing scholars believe that theory-guided practice is the future of nursing. As nursing moves into the 21st century, nurses must place theory-guided practice at the core of nursing, and must integrate relevant outcomes-driven practice with the art and science of caring and healing.

As pointed out in the opening case study, advanced practice nurses like Emily routinely use concepts, principles, and theories from many disciplines, including nursing, to meet the health needs of their clients. To provide comprehensive, holistic, and effective interventions, nurses should rely on sound theoretical principles to develop and implement the plan of care.

Beginning in their basic nursing education program, all nurses should be encouraged to recognize the theoretical basis for practice and seek ways to enhance the knowledge base that supports practice. In addition, there should be an increased emphasis on enhancing the reciprocal interaction among theory, research, and practice with a concerted effort to bridge the theory–practice gap. Through these efforts, nursing can continue to develop and use a unique knowledge base and further contribute to autonomous and professional practice.

## LEARNING ACTIVITIES

1. Obtain a copy of the NIC (Bulechek et al., 2008). Select several interventions and try to identify the possible theoretical bases of each.

2. Debate the pros and cons of EBP with several classmates. Why would a focus on EBP be good for nursing? What are some drawbacks?

3. Obtain copies of recent mainstream nursing journals (e.g., *American Journal of Nursing*, *Nursing*, *RN*). Examine practice-focused articles and try to identify theories that affect the suggested nursing interventions and nursing implications.

4. Review theories and concepts described in previous chapters. Identify how they have been or could be applied in nursing practice.

## INTERNET RESOURCES

### Nursing Interventions

Center for Nursing Classification and Clinical Effectiveness Interventions—provides information on the development and dissemination of materials related to the Nursing Interventions Classification system and Nursing Outcomes Classification.

http://www.nursing.uiowa.edu/excellence/nursing_knowledge/clinical_effectiveness/index.htm

### Evidence-Based Practice

Cochrane Collaboration—produces and disseminates systematic reviews of health care interventions and promotes the search for evidence in the form of clinical trials and other studies.

http://www.cochrane.org/

Agency for Healthcare Research and Quality's National Guideline Clearinghouse—provides best practice and research-based guidelines for the public and health practitioners.

http://www.guideline.gov/

Worldviews—A new journal published by Sigma Theta Tau providing articles and information on EBP.

http://www.nursingsociety.org/Publications/Journals/Pages/worldviews.aspx

## REFERENCES

Allmark, P. (1995). A classical view of the theory-practice gap in nursing. *Journal of Advanced Nursing, 22*(1), 18–22.

Barnum, B. S. (1998). *Nursing theory: Analysis, application, evaluation* (5th ed.). Philadelphia: Lippincott Williams & Wilkins.

Billings, D. M., & Kowalski, K. (2006). Bridging the theory-practice gap with evidence-based practice. *Journal of Continuing Education in Nursing, 37*(6), 248–249.

Bulechek, G. M., Butcher, H. K, & Dochterman, J. M. (2008). *Nursing interventions classification (NIC)* (5th ed.). St. Louis: Elsevier.

Chinn, P. L., & Kramer, M. K. (2008). *Theory and nursing: Integrated knowledge development* (7th ed.). St. Louis: Mosby.

Cleveland, L. M., Minter, M. L., Cobb, K. A., Scott, A. A., & German, V. F. (2008). Lead hazards for pregnant women and children: Part 2. *The American Journal of Nursing, 108*(11), 40–48.

Clingerman, E. (2007). A situation-specific theory of migration transition for migrant farmworker women. *Research and Theory for Nursing Practice, 21*(4), 220–235.

Cody, W. K. (2003). Nursing theory as a guide to practice. *Nursing Science Quarterly, 16*(3), 225–231.

Dale, A. E. (1994). The theory–practice gap: The challenge for nurse teachers. *Journal of Advanced Nursing, 20*, 521–524.

Davidson, P. M., Dracup, K., Phillips, J., Padilla, G., & Daly, J. (2007). Maintaining hope in transition: A theoretical framework to guide interventions for people with heart failure. *Journal of Cardiovascular Nursing, 22*(1), 58–64.

DiCenso, A., Guyatt, G., & Ciliska, D. (2005). Introduction to evidence-based nursing. In A. DiCenso, D. Ciliska, & G. Guyatt (Eds.), *Evidence-based nursing: A guide to clinical practice* (pp. 3–19). St. Louis: Elsevier.

Doane, G. H., & Varcoe, C. (2005). Toward compassionate action: Pragmatism and the inseparability of theory/practice. *Advances in Nursing Science, 28*(1), 81–90.

Dreyfus, H. L., & Dreyfus, S. E. (1996). The relationship of theory and practice in the acquisition of skill. In P. Benner, C. A. Tanner, & C. A. Chesla (Eds.), *Expertise in nursing practice: Caring, clinical judgment and ethics* (pp. 29–47). New York: Springer.

Fawcett, J. (1992). Conceptual models and nursing practice: The reciprocal relationship. *Journal of Advanced Nursing, 17*, 224–228.

Fawcett, J., Watson, J., Neuman, B., Walker, P. H., & Fitzpatrick, J. J. (2001). On nursing theories and evidence. *Journal of Nursing Scholarship, 33*(2), 115–119.

French, P. (1999). The development of evidence-based nursing. *Journal of Advanced Nursing, 29*(1), 72–78.

Gallagher, P. (2004). How the metaphor of a gap between theory and practice has influenced nursing education. *Nurse Education Today, 24*(5), 263–268.

Hannon-Engel, S. L. (2008). Knowledge development: The Roy Adaptation Model and bulimia nervosa. *Nursing Science Quarterly, 21*(2), 126–132.

Hudson, K., Duke, G., Haas, B., & Varnell, G. (2008). Navigating the evidence-based practice maze. *Journal of Nursing Management, 16*(6), 409–416.

Im, E. O. (2005). Development of situation-specific theories: An integrative approach. *Advances in Nursing Science, 28*(2), 137–151.

Im, E. O. (2006). A situation-specific theory of Caucasian cancer patients' pain experience. *Advances in Nursing Science, 29*(3), 232–244.

Im, E. O., & Meleis, A. I. (1999). Situation-specific theories: Philosophical roots, properties and approach. *Advances in Nursing Science, 22*(2), 11–24.

Ingersoll, G. L. (2000). Evidence-based nursing: What it is and what it isn't. *Nursing Outlook, 48*(4), 151–152.

Jennings, B. M., & Loan, L. A. (2001). Misconceptions among nurses about evidence-based practice. *Journal of Nursing Scholarship, 33*(2), 121–127.

Jerlock, M., & Severinsson, E. (2003). Academic nursing education guidelines: Tool for bridging the gap between theory, research and practice. *Nursing and Health Sciences, 5*(3), 219–228.

Johnson, B. M., & Webber, P. B. (2005). *An introduction to theory and reasoning in nursing.* Philadelphia: Lippincott Williams & Wilkins.

Kavanaugh, K., Moro, T. T., Savage, T., & Mehendale, R. (2006). Enacting a theory of caring to recruit and retain vulnerable participants for sensitive research. *Research in Nursing and Health, 29*(3), 244–252.

Kenney, J. W. (1995). Relevance of theory-based nursing practice. In P. J. Christensen & J. W. Kenney (Eds.), *Nursing process: Application of conceptual models* (4th ed., pp. 3–17). St. Louis: Mosby.

Kenney, J. W. (2006). Theory-based advanced nursing practice. In W. K Cody (Ed.), *Philosophical and theoretical perspectives for advanced nursing practice* (4th ed., pp. 295–310). Sudbury, MA: Jones & Bartlett.

Kidner, M. C., & Flanders-Stepans, M. B. (2004). A model for the HELLP Syndrome: The maternal experience. *Journal of Obstetric, Gynecologic, and Neonatal Nursing, 33*(1), 44–53.

Kikuchi, J. F. (2004). Towards a philosophic theory of nursing. *Nursing Philosophy, 5*(1), 79–83.

Kim, H. S. (1994). Practice theories in nursing and a science of nursing practice. *Scholarly Inquiry for Nursing Practice, 8*(2), 145–158.

Larsen, K., Adamsen, L., Bjerregaard, L., & Madsen, J. K. (2002). There is no gap "per se" between theory and practice: Research knowledge and clinical knowledge are developed in different contexts and follow their own logic. *Nursing Outlook, 50*(5), 204–212.

Liaschendo, J., & Fisher, A. (1999). Theorizing the knowledge that nurses use in the conduct of their work. *Scholarly Inquiry for Nursing Practice, 13*(1), 29–41.

LoBiondo-Wood, G., & Haber, J. (2006). The role of research in nursing. In G. LoBiondo-Wood & J. Haber (Eds.), *Nursing research: Methods, critical appraisal, and utilization* (6th ed., pp. 5–26). St. Louis: Mosby.

Manning, M. (2004). The advanced practice nurse in gastroenterology serving as patient educator. *Gastroenterology Nursing, 27*(5), 220–225.

Marrs, J. A., & Lowry, L. W. (2006). Nursing theory and practice: Connecting the dots. *Nursing Science Quarterly, 19*(1), 44–50.

Martinez, L. A. (2005). Self-care for stoma surgery: Mastering independent stoma self-care skills in an elderly woman. *Nursing Science Quarterly, 18*(1), 66–69.

McCloskey, R. M. (2004). Caring for patients with dementia in an acute care environment. *Geriatric Nursing, 25*(3), 139–144.

McKenna, H. P., & Slevin, O. D. (2008). *Nursing models, theories and practice*. West Sussex, UK: Blackwell Publishing.

Mefford, L. C. (2004). A theory of health promotion for preterm infants based on Levine's conservation model of nursing. *Nursing Science Quarterly, 17*(3), 260–266.

Meleis, A. I. (2007). *Theoretical nursing: Development and progress* (4th ed.). Philadelphia: Lippincott.

Melnyk, B. (2004). Sparking a change to evidence-based practice in health care organizations. *Evidence-Based Nursing, 1*(2), 83–84.

Melnyk, B. M., & Fineout-Overholt, E. (2005). Making the case for evidence-based practice. In B. M. Melnyk and E. Fineout-Overhold (Eds.), *Evidence-based practice in nursing and healthcare: A guide to best practice* (pp. 3–24). Philadelphia: Lippincott Williams & Wilkins.

Mitchell, G. J. (1999). Evidence-based practice: Critique and alternative view. *Nursing Science Quarterly, 12*(1), 30–35.

Morton, J. L. (2008). "I Feel Good!" A weekly wellness radio broadcast for elementary school children. *The Journal of School Nursing, 24*(2), 83–87.

Nelson, A. M. (2006). Toward a situation-specific theory of breastfeeding. *Research and Theory for Nursing Practice, 20*(1), 9–27.

Nicoten, J. A., & Andrews, C. (2003). The discovery of unique nurse practitioner theory in the literature: Seeking evidence using an integrative review approach. *Journal of the American Academy of Nurse Practitioners, 15*(11), 494–500.

Parker, M. E. (2006). Introduction to nursing theory. In M. E. Parker (Ed.), *Nursing theories and nursing practice* (2nd ed., pp. 3–13). Philadelphia: F.A. Davis.

Perry, D. J. (2004). Self-transcendence: Lonergan's key to integration of nursing theory, research, and practice. *Nursing Philosophy, 5*(1), 67–74.

Reilly, T., & Humbrecht, D. (2007). Fostering Synergy: A nurse-managed remote telemetry model. *Critical Care Nurse, 27*(3), 22–33.

Rew, L. (2004). A theory of taking care of oneself grounded in experiences of homeless youth. *Nursing Research, 52*(4), 234–240.

Rolfe, G. (1998). The theory–practice gap in nursing: From research-based practice to practitioner-based research. *Journal of Advanced Nursing, 28*(3), 672–679.

Rosswurm, M. A., & Larrabee, J. H. (1999). A model for change to evidence-based practice. *Image: Journal of Nursing Scholarship, 31*(4), 317–322.

Runquist, J. (2007). Persevering through postpartum fatigue. *Journal of Obstetric, Gynecologic, and Neonatal Nursing, 36*(1), 28–37.

Rycroft-Malone, J. (2004). The PARIHS framework— A framework for guiding the implementation of evidence-based practice. *Journal of Nursing Care Quality, 19*(4), 297–304.

Sams, L., Penn, B. K., & Facteau, L. (2004). The challenge of using evidence-based practice. *Journal of Nursing Administration, 34*(9), 407–414.

Sigma Theta Tau International. (2005). Position statement on evidence based nursing. Available at: http://www. nursingsociety.org/aboutus/Position Papers/Pages/ EBN_positionpaper.aspx Accessed March 8, 2009.

Skelly, A. H., Leeman, J., Carlson, J., Soward, A. C. M., & Burns, D. (2008). Conceptual model of symptom-focused diabetes care for African Americans. *Journal of Nursing Scholarship, 40*(3), 261–267.

Smith, A. R. (2006). Using the Synergy Model to provide spiritual nursing care in critical care settings. *Critical Care Nurse, 26*(4), 41–47.

Suh, E. E. (2008). The sociocultural context of breast cancer screening among Korean immigrant women. *Cancer Nursing, 31*(4), E1–E10.

Titler, M. G. (2006). Developing an evidence-based practice. In G. LoBiondo-Wood & J. Haber (Eds.), *Nursing research: Methods, critical appraisal, and utilization* (6th ed., pp. 439–480), St. Louis: Mosby.

Tod, A., Palfreyman, S., & Burke, L. (2004). Evidence-based practice is a time of opportunity for nursing. *British Journal of Nursing, 13*(4), 211–216.

Upton, D. J. (1999). How can we achieve evidence-based practice if we have a theory–practice gap in nursing today? *Journal of Advanced Nursing, 29*(3), 549–555.

Wilson, J. (2008). Bridgin the theory practice gap. *Australian Nursing Journal, 16*(4), 25.

Wilson, L., & Kolcaba, K. (2004). Practical application of comfort theory in the perianesthesia setting. *Journal of PeriAnesthesia Nursing, 19*(3), 164–173.

Young, A., Taylor, S. G., & Renpenning, K. M. (2001). *Connections: Nursing research, theory and practice*. St. Louis: Mosby.

Ziegler, S. M. (2005). Introduction to theory-based nursing practice. In S. M. Ziegler (Ed.), *Theory-directed nursing practice* (2nd ed.). New York, NY: Springer.

# 18

# Application of Theory in Nursing Research

## Melanie McEwen

*P*eter Jacobson is in his second semester of a master's program in nursing. He is currently a supervisor on a general medical floor of a large teaching hospital and wants to advance in nursing administration after his graduation.

Peter's program requires that all students complete either a thesis or a formal research application project, and he wants to get an early start on developing this project. During a theory course in his first semester, Peter read about Pat Benner's work detailing the process of moving from novice to expert practice in nursing, and this work intrigued him. After talking about possible research topics with one of his professors, he decided that he wanted to use concepts from this theory to develop and test an orientation schedule for new graduates using selected "expert" nurses as mentors.

To better conceptualize the research study, he obtained a copy of Benner's most recent work. He also collected articles from nursing journals describing application of the novice to expert framework in different situations including nursing practice, nursing education, and nursing research. From this information, he was able to develop an outline for his research project that used the model as the conceptual framework.

In any discipline, science is the result of the relationship between the process of inquiry (research) and the product of knowledge (theory). The purpose of research is to build knowledge in a discipline through the generation and/or testing of theory. To effectively build knowledge, the research process should be developed within some theoretical structure that facilitates analysis and interpretation of findings. This will ultimately result in development of scientific theory. When a study is placed within a theoretical context, the theory guides the research process, forms the research questions, and aids in design, analysis, and interpretation. Thus, a theory, conceptual model, or framework provides parameters for a research study and enables the scientist to weave the facts together.

For the past several decades, nursing leaders have called for research to develop and confirm nursing knowledge and for theory to organize it. They have recognized the need to link nursing research and theory, because it has been observed that research without theory results in discrete information or data, which does not add to the accumulated knowledge of the discipline (Bishop & Hardin, 2006; Chinn & Kramer, 2008).

However, it has been pointed out that the relationship between research and theory in nursing is not well understood. This may be the result of several factors, including the relative youth of the discipline and debates over philosophical worldviews (i.e., empiricism, constructivism, phenomenology) as described in Chapter 1.

There are also concerns regarding whether nursing should form a discrete body of knowledge without using theories from other disciplines. Nursing science is a blend of knowledge that is unique to nursing and knowledge that is imported from other disciplines (e.g., psychology, sociology, education, biology), but there has been considerable debate about whether the use of borrowed theory has hindered the development of the discipline. This has contributed to problems connecting research and theory in nursing.

This chapter examines a number of issues related to the interface of research and theory in the discipline of nursing. Topics covered include the relationship between research and theory, types of theory and corresponding research, how theory is used in the research process, and the issue of borrowed versus unique theory for nursing. The chapter concludes with discussions of how theory should be addressed in a research report and the discipline's research agenda.

## Historical Overview of Research and Theory in Nursing

In the discipline of nursing, research and theory were first integrated in the works of Florence Nightingale. In *Notes on Nursing*, she identified the need to organize nursing knowledge through observation, recording, and statistical inferences. Nightingale also supported her theoretical propositions through research, as statistical data, and prepared graphs were used to depict the impact of nursing care on the health of British soldiers (Kalisch & Kalisch, 2004).

After Nightingale's time, for almost a century, reports of nursing research were rare. For the most part, research and theory developed separately in nursing. Blegen and Tripp-Reimer (1994) explained that between 1928 and 1959, only 2 of 152 studies published in nursing journals reported a theoretical basis for the research design.

The amount and quality of nursing research grew dramatically, however, beginning with the initial publication of *Nursing Research* in 1952. During the last half of the 20th century, the number of nursing journals focusing on research grew to include *Research in Nursing and Health*, *Western Journal of Nursing Research*, and *Advances in Nursing Science*. Many other nursing journals, both general (e.g., *Journal of Nursing Scholarship*, *Journal of Advanced Nursing*) and specialty based (e.g., *MCN: American Journal of Maternal Child Nursing*, *Heart and Lung: The Journal of Critical Care*, *AORN Journal*), also devote significant portions of each issue to nursing research.

In the early years, research in nursing focused on education and characteristics of nurses rather than on aspects of nursing practice and nursing interventions. However, by the 1990s, clinical studies comprised over 75% of articles in research journals (Blegen & Tripp-Reimer, 1994).

Beginning in the 1970s, nurse scholars encouraged researchers to provide a theoretical or conceptual framework for research studies. At about the same time, a growing number of nurse theorists were seeking researchers to explore ways to test their models in research and clinical application. As a result, there was a push to combine research and nursing models. This emphasis on using nursing models as the framework for research was proposed to provide research into the unique perspective of nursing (Chinn & Kramer, 2008; Fawcett, 2005).

Despite this encouragement, however, the vast majority of research studies in nursing do not test aspects of grand nursing theories or use them as a research framework. Rather, they examine concepts, principles, and theories from a number of theoretical perspectives and disciplines. This trend persisted throughout the 1990s and into the 21st century, as the focus of research and theory has moved more toward middle range and practice theories (see Chapters 10, 11, and 17).

## Relationship Between Research and Theory

Knowledge development is cumulative, and knowledge generated from separate research studies should be integrated into a more comprehensive understanding of the subject or phenomenon being studied. The value of any research study is derived as much from how it fits with, and expands on, previous work as from the study itself. Thus, research gains its significance from the context within which it is placed—specifically from its theoretical context. The theoretical context, therefore, is the structure and system of important concepts, theoretical propositions, and theories that comprise the existing knowledge of the discipline (Chinn & Kramer, 2008; Fawcett, 2005).

Moody (1990) explained that knowledge development in nursing science has lagged due to three major factors: (1) a limited theoretical base to guide practice; (2) an abundance of isolated studies that have not been tied to an integrating theoretical framework or placed in a theoretical context; and (3) inadequate efforts to link theory, measurement, and data interpretation during the research process. To further develop nursing science and strengthen the discipline, it is essential that nurse researchers and nurse scholars address these issues. This requires recognizing the relationship between research and theory and developing an understanding of how theory is used in, and developed through, research. The following sections describe this relationship.

### NURSING RESEARCH

Research is the "systematic inquiry that uses disciplined methods to answer questions or solve problems" (Polit & Beck, 2008, p. 3). Research is conducted to describe, explain, or predict variables, and in a practice discipline such as nursing, research is assumed to contribute to the improvement of care. The research process consists of several essential steps that are followed in planning, implementing, and analyzing a research study (Box 18-1).

Nursing research has been defined as a "scientific process that validates and refines existing knowledge and generates new knowledge that directly and indirectly influences nursing practice" (Burns & Grove, 2009, p. 4). It is concerned with the study of individuals in interaction with their environments, and with discovering interventions that promote optimal functioning and wellness across the lifespan. In nursing, researchers have studied principles and laws governing life processes, the well-being and optimum functioning of human beings, patterns of behavior as individuals interact with their environment during critical life situations (e.g., birth, loss, illness,

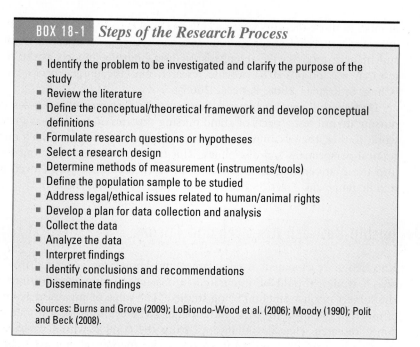

Sources: Burns and Grove (2009); LoBiondo-Wood et al. (2006); Moody (1990); Polit and Beck (2008).

death), and processes that bring about positive changes in a person's health status. Furthermore, nursing research measures the impact of nursing interventions on client outcomes to provide a rational basis for practice.

## PURPOSE OF THEORY IN RESEARCH

Theory is integral to the research process. It is important to use theory as a framework to provide perspective and guidance to a research study. Indeed, theoretical frameworks provide direction regarding selection of the research design, identify approaches to measurement and methods of data analysis, and specify criteria for acceptability of findings as valid (Fitzpatrick, 1998).

Fitzpatrick (1998) summarized how theory can be used to guide the research process. In the process of generating and testing phenomena of interest to nursing, theory can (1) identify meaningful and relevant areas for study, (2) propose plausible approaches to health problems to examine, (3) develop or reformulate middle range theory linked to research, (4) define the concepts and propose relationships among concepts, (5) interpret research findings, (6) develop clinical practice protocols, and (7) generate nursing diagnoses based on research findings.

## THE RESEARCH FRAMEWORK

As shown in Box 18-1, an essential step of the research process is selection of a theoretical or conceptual model that serves as a research framework. The investigator uses the conceptual model to view situations and events through a particular frame of reference, the researcher's perspective about how the concepts and variables of interest in the study fit together. The research framework describes the phenomena and problems to be studied, as well as the purposes to be fulfilled by the research. It identifies the source of the data (e.g., individuals, groups, animals, documents) and the settings in which data are to be gathered. It contributes to selection of the research design and instruments, determines procedures to be used, and identifies the methods to be used for data analysis. Finally, the framework determines the contributions of the research to the advancement of knowledge by placing the findings within the context of previous knowledge (Fawcett, 1999).

Norwood (2000) believes that using a formal and explicit framework facilitates generalizing a study's findings. This can contribute to nursing science development and promote evidence-based practice. She points out that frameworks have a reputation for being abstract, meaningless, and impractical, when in reality using a framework can simplify and provide direction to the research process. Unfortunately, in many published nursing research studies, especially studies involving clinical practice problems, a study's framework is implicit rather than explicit. It may be hidden or implied in the literature review, and the reader must "tease it out."

# Types of Theory and Corresponding Research

As described in Chapter 2, theory is generally classified as descriptive, explanatory, or predictive. The research designs that generate and test these theories are descriptive, correlational, and experimental, respectively (Fawcett, 1999). Prescriptive theories are also mentioned by a number of authors (Dickoff & James, 1968; Meleis, 2007) and are sometimes related to practice theories (Whall, 2005). Table 18-1 shows the three primary types of theory described in nursing literature (descriptive, explanatory, and predictive) and summarizes the examples from the following discussion.

## DESCRIPTIVE THEORY AND DESCRIPTIVE RESEARCH

A descriptive theory is an integrated set of concepts that focuses on dimensions, characteristics, and commonalities of a phenomenon of interest (Norwood, 2000). A descriptive theory looks at a phenomenon and identifies its major elements or events. It may also note some relationships among the elements, but it does not examine why

TABLE 18-1 *Types of Theory and Corresponding Research*

| Type of Theory | Type of Research | Examples from Nursing Literature |
|---|---|---|
| Descriptive | Descriptive or exploratory | Development of a model to describe how mothers assist their adult children who are mentally ill and violent (Copeland & Heilemann, 2008) |
| | | Development of the Theory of Genetic Vulnerability (Hamilton & Bowers, 2007) |
| Explanatory | Correlational | Explaining school nurses' perceived self-efficacy in providing diabetes care and identifying factors that correlate with higher self-efficacy levels (Fisher, 2006) |
| | | Explaining the effect of social support on positive health practices among adolescents (Mahon et al., 2004) |
| Predictive | Experimental | Comparing healing touch, coaching and combined interventions on comfort and stress among college students (Dowd et al., 2007) |
| | | Using creativity enhancement to positively influence positive aging (Flood & Scharer, 2006) |

the phenomenon has those elements, how they relate to each other, or how changes in the elements affect each other (Barnum, 2005).

Descriptive research involves observation of a phenomenon in its natural setting. Data are gathered by participant or nonparticipant observation and by open-ended or structured interview schedules or questionnaires. Data may be qualitative or quantitative or both. Descriptive research uses many different methods, including concept analysis, psychometric analyses, case studies, surveys, phenomenology, ethnography, grounded theory, and historical inquiry (McKenna & Slevin, 2008).

Descriptive research (exploratory research) answers questions such as: What are the characteristics of the phenomenon? What is the prevalence of the phenomenon? What is the process by which the phenomenon is experienced? (Fawcett, 2005). Through systematic study of these or similar questions with a defined population or in a defined setting, a descriptive theory may result.

### Nursing Studies

There are many excellent examples of descriptive theory and explanatory and descriptive research in the nursing literature. For example, Hamilton and Bowers (2007) used grounded theory methods to develop the Theory of Genetic Vulnerability to explain the experience of undergoing genetic testing for certain adult onset diseases (i.e., Huntington's disease or hereditary breast and ovarian cancer). From detailed interviews with 29 participants undergoing genetic testing, they identified five key concepts comprising the basis of the theory: experiencing the family disease, testing for a mutation, foregrounding inherited disease risk, responding to knowledge of genetic vulnerability, and altering or avoiding the family experience of the disease. Implications for nursing practice and related interventions were described based on Roy's Adaptation Model.

Sun, Long, Boore, and Tsao (2006) also used grounded theory methods to interview 15 psychiatric nurses and 15 patients who had either suicidal ideas or had attempted suicide. They determined that providing "safe and compassionate care via . . . the therapeutic relationship" (p. 683) was a key concept. This included such elements as providing holistic assessment, providing protection, providing basic care, and promoting healing. Outcomes of care are to assist the patient to regain the desire to live, resist recurrent suicide thoughts, and prevent future attempts. From these data, they generated the "theory for the nursing care of patients at risk of suicide."

Last, Weiss and others (2008) conducted a grounded theory study of 19 incarcerated adolescent females to elicit information related to sexual decision making. They learned that these young women were bombarded with seductive influences, and as a result they determined that sex was routine by perceiving that "everybody's doing it." The Theory of Normalizing Risky Sexual Behaviors was the result of this work.

## EXPLANATORY THEORY AND CORRELATIONAL RESEARCH

Explanatory theories specify relationships between dimensions or characteristics of individuals, groups, situations, or events. They explain why, and the extent to which, one phenomenon is related to another. Explanatory theories are composed of concepts and propositions (Norwood, 2000).

Explanatory theories are typically generated and tested by correlational research. Correlational research requires measurement of the dimensions or characteristics of phenomena in their natural states. Data are usually gathered by nonparticipant observation or a self-report instrument. Instruments can include fixed-choice, open-ended questionnaires, or interview schedules. Correlational research yields qualitative or quantitative data or both. Statistical analysis uses various nonparametric or parametric measures of association (LoBiondo-Wood, Haber, & Krainovich-Miller, 2006).

### Nursing Studies

Using a correlational study design, Mahon, Yarcheski, and Yarcheski (2004) examined the relationship between social support and positive health practices during adolescence. In this study, 134 adolescents were surveyed using instruments that measured social support, loneliness, hopefulness, and positive health practices. In testing two models describing the relationships between the variables, in terms of theory building, the researchers concluded that loneliness and hopefulness were mediators of the relationship between social support and positive health practices among adolescents, and described the "loneliness mediation model."

Another study (Dunn, 2005) used a correlational design to examine chronic pain among 200 community-dwelling elders. The purpose of the study was to test and continue to develop a theory developed from the Roy Adaptation Model. Path analysis revealed that elders reported similar chronic pain intensities, regardless of gender or race/ethnicity, and that elders with higher pain intensity reported higher levels of functional disability and were more depressed than elders with less chronic pain. Although religious and nonreligious coping strategies were employed to adapt to chronic pain, neither showed superior effect on levels of functional ability or development of depression. The original model of adaptation to chronic pain was modified somewhat, based on study findings.

Finally, Peters (2006) reported on a correlational study undertaken to develop, test and refine the middle range theory of chronic stress emotions based on Lazarus' stress and coping model. The research specifically measured the effect of stress on physiological health (blood pressure) among 162 community-dwelling African-American adults. Structural equation modeling was used to examine the causal and correlational links of the model variables. It was determined that although stress, as indicated by perceived racism and emotion-focused coping contributed to reports of chronic stress, they did not result in increases in blood pressure.

## PREDICTIVE THEORY AND EXPERIMENTAL RESEARCH

Predictive theories move beyond explanation to the prediction of relationships between characteristics or phenomena among different groups. Predictive theories are generated and tested by experimental research.

Experimental research involves the manipulation of some phenomenon to determine how it affects or changes some dimension or characteristic of another phenomenon. Experimentation encompasses many different designs, including pretest–posttest–noncontrol group design, quasi-experiments, time series analyses, and true experiments. Experimental research requires quantifiable data. Statistical analyses, involving various nonparametric and parametric tests, are used to measure differences. Qualitative data can be collected, but generally must be coded to be tested statistically (LoBiondo-Wood et al., 2006).

### Nursing Studies

Experimental research studies, and corresponding predictive theories, are relatively uncommon in nursing literature. Examples from recent nursing literature include a study by Hall and colleagues (2005) which used an experimental, posttest, control group design to evaluate the effectiveness of a culturally sensitive breast cancer education program for African-American women. In the work guided by the Health Belief

Model, the researchers concluded that participants who participated in the multi-faceted educational program reported significantly higher knowledge about breast cancer and screening options.

A second example using an experimental design is a study by Lewandowski (2004). The researcher used Rogers' science of unitary human beings theory as a framework and employed a random assignment with repeated measures design. The aim was to compare the impact of using guided imagery as an intervention to manage chronic pain comparing experimental and control groups. After controlling for potential for differences in imaging ability, it was determined that the treatment group had significantly less pain at the fourth and fifth measures, indicating that these subjects experienced less pain than the control group during the last 2 days of the study.

Then, Dowd, Kolcaba, Steiner, and Fashinpaur (2007) used an experimental design to compare interventions of healing touch, coaching, and a combination of the two on reported stress and comfort in college students. Kolcaba's Comfort Theory was the conceptual framework for the interventions which appeared to reduce stress among those receiving them. Last, Roy's Adaptation Model served as a framework for an experimental study examining the influence of functional performance and creativity on successful aging. Using a pretest–posttest experimental design, Flood and Scharer (2006) learned that striving to enhance creativity among elders contributes to successful aging.

# How Theory Is Used in Research

Theory brings organization to the variables of interest and the concepts reflected in a study. It provides a guide for developing a study and allows the findings to be placed in, or linked to, a larger body of knowledge. Therefore, a theoretical perspective increases the scientific value of a study's findings.

Both nursing and nonnursing theories have relevance for problems studied by nursing researchers, and theories tend to show up in the research process in one of three ways. A theory can be generated as the outcome of a study. In other cases, a research project is undertaken for the specific purpose of testing a theory. Most frequently, a theory is used in a research framework as the context for a study (Norwood, 2000). Each of these three ways that theory is used in research is described in the following sections.

## THEORY-GENERATING RESEARCH

Research that generates theory (i.e., descriptive research) is designed to develop and describe relationships between and among phenomena without imposing preconceived notations of what these phenomena mean (Chinn & Kramer, 2008). It is inductive and includes grounded theory, field observations, and phenomenology. During the theory-generating process, the researcher moves by logical thought from fact to theory by means of a proposition stated as an empirical generalization.

Norwood (2000) explained that there are several steps in the process of theory generation. First, the researcher identifies observations that have shared characteristics or common themes in an identified group or in a particular setting. Second, the researcher translates these observations into more abstract concepts by determining what general phenomenon these observations represent, and identifying patterns of relationships between observations and concepts. Third, the researcher translates observations of relationships into propositional statements and weaves the concepts and propositions together into a framework or tentative theory. In some cases, the researcher may identify an existing theory that these concepts and relationships repre-sent. Nursing Exemplar 1 analyzes a grounded theory study to further illustrate the steps involved in theory-generating research.

## NURSING EXEMPLAR 1: THEORY-GENERATING RESEARCH

The following study is a good example of theory generation using grounded theory research techniques. The study is analyzed using criteria described by Norwood (2000).

Hamilton, R. J., & Bowers, B. J. (2007). The theory of genetic vulnerability: A Roy Model exemplar. *Nursing Science Quarterly, 20*(3), 254–264.

*Common themes in an identified group:* The researchers provided background information explaining the potential emotional problems and concerns related to undergoing genetic testing for adult onset diseases cause by genetic mutations—specifically Huntington's disease (HD) or hereditary breast and ovarian cancer (HBOC). They observed that new advances in genetic testing, combined with the patient's family experiences with the disease in question, will lead to questions related to risk and choices that those with a family history will make to address their risk.

*Observations of general phenomenon:* The researchers explained that individuals who are at risk for HD or HBOC are "acutely aware of their family's history with the disease" (p. 255). Further, they point out that medical anthropologists have observed that genetic testing has resulted in at risk families being "medicalized." Understanding the phenomenon of "genetic vulnerability," the researchers explain has implications for patient counseling and education regarding the family's experience of an inher-ited disease, the medical option of genetic testing, and subsequent actions of individuals after they receive the results.

*Patterns of relationships identified:* From their discussions with 29 individuals undergoing testing for either HD or HBOC (24 who had completed genetic testing and 5 who declined testing), the researchers identified five basic constructs comprising the theory. These are: "experiencing the family disease" (a common, specific understanding about the disease and chances of inheritance); "personal vulnerability" (which combines resemblance to a family member with the disease and history of the disease in the family); "foregrounding inherited disease risk" (sharing the results with family members); "responding to knowledge of genetic vulnerability" (deciding whether or not to take action based on the findings from genetic testing); and "altering or avoiding the family experience of inherited disease" (making choices to avoid the family experience of the disease or to alter personal experience with the disease).

*Translation into prepositional statements:* The researchers described how they used elements of the Roy Adaptation Model to explain the relationships of many of the constructs. They observed that the coping processes of the individuals are influenced by their experience and perceptions, as well as their understanding of the genetic facts. The theory goes on to explain how the individuals under-stood their risk and how their personal experiences of the disease within their family influenced both their understanding and their choices.

### Nursing Studies

Theory-generating research studies can readily be found in nursing literature. As men-tioned, a number of nursing theories have been developed using grounded theory re-search techniques. For example, Copeland and Heilemann (2008) used grounded theory methods to develop a theoretical explanation to explore and analyze mothers' experi-ences of violence perpetrated by adult children with mental illness. Olshansky (2003) used a multiphased grounded theory approach to develop a theoretical explanation for previously infertile mothers' vulnerability to depression. Likewise, Turkel and Ray (2001) used multiple stages to develop and test a theory of "relational complexity," which describes "the nurse–patient relationship within an economic context" (p. 283).

Often new theories are developed from existing theories. For example, Mefford (2004) reportedly developed her theory of health promotion for preterm infants based on Levine's Conservation Model of Nursing. Similarly, the Theory of Dependent Care was derived from Orem's Self-Care Deficit Theory of Nursing (Taylor Renpenning, Geden, Neuman, & Hart, 2001). This theory was designed to describe how individuals provide care to dependents (e.g., infants and the feeble elderly), either on a continuing or intermittent basis.

## THEORY-TESTING RESEARCH

Sometimes a study is conducted for the purpose of testing a theory or assessing its explanatory value in a specific situation. In theory-testing research, theoretical statements are translated into questions and hypotheses. Theory testing requires a deductive reasoning process that also follows several steps (Chinn & Kramer, 2008).

First, the researcher chooses a theory of interest and selects a specific propositional statement from the theory (rather than the entire theory) to be tested. Second, the researcher then develops a hypothesis or hypotheses that must have specific measurable variables that reflect the propositional statement. Third, the researcher conducts the study and interprets findings. The interpretation determines if the study supports or contradicts the propositional statement and, thus, the theory. Finally, the researcher determines if there are any implications for further use of the theory in nursing practice (Norwood, 2000).

Little progress has been made in testing theories in nursing (McQuiston & Campbell, 1997). One reason for this is the lack of clarity about what constitutes theory testing. Silva (1986) pointed out that serious misconception exists among some researchers and theorists that if a conceptual model has been used as a theoretical framework for research, then this constitutes theory testing. It does not, however, because theory testing requires detailed examination of theoretical relationships and necessitates that the study be designed to accept or refute these relationships.

Another reason there has been little theory-testing research relates to interpretation and evaluation of the research. Acton, Irvin, and Hopkins (1991) developed criteria for evaluating theory-testing research (Box 18-2) that will help those who are interested in conducting this type of study, as well as those using the criteria. In addition, Nursing Exemplar 2 gives an example of the evaluation of a theory-testing study using these criteria.

### NURSING EXEMPLAR 2: THEORY-TESTING RESEARCH

The following is a review of an excellent example of theory-testing research. In this study, portions of Pender's Health Promotion Model (HPM) were tested in low-income Korean elderly women. Here, the research is evaluated using the criteria suggested in Box 18-2.

Shin, K. R., Kang, Y., Park, H. J., Cho, M. O., & Heitkemper, M. (2008). Testing and developing the Health Promotion Model in low-income, Korean elderly women. *Nursing Science Quarterly, 21*(2), 173–178.

*Purpose:* "This study was conducted to test Pender's health promotion model in low-income Korean elderly women" (p. 173).

*Explicit summary of theory:* Pender's HPM is succinctly explained.

*Definitions:* Concepts from the HPM are defined, described, and operationalized; relationships are explained.

*Previous studies:* Review of the literature includes a number of studies that show relationships between the concepts being studied (prior health-related behavior, activity limitations, commitment to a plan of action); many specifically addressed use of the HPM in research of Korean patients. The literature review is thorough and supports the theory as well as placing the current research in context.

*Hypotheses:* Three hypothetical propositions were presented and based on the previous reported studies using the HPM. One, for example, read: "behavior-specific cognitions and affect and environmental influences have indirect influences on health-promoting behaviors through commitment to a plan of action" (p. 174).

*Operational definitions:* Operational definitions are clearly described and derived from Pender's work.

*Study design:* The design was a descriptive, survey using face-to-face interviews. Structural equation modeling (SEM) was employed to test the hypotheses and the model.

*Instruments:* A number of instruments were used in the study. Each instrument is described in the text and includes data on their use in multiple studies and evidence of reliability and validity.

*Sample:* The convenience sample of 400 low-income elderly women from two public health centers in Seoul consented to participate. From this group, 389 interviews were completed and included in the final sample.

*Statistics:* Covariance structural analysis was used to analyze the data.

*Data analysis:* The results did not support the initial hypothetical propositions and the model was adapted using data provided by the SEM and supported by Pender's model. The modified proposition demonstrated a good fit to the empirical data. In all, 73% of the variance in predicting health-promoting behaviors of the sample was accounted for by the study variables (e.g., biological factors, psychological factors, commitment to a plan of action).

*Research report:* The report detailed findings that directly related to Pender's HPM.

*Significance of theory for nursing:* It was concluded that Pender's HPM is useful for explaining relationships among health-promoting behaviors among low-income elderly Korean women. Findings can be used to provide suggestions for future nursing interventions among this aggregate.

*Recommendations:* The researchers suggested studies on nursing interventions to enhance self-esteem, perceived health, interest in health and social support.

---

**BOX 18-2** *Criteria for Evaluating Theory-Testing Research*

- The purpose of the study is to examine the empirical validity of the constructs, concepts, assumptions, or relationship from the identified theory
- The theory is explicitly described and summarized
- The constructs and concepts to be examined are theoretically defined
- An overview of the previous studies that are based on the theoretic framework, or that clearly show the derivation of the concepts being tested, must be included in the review of the literature
- The research questions or hypotheses are logically derived from the definitions, assumptions, and propositions of the theory
- The research questions or hypotheses are specific enough to put the theory at risk for falsification
- The operational definitions are clearly derived from the theory
- The design is congruent with the level of theory described
- The instruments are theoretically valid and reliable
- The theory guides the sample selection
- The statistics used are the most robust possible
- Data analysis provides evidence for supporting, refuting, or modifying the theory
- The research report includes an interpretative analysis of the finding in relation to the theory being tested
- The significance of the theory for nursing is discussed in the report
- The researcher makes recommendations for further research on the basis of the findings
- Researchers should identify theory-testing studies in their abstracts, publication titles, and library retrieval key words

### Nursing Studies

Some studies testing theories were found in recent nursing literature. Not surprisingly, most of those studies identified tested grand or middle range nursing theories or theories derived from grand nursing theories.

Research testing grand nursing theories included a study conducted by Gigliotti (2004). In this work, elements of the Neuman's systems model were tested by examining maternal–student role stress. This study was designed to examine the moderating capabilities of the psychological and sociocultural variables in the flexible line of defense. In the study, 135 women were given questionnaires to measure role stress, maternal and student role involvement, and social support. It was concluded that the effect of student role involvement on maternal–student role stress is contingent upon low network support. Also, the effect of maternal role involvement on maternal–student role stress is significantly enhanced for women age 37 years and older.

Research that tested theories or models derived from grand or middle range nursing theories included Kerr, Lusk, and Ronis (2002), who tested the applicability of using Pender's HPM to predict Mexican-American workers' use of hearing protection devices. Two additional studies (Dunn, 2005; Tsai, Tak, Moore, & Palencia, 2003) reportedly tested a theory of chronic pain derived from the Roy Adaptation Model.

Research that tested nonnursing theories was also identified in the nursing literature. For example, a study by Werner and Mendelsson (2001) tested the theory of planned behavior in examining the nurses' intention to use physical restraints with older people. The theory of planned behavior was also tested in a study designed to predict sexual intercourse and condom use intentions among Latino youths (Villarruel, Jemmott, Jemmott, & Ronis, 2004) and a study that examined childhood fever management (Edwards, Walsh, Courtney, Monaghan, Wilson, & Young, 2007).

## THEORY AS THE CONCEPTUAL FRAMEWORK OR CONTEXT OF A STUDY

The most common way of incorporating a theory into the research process is by using the theory to drive the entire study (Moody, Wilson, Smyth, Schwartz, Tittle, & Van Cott, 1988; Silva, 1986). In these cases, the problem being investigated is fitted into an existing theoretical framework, which guides the study and enriches the value of its findings.

The process of using a theory as a conceptual framework also involves several steps. Typically, during the process of conducting the literature review, the researcher

---

| BOX 18-3 | *Use of a Theory as a Conceptual Framework in a Nursing Study* |

- The research subproblems are derived from and are consistent with the framework
- The conceptual definitions are drawn from the framework
- The data collection instrument is congruent with the framework
- Findings are interpreted in light of explanations provided by the framework
- The researcher determines support for the framework based on study findings
- Implications for advanced practice nursing are based on the explanatory power of the framework
- Recommendations for future research address the concepts and relationships designated by the framework

Source: Norwood (2000).

identifies an existing framework that can be meaningfully applied to the study or develops a conceptual framework that is unique to the study (Norwood, 2000). When a framework is used as the context, it is integrated into the study in a number of ways (Box 18-3). Nursing Exemplar 3 presents an evaluation of a published research study illustrating how a nursing theory is used as a conceptual framework.

## NURSING EXEMPLAR 3: THEORY AS A CONCEPTUAL FRAMEWORK

The following is a good example of using a nursing theory (the Roy Adaptation Model) as the conceptual framework for a research study. The criteria suggested in Box 18-3 were used to evaluate this work.

DeSanto-Madeya, S. (2009). Adaptation to spinal cord injury for families post-injury. *Nursing Science Quarterly, 22*(1), 57–66.

*Research problems consistent with the framework:* The purpose of this study was to "identify individuals' and family members' perspectives of the physical, emotional, functional, and social components of adaptation and their adjustment to spinal cord injury" (p. 58).

*Conceptual definitions derived from the framework:* Concepts studied were derived from the Roy Adaptation Model. Concepts described were: adaptive systems (families) in constant interaction with changing focal stimuli (time since injury) and contextual stimuli (level of injury and factors that help or hinder their adaptation).

*Instruments congruent with the framework:* The research instruments were described in detail. They included the Adaptation to Spinal Cord Injury Interview Schedule (developed by the researcher for a previous study) and a detailed background data sheet.

*Findings interpreted based on the framework:* The findings were interpreted based on explanations of the Roy Adaptation Model.

*Relationship of findings to framework:* The researchers described the findings in relation to the Roy Adaptation Model by explaining how family members' responses fell within Roy's Modes of Adaptation. An "adaptation score" was calculated for spinal cord injured individuals and their family members, and adjustment to spinal cord injury was evaluated at Year 1 and Year 3. Factors that help or hinder adaptation were also assessed.

*Implications for nursing:* It was concluded that family relationships and refocusing of values positively influenced adaptation to spinal cord injury. Additionally, it was noted that depression is common for both the injured person and the family members, an observation that is very important for nurses providing care.

*Recommendations for future research:* The researchers noted that further inquiry should be conducted with a larger sample to determine the utility and adequacy of applying aspects of Roy's model to caring for individuals with spinal cord injury.

---

If the conceptual framework used by the researcher is an existing framework, the process can be termed *theory fitting*. In theory fitting, the researcher formulates a research purpose or research question and then proceeds to the literature to search for a theory to guide the study. The theory that best fits the research study is then selected. There are potential problems with this practice, however. The concepts or relationships from the original theory may be incorrectly applied, the work may appear "forced," or the study may fail to lead to meaningful conclusions. To be effective, theory fitting requires an extensive search of the literature and an understanding of theoretical progress in nursing and other fields (Moody, 1990).

### Nursing Studies

A number of current studies using both nursing and nonnursing theories as the research framework were identified. For example, a recent study that used nursing theory as the conceptual framework was one conducted by Mock and others (2007). This work used Levine's Conservation Model as a conceptual framework to study the effects of exercise on fatigue and physical functioning in cancer patients. Another study (Lancaster, 2005) used Betty Neuman's Systems Model to examine how women with a family history of breast cancer appraise and cope with breast cancer risk.

Orem's theory of self-care was used as the framework to examine whether easy-to-read immunization information could improve vaccination rates among children of low-income, urban mothers (Wilson, Brown, & Stephens-Ferris, 2006). Leininger's Culture Care Diversity Theory was the framework of Anuforo, Oyedele, and Pacquiao's (2004) study of the meanings, beliefs, and practices of female circumcision among Nigerians in the United States and Nigeria.

Nonnursing theories are frequently used as conceptual frameworks and numerous examples are found throughout the nursing literature. For example, Sethares and Elliott (2004) used the Health Belief Model as the framework to use tailored messages to change the benefit and barrier beliefs of persons with heart failure related to taking medications, following a prescribed diet, and self-monitoring for signs of fluid overload. Similarly, Hall and colleagues (2005) used the Health Belief Model as the framework of an experimental study to determine whether a culturally sensitive educational program would improve knowledge, beliefs and practices associated with early detection of breast cancer in African-American women. Last, Buchanan and Likness (2008) used Bandura's Social Learning Theory to design an intervention that was shown to be beneficial in assisting women reduce cardiovascular disease by quitting smoking.

## Nursing and Nonnursing Theories in Nursing Research

As was alluded to in previous chapters, there has been significant debate in the discipline of nursing regarding the source of the theories used in nursing research. Indeed, many scholars have warned of the importance of using only nursing theories for research to ensure that what results is indeed nursing research. But it has also been shown that nurses depend on and use knowledge drawn from various sources in developing nursing research, and that this practice does not negate the importance of the findings to nurses.

In a study of nursing research, Moody and colleagues (1988) determined that from the mid-1970s through the mid-1980s there was a significant increase in the use of the terms *theoretical framework*, *model*, or *conceptual model* in published research studies. Moody concluded that the majority of studies did not actually test a theory, but only cited the theoretical framework or model. In this study, there was mention of some type of theoretical perspective in 55% of the studies, but only 10% reported using a nursing model. The most frequently used nursing models were those of Orem, Rogers, Newman, and Roy. Theories from other disciplines (e.g., psychology, physiology, and sociology) were more commonly used. The most frequently cited theories were those involving coping, health beliefs, and locus of control from social learning. Among a number of education theories used in nursing research; adult learning theory was the most common (Moody, 1990).

### RATIONALE FOR USING NURSING THEORIES IN NURSING RESEARCH

Some nursing theorists and nursing researchers believe that it is essential to use only nursing theories and models in nursing research. They assert that only nursing models truly deal with the scope and direction of nursing interventions; therefore, they provide a sound conceptual framework for nursing research. Additionally, their use as frameworks for research is one way of ensuring that the study will be relevant to the discipline (Fawcett, 2005).

Proponents argue that conceptual models of nursing and nursing theories can be used to guide all forms of nursing research. They believe that nursing theories help nurse researchers identify the phenomena of central interest to the discipline and assist in designing studies that reflect nursing's distinctive perspective of people and their environment in matters of health. Furthermore, they point out that there is concern that nursing research journals are filled with reports of research designed to generate or test theories from disciplines other than nursing, and that very few nurses conduct research using nursing conceptual models and theories (Fawcett, 2000).

Fawcett (2000), in particular, questioned whether using a theory from another discipline resulted in nursing research, even if a nurse conducted the research. To address her concerns about using theories and concepts from other disciplines, she challenged researchers to base studies in the context of conceptual models of nursing and nursing theories.

One common criticism regarding the use of nursing models to direct research is a practice used by the editors of many nursing journals. It has been reported that if a nursing theory is used as a conceptual framework, the authors are often asked (by the journal's editors) to rewrite an article to delete the notation of the nursing theory component. Roberts (1999) concluded that it appears that "editors and reviewers of clinical specialty journals are anxious to protect the reader from nursing theory . . . to make the article more readable" (p. 300).

## CONCERNS OVER RELIANCE ON NURSING MODELS TO DIRECT NURSING RESEARCH

In response to repeated calls to focus research only on nursing theories and models, Brink (2000) wrote that many manuscripts that include a nursing theory or conceptual model treat the model or theory as an appendage. She pointed out that, in many cases, reporting of the conceptual framework consists of a single-paragraph description of the model, which often has nothing to do with the rest of the manuscript (which is consistent with Silva's [1986] findings). She explained that the theory does not direct the literature review, the models, or the problem under study, and never relates to the conclusions, and the author is asked to delete the paragraph. Brink argued that borrowed theories or practice theories can as readily be used to describe and explain phenomena that affect nursing and concluded that to limit nurses to using only nursing theories in nursing research is shortsighted.

Diers (1984) agreed, stating that in many cases, citing a nursing model as a framework appears extraneous both to the design of the study and the eventual conclusions. She pointed out that in many cases the model is not necessary to understand the hypotheses, the findings, or the implications. Further, she noted that it is often unclear what the function of the nursing model is in the context of the research, because the research would have been done precisely the same way, with the same conclusions and implications, without any reference to the model.

Finally, Tripp-Reimer (1984) described the difference between theories "of" nursing and theories "for" nursing. She believed that grand theories are theories "of" nursing and describe the nature and scope of the discipline to assist nurses in their general approach to care. On the other hand, theories "for" nursing identify what nurses should do to achieve the best client care. She noted that too often superimposing a grand theory as a conceptual framework is confusing, and theories or concepts that are being studied do not underlie the nursing models, even though they may be congruent with them. Thus, although the theories are congruent with the nursing models, they do not underlie the models; thus the relationship appears forced.

Tripp-Reimer (1984) wrote that research should develop and test theories "for" nursing practice. Research should focus on testing which interventions work best with certain types of clients in specific clinical situations. This is being accomplished with the increasing interest in the development and testing of middle range nursing theories (see Chapters 10 and 11) and practice theories (see Chapter 17).

## Other Issues in Nursing Theory and Nursing Research

To enhance understanding of the use of theory in nursing research, other issues should be addressed. Two significant issues are:

1. Recognizing the importance of adequately describing the theory in the research report.
2. Examining how theory fits into the discipline's research agenda.

### THE RESEARCH REPORT

To clearly illustrate the impact of the theoretical framework in developing the research study, and to show the context within which the findings should be interpreted, discussion of the theoretical framework should be incorporated into several sections of the research report (Norwood, 2000). First, the framework should be introduced and briefly described in the problem statement.

Second, the framework is usually described in detail under its own heading at the end of the literature review. In this section, the description of the theory or concepts should be drawn from primary sources. The concepts should be clearly defined and proposed relationships need to be described. A model or diagram that depicts both the framework and how it is being translated or applied to the present study may be added. Additionally, if the study is using an existing framework, the section should describe previous research application of the framework.

Third, how the framework is operationalized should be delineated in the methodology section. This will explain how the framework influences or is reflected in the study's design, data collection strategies, and data analysis methods. If an instrument has been developed for the study, the specific items that are used as indicators of the concepts in the framework need to be identified (Norwood, 2000).

Fourth, the framework needs to be referred to in the discussion section of the research report. The findings should be discussed in terms of how they illustrate, support, challenge, or contradict the framework.

Finally, suggestions for changing nursing practice or conducting further research that are consistent with the framework's concepts and propositions, should be offered in the report's conclusion (Norwood, 2000). Box 18-4 presents an outline for inclusion of the theoretical framework in the research report.

### NURSING'S RESEARCH AGENDA

There is a need for nurses to increase research that addresses significant clinical problems and adds to the knowledge base of the discipline. To accomplish this, research themes must be significant to the discipline's theory and practice, and research must build on previous knowledge to lead to knowledge accumulation. Recommendations for future nursing research are to move beyond descriptive studies to explanatory and

| BOX 18-4 | *Guidelines for Writing About a Research Study's Theoretical Framework* |
|---|---|

**IN THE STUDY'S PROBLEM STATEMENT**

- Introduce the framework
- Briefly explain why it is a good fit for the research problem area

**AT THE END OF THE LITERATURE REVIEW**

- Thoroughly describe the framework and explain its application to the present study
- Describe how the framework has been used in studies about similar problems

**IN THE STUDY'S METHODOLOGY SECTION**

- Explain how the framework is being operationalized in the study's design
- Explain how data collection methods (such as questionnaire items) reflect the concepts in the framework

**IN THE STUDY'S DISCUSSION SECTION**

- Describe how study findings are consistent (or inconsistent) with the framework
- Offer suggestions for practice and further research that are congruent with the framework's concepts and propositions

Source: Norwood (2000).

predictive studies, to promote study replication, and to conduct meta-analyses in areas where experimental studies have been conducted. Finally, it is important that nurses explicate the theoretical perspective of the research design in the research report to demonstrate how the study fits into the current body of knowledge.

The National Institute for Nursing Research (NINR) began as a "center" within the National Institutes of Health in 1986 and became an "institute" in 1993. The NINR supports clinical and basic research to establish a scientific basis of the care of individuals across the life span. This includes caring for individuals during illness and recovery, reduction of risks for disease and disability, promotion of healthy lifestyles, promotion of quality of life in those with chronic illness, and care for individuals at the end of life. Research priorities of the NINR for 2008 were:

- Low birth weight: mothers and infants
- HIV infection: prevention and care
- Long-term care for older adults
- Symptom management: pain
- Nursing informatics: enhancing patient care
- Health promotion for older children and adolescents
- Technology dependency across the lifespan (NINR, 2009).

To build the body of nursing knowledge, nurses must consider these issues from a theoretical perspective and must avoid looking at them in isolation.

In a well-supported essay, Hinshaw (2000) identified "areas of evolving nursing science" (p. 119) that should be targeted for directed nursing research (Box 18-5). These areas should receive priority attention in nursing theory and nursing research in the 21st century. Additionally, according to Hinshaw, research programs should focus on intervention research to provide a stronger, more predictable base for nursing practice.

Hinshaw (2000) also called for interdisciplinary collaboration and multidisciplinary research partners. She wrote that this will more effectively address complex problems

BOX 18-5 | *Areas of Evolving Nursing Science*

- Critical health needs of communities and vulnerable populations
- Practice strategies and outcomes
- Family health and transitions
- Health promotion/risk reduction
- Biobehavioral manifestations of health and illness
- Women's health
- Health and illness of older adults
- Environments for optimizing client outcomes
- Genetics research
- End-of-life research

TABLE 18-2 *Examples of Research Priorities in Nursing Practice, Nursing Administration/Management, and Nursing Education*

| Nursing Practice | Nursing Administration and Management | Nursing Education |
|---|---|---|
| Client needs related to health and illness (e.g., health promotion/illness prevention; symptom management; enhancing quality of life) | Development and evaluation of new patient care delivery models | Use of instructional technology (e.g., new approaches to laboratory and simulated learning) |
| Providing and testing nursing care interventions and measuring outcomes of care | Provision and maintenance of healthful work/practice environments | Development, implementation, and evaluation of new pedagogies |
| Evidence-based nursing practice (multiple areas) | Development of provider and patient safety guidelines | Development, implementation, and evaluation of flexible curriculum designs |
| Identification, prevention, and management of common health problems/threats in specific community-based settings (e.g., worksites, homes, schools) | Implementation and evaluation of use of technology to complement patient care | Development of new models for teacher preparation and faculty development |
| Reducing health disparities (e.g., delivery of culturally competent care, enhancing access to and utilization of health care) | Evaluation of outcomes of care related to cost effectiveness and quality | Methods for teaching evidence-based practices |
| Enhancing nursing care provision related to specific health problems or issues (by specialty area, setting or other) (e.g., pain management; reducing incidence of low-birth-weight infants; improving immunization compliance; prevention of nosocomial infection; reduction of HIV infection; prevention of lower back strain) | Program planning, implementation, and evaluation | Evaluation of processes for grading, testing, and evaluation of students, faculty, and curricula |
| Examination of appropriate application of genetics information and knowledge in nursing practice | Strategies to improve nurse retention and satisfaction | Strategies to enhance community-based learning and service strategies |

Sources: Websites of American Organization of Nurse Executives; International Council of Nurses; National League for Nursing; American Association of Operating Room Nurses.

and provide a global perspective for care. However, it is important to recognize that interdisciplinary and multidisciplinary research will necessitate familiarity with theories, concepts, and principles of other disciplines.

In addition to the research priorities listed in Box 18-5, nursing knowledge must be developed that will direct nursing practice, nursing administration and management, and nursing education. Table 18-2 gives suggestions for further research in these three areas that will be beneficial for the development of the discipline.

## Summary

The relationship between research and theory is undeniable, and it is important to recognize the impact of this relationship on the development of nursing knowledge. This chapter has provided details on the interface of theory and research and given examples of when, where, and how theory and research interface.

In the discipline of nursing, research may be theory generating or theory testing. Or, as in the opening case study, a theory may be used as the conceptual framework that drives the study. The source of the theory for a research study may be unique to nursing (such as using Benner's Novice to Expert model by the student in the case study) or borrowed from another discipline, but the theoretical base should be explicit and appropriate.

As an evolving science, nurses should avoid research in isolation. It is imperative that nursing research respond to important questions and issues from nursing practice, administration and management, and education. This will provide a sound base of knowledge, which will further strengthen the discipline.

## LEARNING ACTIVITIES

1. Search recent issues of a prominent research journal (e.g., *Nursing Research, Research in Nursing and Health, Western Journal of Nursing Research*) for notations of conceptual frameworks of the published studies. Tally information about the conceptual or research frameworks. How many studies did not mention any theoretical framework? How many used grand nursing theories as a framework? How many used borrowed theories as a framework? How many studies were theory generating? How many were theory testing? Share findings with classmates.

2. Find a research article from a recent journal that purports to test a theory. Use the guidelines from Box 18-2 to evaluate the research study (see the example in Nursing Exemplar 2).

3. Find a research article from a recent nursing journal that uses a grand or middle range theory as a conceptual framework. Use the guidelines from Box 18-3 to evaluate how well the conceptual framework is used to guide the research project (see the example in Nursing Exemplar 3).

## INTERNET RESOURCES

National Institute of Nursing Research:

http://ninr.nih.gov/ninr/

National League for Nursing:

http://www.nln.org/

American Association of Colleges of Nursing:

http://www.aacn.nche.edu/

International Council of Nurses:

http://www.icn.ch/

American Organization of Nurse Executives:

http://www.aone.org/aone/index.jsp

American Association of Operating Room Nurses:

http://www.aorn.org/

# REFERENCES

Acton, G. J., Irvin, B. L., & Hopkins, B. A. (1991). Theory-testing research: Building the science. *Advances in Nursing Science, 14*(1), 52–61.

Anuforo, P. O., Oyedele, L., & Pacquiao, D. F. (2004). Comparative study of meanings, beliefs and practices of female circumcision among three Nigerian tribes in the United States and Nigeria. *Journal of Transcultural Nursing, 15*(2), 103–113.

Barnum, B. S. (2005). *Nursing theory: Analysis, application, evaluation* (5th ed.). Philadelphia: Lippincott Williams & Wilkins.

Bishop, S. M., & Hardin, S. R. (2006). History and philosophy of science. In A. M. Tomey & M. R. Alligood (Eds.), *Nursing theorists and their work* (6th ed., pp. 16–24). St. Louis: Mosby.

Blegen, M. A., & Tripp-Reimer, T. (1994). The nursing theory–nursing research connection. In J. C. McCloskey & H. K. Grace (Eds.), *Current issues in nursing* (4th ed., pp. 87–91). St. Louis: Mosby.

Brink, P. J. (2000). A response to Fawcett. *Western Journal of Nursing Research, 22*(6), 653–655.

Buchanan, L., & Likness, S. (2008). Evidence-based practice to assist women in hospital settings to quit smoking and reduce cardiovascular disease risk. *Journal of Cardiovascular Nursing, 33*(5), 397–406.

Burns, N., & Grove, S. K. (2009). *The practice of nursing research: Appraisal, synthesis and generation of evidence* (6th ed.). St. Louis: Elsevier.

Chinn, P. L., & Kramer, M. K. (2008). *Theory and nursing: Integrated knowledge development* (7th ed.). St. Louis: Mosby.

Copeland, D. A., & Heilemann, M. V. (2008). Getting "to the point": The experience of mothers getting assistance for their adult children who are violent and mentally ill. *Nursing Research, 57*(3), 136–143.

Dickoff, J., & James, P. (1968). A theory of theories: A position paper. *Nursing Research, 17*(3), 197–203.

Diers, D. (1984). Commentaries. *Western Journal of Nursing Research, 6*(2), 191–192.

Dowd, T., Kolcaba, K., Steiner, R., & Fashinpaur, D. (2007). Comparison of a healing touch, coaching, and a combined intervention on comfort and stress in younger college students. *Holistic Nursing Practice, 21*(4), 194–202.

Dunn, K. S. (2005). Testing a middle-range theoretical model of adaptation to chronic pain. *Nursing Science Quarterly, 18*(5), 146–156.

Edwards, H., Walsh, A., Courtney, M., Monaghan, S., Wilson, J., & Young, J. (2007). Promoting evidence-based childhood fever management through a peer education programme based on the Theory of Planned Behaviour. *Journal of Clinical Nursing, 16*(10), 1966–1979.

Fawcett, J. (1999). *The relationship of theory and research* (3rd ed.). Philadelphia: Davis.

Fawcett, J. (2000). But is it nursing research? *Western Journal of Nursing Research, 22*(5), 524–525.

Fawcett, J. (2005). *Contemporary nursing knowledge: Analysis and evaluation of nursing models and theories* (2nd ed.). Philadelphia: F.A. Davis.

Fisher, K. L. (2006). School nurses' perceptions of self-efficacy in providing diabetes care. *Journal of School Nursing, 22*(4), 223–228.

Fitzpatrick, J. J. (1998). *Encyclopedia of nursing research.* New York: Springer.

Flood, M., & Scharer, K. (2006). Creativity enhancement: Possibilities for successful aging. *Issues in Mental Health Nursing, 27*, 939–959.

Gigliotti, E. (2004). Etiology of maternal–student role stress. *Nursing Science Quarterly, 17*(2), 156–164.

Hall, C. P., Wimberley, P. D., Hall, J. D., Pfriemer, J. T., Hubbard, E. M., Stacy, A. S., & Gilbert, J. D. (2005). Teaching breast cancer screening to African American women in the Arkansas Mississippi river delta. *Oncology Nursing Forum, 32*(4), 857–862.

Hamilton, R. J., & Bowers, B. J. (2007). The theory of genetic vulnerability: A Roy Model exemplar. *Nursing Science Quarterly, 20*(3), 254–264.

Hinshaw, A. S. (2000). Nursing knowledge for the 21st century: Opportunities and challenges. *Image: Journal of Nursing Scholarship, 32*(2), 117–123.

Kalisch, P. A., & Kalisch, B. J. (2004). *The advance of American nursing* (4th ed.). Philadelphia: Lippincott Williams & Wilkins.

Kerr, M. J., Lusk, S. L., & Ronis, D. L. (2002). Explaining Mexican-American workers' hearing protection use with the health promotion model. *Nursing Research, 51*(2), 100–109.

Lancaster, D. R. (2005). Coping with appraised breast cancer risk among women with family history of breast cancer. *Research in Nursing and Health, 28,* 144–158.

Lewandowski, W. A. (2004). Patterning of pain and power with guided imagery. *Nursing Science Quarterly, 17*(3), 233–241.

LoBiondo-Wood, G., Haber, J., & Krainovich-Miller, B. (2006). The research process: Integrating evidence-based practice. In G. LoBiondo-Wood & J. Haber (Eds.), *Nursing research: Methods, critical appraisal, and utilization* (6th ed., pp. 27–44). St. Louis: Mosby.

Mahon, N. E., Yarcheski, A., & Yarcheski, T. J. (2004). Social support and positive health practices in early adolescents. *Clinical Nursing Research, 13*(3), 216–236.

McKenna, H. P., & Slevin, O. D. (2008). *Nursing models, theories and practice.* Oxford, UK: Blackwell Publishing.

McQuiston, C. M., & Campbell, J. C. (1997). Theoretical substitution: A guide for theory testing research. *Nursing Science Quarterly, 10*(3), 117–123.

Mefford, L. C. (2004). A theory of health promotion for preterm infants based on Levine's Conservation Model of Nursing. *Nursing Science Quarterly, 17*(3), 260–266.

Meleis, A. I. (2007). *Theoretical nursing: Development and progress* (4th ed.). Philadelphia: Lippincott Williams & Wilkins.

Mock, V., St. Ours, C., Hall, S., Bositis, A., Tillery, M., Belcher, A., Krumm, S., & McCorkle, R. (2007). Using a conceptual model in nursing research—mitigating fatigue in cancer patients. *Journal of Advanced Nursing, 58*(5), 503–512.

Moody, L. E. (1990). Developing a theoretical design for research. In L. E. Moody (Ed.), *Advancing nursing science through research* (pp. 211–248). Newbury Park, CA: Sage.

Moody, L. E., Wilson, M. E., Smyth, K., Schwartz, R., Tittle, M., & Van Cott, M. L. (1988). Analysis of a decade of nursing practice research: 1977–1986. *Nursing Research, 37*(6), 374–379.

National Institute for Nursing Research (NINR). (2009). 2008 Areas of Research Opportunity. http://www.ninr.nih.gov/NR/rdonlyres/5AC1595B-08BF-4A6C-A08B-3B2B2FF82829/4750/ExecutiveSummary.pdf. Retrieved April 2, 2009.

Norwood, S. L. (2000). *Research strategies for advanced practice nurses.* Upper Saddle River, NJ: Prentice-Hall Health.

Olshansky, E. (2003). A theoretical explanation for previously infertile mothers' vulnerability to depression. *Journal of Nursing Scholarship, 35*(3), 263–268.

Peters, R. M. (2006). The relationship of racism, chronic stress emotions and blood pressure. *Journal of Nursing Scholarship, 38*(3), 234–240.

Polit, D. F., & Beck, C. T. (2008). *Nursing research: Generating and assessing evidence for nursing practice* (8th ed.). Philadelphia: Lippincott Williams & Wilkins.

Roberts, K. L. (1999). Through a looking glass: Nursing theory and clinical nursing research. *Clinical Nursing Research, 8*(4), 299–301.

Sethares, K. A., & Elliott, K. (2004). The effect of a tailored message intervention on heart failure readmission rates, quality of life and benefit and barrier beliefs in persons with heart failure. *Heart and Lung, 33*(4), 249–260.

Silva, M. C. (1986). Research testing nursing theory: State of the art. *Advances in Nursing Science, 9*(1), 1–11.

Sun, F. K., Long, A., Boore, J., & Tsao, L. I. (2006). A theory for the nursing care of patients at risk of suicide. *Journal of Advanced Nursing, 53*(6), 680–690.

Taylor, S. G., Renpenning, K. E., Geden, E. A., Neuman, B. M., & Hart, M. A. (2001). A theory of dependent-care: A corollary theory to Orem's theory of self-care. *Nursing Science Quarterly, 14*(1), 39–47.

Tripp-Reimer, T. (1984). Commentaries. *Western Journal of Nursing Research, 6*(2), 195–197.

Tsai, P. F., Tak, S., Moore, C., & Palencia, I. (2003). Testing a theory of chronic pain. *Journal of Advanced Nursing, 43*(2), 158–169.

Turkel, M. C., & Ray, M. A. (2001). Relational complexity: From grounded theory to instrument development and theoretical testing. *Nursing Science Quarterly, 14*(4), 281–287.

Villarruel, A., Jemmott, J. B., Jemmott, L. S., & Ronis, D. L. (2004). Predictors of sexual intercourse and condom use intention among Spanish-dominant Latino youth: A test of the Planned Behavior Theory. *Nursing Research, 53*(3), 172–181.

Weiss, J. A., Jampol, M. L., Lievano, J. A., Smith, S. M., & Wurster, J. L. (2008). Normalizing risky sexual behaviours: A grounded theory study. *Pediatric Nursing, 34*(2), 163–169.

Werner, P., & Mendelsson, G. (2001). Nursing staff members' intentions to use physical restraints with older people: Testing the theory of reasoned action. *Journal of Advanced Nursing, 35*(5), 784–791.

Whall, A. L. (2005). The structure of nursing knowledge: Analysis and evaluation of practice, middle range and grand theory. In J. J. Fitzpatrick & A. L. Whall (Eds.), *Conceptual models of nursing: Analysis and application* (3rd ed., pp. 13–26). Norwalk, CT: Appleton & Lange.

Wilson, F. L., Brown, D. L., & Stephens-Ferris, M. (2006). Can easy-to-read immunization information increase knowledge in urban low-income mothers? *Journal of Pediatric Nursing, 21*(1), 4–14.

# 19

# Application of Theory in Nursing Administration and Management

## Melinda Granger Oberleitner

*G*reta Martin is a family nurse practitioner who has been employed for several years as part of a multiphysician practice. The majority of her practice has been focused on managing the care of adults with chronic illnesses, such as congestive heart failure and diabetes.

Although she enjoys her work very much, Greta has always been interested in exploring one of the entrepreneurial opportunities that a career in nursing has to offer. Recently, she has focused on combining her interests in computers and the internet with her expertise as an advanced practice nurse (APN). Along with several investors, she is in the process of creating a disease management company that is to be operated solely via the internet. As envisioned, the company will focus on the needs of older adults and will hire APNs and other registered nurses (RNs) to provide clinical services and to serve as case managers for plan members diagnosed with chronic illnesses.

As she began the planning process for the project, Greta found that she had much to learn in regard to applying management and administration principles. In particular, she needed to learn more about organizational design. As the company is established, she must examine issues such as chain of command, control, authority, and responsibility. The group must determine how the company will be structured and who will be responsible for day-to-day operations.

The group is also looking at case management models to select or modify one that is appropriate for use with its anticipated clientele and the method of delivery. Finally, Greta realized that she should learn about her leadership style and develop her leadership abilities to direct the new company. Recognizing her deficiencies in administration and management, Greta sought information from a number of sources to learn about administration theories and how to apply them in her new enterprise.

Nursing practice, including advanced nursing practice, occurs within a larger context and framework that is shaped by traditional and prevailing theories, models, and frameworks of administration and management. Even if only one nurse is employed by an organization, that nurse's practice is shaped and influenced by models and principles of leadership, management, and administration used by the leaders of the organization. To be most effective in the advanced practice role, an APN should be able to recognize and adapt to the specific organizational characteristics that define the organization in which she or he practices.

This chapter expands on concepts and principles presented in Chapter 15. It explores specific applications of administration and management theories, models, and frameworks in nursing and health care. These concepts include organizational design; shared governance; transformational leadership; patient care delivery models; case management; disease/chronic illness management; quality management (QM)/performance improvement processes, tools, and techniques; and evidence-based practice (EBP).

# Organizational Design

The structure of an organization provides a formal framework in which management processes occur. This formal framework historically serves many purposes, including provision of a chain of administrative command or authority that should be evident to all employees, a formal system of communication between management and staff, and a method to accomplish the work of the organization effectively and efficiently. The right structure enables the organization to reach its organizational goals.

Six elements of structure that were formulated by management theorists in the 1900s still provide a guide to the design of organizations in the 21st century. These six elements are listed in Box 19-1, and each is discussed briefly in the following sections (Robbins & Judge, 2009).

## WORK SPECIALIZATION

*Work specialization* is having each step of the work process performed by a different individual rather than the whole process being done by one person. Proponents of work specialization argue that it makes the most efficient use of worker skills, attributes, and characteristics. Medication administration can be used to illustrate the concept of work specialization. Physicians determine the need for a medication order and determine the composition of that order; hospital pharmacists then review the order and fill the prescription as directed by the physician. The nurse on the unit administers the medication ordered by the physician and prepared by the pharmacist. In the traditional hospital structure, pharmacists work in an isolated group to prepare all medications to be delivered by nurses to patients in the facility.

---

**BOX 19-1** *Elements of Organizational Structure*

1. Work specialization
2. Chain of command
3. Span of control
4. Authority and responsibility
5. Centralization versus decentralization
6. Departmentalization

In recent years, recognition that work specialization can lead to boredom, low productivity, and poor quality has led to a reexamination of the concept. In many cases, this has resulted in assigning employees a variety of activities to accomplish and encouraging employees to work in teams. In some hospitals, a clinical pharmacist is part of a team of health care workers assigned to accomplish the work of the unit and resides, along with the traditional nursing staff, on the clinical unit. Some unit-based clinical pharmacists engage in tasks such as medication administration, which was once considered the exclusive domain of nursing.

The usual configuration of clinical nurse specialists (CNSs) is perhaps the most vivid representation of work specialization. For example, a neuroscience CNS would not be considered interchangeable with a cardiovascular CNS because of the extreme degree of work specialization in the role of the CNS. The CNS is educationally prepared as an expert in a specific specialty area and is not considered a generalist.

## CHAIN OF COMMAND

Fayol (1949), Weber (1970), and Taylor (1911) (see Chapter 15) advocated that an employee should be administratively responsible to, or report to, only one supervisor. This arrangement is termed the chain of command. Chain of command refers to formal lines of communication and authority and can usually be determined by looking at an organizational chart. However, as organizations have become increasingly complex, individuals in organizations may find themselves administratively responsible to more than one individual.

Although the nurse working on the 7 PM to 7 AM shift in the intensive care unit (ICU) is ultimately administratively responsible to the ICU director, there is usually a different chain of command on the night shift; this may include the night charge nurse and the night house supervisor.

APNs in today's health care organizations may be administratively responsible to a variety of individuals, some of whom may not be nurses, such as product or service line managers. Some APNs may also assume managerial roles, as in the case of a nurse anesthetist who is administratively in charge of a group of nurse anesthetists.

## SPAN OF CONTROL

The third element of management, span of control, can also be determined from the organizational chart. Span of control refers to the number of employees directed by a manager. The classical management theorists recommended narrow spans of control for workers performing complex jobs. There is no consensus regarding the optimal number of employees one manager should have in his or her span of control—suggested ranges are from 3 to 50 employees. Several contingencies play a role in the variability of the range of numbers of employees in span of control. These contingencies include the quality and experience of the manager, the abilities and maturity of the employees, the complexity of the task and, in some cases, the geographic location of the work setting. The most recent research results indicate a significant level of improvement in nurse engagement when the manager is responsible for 50 or fewer direct reports (Cathcart, 2004).

In recent years because of cost-cutting initiatives in health care and other organizations, management layers have been decreased and span of control for managers has increased. Communication patterns between manager and employees and between employee and employee change when span of control changes. Graicunas (1937) developed a mathematical model to illustrate the changes in numbers of communication patterns when span of control is changed. This mathematical model demonstrated that as the number of employees reporting to a manager increases, the number of interactions increases geometrically. As a result of this geometric increase, Graicunas recommended that a span of six or seven employees was the maximum that a manager could handle effectively. In his mathematical computations, Graicunas did not consider contingency factors or variables, such as the manager's experience, the maturity of the employees, or the stability or predictability of the work being performed, which may also influence the effectiveness of a manager with a given span of control.

Several factors should be considered when contemplating altering managerial span of control on inpatient nursing units. These factors include skill mix and expertise of the unit staff, duties of first-level managers (i.e., charge nurses) when the middle-level manager is not present, and the potential savings in salary expenses.

## AUTHORITY AND RESPONSIBILITY

*Line authority* and *staff authority* are two distinctions that describe formal relationships in an organization. When looking at an organizational chart, line authority refers to chain of command, superior–subordinate, and leader–follower relationships. For example, the chief nursing officer delegates authority to the unit manager, who then delegates to a subordinate, the charge nurse. The command relationship is a direct "line" between supervisor and subordinate.

In larger organizations, managers can be designated as top-level, middle-level, or first-level managers. Top-level managers include the organization's chief executive officer (CEO) and the highest nursing administrator. Middle-level managers, as the name implies, coordinate management activities between the top management level and first-level managers. Middle-level managers are usually involved in long-range planning and in policy decisions that affect one unit or multiple units. This manager is usually responsible for day-to-day activities of the units. Titles in nursing that represent middle-level managers include unit managers, unit directors, unit supervisors, and head nurses. First-level managers are assigned to one unit and are concerned with that specific unit's work. First-level managers such as charge nurses, team leaders, and primary care nurses are crucial to the success of the unit's work. APNs are most often administratively responsible to either top-level or middle-level managers. APNs who assume administrative responsibilities in the organization may be top-level or middle-level managers.

In some organizations APNs are in *staff* positions, as opposed to *line* positions. Staff authority supports the work of the line manager without having any line authority or responsibility. Employees in staff positions support, assist, and advise those in line authority positions. In a staff position the APN is not responsible for the hiring, firing, directing, or disciplining of other employees. This lack of authority could be a disadvantage to the APN in accomplishing the tasks of the role because the APN often must work through others to accomplish goals. Even when the APN is in a staff position, the APN is responsible to a line manager, who is either a top-level or middle-level manager.

## CENTRALIZATION VERSUS DECENTRALIZATION

*Centralization* and *decentralization* are degrees of how decision making is dispersed or diffused throughout the organization. In organizations with centralized decision making, decisions are made by one individual or a small group of individuals at the top of the organizational structure. Decentralization refers to decision making that occurs at the lowest levels feasible. Most of today's organizations are really neither totally centralized nor decentralized, but are a combination of the two. With the advent of performance improvement initiatives over the past 30 to 40 years, the trend in American organizations has been toward decentralization in an effort to involve employees directly responsible for the work product in the decision-making process. In nursing, organizational designs such as shared governance have gained popularity as a method to empower and engage staff in the decision-making process.

## DEPARTMENTALIZATION

The primary purpose of *departmentalization* is to subdivide the work of the organization so that specialization of the work can be accomplished. Departmentalization emphasizes specialization of skills. Hospitals have historically implemented departmentalization with traditional departments, such as central supply, pastoral care, and patient care departments, among others. A typical manufacturing plant, although different from a hospital, is probably organized in much the same way as the hospital. For example, both probably have marketing, accounting, and human resources departments. Grouping activities in this manner is known as functional departmentalization.

Other types of departmentalization include product, customer, geographic, and process departmentalization. Today, hospitals and other organizations use cross-disciplinary teams to accomplish the organization's performance initiatives that transcend traditional departmental boundaries to better focus on customer needs (Robbins & Judge, 2009).

## Shared Governance

*Shared governance* is "a structural model through which nurses can express and manage their own practice with a higher level of professional autonomy" (Porter-O'Grady, 2003, p. 251). Nursing shared governance, an organizational structure and process, was introduced in the late 1970s as an alternative to traditional or industrial bureaucratic organizational design (Christman, 1976; Cleland, 1978; Laschinger & Finegan, 2005). In this design, professional nurses use self-directed work teams at the unit level to make professional practice decisions and to accomplish the work of the unit.

Porter-O'Grady, Hawkins, and Parker (1997) described the major components of shared governance as the creation of partnerships, equity, accountability, and ownership. Much of the effort directed at restructuring the nursing organization to implement shared governance was done to empower nurses to join with each other and with other health care decision makers to better confront issues affecting the practice of professional nursing (Porter-O'Grady, 1994). In the shared governance model, staffs, not managers, are empowered to make patient care decisions at the staff level (Kramer et al., 2008).

Implementation of shared governance is usually accompanied by the simultaneous implementation of participation and decentralization. Participation and decentralization are not substitutes for shared governance and should not be used synonymously with the term *shared governance*. Participative models call for employees to be involved in the decisions that involve them. However, management still determines the breadth and depth of employee participation. Decentralization allows employees at lower levels of the hierarchical structure to have greater involvement in decision making and to have some authority to implement the decisions. However, management usually retains the real authority and power in terms of which decisions are to be implemented. In short, both participation and decentralization rely on management discretion to determine the amount of employee involvement in decision making, whereas shared governance does not.

Nursing shared governance models have always focused on nurses controlling their professional practice. A comparative analysis by Kramer and Schmalenberg (2003), who interviewed 279 nurses at 14 magnet hospitals, found the highest staff nurse ownership of practice issues and outcomes occurred when there were visible, viable, and recognized structures devoted to nursing control over practice. To be able to control practice, nurses must have control over resources that impact professional practice and they must also have influence over themselves as a professional group (Lake, 2007).

Three general models of shared governance are:

1. Councilor model—the most common model; utilizes a coordinating council to integrate decisions made by staff and managers in subcommittees that report to the coordinating council;
2. Administrative model—the organizational chart is split to resemble two tracks—a management track and a clinical track; membership in both tracks includes managers and staff;
3. Congressional model—uses a democratic process to empower nurses to vote on issues.

Structure of the models is not important; what is important is control over practice that leads to improved patient, nurse, and organizational outcomes (Anthony, 2004; Hess, 2004; Kramer et al., 2008; Weston, 2008).

Research-based studies have attempted to evaluate the outcomes of shared governance from the perspectives of the organization, the nurse, and the patient. From an organizational perspective, in general, research supports the finding of an improved financial posture for the organization after implementation of shared governance. The improved finances stem from either cost savings or cost reductions. Reported examples of cost savings and reductions range from a decrease in overall meeting time for staff to multimillion dollar reductions in the use of temporary or agency nurses once shared governance has been fully implemented. Research studies indicate implementation of shared governance has resulted in improving the work environment of nurses, which could lead to increased nurse satisfaction and ultimately to improved nurse retention.

Detractors of the shared governance model point to the expense of introducing and maintaining the model, the longer time it takes to arrive at decisions using the model, and the fact that not all nurses want to have a role in decision making or want accountability for decisions.

## Transformational Leadership in Nursing and in Health Care

Historically, nursing and health care organizations were built on old paradigm beliefs of hierarchical structures with an emphasis on rationality and logical decision making. The old paradigm is evolving to a new paradigm that values mutuality, affiliation, cooperation, networking, and an emphasis on human relations. In nursing, the shift has led to decentralization, participative management and decision making, and self-governance.

In transformational leadership, the leader and the follower have the same purpose. Barker (1994) proposed that it is easier to study the *results* of transformational leadership than the *process*. Transformational leadership is moral and philosophical leadership rather than technical leadership. Bennis and Nanus (1985) conceptualized four strategies for transformational leadership: creating a vision, building a social architecture that provides the framework for generating commitment to the vision and for establishing an organizational identity, developing and sustaining organizational trust,

nursing assistants. The team is responsible for the provision of care to a group of patients on a nursing unit.

The team leader is the coordinator of the group and is responsible for assigning team members to specific patient assignments. The team leader may or may not have a patient assignment. The team leader is responsible for knowing about the conditions and needs of all of the patients assigned to the team and for communicating with physicians. Duties that cannot be performed by other team members, because of lack of skill, expertise, or licensure, are performed by the team leader. Team members report to the team leader, who in turn reports to the unit manager.

Advantages of team nursing are the democratic nature of the method, the focus on the entire patient rather than on specific tasks to be accomplished, the autonomy provided to the team to accomplish the work, and increased satisfaction with the method by workers and patients. Disadvantages of team nursing include the high degree of coordination and planning required and the dependence on the unique skills of the team leader to make the concept work efficiently and effectively. Team nursing has rarely been implemented in its purest form. Instead, a combination of team and functional nursing has most frequently been implemented.

## PRIMARY NURSING

Primary nursing was initiated in the late 1960s and early 1970s in response to professional nurses who decried the lack of personal contact with patients and who were unhappy with the provision of fragmented care. Primary nursing uses some of the concepts on which total patient care was based (i.e., during work hours the primary nurse, an RN, would be responsible for planning care and providing total patient care to a group of patients). When the primary nurse was not on duty, an associate nurse (another RN) would provide care to the patients based on a care plan developed by the primary nurse. However, the primary nurse retained responsibility for the assigned patient load 24 hours a day while the patient was hospitalized.

Job satisfaction is high in primary nursing because of the high degree of autonomy and responsibility afforded to the primary nurse. Continuity of care is greatly facilitated by the primary nursing model. Disadvantages to primary nursing include the numbers of RNs required to implement primary nursing and the high degree of coordination and professional nursing expertise required for the role. Primary nurses who are inadequately trained or incompetent to implement the role may be incapable of fulfilling the primary nurse role.

## PATIENT-FOCUSED CARE/PATIENT-CENTERED CARE

The PFC model was developed in an effort to decrease the cost of providing health care while improving the quality of the service (Myers, 1998). The principles of PFC are derived from total QM/continuous quality improvement in that PFC brings patient care needs as close as possible to the bedside. A goal of PFC is to decrease the number of health care workers needed, while simultaneously increasing the time nurses would have to spend with patients. Theoretically, the cost of care should decrease while quality of care increases.

Mang (1995) described principles of implementation of PFC. These principles are summarized in Box 19-3 and are discussed briefly in the following text. *Patient redeployment* involves placing patients with similar needs and diagnoses in the same geographic location. The optimal number of patients with similar needs and diagnoses on a unit should be between 50 and 100 to create an economy of scale and to ensure

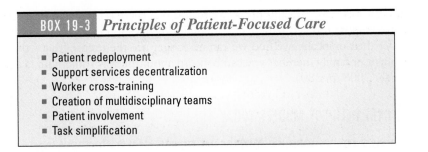

predictable census and workload. *Decentralization of support services* refers to relocation of ancillary services (i.e., pharmacy, radiology, admissions, and laboratory) closer to the patient to allow for more efficient use of personnel.

Creation of *multiskilled workers,* or cross-trained workers, is accomplished by combining appropriate types of tasks. For example, the multiskilled worker would be responsible for housekeeping, food service, and other unskilled tasks for a group of patients. However, Mang (1995) does not advocate training unskilled workers to perform tasks that traditionally would require a worker to be licensed. The goal of creating the multiskilled worker is to decrease the number of workers the typical patient comes in contact with by up to 75% (Clouten & Weber, 1994).

Over time, patient-focused care evolved into a model in which patients and families are active participants in decision making about care. Four concepts are associated with contemporary patient and family focused care models: dignity and respect; information sharing; participation; and collaboration (Johnson et al., 2008). Indeed, in this model, patients must be well informed and included in all decision making related to the plan of care. In addition, *task simplification* would be applied to every aspect of the patient's care to allow for greater efficiency and time savings, which results in earlier discharge for the patient.

The goals of PFC are to (1) transform the health care organization into a customer-focused organization; (2) improve continuity of care for patients; (3) improve professional relationships among doctors, nurses, and other caregivers; (4) minimize the movement of patients throughout hospitals; (5) increase the proportion of direct care activities as compared to other activities in the organization; (6) reconfigure the clinical environment to truly meet the needs of the patients; and (7) empower direct caregivers to plan and implement work in ways that are most responsive to the needs of patients (Zarubi, Reiley, & McCarter, 2008).

The results of some studies evaluating the PFC model indicate that patient and staff satisfaction improve after implementation of PFC, as does physician satisfaction with relationships with nursing staff. In terms of savings, some institutions reported a decrease in time of the admission process, a decrease in inventory, and an improvement in costs. Quality indicators, such as direct patient care time, patient satisfaction, continuity of care, and nosocomial infection rates, revealed positive trends after implementation of PFC. Zarubi and colleagues (2008) describe adoption of patient and family centered care (PFCC) as the model for patient care delivery in a health system in Arizona. One goal of the health system was to provide greater opportunities for patients and families to be involved in decision making at all organizational levels. As a result, the health system adopted a philosophy that integrates key concepts and principles of PFCC as identified by the Institute for Family-Centered Care (2009). An example of a change that reflected a focus on PFCC was the elimination of the standard, preset 10 AM to 8 PM hospital visiting policy so that visiting hours could be determined by patients and family according to their wishes and needs. Since implementation in 2006 the authors state, "At this point, we realize that there is no turning back. Now that we have empowered our patients and families to question our policies and practices and offer their opinions, we find we can no longer use the excuse 'that's the rule' when a patient or family member voices a concern about the way something is done." (Zarubi et al., 2008, p. 280).

## USE OF PATIENT CARE DELIVERY MODELS TODAY

Rarely do pure forms of any of the patient care delivery methods described earlier exist in practice today. Typically, components of several of the methods, or a combination of the methods, are used to accomplish patient care. Delivery methods usually differ between inpatient and outpatient areas, and from unit to unit, depending on the nature of the patient care unit and the skill mix of the staff assigned to the unit.

Kangas, Kee, and McKee-Waddle (1999) explored the differences and relationships among job satisfaction of RNs, patient satisfaction with nursing care, nursing care delivery models, organizational structure, and organizational culture. In this study there were no differences in nurse job satisfaction or patient satisfaction with nursing care in different organizational structures (i.e., shared governance) or where different nursing care delivery methods (i.e., primary, team, functional) were used. A "supportive" environment was most crucial to the job satisfaction of the RNs. More recently, a growing body of research related to organizational attributes of health care organizations which support clinical practice has been conducted. Organizational attributes that support professional clinical practice include elements, such as decentralization of authority, support from management, interdisciplinary collaboration, effective communication, access to adequate resources for the provision of patient care, and control over professional practice (Flynn, 2007). Support of clinical practice translates to improved patient care and quality clinical outcomes.

The Nursing Work Index-Revised (Aiken & Patrician, 2000) has been used to measure attributes of the work environment of professional nurses that support professional clinical practice. These attributes include organizational support for nursing practice, specifically, adequacy of resources to support the practice of professional nursing including adequate RN staffing, autonomy for nurses, nurse control of nursing practice, and collegial nurse–physician relationships. When these attributes are present to a sufficient degree, nurse job satisfaction is higher and burnout rates and physical disability rates are lower. Improved patient-related outcomes, such as decreased adverse events, lower mortality, and higher levels of patient satisfaction with care, are noted (Flynn, 2007).

Aiken, Clarke, Sloane, Sochalski, and Silber (2002) attempted to explicate the evidence linking nurse staffing to patient outcomes. In a study that was based on an analysis of outcomes of 232,342 patients in 168 Pennsylvania hospitals over a 20-month period, risk of death following common surgical procedures increased by 7% for each patient added to the nurse's workload over a nurse-to-patient ratio of 1:4. The difference in mortality for surgical patients in hospitals in which nurses cared for an average of eight patients was 30% higher than in hospitals in which nurses cared for four patients or fewer. Failure-to-rescue rates for patients with complications were 30% higher in the hospitals in which nurses cared for an average of eight patients as compared to the hospitals in which the nurses cared for four or fewer patients (Clarke & Aiken, 2003). The result is that nurses employed by hospitals that enforce large patient loads are significantly less likely to save the life of a patient who develops a serious complication. In addition, increased needlestick injuries for nurses (Clarke, Sloane, & Aiken, 2002), increased patient and family complaints, falls with injuries, medication errors, and hospital-acquired infections are more likely to occur when the nurse-to-patient ratio is higher (Aiken, Clarke, & Sloane, 2002; Cho, Ketefian, Barkauskas, & Smith, 2003).

Needleman, Buerhaus, Mattke, Stewart, and Zelevinsky (2002), in a study of administrative data for 799 hospitals in 11 states, examined the relationship between the amount of care provided by nurses in the hospitals and patients' outcomes. A higher proportion of hours of nursing care provided by RNs and a greater number of hours of care per day provided by RNs were associated with better care for hospital patients. Specifically, among medical patients, a higher proportion of hours of care per day provided by RNs was associated with shorter lengths of stay and lower rates of urinary tract infections and gastrointestinal bleeding. A higher proportion of hours of care provided by RNs was also associated with lower rates of pneumonia, shock, and cardiac arrest, and with lower rates of failure-to-rescue that was defined as death from complications, such as pneumonia, shock, or cardiac arrest, upper gastrointestinal bleeding, sepsis, or deep venous thrombosis. Among surgical patients, a higher proportion of care provided by RNs was associated with lower rates of urinary tract infections. A greater number of hours of care per day by RNs was associated with lower failure-to-rescue rates.

Higher patient-to-nurse ratios are also associated with increased nurse burnout and job dissatisfaction rates. Each patient over a 4:1 ratio increased nurse burnout by 235 and job dissatisfaction by 15% (Aiken et al., 2002). In 1999, California was the first state in the United States to pass legislation to enforce minimum nurse staffing levels in hospitals. Implementation of the legislation began in 2004. The stated goal of the legislation was to improve the quality of care for patients in California hospitals. Spetz (2008) conducted research to examine whether nurses who work in hospitals in California are more satisfied with staffing levels and other job attributes since minimum staffing levels have been enacted. The results of this research indicate that nurse satisfaction did increase from 2004 to 2006. Nurse satisfaction with the adequacy of RN staffing, time for patient education, benefits and amount of clerical support was increased. At this time it is not known whether the legislation to provide minimum nurse staffing levels in California has improved the care of hospitalized patients in that state. However, it is postulated that if nurse satisfaction is improved, nurse turnover will be decreased. High nurse turnover rates have been correlated with decreases in quality of patient care. Job dissatisfaction is a major cause of nurse turnover, which can then exacerbate a nursing shortage.

Aiken and colleagues (2008) empirically examined whether better hospital nurse care environments resulted in lower patient mortality and better nurse outcomes independent of nurse staffing levels and the educational level of the RN workforce in the hospital. Results of this study indicate that attributes of the care environment must be optimized, in addition to nurse staffing and nurse educational levels, to achieve the highest level of quality care. Specifically, the researchers state "it seems reasonable to assume that the actual number of patient deaths that could be averted annually by improved care environments, nurse staffing, and nurse education is somewhere in the range of 40,000 per year" when extrapolating study results across the United States. The results of this study imply that if all hospitals had better care environments, a 4:1 patient-to-nurse ratio and if 60% of staff nurses were BSN-prepared, the overall mortality rate would be significantly decreased as would the failure-to-rescue rate.

## AMERICAN NURSES CREDENTIALING CENTER (ANCC) MAGNET RECOGNITION PROGRAM

The Magnet Recognition Program originated as a result of a 1983 landmark policy study (McClure, Poulin, Sovie, & Wandelt, 1983) conducted by the American

Academy of Nursing to identify characteristics common to hospitals with environments of nurse recruitment and retention. At that time during a national nursing shortage, 41 hospitals became the focus of intensive research efforts. The characteristics identified were referred to as the "Forces of Magnetism" (Wolf, Triolo, & Ponte, 2008).

The Magnet Recognition Program was developed by the American Nurses Credentialing Center (ANCC) in the early 1990s to recognize health care organizations that provide exemplary nursing care and that uphold the traditions within nursing of professional nursing practice. The program also serves as a method or means to disseminate successful best practices and strategies in nursing among institutions. Magnet hospitals have incorporated proven solutions to address nurse recruitment and retention and to foster nursing leadership (Kirkley, Johnson, & Anderson, 2004).

In 2005, the Commission on Magnet (COM) approved 26 recommendations for change to the Magnet program. The recommendations were primarily focused on changes to the appraisal process. Once these changes were ratified, the Commission began work on a new conceptual model of the forces of magnetism in an effort to clarify the role of the forces in pursuit of excellence in nursing practice. Research related to the 14 forces revealed there was redundancy among the forces which have been reconfigured into seven domains or clusters of evidence: leadership; resource utilization and development; nursing model; safe and ethical practice; autonomous practice; research; and quality processes. In addition, an eighth domain, focusing on outcomes or results, was added in recognition of the importance of outcomes of care when referring to a culture of excellence and innovation, such as Magnet recognition (Triolo, Scherer, & Floyd, 2006; Wolf et al., 2008).

The new model for Magnet which was adopted by the COM comprises five components which lead to empirical quality outcomes. Overarching the five components is the concept of global issues in nursing and health care. The five components are presented in Box 19-4.

The Magnet Recognition Program is based on quality indicators and standards of nursing practice as defined in the American Nurses Association's *Scope and Standards for Nursing Administrators* (2004). The Magnet designation process includes the appraisal of both qualitative and quantitative factors in nursing. As of early 2009, a total of 310 health care organizations in 45 states and 1 organization in Australia and New Zealand each have achieved Magnet designation. Magnet hospitals have low nurse turnover (Janzen, 2003; McClure & Hinshaw, 2002); are safer workplaces (Aiken, Sloane, Lake, Sochalski, & Weber, 1999); have better patient outcomes (Aiken, Havens, & Sloane, 2000); shorter lengths of stay (Aiken et al., 1999); and higher patient satisfaction and lower Medicare patient mortality rates (Aiken, Smith, & Lake, 1994) than non-Magnet designated hospitals. A high degree of staff nurse control over nursing practice, which is highly correlated with job satisfaction (Kramer & Schmalenberg, 2003), has consistently been reported in research conducted in Magnet hospitals (Aiken, Sloane, & Lake, 1997;

---

**BOX 19-4** *Components of the Magnet Model*

- Transformational leadership
- Structural empowerment
- Exemplary professional nursing practice
- New knowledge, innovations, and improvements
- Empirical quality results

Aiken et al., 1994; Buchan, 1999; Havens & Aiken, 1999; Kramer & Hafner, 1989; Kramer & Schmalenberg, 1988a, 1988b, 1993; Kramer, Schmalenberg, & Hafner, 1989; Laschinger & Havens, 1996).

# Case Management

The Case Management Society of America (CMSA) defines case management as "a collaborative process that assesses, plans, implements, coordinates, monitors, and evaluates options and services to meet an individual's health needs through communication and available resources to promote quality cost-effective outcomes" (Yamamoto & Lucey, 2005). Case management is a role developed in the late 1980s and early 1990s in response to the prospective payment system and diagnosis-related groups (DRGs). An expansion of the total patient care system, case management originated in outpatient settings. For example, community and public health nurses carry a caseload of patients for which they plan, coordinate, and evaluate care. Rarely do these nurses implement the care personally; however, they retain responsibility for patient outcomes.

As a result of the proliferation of managed care in hospitals, case management was also adopted in inpatient facilities, which is sometimes referred to as "within the walls" case management (Yamamoto & Lucey, 2005). Most inpatient case management systems are based on one of two models: the New England Medical Center Model, which focuses primarily on managing patient care to control resources; or the St. Mary's (or Carondelet) Model, in which the role of the case manager is to control or lower costs associated with patient stays, while simultaneously reducing the length of stay and producing optimal patient outcomes.

The minimal recommended educational requirement for nurse case manager roles is the baccalaureate degree in nursing. However, although not all case managers may need to perform case management duties at the advanced level, many organizations prefer advanced educational preparation and specialization for nurses in the role of case manager. Advantages of the APN as opposed to the BSN in the case management role include recognition of the APN as expert practitioner, change agent, researcher, manager, teacher, and consultant—roles for which the BSN nurse has not been educated in a comprehensive fashion (Benoit, 1996; Blass & Reed, 2003; Stanton, Swanson, Sherrod, & Packa, 2005).

Although case management implementation varies from institution to institution, one variation is to assign a case manager to a group of high-risk patients within a specific population. For example, one hospital may have case managers in pediatrics, neuroscience, oncology, cardiovascular, orthopedics, and other specialty areas. The case manager does not coordinate the care of all the patients in a specialty. Instead, coordination of care by a case manager occurs only for those patients who have been designated as "high risk" because of age, comorbidities, and other factors that would place that patient at risk for greater consumption of resources or prolonged length of stay.

Ideally, the case manager coordinates the care of the patient from preadmission to the time of discharge and perhaps beyond discharge. This coordination of care requires interdisciplinary collaboration and cooperation. The case manager's role in this model transcends geographic or unit boundaries. The neuroscience case manager, for example, may first meet the patient in the neurosurgery clinic or at the neurosurgeon's office and would play a role in coordinating preadmission testing. Following surgery, the case manager would track the progress of the patient from the ICU, to an intermediate care unit, to the neurology floor, then to a rehabilitation unit if required. The case manager would then be involved in establishing postdischarge home care if necessary.

## CLINICAL PATHWAYS

Clinical pathways (also called critical paths) are used by some case managers as frameworks and guides that describe a sequence of events and processes that move the patient toward a goal (usually discharge) and that can help achieve better control, quality care, and lower cost outcomes for the patient and the institution (Poirrier & Oberleitner, 1999). Ideally, the pathway is developed in a collaborative fashion by all members of the interdisciplinary health care team involved in the patient's care. The clinical pathway can also serve as a documentation tool for health care providers. Clinical pathways foster improved communication and enhance the ability of a multitude of health care providers to track and monitor patient progress toward a predetermined goal. Although clinical pathway formats vary from institution to institution, four core components should be included in every pathway: comprehensive aspects of care, time references, multidisciplinary interventions, and expected patient outcomes (Box 19-5) (Poirrier & Oberleitner, 1999).

The literature is replete with reports of improved patient outcomes, coupled with reduced costs, as a result of the implementation of case management processes. Organizations are now using aggregate data derived from case management activities for benchmarking purposes as part of overall performance improvement initiatives. As the caseloads of individuals with chronic illnesses increase in conjunction with the increase in the aging population, case management holds even greater promise for patients as well as for health care providers (Harrison et al., 2004).

A recent issue of *Case Management Advisor* (2008) details the success of an intensive nurse case management program targeted to patients diagnosed with end-stage renal disease (ESRD). Implementation of the program resulted in an 83% drop in hospitalization rates of patients with ESRD in just 6 months. Nurse case managers, who make home visits to patients with ESRD, are available to patients 24 hours daily, 7 days per week via a call line. They make at least monthly visits to dialysis clinics and target patients who are deemed to be at highest risk for hospitalization and who are in most need of assistance with treatment plan adherence. The face-to-face meetings and intensive one-on-one support appear to be the key to this initiative's success rates.

The Aurora Health Care Community-Based Case Management (CBCM) program, implemented in 1997, serves clients diagnosed with chronic health problems that predispose them to recurrent hospitalizations and costly adverse medical events. In this system, the nurse case manager is an APN whose role is to work with complex clients with demonstrated risk for poor health outcomes, high cost, high utilization of health care

---

**BOX 19-5** *Core Components of Clinical Pathways*

*Comprehensive aspects of care:* Subjective and objective assessment data, the plan of care, relevant medical and nursing diagnoses, medications, treatments, diet, activity level, and other needs such as teaching needs and discharge planning.

*Time references:* Realistic information relevant to the sequencing of interventions; may be hour-to-hour in an intensive care unit, day-to-day on an inpatient hospital unit, or visit-to-visit in home health care.

*Multidisciplinary interventions:* Collaborative efforts of various health care disciplines in developing and implementing the pathway (include relevant time references).

*Expected patient outcomes:* A guide to all care providers about the patient's actual status versus expected status at a point in time. Outcomes can be developed on an hour-by-hour, day-by-day, or visit-by-visit time frame as appropriate. Discharge outcomes should always be individualized and included on the clinical pathway.

services, suboptimal self-management practices, and poor coordination of services. The plan of care, developed by the client, APN, physician, pharmacist, and social worker, supports the client's self-management in the community. The primary roles of the APN case manager are collaborator, interpreter, advocate, and surveillance.

A review of data pre- and postimplementation of case management intervention reveals CBCM has been effective in both clinical and financial outcomes for high-risk patients with complex disease. Before case management implementation, the total cost for care of 56 clients was $2,511,692 with an annualized monthly cost of $209,307. After implementation, the cost was reduced to $1,738,294 with an annualized monthly cost of $144,857. Also, after implementation of case management, the average monthly length of stay in the hospital was reduced by 40%; a 20% reduction in emergency room visits was realized as well (Schifalacqua, Ulch, & Schmidt, 2004).

Stanton and Packa (2001) describe a Rural Practice Model of Case Management that incorporates concepts from rural nursing and case management theories. APNs practicing as case managers in rural communities must be expert generalists because of the diversity found in rural communities in terms of health problems encountered, age groups, and community characteristics. The authors contend that nurse case managers in rural communities have a broader and more diverse scope of practice than case managers in nonrural practice settings. Nursing case management in rural settings encompasses both individual and disease-management approaches.

Case managers are employed not only by hospitals but also by health maintenance organizations (HMOs), other managed care organizations, insurance companies, and disease management companies. Case managers serve as the liaison between patients and families, health plans, care providers, and purchasers to determine the extent of coverage and probable costs and to coordinate treatment at a lower cost and outside of inpatient care if possible.

Although RNs constitute the largest professional group in case management, the role is becoming increasingly multidisciplinary, with social workers, respiratory therapists, physical therapists, and other health care professionals joining organizations as case managers. However, many recognize the unique capabilities of the RN in optimizing the role of case manager. Indeed, it is thought that RNs who are experienced in management are best able to achieve the desired goals of consumer satisfaction and cost savings (Caldwell, 2000).

## Disease/Chronic Illness Management

The onset and eventual progression of many chronic illnesses is considered by many to be preventable. *Disease management* has been defined in the literature as a patient care approach that emphasizes comprehensive, coordinated care along a disease continuum and across health care delivery systems (Ellrodt, Cook, Lee, Cho, Hunt, & Weigarten, 1997). Disease management is the redirection of patient care services from inpatient to outpatient settings and is viewed as a proactive rather than a reactive approach to providing health care services (Rossiter et al., 2000). In essence, disease management programs use medical, prescription drug, and other health-related data to identify individuals with chronic illnesses who are at high risk of experiencing serious health problems and to provide early intervention to avoid or minimize those problems (Marlowe, 2000).

People diagnosed with chronic illnesses (e.g., asthma, diabetes mellitus, congestive heart failure [CHF], AIDS, lower back pain, and certain forms of cancer) are potential candidates for disease management interventions. Kongstvedt (1997) offered

> **BOX 19-6** *Criteria for Evaluating Need for Disease Management Services*
>
> - A high percentage of complications associated with the disease are preventable
> - The effect of a disease management program would be evident within 1 to 3 years after implementation
> - The conditions that are manifested can be managed in a nonsurgical, outpatient setting
> - There is a high rate of noncompliance with treatment protocols; however, the noncompliance is amenable to change
> - Practice guidelines are available (or there is potential to develop such guidelines) that outline optimal treatments of the disease

a set of criteria by which to evaluate what types of chronic illnesses are appropriate for disease management (Box 19-6).

The potential of disease management to reduce health care costs associated with common chronic illnesses seems significant. With the aging of the large "baby boomer" cohort of the population, a precipitous rise in the incidence of chronic illnesses, such as diabetes and CHF, seems to be a foregone conclusion. At current rates, the economic burden related to the treatment of just three chronic illnesses (heart disease, diabetes mellitus, and asthma) in the United States is staggering, with an estimated 80% of all health care dollars in the United States spent on managing a relatively small number of chronic illnesses (Wojcik & Bradford, 2000).

## DISEASE MANAGEMENT MODELS

Historically, disease management programs were developed by pharmacy benefits management (PBM) organizations, which were mainly owned by pharmaceutical companies who had a financial stake in management of diseases. The theory was that if disease management programs were successful, the drug manufacturing company sponsoring the program would sell more drugs to the individual. As interest in disease management has grown, PBMs, as disease management program sponsors, represent only a small segment of the business. Other more recent sponsors and advocates of disease management programs include managed care companies, individual state Medicaid agencies, provider organizations, and independent vendors. Independent disease management vendors are the most rapidly growing segment in the disease management arena because of the potential for profitability. Many of the independent vendors are web-based providers of disease management services.

Managed care and managed care organizations (MCOs) evolved in an attempt to control costs associated with traditional fee-for-service insurance reimbursement practices. MCOs are held clinically and financially responsible for health outcomes of their enrolled members on a capitated fee basis. Many MCOs have implemented disease management and wellness programs that utilize a case management approach to improve clinical outcomes (Sackett, Pope, & Erdley, 2004).

The method of disease management implementation in Medicaid and other state programs varies by state and is becoming more widely used, with states reporting disease management programs to cover asthma, diabetes, CHF, and other chronic illnesses. One such program, the Louisiana State University Health Care Services Division (HCSD) utilizes disease management to provide care based on evidence-based guidelines from professional organizations to patients with high-volume, high-cost diseases such as diabetes, asthma, CHF, HIV, and chronic kidney disease.

Other HCSD programs focus on cancer screening, smoking cessation, diet, exercise, and weight control. Programs, which operate at hospital and clinic sites in southern Louisiana, are targeted to clients who are uninsured; however, the program also serves insured clients.

The HCSD program was created approximately 10 years ago. Clinical outcomes have been tracked using disease management indicators since the inception of the program. Examples of disease management indicators related to patients with CHF, for example, include tracking the percent of patients with appropriate use of drugs, such as ACE inhibitors and beta-blockers, inappropriate use of calcium channel blockers and NSAIDS, hospital admission rates, use of emergency departments, and regular primary care or cardiology visits as well as other indicators.

Among the most notable outcomes of this disease management program are increases in the percentages of patients with improved HbA1c levels, improved LDL levels, and the increased use of aspirin in the diabetic population. Clinical improvements were also observed in the CHF population, in patients with asthma and in patients with HIV. Cancer-related screening practices also improved including increased use of mammography, PAP, and PSA testing (Horswell et al., 2008).

Sackett and colleagues (2004) write of the need to demonstrate return on investment (ROI) for disease management programs. Disease management programs that are appropriately designed and implemented can reduce health care costs by controlling utilization of services.

Ritterband (2000) elaborated on some of the challenges facing disease management providers. These challenges include clinical, financial, and regulatory considerations as well as skepticism on the part of patients and providers about disease management motives, particularly if involvement of a drug manufacturer is evident. Physicians and other providers have expressed related concerns that include separating care for the chronic illness from other care the primary care physician provides, duplicating services, and creating a possible source of confusion for the patient over whose instructions to follow. Financial challenges include the management of low-risk groups who have not been as aggressively managed as high-risk members. However, the low-risk members do have the potential to move into the high-risk category at some point. This especially holds true for Medicaid recipients.

The growing need to manage chronic illnesses is creating an unprecedented opportunity for nurses, particularly APNs, who by virtue of their educational credentials and clinical expertise, are uniquely positioned to become leaders in disease management. Roles for APNs include coordination of care for persons with chronic illnesses in for-profit and in not-for-profit health care organizations in which APNs provide an array of direct services to plan members. APNs use published practice guidelines to manage and coordinate care of individuals with chronic illnesses across health care settings. Nurses are the best prepared for the scope of this care coordinator role, particularly those prepared as nurse practitioners (NPs) and CNSs who have specialized in caring for patients with one or more chronic illnesses.

## Quality Management

In 2001, the Institute of Medicine (IOM) released the publication *To Err Is Human*. The release of this document, which asserted that medical errors were responsible for between 44,000 and 98,000 deaths annually in the United States, spurred demands for greater accountability and quality in the U.S. health care system (Kohn, Corrigan, & Donaldson, 2000). Since that time many quality improvement or QM initiatives have been undertaken in health care systems and organizations which directly impact the discipline of nursing.

Although there is some variation in the emphasis placed on specific aspects of QM between organizations, there are seven key principles or elements that are viewed as integral components of all QM programs. These elements include focus on the customer, process improvement, variance analysis, leadership, employee involvement, scientific method, and benchmarking (Baker & Gelmon, 1996).

In the QM environment, quality is defined in terms of what is acceptable to the customer; that is, the customer determines expectations of quality. Comprehensive knowledge of the customer's needs and expectations is integral to providing the best in quality customer service. There are two types of customers: customers who are external to the organization and customers who are internal. In health care, for example, external customers are patients, families, physicians not employed by the organization, payers, and communities. Internal customers are staff members employed by the organization to provide a service to external customers. For example, the staff on a nursing unit is a customer of pharmacy services. The nursing staff relies on the pharmacy staff to provide accurate medications in a timely fashion to the nursing unit to enable the external customer, the patient, to receive medications appropriately and on time.

*Process improvement* involves scrupulously examining work processes involved in achieving a work product. For example, in a hospital setting the process of transferring a patient from an orthopedic unit to a rehabilitation unit may have 20 or more steps and may involve five or six different departments. The more steps (and people) involved, the greater the likelihood that the transfer will be delayed or that an error will be made during the transfer, which leads to increased costs. Process improvement dictates that every aspect of patient transfer must be examined to determine whether each step in the process is really needed to accomplish the transfer. Members of each department or unit involved in the transfer are included on a process improvement team to examine the process for redundancies and lapses in service and to streamline the process.

Monitoring and analysis of variation in processes is crucial, particularly in health care organizations. There are two types of variation, common cause variation, which occurs no matter how well a system operates, and special cause variation. Special cause variation is variation that occurs outside of what is to be expected and can be caused by employee error and equipment or systems failure. The scientific method used to distinguish between common cause and special cause variation is statistical control (Varkey, Reller, & Resar, 2007).

Leadership in a QM environment has two components: comprehensive knowledge and an understanding of concepts and techniques of quality improvement and personal involvement. Leaders must be familiar with the terminology, the concepts, and the statistical techniques used in QM. Essential roles and responsibilities of leaders in QM include being personally committed to the philosophy, providing resources that include training others in the philosophy, reviewing progress on a regular basis, giving recognition, and managing resistance while empowering others.

To initiate and sustain a successful, meaningful quality improvement program, all members of the organization should have education and training related to QM. Employees should come away from the training with a clear understanding of their individual roles and responsibilities related to quality improvement. A broad range of employees should be encouraged to participate on quality improvement teams to design and improve work processes. Organizations that have been successful in implementing QM have empowered employees at all levels to search for better ways to redesign work processes to achieve customer satisfaction.

True quality improvement activities are based on scientific and statistical methods rather than on trial-and-error approaches to problem identification and problem-solving. The scientific method is a precise, systematic, orderly, planned, and organized method of problem solving that can be replicated and understood by employees of the organization. Several problem-solving methods can be used by health care organizations including the most commonly used approach for rapid improvement in healthcare, the plan-do-stay-act (PDSA) cycle (Varkey et al., 2007). Other quality improvement methods utilized in contemporary health care organizations are six sigma and lean strategies. Problem analysis tools (also called statistical process control tools) used in the problem-solving process include flowcharts, cause-and-effect diagrams, and run charts.

Benchmarking, a process originally implemented by the Xerox Corporation in 1979 (Camp & Tweet, 1994), is the identification, adaptation, and dissemination of best practices among competitors and noncompetitors that lead to their superior performance. In other words, quality can be improved in an organization by analyzing and then copying the methods of leaders in a field such as health care. Effective benchmarking involves identifying specific key indicators of a process (i.e., length of endotracheal intubation in postoperative patients), comparing this process with other organizations, determining the best process, and then using knowledge of the best process internally to design new processes or improve existing ones (Baker & Gelmon, 1996).

Many governmental, public and private groups are working to make health care rankings and information available to consumers. For example, the U.S. government's Agency for Healthcare Research and Quality (AHRQ) posts consumer ratings of health plans and some widely used clinical performance ratings on its website (http://www.ahrq.gov/consumer/qnt/qntqlook.htm). This site also provides information regarding health care facility accreditation. From the website a prospective patient can determine whether a health care facility is accredited by the Joint Commission. If so, the consumer can view the facility's most recent performance report which includes the following information: accreditation status; date of the last survey; evaluation of key areas during the survey; areas that require improvement; and comparison with state and national results (benchmarking data).

## QUALITY IMPROVEMENT INITIATIVES IN NURSING

Examples of quality improvement initiatives in nursing and health care abound in the literature and range from simple one-team solutions to complex multisite collaborations. Pappas (2008) describes a quality improvement study whose objective was to establish a methodology for nursing leaders to determine the cost of nurse sensitive adverse events (e.g., medication errors, patient falls, urinary tract infection, pneumonia, and pressure ulcers) from hospital cost accounting systems. A further objective of the study was to determine if relationships existed between the occurrence of nurse-sensitive adverse events in selected medical and surgical patients, the level of nurse staffing, and the actual cost of patient care for an inpatient hospital admission. The results of this study revealed that in both medical and surgical patients the occurrence of an adverse event (although only a small number of adverse events occurred in the study time period) was the best predictor of cost per case. In other words, when an adverse event occurred, the costs for the inpatient visit increased by an average of $659 for medical patients and by an average of $903 for surgery patients.

In this study, the occurrence of pneumonia in the surgery patient study group was the only significant relationship found between quantity of nurse staffing and the occurrence of a nurse-sensitive adverse event. Other implications related to quality improvement included the finding that age and severity were the best predictors of adverse events. The author recommends this information be used to influence staffing decisions at the individual unit level to reduce the risk of future occurrence of adverse events. The results of this research also contribute to the growing body of evidence related to the role of adequate nurse staffing in preventing patient complications, which may lead to increased morbidity and mortality and ultimately to poorer quality outcomes and increased health care costs.

Kleinpell (2007) describes the value of APNs in promoting evidence-based care and acting as champions of quality improvement. Various studies have measured the impact of APN practice on quality of care. One study documented that patients receiving APN care had significantly fewer days with an indwelling urinary catheter, fewer days to tracheostomy placement when intubated, less time in the ICU, and less wait time for post-discharge placement once discharge orders were written (Russell, VorderBruegge, & Burns, 2002). Another study revealed that cardiac surgery patients in the ICU setting who had been cared for by surgeon/NP teams had better outcomes; for example, less time intubated, fewer complications, decreased length of stay, and lower costs of care than comparable patients cared for by a cardiac surgeon alone (Myers & Miers, 2005).

Experts predict that financial pressures for hospitals and health systems will be more intensive in the future than in the past. The only way for MCOs to control costs will be through operational and clinical improvements. Health care institutions that can provide documented successes in quality improvement that result in improved clinical and cost outcomes will be the institutions most heavily courted by MCOs, by private and government insurers, and by consumers.

Also, as a result of new internet-based rating mechanisms, health care consumers are becoming increasingly savvy about checking quality "report cards" of health care facilities and providers. Health care–related sites are among those most sought after among internet users. At the same time, Americans age 50 and older, the segment of the population that uses the most health care services, are using the internet in ever-increasing numbers. Institutions that are implementing best practices, and continually striving to improve performance while decreasing costs, will be the biggest winners in the competitive health care environment of the future (Health Care Strategic Management, 2000).

## EVIDENCE-BASED PRACTICE

Health care consumers expect quality care and most health care practitioners want to provide quality care. Pressure for cost containment compels providers to demonstrate that interventions produce cost-effective outcomes that do not sacrifice the quality of health care. Further, selected interventions must be not only effective but also justified and congruent with acceptable standards (Glanville, Schirm, & Wineman, 2000).

EBP is a problem-solving approach that enables clinicians to provide the highest quality of care to patients and their families by integrating the following approaches:

- Critical appraisal and critique of the most recent and relevant research (evidence)
- Considering the clinician's own clinical expertise
- Considering preferences and values of the patient (Melnyk & Fineout-Overholt, 2005).

EBP allows for the translation of research evidence into direct patient care. Results from research studies indicate that patients who receive care based on the most rigorous and latest evidence from well-designed studies experience 28% better outcomes (Heater, Becker, & Olson, 1988). Balas and Boren (2000) contended that it may take as many as 17 years to translate research findings into actual patient care practice. This unacceptable gap raised the concern of patient advocacy groups, the government, and organizations that represent health care practitioners. As a result, federal funding of EBP centers has been implemented and much greater attention has been focused on implementing EBP in virtually every specialty medical and nursing organization.

For EBP to take root and flourish in an organization there must be institutional support and commitment from administrators. This support stems from the mission, goals, and culture of the organization. Without this support, necessary resources and infrastructure components, such as access to databases, dedicated personnel, and computer support, which are integral to a successful EBP program, may not be allocated or made fully available and accessible (Melnyk & Fineout-Overholt, 2005).

APNs must make clinical decisions on the best evidence available. They must also select interventions that are linked to cost-effective outcomes. This integrated approach allows the APN to use critical thinking skills to determine whether scientific evidence and clinical practice guidelines are relevant and consistent with the applicable health care situation and with the patient's values, preferences and life context (Glanville et al., 2000).

Buchanan (2002), an APN, described the U.S. Department of Health and Human Services clinical practice guideline for treating tobacco use and dependence, and demonstrated how the guideline was used in a small pilot study of pregnant women ($n = 20$) in an effort to help the women decrease smoking. Clinical results showed better outcomes for the women in the pilot program as compared to women in a comparison group. There was a statistically significant difference between the two groups in the average number of cigarettes smoked per day at delivery and 2 weeks after delivery, with women in the pilot program self-reporting less smoking.

In another example, Stacey, DeGrasse, and Johnston (2002), conducted a study to identify the support needs of women at high risk for breast cancer and to enhance an evidence-based service for women at high risk for breast cancer within a new high-risk breast assessment clinic. Most of the women in this study who were under age 50 wanted information related to breast cancer screening, risk of breast cancer, lifestyle options to lower risk, and hormone replacement therapy. Women over age 50 wanted information on risk of breast cancer, lifestyle options, breast cancer screening, and chemoprevention of breast cancer. The satisfaction component of the survey revealed that most women's needs were met. Oncology APNs practicing in this high-risk program required specialized skills in risk communication, behavior modification, and decision support.

Drenning (2006), an APN, describes a collaborative approach that was utilized to implement an EBP change to address the knowledge and comfort level of RNs in discussing advanced directives with patients. Members of the team included staff nurses, nursing managers, directors, an APN with clinical expertise in palliative care, and a doctorally prepared nurse educator and researcher. The team identified the need for a practice change, clarified the practice problem, and identified desired patient and clinical outcomes. The team also researched relevant and evidence-based interventions related to the identified problem and proposed solutions for implementation. Chapter 17 contains additional information about EBP.

## Summary

This chapter has provided examples of the application of specific theories, models, and frameworks in nursing administration and management. The models, which were described along with related historical and contemporary applications, should provide the APN with a foundation for navigating the complex, ever-changing environment of health care organizations today and in the future.

Health care organizations of the future hold great promise for APNs, such as Greta from the opening case study, who are willing to assume entrepreneurial and intrapreneurial roles in providing cost-effective quality health care. A more detailed understanding of some of these models will be necessary in certain circumstances (e.g., as in the case study), but it is hoped that this chapter has provided a basis for further investigation for those who need more detailed information.

## LEARNING ACTIVITIES

1. Interview a middle-level manager in a hospital to determine recent changes in span of control. Has the span of control for the manager decreased or increased in the past 2 to 3 years? What impact has the manager noticed related to decreased or increased span of control? What is the manager's preference in terms of numbers of employees in his or her span of administrative control?

2. What are the roles of APNs employed by health care organizations in quality improvement activities in your community? Are APNs the leaders of quality improvement teams? What significant contributions have occurred as a result of APN involvement on QI teams?

3. Talk with APNs who are employed in hospitals in your area. Determine the following:

   a. Are the APNs unit based? If so, what is the method of patient care delivery on the unit, that is, primary nursing, team nursing, PFC? What are the advantages and disadvantages to the APN role related to each of the different delivery methods?

   b. Do the APNs have staff or line authority? What are the advantages and disadvantages to the role of each type of authority?

   c. Administratively, do the APNs report to a senior or middle-level manager?

   d. Do any of the APNs work in a shared governance environment?

4. What EBP activities have APNs in your area spearheaded? Have health care consumers benefited?

## INTERNET RESOURCE

American Nurses Credentialing Center (2009) ANCC Magnet Program.

http://www.nursecredentialing.org/Magnet.aspx

## REFERENCES

Agency for Healthcare Research and Quality (AHRQ). Your guide to choosing quality health care. A quick look at quality. http://www.ahrq.gov/consumer/qnt/qntlook.htm.

Aiken, L. H., Clarke, S. P., & Sloane, D. M. (2002). Hospital staffing, organization, and quality of care: Cross-national findings. *International Journal of Quality Health Care, 14*(1), 5–13.

Aiken, L. H., Clarke, S. P., Sloane, D. M., Lake, E. T., & Cheney, T. (2008). Effects of hospital care environments on patient mortality and nurse outcomes. *Journal of Nursing Administration, 38*(5), 223–229.

Aiken, L. H., Clarke, S. P., Sloane, D. M., Sochalski, J., & Silber, J. H. (2002). Hospital nurse staffing and patient mortality, nurse burnout and job dissatisfaction. *The Journal of the American Medical Association, 288*(16), 1987–1993.

Aiken, L. H., Havens, D. S., & Sloane, D. M. (2000). The magnet nursing services recognition program: A comparison of two groups of magnet hospitals. *American Journal of Nursing, 100*(3), 26–36.

Aiken, L. H., & Patrician, P. (2000). Measuring organizational attributes of hospitals: The revised Nursing Work Index. *Nursing Research, 49(3)*, 146–153.

Aiken, L. H., Sloane, D. M., Lake, E. T., Sochalski, J., & Weber, A. L. (1999). Organization and outcomes of inpatient AIDS care. *Medical Care, 37*(8), 760–772.

Aiken, L. H., Smith, H. L., & Lake, E. T. (1994). Lower Medicare mortality among a set of hospitals known for good nursing care. *Medical Care, 32*(8), 771–787.

Aiken, L. H., Sloane, H. L., & Lake, E. T. (1997). Satisfaction with inpatient acquired immunodeficiency syndrome care: A national comparison of dedicated and scattered-bed units. *Medical Care, 35*(9), 948–962.

American Nurses Association. (2004). *Scope and standards for nurse administrators* (2nd ed.). Silver Springs, MD: ANA.

Anthony, M. K. (2004). Shared governance models: The theory, practice, and evidence. *Online Journal of Issues in Nursing, 9*(1). Available at: http://www.nursingworld.org/MainMenuCategories/ANAMarketplace/ANAPeriodicals/OJIN/TableofContents/Volume92004/No1Jan04/SharedGovernanceModels.

Baker, G. R., & Gelmon, S. B. (1996). Total quality management in health care. In J. A. Schmele (Ed.), *Quality management in nursing and health care* (pp. 66–87). Boston: Delmar.

Balas, E. A., & Boren, S. A. (2000). Managing clinical knowledge for health care improvements. In J. H. Van Bemmel & A. T. McCray (Eds.), *2000 Yearbook of Medical informatics—Patient-centered systems* (pp. 65–70). Germany: Schattauer Publishing Company.

Barker, A. M. (1994). An emerging leadership paradigm: Transformational leadership. In E. C. Hein & J. M. Nicholson (Eds.), *Contemporary leadership behavior: Selected readings* (4th ed., pp. 81–86). Philadelphia: J. B. Lippincott.

Bennis, W., & Nanus, B. (1985). *Leaders: Strategies for taking charge.* New York: Harper & Row.

Benoit, C. B. (1996). Case management and the advanced practice nurse. In J. V. Hickey, R. Ouimette, & S. L. Venegoni (Eds.), *Advanced practice nursing: Changing roles and clinical applications* (pp. 107–129). Philadelphia: Lippincott-Raven.

Blass, T. C., & Reed, T. L. (2003). Case management serves as an alternative career for advanced practice nurses. *Nursing Management, 34*(10), 81–83.

Brennan, P. F., & Anthony, M. K. (2000). Measuring nursing practice models using multi-attribute utility theory. *Research in Nursing and Health, 23*(5), 372–382.

Buchan, J. (1999). Still attractive after all these years? Magnet hospitals in changing health care environment. *Journal of Advanced Nursing, 30*(1), 100–108.

Buchanan, L. (2002). Implementing a smoking cessation program for pregnant women based on current clinical practice guidelines. *Journal of the American Academy of Nurse Practitioners, 14*(6), 243–250.

Caldwell, B. (2000). Case managers are conduit between patients, providers in quest for quality, cost-effective care. *Employee Benefit Plan Review, 54*(7), 12–14.

Camp, R. C., & Tweet, A. G. (1994). Benchmarking applied to health care. *Journal of Quality Improvement, 20*(5), 229–238.

Cathcart, D. (2004). Span of control matters. *Journal of Nursing Administration, 34*(9), 395–399.

Cho, S. H., Ketefian, S., Barkauskas, V. H., & Smith, D. G. (2003). The effects of nurse staffing on adverse events, morbidity, mortality, and medical costs. *Nursing Research, 52*(2), 71–79.

Christman, L. (1976). The autonomous nursing staff in the hospital. *Nursing Administration Quarterly, 1*(1), 37–44.

Clarke, S. P., & Aiken, L. H. (2003). Failure to rescue: Measuring nurses' contributions to hospital performance. *American Journal of Nursing, 103,* 42–47.

Clarke, S. P., Sloane, D. M., & Aiken, L. (2002). Effects of hospital staffing and organizational climate on needlestick injuries to nurses. *American Journal of Public Health, 92*(7), 1115–1119.

Cleland, V. S. (1978). Shared governance in a professional model of collective bargaining. *Journal of Nursing Administration, 8*(5), 39–43.

Clouten, K., & Weber, R. (1994). Patient-focused care . . . playing to win. *Nursing Management, 25*(2), 34–36.

Cottingham, C. (1988). Transformational leadership: A strategy for nursing. *Today's OR Nurse, 10*(6), 24–27.

Drenning, C. (2006). Collaboration among nurses, advanced practice nurses, and nurse researchers to achieve evidence-based practice change. *Journal of Nursing Care Quality, 21*(4), 298–301.

Ellrodt, G., Cook, D. J., Lee, J., Cho, M., Hunt, D., & Weigarten, S. (1997). Evidence-based disease management. *Journal of the American Medical Association, 278*(20), 1687–1692.

Fayol, H. (1949). *General and industrial management.* London: Pitman & Sons. (Original work published in 1918).

Flynn, L. (2007). Extending work environment research into home health settings. *Western Journal of Nursing Research, 29*(2), 200–212.

Glanville, I., Schirm, V., & Wineman, N. M. (2000). Using evidence-based practice for managing clinical outcomes in advanced practice nursing. *Journal of Nursing Care Quality, 15*(1), 1–11.

Graicunas, A. (1937). Relationships in organizations. In L. Gullick & L. Urwick (Eds.), *Papers on the science of administration* (pp. 181–188). New York: Institute on Public Administration.

Harrison, J. P., Nolin, J., & Suero, E. (2004). The effect of case management on U.S. hospitals. *Nursing Economics, 22*(2), 64–70.

Havens, D., & Aiken, L. (1999). Shaping systems to promote desired outcomes. *Journal of Nursing Administration, 29*(2), 14–20.

Health Care Strategic Management (2000). While quality, best outcomes have been "nice to do," they will become essential for survival in coming years. *Health Care Strategic Management* (Suppl.), 11–13.

Heater, B., Becker, A., & Olson, R. (1988). Nursing interventions and patient outcomes: A meta-analysis of studies. *Nursing Research, 37*(5), 303–307.

Hess, R. G. (2004). From bedside to boardroom—nursing shared governance. *Online Journal of Issues in Nursing, 9*(1), 2.

Horswell, R., Butler, M. K., Kaiser, M., Moody-Thomas, S., McNabb, S., Besse, J., & Abrams, A. (2008). Disease management programs for the underserved. *Disease Management, 11*(3), 145–152.

Institute for Family-Centered Care. http://www.familycenteredcare.org/faq.html. Accessed January 13, 2009.

Janzen, S. K. (2003). Testimony before the House of Representatives Committee on Veteran Affairs, Subcommittee on Oversight and Investigation.

Johnson, B., Abraham, M., Conway, J., Simmons, L., Levitan, S. E., Sodomka, P., Schlucter, J., & Ford, D. (2008). *Partnering with patients and families to design a patient-and-family-centered health care systems. Recommendations and promising practices.* Bethesda, MD: Institute for Family-Centered Care in Collaboration with the Institute for Healthcare Improvement. http://www.familycenteredcare.org/tools/downloads.html. Accessed January 13, 2009.

Kangas, S., Kee, S., & McKee-Waddle, R. (1999). Organizational factors, nurses' job satisfaction, and patient satisfaction with nursing care. *Journal of Nursing Administration, 29*(1), 32–42.

Kirkley, D., Johnson, A. P., & Anderson, M. A. (2004). Technology support of nursing excellence: The magnet connection. *Nursing Economics, 22*(2), 94–98.

Kleinpell, R. M. (2007). APNs—Invisible champions? *Nursing Management, 38*(5), 19–22.

Kohn, L. T., Corrigan, J. M., Donaldson, M. S. (Eds.). (2000). *To err is human: Building a safer health system.* Washington, D.C.: National Academy Press.

Kongstvedt, P. R. (1997). *Essentials of managed health care* (2nd ed.). Gaithersberg, MD: Aspen.

Kramer, M., & Hafner, L. P. (1989). Shared values: Impact on staff nurse job satisfaction and perceived productivity. *Nursing Research, 38*(3), 172–177.

Kramer, M., & Schmalenberg, C. E. (1988a). Magnet hospitals: Part I: Institutions of excellence. *Journal of Nursing Administration, 18*(1), 13–24.

Kramer, M., & Schmalenberg, C. E. (1988b). Magnet hospitals: Part II: Institutions of excellence. *Journal of Nursing Administration, 18*(2), 11–19.

Kramer, M., & Schmalenberg, C. E. (1993). Learning from success: Autonomy and empowerment. *Nursing Management, 24*(5), 58–64.

Kramer, M., & Schmalenberg, C. E. (2003). Magnet hospital nurses describe control over nursing practice. *Western Journal of Nursing Research, 25*(4), 424–452.

Kramer, M., Schmalenberg, C. E., & Hafner, L. P. (1989). What causes job satisfaction and productivity of quality nursing care? In T. Moore & M. Mundinger (Eds.), *Managing in the nursing shortage: A guide to recruitment and retention* (pp. 12–32). Rockville, MD: Aspen.

Kramer, M., Schmalenberg, C. E., Maguire, P., Brewer, B. B., Burke, R., Chmielewski, L., Cox, K., Kishner, J., Krugman, M., Meeks-Sjostrom, D., & Waldo, M. (2008). Structures and practices enabling staff nurses to control their practice. *Western Journal of Nursing Research, 30*(5), 539–559.

Lake, E. T. (2007). The nursing practice environment: Measurement and evidence. *Medical Care Research and Review, 64,* 1045–1225.

Laschinger, H. K., & Finegan, J. (2005). Empowering nurses for work engagement and health in hospital settings. *Journal of Nursing Administration, 35*(10), 439–448.

Laschinger, H. K. S., & Havens, S. (1996). Staff nurse work empowerment and perceived control over nursing practice: Conditions for work effectiveness. *Journal of Nursing Administration, 26*(9), 27–35.

Mang, A. L. (1995). Implementation strategies of patient-focused care. *Hospital and Health Services Administration, 40*(3), 426–435.

Marlowe, J. F. (2000). Disease management: Managed care's new thing. *Journal of Compensation and Benefits, 16*(3), 48–55.

Marriner-Tomey, A. (2009). *Guide to nursing management and leadership* (8th ed.). St. Louis: Mosby Elsevier.

McClure, M. L., & Hinshaw, A. S. (2002). *Magnet hospitals revisited: Attraction and retention of professional nurses.* Washington, DC: American Nurses Publishing.

McClure, M. L., Poulin, M. A., Sovie, M. D., & Wandelt, M. A. (1983). *Magnet hospitals: Attraction and retention of professional nurses.* Washington, DC: American Nurses Publishing.

McGuire, E., & Kennerly, S. M. (2006). Nurse managers as transformational and transactional leaders. *Nursing Economics, 24*(4), 179–185.

Medley, F., & Larochelle, D. R. (1995). Transformational nursing leadership and job satisfaction. *Nursing Management, 26*(9), 64JJ–64LL.

Melnyk, B. M., & Fineout-Overholt, E. (2005). *Evidence-based practice in nursing and health care.* Philadelphia: Lippincott Williams & Wilkins.

Moss, R., & Rowles, C. J. (1997). Staff nurse job satisfaction and management style. *Nursing Management, 28*(1), 32–34.

Myers, S. (1998). Patient-focused care: What managers should know. *Nursing Economics, 16*(4): 180–188.

Myers, S. C., & Miers, L. J. (2005). Cardiovascular surgeon and acute care nurse practitioner collaboration on postoperative outcomes. *AACN Clinical Issues, 16*(2), 149–158.

Needleman, J., Buerhaus, P., Mattke, S., Stewart, M., & Zelevinsky, K. (2002). Nurse staffing levels and the quality of care in hospitals. *The New England Journal of Medicine, 346*(22), 1715–1722.

Pappas, S. H. (2008). The cost of nurse-sensitive adverse events. *Journal of Nursing Administration, 38*(5), 230–236.

Poirrier, G. P., & Oberleitner, M. G. (1999). *Clinical pathways in nursing: A guide to managing care from hospital to home.* Springhouse, PA: Springhouse.

Porter-O'Grady, T. (1992). Transformational leadership in an age of chaos. *Nursing Administration Quarterly, 17*(1), 17–24.

Porter-O'Grady, T. (1994). Whole systems shared governance: Creating the seamless organization. *Nursing Economics, 12*(4), 187–195.

Porter-O'Grady, T. (2003). Researching shared governance: A futility of focus. *Journal of Nursing Administration, 33*(4), 251–252.

Porter-O'Grady, T., Hawkins, M., & Parker, M. (1997). *Whole systems shared governance: Architecture for integration.* Gaithersburg, MD: Aspen.

Ritterband, D. R. (2000). Disease management: Old wine in new bottles? *Journal of Health Care Management, 45*(4), 255–266.

Robbins, S. P., & Judge, T. A. (2009). *Organizational behavior* (13th ed.). Upper Saddle River, NJ: Prentice-Hall.

Rossiter, L. F., Whitehurst Cook, M. Y., Small, R. E., Shasky, C., Bovbejerg, B. E., Penberthy, L., Okasha, A., Green, J., Ibrahim, I. A., Yang, S., & Lee, K. (2000). The impact of disease management on outcomes and cost of care: A study of low income asthma patients. *Inquiry—Blue Cross and Blue Shield Association, 37*(2), 188–202.

Russell, D., VorderBruegge, M., & Burns, S. (2002). Effect of an outcomes-managed approach to care of neuroscience patients by acute care nurse practitioners. *American Journal of Critical Care, 11*(4), 353–364.

Sackett, K., Pope, R. K., & Erdley, W. S. (2004). Demonstrating a positive return on investment for a prenatal program at a managed care organization: An economic analysis. *Journal of Perinatal and Neonatal Nursing, 18*(2), 117–127.

Schifalacqua, M. M., Ulch, P., & Schmidt, M. (2004). How to make a difference in the health care of a population one person at a time. *Nursing Administration Quarterly, 28*(1), 29–35.

Spetz, J. (2008). Nurse satisfaction and the implementation of minimum nurse staffing requirements. *Policy, Politics, and Nursing Practice, 9*(1), 15–21.

Stacey, D., DeGrasse, C., & Johnston, L. (2002). Addressing the support needs of women at high risk for breast cancer: Evidence-based care by advanced practice nurses. *Oncology Nursing Forum, 29*(6), 77–84.

Stanton, M. P., & Packa, D. (2001). Nursing case management: A rural practice model. *Lippincott's Case Management, 6*(3), 96–103.

Stanton, M. P., Swanson, M., Sherrod, R. A., & Packa, D. R. (2005). Case management evolution: From basic to advanced practice role. *Lippincott's Case Management, 10*(6), 274–286.

Taylor, F. W. (1911). *The principles of scientific management.* New York: Harper.

Thomas, M. B. (Ed.). (2008). Case management program slashes hospital stays for the ESRD patients. *Case Management Advisor, 19*(10), 109–111. Available at http://www.ahcpub.com

Triolo, P. K., Scherer, E. M., & Floyd, J. M. (2006). Evaluation of the magnet recognition program. *Journal of Nursing Administration, 36*(1), 42–48.

Trott, M. C., & Windsor, K. (1999). Leadership effectiveness: How do you measure up? *Nursing Economics, 17*(3), 127–130.

Varkey, P., Reller, M. K., & Resar, R. K. (2007). Basics of quality improvement in health care. *Mayo Clinic Proceedings, 82*(6), 735–739.

Weber, M. (1970). Bureaucracy. In W. Sexton (Ed.), *Organization theories* (pp. 39–43). Columbus, OH: Charles E. Merrill.

Weston, M. J. (2008). Defining control over nursing practice and autonomy. *Journal of Nursing Administration, 38*(9), 404–408.

Wojcik, J., & Bradford, M. (2000). Online disease management. *Business Insurance, 34*(45), 23.

Wolf, G., Triolo, P., & Ponte, P. R. (2008). Magnet Recognition Program: The next generation. *Journal of Nursing Administration, 38*(4), 200–204.

Yamamoto, L., & Lucey, C. (2005). Case management "within the walls". *Critical Care Nursing Quarterly, 28*(2), 162–178.

Zarubi, K. L., Reiley, P., & McCarter, B. (2008). Putting patients and families at the center of care. *Journal of Nursing Administration, 38*(6), 275–281.

# CHAPTER

# 20

# Application of Theory in Nursing Education

## Evelyn Wills and Melanie McEwen

*L*inda Washington is a supervisor on a surgical floor of a large teaching hospital. Her responsibilities require her to work closely with the faculty from two area nursing schools and help place students with preceptors. Linda enjoys working with students and decided that she would like to become a nursing instructor.

Linda is currently enrolled in a master's degree program. This semester she is taking a course on nursing education, and she is learning a great deal about how nursing programs are structured and why. The course requires a project in which a small group of students designs a nursing program that will meet the changing needs of the health care system and the changing profile of nursing students at the beginning of the 21st century. This project was daunting for Linda and her colleagues, and they were unsure where to begin.

During one class period, Linda's professor explained how a curriculum is derived from the faculty's philosophy of nursing and nursing education. She taught that a conceptual framework is then developed from the philosophy, and it is from this framework that the curriculum is built. The students also learned that in most nursing programs, the conceptual framework is an eclectic blend of concepts and processes, although some programs use grand nursing theories as a basis.

In a brainstorming session, Linda and her group agreed on a philosophy of nursing education, describing what they saw as the interplay of the metaparadigm concepts and concepts of teaching and learning. But there was considerable discussion, and significant differences among group members, about what additional concepts or theories should be used as the basis for the curriculum framework. In addition, there was disagreement on what would be the best teaching strategies to meet the needs of older nursing students and students from diverse backgrounds. Some members of the group favored a structured, traditional type of program, in which the faculty member was responsible for directing learning experiences, whereas other group members preferred to focus on less rigid instructional techniques, and incorporate more web-based options and computer-assisted instruction.

The discussions were enlightening, and finally Linda's group compromised. They would use "caring" as a central concept and draw heavily from Jean Watson's (1996) work to *structure the curriculum. They would also incorporate adult learning principles and technologically based instructional strategies into their program. With these parameters in place, the group began to describe courses, write objectives, outline course sequencing, discern outcome measures, identify teaching strategies, and set up evaluation methods.*

---

The health care delivery system has changed dramatically during the past 15 years. Nursing practice has also changed, requiring it to adapt to a move from institution-based acute care to community-based care with an enhanced focus on persons with chronic conditions. Nursing education has been somewhat slow to respond to changes and anticipated trends in health care, however. This is contrary to assertions by nursing leaders and nursing organizations, who feel that "it is the responsibility of nursing education, in collaboration with practice settings, to shape practice, not merely respond to changes in the practice environment" (American Association of Colleges of Nursing [AACN], 1999, p. 60).

The literature is awash with "buzz words" for nursing education. Problem-based learning, caring, lifelong learning, informatics competency, evidence-based education, quality/performance improvement, culturally relevant care, interpersonal communication, and excellence are only a few. Furthermore, new models for curricula reflect "humanistic" approaches to teaching, learning, and practice, and highlight caring relationships, student–faculty shared responsibilities for learning, and multiple ways of knowing (Cook & Cullen, 2003; Rentschler & Spegman, 1996). Other evolving emphases in nursing education include enhanced attention to nursing values, meanings, and experiences (Mawn & Reece, 2000; Webber, 2002), a greater focus on community-based curricular threads (Hamner & Wilder, 2001), and more attention to multidisciplinary, interdisciplinary, and transdisciplinary educational collaborations (Dyer, 2003).

A well-developed and articulated theoretical basis gives a nursing program the perspective that shapes the content and the methods that guide students' learning; eventually these methods have an impact on nursing practice (Mawn & Reece, 2000). A theoretical basis provides a framework that helps nursing students define their professional philosophies and values. It identifies and describes essential concepts and significant problems and suggests approaches to structure and methods that the student may use in continuing to develop her or his knowledge. Additionally, the theoretical basis of the nursing program influences the means by which material is presented and the methods by which learning is evaluated.

Barnum (1998) stated that theoretical principles drawn from a number of sources directly affect a curriculum whether faculty members recognize it or not. Indeed, a nursing curriculum conveys a theory (or theories) of nursing by virtue of the content selected. She explained that a program's curricular framework may be a specific nursing theory adopted (or adapted) from a given nurse theorist, it may be a model designed by the faculty, or it may be an intuited image of nursing. Likewise, the means of presenting the content, the structure of courses, and evaluation methods are heavily theoretically based.

In general terms, theoretical principles, concepts, and models are used in two major ways in nursing education. First, they are used to determine the content and structure of a program's curriculum. Second, they are used to determine the instructional processes and strategies used by faculty to teach students. Both of these contributions of theory to nursing education are discussed in this chapter.

# Theoretical Issues in Nursing Curricula

Curriculum refers to the content and processes by which learners gain knowledge and understanding, develop skills, and alter attitudes, appreciation, and values under the auspices of a given school or program. The curriculum of a school of nursing typically includes philosophy and mission statements; an organizational or conceptual framework; lists of outcomes, competencies, and objectives for the program; and individual courses; course outlines and syllabi; educational activities; and evaluation methods (Dillard & Siktberg, 2009). Furthermore, most curricula specify essential nursing content and means of application in clinical practice (Webber, 2002). Specific components of the curriculum of a given program of study are summarized in Box 20-1.

Several issues that relate to the incorporation of theoretical principles and frameworks into nursing curricula are reviewed in this section. These include basic curriculum design, the impact of regulating organizations on nursing curricula, components of curricular conceptual/organizational frameworks, and the processes involved in designing and organizing nursing curricula. The section concludes with a short discussion of current issues in nursing curriculum development.

## CURRICULUM DESIGN IN NURSING EDUCATION

A *curriculum* is a "formal plan of study that provides the philosophical underpinnings, goals, and guidelines for the delivery of a specific educational program" (Keating, 2006a, p. 2). The curriculum provides faculty with a means of conceptualizing and organizing the knowledge, skills, values, and beliefs critical to the delivery of a coherent program of study that facilitates the achievement of the desired outcomes (Boland, 2009).

The curricula of most nursing programs are based on the Tyler Curriculum Development Model, which was published in 1949. Bevis (1989a, 1989b) stated that the incorporation of the Tyler model within nursing curricula began in the 1950s and continued throughout the 1960s and 1970s. According to Bevis (1989b), introduction of Tyler's concepts in the 1950s, along with her first book on curriculum development (Bevis, 1973), and Mager's (1962) publication of *Preparing Instructional Objectives*, led to the development of Tyler-type curricula throughout nursing education. Eventually, the Tyler model became the only model used in developing nursing curricula for all levels of nursing education—diploma, associate degree, and baccalaureate.

The Tyler model begins with identification of the educational purposes or objectives for the program. It then differentiates what learning experiences should be selected to

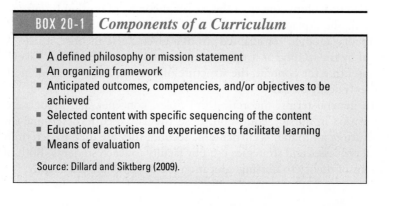

**BOX 20-1** *Components of a Curriculum*

- A defined philosophy or mission statement
- An organizing framework
- Anticipated outcomes, competencies, and/or objectives to be achieved
- Selected content with specific sequencing of the content
- Educational activities and experiences to facilitate learning
- Means of evaluation

Source: Dillard and Siktberg (2009).

attain the objectives. The third issue addressed by the Tyler model is how to organize learning experiences for effective instruction. Finally, the model focuses on evaluation of behaviors to determine if objectives have been met (Bevis, 1989b). The Tyler model values effectiveness, efficiency, and predictability, and it emphasizes individualism and competition. It assumes that knowledge consists of facts, generalizations, principles, and theories and that events or phenomena can be explained by cause-and-effect relationships that can be deductively examined (Diekelmann, 1987).

## NURSING CURRICULA AND REGULATING BODIES

The impact of the Tyler model on nursing curricula and nursing education cannot be overstated; it has directly influenced both state boards of nursing and the accreditation process. State boards of nursing set rules and requirements regarding nursing educational programs and curricula; these boards eventually based criteria for licensure of nursing programs on the Tyler model (Bevis, 1987; Rentschler & Spegman, 1996).

According to Bevis (1989b), the Tyler-based curriculum development process has been translated into essential curricular components, and without evidence of these components, state boards will not grant program approval. The rules and regulations set by state boards of nursing typically specify content areas that must be covered, minimum hours that must be spent by all students in clinical settings, and competencies or skills that all students must possess at the completion of the nursing program (Boland & Finke, 2009). A stated or defined conceptual framework is required for program approval by many state boards of nursing (National Council of State Boards of Nursing [NCSBN], 2005).

Similar to the impact on state board criteria, the Tyler model has heavily influenced the framework for accreditation by the National League for Nursing (NLN). Through the accreditation process, the NLN has had a great impact on the development, implementation, and evaluation of undergraduate nursing curricula (Boland & Finke, 2009). The first NLN accreditation visits were in 1939, and soon NLN accreditation requirements became the standard for nursing education (Bevis, 1989a; Flood, 2006). Beginning in 1972, the NLN criteria for bachelor's (BSN) programs included a criterion requiring that the curriculum be based on a conceptual framework that was consistent with the stated philosophy, purposes, and objectives of the program (Kelley, 1975; NLN, 1972; Wu, 1979). Likewise, in the 1970s, accreditation requirements for associate degree (ADN) programs required that the "conceptual framework of the program of learning is clearly stated and implemented" (NLN, 1977, p. 14).

Meleis (2005) observed that the recognition of the potential of nursing theories to be used as guidelines for the conceptual frameworks of nursing curricula and programs in the 1960s and 1970s coincided with the development of most of the nursing theories. Indeed, nursing education promoted theory development in the search for a coherent presentation of nursing to guide and structure curricula.

Over the ensuing years, accreditation criteria changed somewhat. During this time, "the requirements for a conceptual framework were a major source of confusion and concern among nurse educators" (Tanner, 1989, p. 8). Because of this confusion, guidelines were changed, and since the mid-1980s, they have been more flexible. The NLNAC's accreditation standards, for example, state that the curriculum must follow an "organizing framework" that outlines a logical progression of objectives and learning activities. *Organizing framework* is defined as "a set of concepts derived from program philosophy that are ordered in a logical and meaningful manner so as to direct the delivery of the curriculum" (National League for Nursing Accrediting Committee [NLNAC],

2004 p. 97). Thus, while not explicitly requiring a defined conceptual framework, some type of specific organizational strategy must be used to structure the program.

Since the mid-1990s, the AACN Commission on Collegiate Nursing Education (CCNE) has also been accrediting baccalaureate and master's nursing programs. In its accreditation standards, like the NLNAC, the CCNE does not specify an organizing framework. Rather, the need for a curricular framework is implied as Standard III states that the "curriculum is . . . consistent with professional nursing standards and guidelines and congruent with the program's mission and goals. . . . The curriculum is logically structured to meet expected program outcomes" (CCNE, 2003, Standard III).

## CONCEPTUAL/ORGANIZATIONAL FRAMEWORKS FOR NURSING CURRICULA

The conceptual or organizational framework of a nursing program must be an outgrowth of the philosophy of the faculty, which typically reflects the faculty's philosophical beliefs about the metaparadigm concepts (Boland, 2009; Keating, 2006b). Scales (1985) explained that the interrelationship of these concepts is the basic organizational framework of the curriculum, and as the concepts are further defined within the framework, the curriculum becomes established. Additional concepts and theories selected to comprise the conceptual framework are likewise taken from the philosophy (Boland, 2009).

According to Bevis (1989a), a curriculum conceptual framework is an "interrelated system of premises that provides guidelines or ground rules for making all curricular decisions—objectives, content, implementation, and evaluation" (p. 26). The conceptual framework may be referred to as the curriculum framework, the framework for curriculum development, the conceptual system, the curriculum theory, a theory of education, or the theoretical framework, but regardless of the name, it is the conceptualization and articulation of concepts, facts, propositions, postulates, theories, and variables relevant to the specific nursing program.

### Purposes of the Conceptual Framework
The conceptual or organizational framework for a curriculum serves several purposes. First, it allows faculty to determine what knowledge is important to nursing (i.e., the concepts, principles, skills, and theories to be covered) and how that knowledge should be defined, categorized, and linked with other knowledge. It also helps explain how these ideas or concepts apply to nursing practice. Second, the conceptual framework facilitates the sequencing and prioritizing of knowledge in a way that is logical and internally consistent (Boland, 2009). Finally, "conceptual frameworks provide faculty with a defined, cohesive curriculum to give students planned, organized, consistent, and cohesive learning experiences. This assists in achieving the proposed educational outcomes (Dillard & Siktberg, 2009, p. 82).

### Research Studies of Conceptual Frameworks
Three studies describing various aspects of conceptual frameworks in nursing education were identified in the nursing literature. Hall (1979) surveyed BSN programs to identify the conceptual frameworks on which they based their curricula. Of those responding, 41% of the BSN programs based their curricula on one or more of a researcher-provided list of nursing theorists (i.e., Orem, Rogers, Levine, King, Roy, and Johnson). Hall reported that other programs indicated that other nursing theorists (i.e., Henderson and M. Newman) were used. Nonnurse theorists and models were also identified as directing nursing programs. These included the works of Dunn and Blum, as well as theories of stress, adaptation, and systems.

Hall (1979) stated that "only in rare instances in any of the programs, where a particular theorist's framework was being used, was the framework employed without modification" (p. 28). She concluded that most nursing educators are developing their own conceptual frameworks that are consistent with the program's philosophy and objectives.

Quiring and Gray (1982) conducted a survey to "determine which organizing approaches were employed most frequently" in BSN programs (p. 39). They reported that 91 of 144 survey questionnaires were returned, and findings indicated that most programs used a combination of concepts, "threads," and the nursing process as organizers of their curricula. They concluded that the nursing process "is an integral part of most programs" (p. 41). The concepts of health and illness, life cycle, stress–adaptation, socialization–professionalization, and man–environment were also commonly used threads.

More recently, McEwen and Brown (2002) completed a large-scale, nationwide study that examined the curricular frameworks of BSN, ADN, and diploma nursing programs. Responses were received from 160 programs (from a sample of 300), and the findings illustrated current trends in structuring the conceptual frameworks of nursing curricula. Although there were a few differences based on type of program, in general, the nursing process was the most commonly used component of conceptual frameworks for nursing curricula, being used by 55% of all programs. Simple-to-complex organization (37% of all programs), a biopsychosocial model (36% of all programs), and nursing theorists (33% of all programs) were the other most frequently reported components.

The most commonly reported nursing theorists for incorporation into nursing curricula were Orem (11 of 160 programs) and Roy (10 of 160 programs). Watson (6 programs), Betty Neuman (5 programs), and Benner (4 programs) were nursing theorists whose works were used in the curriculum frameworks of more than three responding schools. Nonnursing theories that were reported were systems theory, Maslow's and Erickson's theories, and adaptation, although each was relatively infrequent. An interesting finding was a move away from using nursing theorist-based curricula, because 20 different programs indicated that they had changed from a theorist-based framework to a nontheorist focus in their last curricular change (McEwen & Brown, 2002). One contributing factor to this shift is the notion that using a nursing theory or conceptual model as the curricular framework makes concepts and processes difficult for new students to understand. Indeed, the language and degree of abstraction of many of the nursing theories can be very confusing for beginners (Boland, 2009; Secrest, 2008). McEwen and Brown (2002) also examined how the conceptual framework was used in the curriculum. The most common responses and percentages of programs were as follows: "determines objectives" (85%), "determines outcomes" (78%), "directs assessment" (64%), and "directs nursing interventions" (59%).

### Designing a Curriculum Conceptual Framework

Boland (2009) stated that there are two approaches to determining or developing an organizational framework for a nursing curriculum. Faculty members may choose a single, specific nursing theory or model on which to build the framework, or they may choose a more eclectic approach, selecting concepts from multiple theories or models. She explained that use of a single theory to develop the conceptual framework helps by providing a single image with a defined vocabulary that is shared by both the learner and the teacher. In some cases, however, it was observed that the language of the theory and the definitions of the central concepts may be too abstract to be helpful. If a single theory is used as the framework, the faculty will adopt the theory and use its definitions and relationships to structure and organize content.

Several articles in recent nursing literature describe the use of nursing theories as the basis for the curriculum framework of nursing programs. Secrest (2008) described the role of tool development in an Orem-based curriculum and the role of faculty in bringing the revision to fruition. Seng, Mirenda, and Lowry (1996) examined the implementation of a curriculum using Neuman's Systems Model in both a BSN program and an ADN program. Finally, Cook and Cullen (2003) described the use of Watson's work as a theoretical framework at an ADN program.

To avoid being constrained by a single nursing theory or model, many faculty choose an eclectic approach, which combines many theories and concepts in framework development (McEwen & Brown, 2002). Often two or three organizing themes are used to build a curriculum grid. These themes can be variables such as life phases, body systems, and the nursing process.

A criticism of the eclectic approach to constructing conceptual frameworks is that it impedes the development of a body of knowledge that is uniquely nursing. If the eclectic approach is taken, a combination of many theories or concepts is used, and borrowed concepts must be specifically defined for the program. Relationships between and among the concepts must also be explained. On the other hand, an advantage to an eclectic approach is the ability to "borrow" concepts and definitions that best fit the faculty's beliefs and values (Boland, 2009).

### Components of the Curricular Conceptual Framework

The two major areas to be addressed during development of a curriculum framework are as follows: (1) What concepts will be covered? (2) What will be the structure, ordering, or sequencing for introducing the concepts and delineating the relationships between and among them?

#### Curriculum Concepts

Once a conceptual framework for a nursing program is agreed on, the task is to identify the major elements or concepts that will appear and reappear at each level of the curriculum, and thus provide a basis for the organization and sequencing of content. Most undergraduate nursing conceptual frameworks minimally describe the concepts of health, person, environment, and nursing. Other concepts, such as caring, self-care, growth and development, nursing process, and adaptation, may be added to expand or clarify the framework. Each of the central concepts should be defined, and the linkages between and among the concepts should be explained to unify or interrelate the details.

The conceptual framework may then use additional constructs or devices to help structure or organize the material. It may use developmental stage, acute/chronic concepts, health/illness continuum, settings, or the nursing process as the chief organizer. In addition, "process threads" are usually present throughout the curriculum. These might include the nursing process, problem-solving, interpersonal relationships, communication, research, change, and teaching. Each of these constructs or devices should also be defined and explained.

#### Curriculum Structure or Sequencing

The curriculum is designed to provide a sequence of learning experiences that will enable students to achieve desired educational outcomes. Content may be structured or organized based on such variables as location (i.e., hospital, clinics, community), developmental stage (i.e., infant, child, adolescent, adult, elder), or physiologic systems (i.e., musculoskeletal, gastrointestinal, cardiovascular, reproductive). Factors to be

TABLE 20-1 *Methods for Sequencing Used in Nursing Curricula*

| Basis of Sequencing | Beginning Level | Intermediate Levels | Final Level |
|---|---|---|---|
| Sequencing based on metaparadigm concepts | Introduction to the concepts and discussion that there are interrelationships | Focus on relationship between person(s) and nursing; move toward focus on interrelationships of person(s), nursing, and health | Focus on interrelationship of all concepts (persons, nursing, health, environment) |
| Sequencing based on the attributes of person(s) | Concept of personhood established (individual, family, community) | Focus on individual; move to focus on family and groups | Focus on community |
| Sequencing based on relationships of concepts | Person (individual, family, community) identified; nursing focused on restoration, maintenance, or promotion; health on a continuum; environment controlled | Focus on relationship of individual and the nursing goal of health restoration; environment is controlled. Move to focus on nursing of family and/or groups and the goal of health maintenance; environment is less controlled | Focus on relationship of community and the nursing goal of health promotion; environment is open and less confined |
| Sequencing based on activities | Student is an observer | Student is an observer–participant | Student is a participant–practitioner |
| Sequencing based on complexity | Examines health care environments with few variables | Examines health care environments with many variables | Examines health care environments with complex variables |

Source: Scales (1985).

considered in sequencing the curriculum include consideration of the relationships among the concepts and the sequences in which the content should be ordered so that the organization supports the selected relationships. The conceptual properties (attributes) of the concepts to be learned, and the sequence in which the content is ordered, should be logically consistent. Table 20-1 gives examples of how sequencing can be used to organize courses based on several parameters (i.e., metaparadigm concepts, attributes of the person, subconcepts, activities, and complexity).

In most programs, sequencing moves from concepts that are relatively simple to concepts that are more complex, or from wellness to progressively serious illnesses. It has been noted that both of these organizational strategies can be problematic, because the self-evident needs of the ill may be easier for the novice nurse to recognize and understand than the more subtle health needs of the well (Scales, 1985).

### Patterns of Curricular Conceptual Frameworks

There are two common patterns of curriculum organization in nursing programs. Probably the more common one is that of *blocking* course content. When courses are blocked, content is generally structured around a particular clinical specialty area, client population, or body systems. In this organizational scheme, content can be organized according to specific practice settings (e.g., medical-surgical nursing, mental health nursing, critical care nursing), developmental stages (birth, infancy, childhood, adulthood, older adult), or body systems (respiratory system, circulatory system, digestive system). This approach produces a curriculum that is highly structured (Boland & Finke, 2009).

## THEORY-BASED TEACHING STRATEGIES

To best meet the learning needs of students at the beginning of the 21st century, nursing educators are encouraged to move beyond reliance on traditional techniques of lecture and reading assignments to incorporate other teaching strategies, which are based on sound theoretical principles. Some theories suggested by Barnum (1998) are dialectic learning, problem-based learning, operational instruction, and logistic teaching. Each of these strategies is presented in this section, along with examples from the nursing literature showing how they have been applied in education.

### Dialectic Learning

Traditional dialectic teaching leads students to develop and expand their own thoughts on a given subject, primarily through the use of well-constructed questions. Questioning can lead to demonstration of inconsistencies in, or contradictions to, the student's position. In dialogue, the student moves from a narrow conception of the subject matter to a broader and more comprehensive understanding that encompasses more events and more complexities. Dialogue often results in self-revelation, because the student is required to think through issues while considering answers to complex questions (Barnum, 1998).

*Application to Nursing*

Dialectic teaching is used frequently in nursing education. For example, it is commonly used in clinical situations and postclinical conferences. Dialectic teaching has shown to be effective, as Ironside (1999) described how questioning and dialogue techniques used by nursing faculty promote critical thinking in nursing students.

Online discussions provide an environment for dialectic learning. Anderson and Tredway (2009) designed an online critical-thinking course using problem-based learning methods. The students were cast as stakeholders in the project. Outcomes were that redesigning traditional courses presents obstacles and may be difficult, but the outcomes were: the students were engaged in the content; and faculty were able to enact new teaching–learning methods.

### Problem-Based Learning Strategies

Problem-based learning (PBL) involves the use of predefined clinical situations and case studies to enhance or stimulate students to acquire specific skills, knowledge and abilities (Rowles & Russo, 2009). Simulated clients may be used, or the student might be given a real problem in an actual clinical case; the objective of PBL is to determine how to manage the person's care.

PBL allows the instructor to manipulate multiple variables to add increasingly complex issues or circumstances that must be considered in problem resolution. For beginning students, the teacher may identify the problems, but let the students seek solutions. Or the teacher may use the case as a problem-seeking exercise, teaching students how to find the important facts among the array of available data (Barnum, 1998).

PBL is innovative and encourages self-direction, interpersonal communication, and use of information technology. Typically, small groups of students work together in self-directed teams; the case studies challenge them to improve their critical-thinking capabilities, learn self-evaluation strategies, and promote communication among peers (Bently, 2004; Rowles & Russo, 2009). Although it is an effective learning strategy, PBL can be time-intensive to implement, as it requires faculty to develop realistic scenarios that usually focus on problems encountered by a single individual and/or family in a changeable clinical situation (Bently, 2004; Kane, 2004).

*Application to Nursing*

PBL techniques are commonly used in nursing education. For example, Wong et al. (2008) devised and tested a PBL framework in a simulated clinical setting. They noted that PBL is difficult in the real clinical setting because the needs of the patient take precedence; however, they found a simulated PBL situation successful. Papastrat and Wallace (2003) described using PBL to teach students to prevent medication errors and Kleiman, Frederickson, and Lundy (2004) used PBL to promote cultural awareness and sensitivity in undergraduate students.

Several reports were identified that evaluated students response to PBL. Choi (2003) determined that incorporating PBL enhanced student satisfaction and learning effectiveness. Richardson and Trudeau (2003) found that student evaluations of PBL exercises were both positive and negative. The consensus among the students was that although it took considerable effort to complete the case studies, the technique promoted their experiential learning. Finally, Dowd and Davidhizar (1999) reported on the use of case studies in the classroom to teach clinical problem-solving skills. They described positive reception by the students and significant progress in developing the critical-thinking abilities of the students.

## Operational Teaching Strategies

Operational teaching strategies focus on presenting various perspectives regarding an agent or issue. A symposium that uses speakers with different perspectives on the same subject matter or a debate is an example. Other operational strategies focus on providing different or atypical activities for the learner. Using educational games or viewing nonmedical videos for illustration are considered to be operational teaching activities (Barnum, 1998).

*Application to Nursing*

Many nursing faculty use operational teaching techniques to make learning more interesting and enjoyable and to provide a different perspective on a particular topic (Rhorer, 2000). Use of games to enhance students' understanding of ethical situations was described by Metcalf and Yankou (2003). They used a debate-type gaming strategy to address ethical issues including responsibilities, ethical principles, and legal implications. In other examples, Youseffi, Caldwell, Hadnot, and Blake (2000) described how a game using cards was creative, fun, and effective in teaching nursing skills; and Batscha (2002) designed a computerized game that was reported to be effective in helping students review pharmacology concepts.

## Logistic Teaching Strategies

Logistic teaching strategies are based on the concept of mastery of sequential learning. Logistic teaching techniques generally divide the material to be learned into learning sequences, where acquisition of one section of the material is a necessary prerequisite to acquisition of another component. Logistic strategies teach the student clearly defined components and provide for reinforcement and testing of each component as the program progresses. As sections of the material are added and related to each other, knowledge accumulates (Barnum, 1998).

Formative testing is a logistic teaching strategy, because a course is conceived as consisting of separate and definite units, and tests are constructed to measure attainment of each unit. Other strategies include use of self-instructional modules and portfolios; these are typically logistic in nature because they follow a pattern of assembling information that is built on previously explained material (Rowles & Russo, 2009).

*Application to Nursing*

Logistic or sequential teaching is common in nursing curricula and has been effective because courses are sequenced and must be passed, and objectives or outcomes met, before students can progress to the next course or level. Examples from recent nursing literature include a work by Ramey and Hay (2003), which described a mechanism in which students were required to maintain and periodically submit electronic portfolios to document academic progress. Use of modules to promote learning was described in several situations. Examples include using a modular format to teach: nursing research statistics (Messecar, Van Son, & O'Meara, 2003), "nursing as human caring" (Hoover, 2002), and information literacy (Jacobs, Rosenfeld, & Haber, 2003).

## USE OF TECHNOLOGY IN NURSING EDUCATION

The use of technology-based distance learning methods, such as the Internet and interactive video conferencing, has recently been introduced into nursing programs. In addition, computer-assisted instruction, which has been available since the early 1990s, is becoming more sophisticated and more widely used (Zwirn & Muehlenkord, 2009).

Three main types of technology-based educational methods are available to nursing educators at this time in the 21st century. Interactive distance learning includes the use of two-way video and audio broadcasts carried over telephone lines to video classrooms in widely dispersed geographic locations. This technology requires that teacher and student be available to each other simultaneously, and is termed synchronous delivery. Another interactive distance learning technique uses virtual classrooms that are available to students who have Internet carriers. These interactive virtual classrooms are available at all hours via a server. Finally, computer-based virtual reality simulations allow students under the guidance of the nursing educator to rehearse psychomotor interventions in realistic nursing situations prior to placing the patient into the learning situation as happens in a practicum (Leigh & Hurst, 2008; Lupien & George-Gay, 2004).

Familiarity with both synchronous (immediate or real-time access) and asynchronous (delayed access) technology makes it possible to use multiple teaching strategies (Peterson, Hennig, Dow, & Sole, 2001). Virtual classrooms may combine both synchronous and asynchronous technology. Synchronous technology (i.e., video conferencing and chat rooms) allows students to have personal contact with the instructor with immediate feedback, similar to face-to-face instruction, although the depth of the discussion may suffer. Asynchronous methods (i.e., listservs, discussion boards, and bulletin boards) permit students to fit learning into their busy lifestyles. Asynchronous methods allow students to answer in greater depth because they have time to consider an answer.

Synchronous methods such as video conferencing offer slightly more traditional pedagogy than strict reliance on Internet delivery, as the instructor is seen and heard, and through multiple media, can present a broad and diverse lecture format. Depending on the depth and difficulty of the materials, students may respond less frequently in the video classroom than on a chat facility in the virtual classroom.

Use of both synchronous and asynchronous methods supports adult learning more effectively than any single method alone. Peterson and colleagues (2001) believe that a combination of methods is preferable to students, who express greater satisfaction with both methods than with either method alone.

Virtual reality simulation is an innovation in clinical skills education and often employs use of high-fidelity human patient simulators. Some of these computerized mannequins produce motion and sounds that allow realistic situations as students practice assessing, planning, and carrying out interventions. The faculty preprogram the simulator with clinical situations to allow students to practice skills in a patient safe environment (Leigh & Hurst, 2008; Lupien & George-Gay, 2004).

The high-fidelity patient simulator is the closest thing to virtual reality currently in existence for nursing education. It consists of a mannequin, the apparatus within which is programmed and accessed using a laptop, desktop, or handheld computer. Several current models simulate patients of all ages providing students with opportunities to assess heart, lung, and bowel sounds, and initiate interventions to deal with multiple situations and patient responses (Leigh & Hurst, 2008).

### Issues in Technology-Based Teaching

Several issues should be considered when applying technological innovations in nursing instruction. Institutional issues include the provision of the technology, software, and facilities for its use (Hodson-Carlton, 2009; Zwirn & Muelenkord, 2009). Faculty responsibilities include design or modification of the curriculum and the course content to reflect technology-based delivery. Other faculty concerns are the type of media to be used, faculty–student interaction, technology management, student evaluation, and faculty and course evaluation (Anderson & Tredway, 2009; Halstead & Coudret, 2000; Kessler & Lund, 2004; Peterson et al., 2001).

Recent changes in legislation have strengthened the acceptance of distance education as an educational strategy. The Telecommunications Act of 1996 made educational modalities transmitted by telephone lines (i.e., video conferencing and Internet-based education) available to the general public (Beason, 1997). The changes resulting from this support are far reaching, and instructors who use distance education by electronic modalities should be familiar with the technology at the user level and must carefully design courses for students involved in self-paced, independent study. Further, faculty using electronic educational methods should be familiar with principles of adult learning (Knowles, 1980) when constructing the curricula and the course work for electronic delivery.

Numerous commercial programs are available to educators that permit multiple methods of interface between the teacher and student. Many of these programs allow students to gain access to the course materials on their own schedule and to have real-time experiences with the instructor, such as is found in a chat facility. Some also allow testing and provide security parameters to authorize only the teacher and student to have access to the student's records. E-mail and bulletin boards permit messages between instructor and students and among students or groups of students.

To take full advantage of up-to-date electronic teaching methods, the instructor needs to become proficient in multiple methods of conveying content and needs to apply learning theories. Technology-based distance education embraces adult educational principles. Indeed, the content is presented in useful form, the immediacy of the student's need for knowledge is supported, and the student's ability to rely on previous knowledge base to provide a foundation for her or his questioning are all present in the typical interactive web-based classroom. The use of multiple ways of presenting the material in a course conducted using interactive technology-based education/learning creates the stimulus for learning and expands the educator's abilities in conveying course content.

Although the rewards of teaching by electronic methods are many, there are also issues of which faculty who are teaching web-based and online courses should be made aware. Distance methods such as web-based teaching–learning require considerably more time than in-class face-to-face strategies (Anderson & Avery, 2008; Halstead & Billings, 2009). The necessary time to spend on this activity is becoming more recognized, but has still not been adequately addressed by educational administrators. The usual 6 hours of preparation to 1 hour of class time for face-to-face classroom instruction may expand to as much as 12 or more hours to each hour of web-based class time as the educator learns new electronic teaching methods. Indeed, the time that instructors invest in teaching web-based and online courses can be overwhelming to both novices and experienced educators.

The advantage of the method is that communication can be carried on all hours of the day, 7 days weekly, by web-based classroom, virtual chat, discussion boards, e-mail, fax, and telephone (Halstead & Billings, 2009). Although the educator becomes a facilitator of adult education and the strategies are organized to take advantage of the self-directed, independent nature of the learners, the educator involved in this strategy soon learns it is important to manage time so as to avoid becoming overwhelmed and burned out (Ramsey & Clark, 2009; Halstead & Billings, 2009). Although electronic web-based online learning frees students from travel and necessity of reorganizing their already busy lives, it does not lighten the instructor's load and adds hours to preparation and teaching activities (Anderson & Avery, 2008). The immediacy of the needs of the students who have continuous access to educators may tempt faculty members to spend excessive time reading e-mail and in other communication efforts.

Faculty recognition for their innovations in web-based education is an issue that is being addressed by authors (Halstead & Billings, 2009; Ramsey & Clark, 2009; Salzer, 2004). Such recognition from supervisors and administrators is often lacking. Faculty's innovative teaching strategies and rights to their intellectual property are often ignored (Salzer, 2004).

Faculty may entertain a new web-based teaching opportunity with high hopes and expectations only to learn that this mode of teaching demands a great deal more from them without the hope of recognition for their time and talents (Salzer, 2004). Educators who are contemplating using web-based teaching–learning strategies should consult with seasoned faculty mentors. They should be encouraged to take advantage of their experience with the methods of delivery for electronic education; peruse the literature about the issues of time and recognition; and negotiate from a position of knowledge to obtain the required time and promise of recognition.

### Application to Nursing

Although technology-based instruction in nursing is relatively new, an increasing number of examples have appeared in the literature describing how technology is being used in nursing education and discussing successes and lessons learned. Billings and Kowalski (2007) defined podcasting as a nursing educational tool. They found that implementing podcasting is a means of accessing the current generation of learners that allows educators to "take the learning to the learners" (p. 57). Fetter (2009) found that competencies in information technology could be integrated into an undergraduate curriculum. Lewis and Price (2007) studied distance education and the integration of e-learning into a New Zealand graduate program. They found that the students were enthusiastic for the online courses regardless of the "frailty" (p. 143) of the technology.

Dauffenbach, Murphy, and Zellner (2004) reported on the outcomes of teaching novice faculty to use distance learning in newly organized web-based courses. They reported that three major themes pervaded their evaluations: (1) the need for sufficient technical support; (2) the need for sufficient time to prepare for learning activities; and (3) the variability in the technological abilities of the members of the faculty. They concluded that administration should make efforts to provide user-friendly equipment and technical support, time for development, and faculty education to bring all users to an optimal level of ability early in the process.

Several articles were found that described use of high-tech simulators. Leigh and Hurst (2008) provided information on the realities high-fidelity simulator use in nursing education, and faculty needs for time and support. In an earlier work, Lupien and George-Gay (2004) provided historical, theoretical, and educational grounding for the use of virtual reality simulations. They support using a seven-step process for developing clinical simulations for the use of high-fidelity patient simulations. They found that although the clinical simulators were developed for medical education originally, they have definite use in nursing education. Leigh and Hurst (2008) found that incorporating high-fidelity patient simulation into the curriculum was not always easy, and the time needed by faculty exceeded that for face-to-face teaching, but it provided a "safe" means of teaching acute care skills while allowing students to correct their errors free from fear of endangering living patients.

## Summary

This chapter has presented two major areas relevant to the use of theoretic principles and models in nursing education: curriculum design and instruction. In the opening case study, Linda and her classmates learned that it is necessary to have a sound, identified theoretical base to serve as the framework for a nursing program. They also recognized that it is important to select multiple teaching strategies to deliver the material in a manner that will best support student learning.

Likewise, it is essential that all nurse educators be aware of how theoretical principles are used in education. They should be able to articulate the conceptual framework of their program and recognize how the framework shapes the program. Nursing educators should also use multiple strategies and techniques for instruction to enable students to develop their knowledge base and to develop critical-thinking abilities and problem-solving skills. Finally, nursing educators should recognize that technology will play an increasingly important role in nursing education and be prepared to incorporate distance education methods and virtual reality simulation into instruction. Distance education has rewards for both students and faculty. For students and faculty both the opportunity to make contacts with individuals who would not ordinarily be in the classroom is a great opportunity. There are, however, issues that should be confronted as these new and innovative strategies are adopted. Faculty should obtain mentoring and sufficient information to make educated decisions about teaching in web-based, online, electronic, and virtual classrooms. They must be aware that what they are contemplating will not be a labor- or time-saving strategy; rather it is time consuming, along with being a most fascinating way to provide education.

Whether the focus is continuing education of practicing nurses or fundamental education of students of the discipline, modern teaching and learning methods make educational efforts more available to a wide variety of individuals with a variety of educational and learning needs. It is therefore imperative that nursing educators understand relevant principles and theories to address these needs.

## LEARNING ACTIVITIES

1. Develop a curriculum framework for a nursing program and explain the rationale for the framework. Describe how the framework will be used in the curriculum. From this, outline a curriculum for a nursing program.

2. Design a nursing course that incorporates several teaching strategies other than lecture, discussion, and assigned readings. Write course objectives/outcomes and specify methods to assess if the objectives/outcomes are met.

3. Select one of the courses in a nursing program and modify it to be delivered using some type of distance learning (e.g., internet delivery, such as podcasting, or any other innovative online method). How will presentation of the material be accomplished? How will students interact with each other and with the instructor? What activities will be added? What activities will be deleted?

4. Search recent nursing literature for research on technology-based nursing education. Do these techniques appear to be as effective as traditional classwork in ensuring that students achieve the goals or competencies of the nursing program?

5. Discuss the use of virtual reality simulations in clinical nursing staff education. Consider the cost and upkeep of the equipment for virtual reality simulations, the need for technical support of the equipment, the learning needs of the educator, and the expenditure of time to learn to program and to use the equipment. Make an educated decision as to whether the initial expense and the continued maintenance and faculty time expenditure warrant the use of virtual reality for continuing clinical education in your institution.

## INTERNET RESOURCES

National Council of State Boards of Nursing (NCSBN):

**http://www.ncsbn.org/regulation/boardsofnursing.asp**

## REFERENCES

American Association of Colleges of Nursing (AACN). (1999). A vision of baccalaureate and graduate nursing education: The next decade. *Journal of Professional Nursing, 15*(1), 59–65.

Anderson, K. M., & Avery, M. D. (2008). Faculty teaching time: A comparison of web-based and face-to-face graduate nursing courses. *International Journal of Nursing Education Scholarship, 5*(1), 1–12, article 2.

Anderson, M. S., & Tredway, C. A. (2009). Transforming the nursing curriculum to promote critical thinking online. *Journal of Nursing Education, 48*(2), 111–115.

Barba, B. E., & Gendler, P. (2006). Education/Community collaboration for undergraduate nursing gerontological clinical experiences. *Journal of Professional Nursing, 22*(2), 107–111.

Barnum, B. S. (1998). *Nursing theory: Analysis, application, evaluation* (5th ed.). Philadelphia: Lippincott Williams & Wilkins.

Batscha, C. (2002). The pharmacology game. *Computers in Nursing, 5*(3), 1–5.

Beason, C. F. (1997). Distance learning—Education to prepare nurses for practice in the 21st century. In V. D. Ferguson (Ed.), *Educating the 21st century nurse: Challenges and opportunities* (publication no. 14-7467, pp. 219–244). New York: National League for Nursing Press.

Bently, G. W. (2004). Problem-based learning. In A. J. Lowenstein & M. J. Bradshaw (Eds.), *Fuszard's innovative teaching strategies in nursing* (3rd ed., pp. 83–106). Sudbury, MA: Jones & Bartlett.

Bevis, E. O. (1973). *Curriculum building in nursing: A process.* New York: National League for Nursing Press.

Bevis, E. O. (1987). History of curriculum development. In National League for Nursing, *Curriculum revolution: Mandate for change* (publication no. 15-2224, pp. 27–40). New York: National League for Nursing Press.

Bevis, E. O. (1989a). *Curriculum building in nursing: A process* (3rd ed., publication no. 15-2277). New York: National League for Nursing Press.

Bevis, E. O. (1989b). Illuminating the issues: Probing the past, a history of nursing curriculum development—The past shapes the present. In E. O. Bevis & J. Watson (Eds.), *Toward a caring curriculum: A new pedagogy for nursing* (publication no. 15-2278, pp. 13–35). New York: National League for Nursing Press.

Billings, D. M., & Kowalski, K. (2007). Using podcasts for nursing education. *Journal of Continuing Education in Nursing, 38*(2), 56–57.

Boland, D. L. (2009). Developing curriculum: Frameworks, outcomes and competencies. In D. M. Billings & J. A. Halstead (Eds.), *Teaching in nursing: A guide for faculty* (3rd ed., pp. 137–153). St. Louis: Elsevier.

Boland, D. L., & Finke, L. M. (2009). Curriculum designs. In D. M. Billings & J. A. Halstead (Eds.), *Teaching in nursing: A guide for faculty* (3rd ed., pp. 119–136). St. Louis: Elsevier.

Brajtman, S., Fothergill-Bourbonnaise, F., Casey, A., Alain, D., & Fiset, V. (2007). Providing direction for change: Assessing Canadian nursing students' learning needs. *International Journal of Palliative Nursing, 13*(5), 213–221.

Choi, H. (2003). A problem-based learning trial on the Internet involving undergraduate nursing students. *Journal of Nursing Education, 42*(8), 359–363.

Commission on Collegiate Nursing Education (CCNE). (2003). *Standards for accreditation of baccalaureate and greater nursing education programs.* Washington, DC: American Association of Colleges of Nursing. Available at: http://www.aacn.nche. edu/Accreditation/ NEW_STANDARDS.html. Accessed March 4, 2005.

Cook, P. R., & Cullen, J. A. (2003). Caring as an imperative for nursing education. *Nursing Education Perspectives, 24*(4), 192–197.

Dalley, K., Candela, L., & Benzel-Lindley, J. (2008). Learning to let go: The challenge of de-crowding the curriculum. *Nurse Education Today, 28*(1), 62–69.

Dauffenbach, V., Murphy, L., & Zellner, K. (2004). Distance education experiential learning activity for novice faculty. *Nurse Educator, 29*(2), 71–74.

Diekelmann, N. (1987). Curriculum revolution: A theoretical and philosophical mandate for change. In National League for Nursing, *Curriculum revolution: Mandate for change* (publication no. 15-2224, pp. 137–157). New York: National League for Nursing Press.

Dillard, N., & Siktberg, L. (2009). Curriculum development: An overview. In D. M. Billings & J. A. Halstead (Eds.), *Teaching in nursing: A guide for faculty* (3rd ed., pp. 75–91). St. Louis: Elsevier.

Dowd, S. B., & Davidhizar, R. (1999). Using case studies to teach clinical problem-solving. *Nurse Educator, 24*(5), 42–46.

Dyer, J. A. (2003). Multidisciplinary, interdisciplinary and transdisciplinary educational models and nursing education. *Nursing Education Perspectives, 24*(4), 186–188.

Fetter, N. S. (2009). Curriculum strategies to improve baccalaureate nursing information technology outcomes. *Journal of Nursing Education, 48*(2), 78–85.

Flood, M. E. (2006). Best laid plans: A century of nursing curricula. In S. B. Keating (Ed.), *Curriculum development and evaluation in nursing* (pp. 5–30). Philadelphia: Lippincott Williams & Wilkins.

Hall, K. B. (1979). Current trends in the use of conceptual frameworks in nursing education. *Journal of Nursing Education, 18*, 26–29.

Halstead, J. A., & Billings, D. M. (2009). Teaching and learning in online learning communities. In D. M. Billings & J. A. Halstead (Eds.), *Teaching in nursing: A guide for faculty* (3rd ed., pp. 369–387). St. Louis: Elsevier.

Halstead, J. A., & Coudret, N. A. (2000). Implementing Web-based instruction in a school of nursing: Implications for faculty and students. *Journal of Professional Nursing, 16*(5), 273–281.

Hamner, J., & Wilder, B. (2001). A new curriculum for a new millennium. *Nursing Outlook, 49*(2), 127–131.

Heller, B. R., Oros, M. T., & Durney-Crowley, J. (2000). The future of nursing education: 10 trends to watch. *Nursing and Health Care Perspectives, 21*(1), 9–13.

Hodson-Carlton, K. E. (2009). The learning resource center. In D. M. Billings & J. A. Halstead (Eds.), *Teaching in nursing: A guide for faculty* (3rd ed., pp. 303–321). St. Louis: Elsevier.

Hoover, J. (2002). The personal and professional impact of undertaking an educational module on human caring. *Journal of Advanced Nursing, 37*(1), 79–86.

Horner, S. D., Abel, E., Taylor, K., & Sands, D. (2004). Using theory to guide the diffusion of genetics content in nursing curricula. *Nursing Outlook, 52*(2), 80–84.

Ironside, P. M. (1999). Thinking in nursing education: Part I: A student's experience learning to think. *Nursing and Health Care Perspectives, 20*(5), 238–242.

Jacobs, S. K., Rosenfeld, P., & Haber, J. (2003). Information literacy as the foundation for evidence-based practice in graduate nursing education: A curriculum-integrated approach. *Journal of Professional Nursing, 19*(5), 320–328.

Jenkins, J. F., Dimond, E., & Steinberg, S. (2001). Preparing for the future through genetics nursing education. *Journal of Nursing Scholarship, 33*(2), 191–195.

Kane, V. (2004). Example: Problem-based learning: The use of the exemplar family as the basis for learning health promotion and illness/injury prevention. In A. J. Lowenstein & M. J. Bradshaw (Eds.), *Fuszard's innovative teaching strategies in nursing* (3rd ed.). Sudbury, MA: Jones & Bartlett.

Keating, S. B. (2006a). Introduction to the history of curriculum development and faculty role. In S. B. Keating (Ed.), *Curriculum development and evaluation in nursing* (pp. 1–3). Philadelphia: Lippincott Williams & Wilkins.

Keating, S. B. (2006b). Components of the curriculum. In S. B. Keating (Ed.), *Curriculum development and evaluation in nursing* (pp. 163–207). Philadelphia: Lippincott Williams & Wilkins.

Kelley, J. (1975). The conceptual framework in nursing education. In National League for Nursing, *Curriculum development, part VI: Curriculum revision in baccalaureate nursing education* (publication no. 15-1576, pp. 15–20). New York: National League for Nursing Press.

Kessler, P. D., & Lund, C. H. (2004). Reflective journaling: Developing an online journal for distance education. *Nurse Educator, 29*(1), 20–24.

Kim, S. S., Erlen, J. A., Kim, K. B., & Sok, S. R. (2006). Nursing students' and faculty members' knowledge of, experience with, and attitudes toward complementary and alternative therapies. *Journal of Nursing Education, 45*(9), 375–378.

Kleiman, S., Frederickson, K., & Lundy, T. (2004). Using an eclectic model to educate students about cultural influences on the nurse–patient relationship. *Nursing Education Perspectives, 25*(5), 249–253.

Knowles, M. S. (1980). *The modern practice of education: From pedagogy to andragogy* (2nd ed.). New York: Cambridge Books.

Leigh, G., & Hurst, H. (2008). We have a high-fidelity simulator, Now what? Making the most of simulators. *International Journal of Nursing Education Scholarship, 5*(1), 1–9. Article 33.

Lewis, P. A., & Price, S. (2007). Distance education and the integration of e-learning in a graduate program.

*The Journal of Continuing Education in Nursing, 38(3),* 139–143.

Lupien, A. E., & George-Gay, B. (2004). High-fidelity patient simulation. In A. J. Lowenstein & M. J. Bradshaw (Eds.), *Fuszard's innovative teaching strategies in nursing* (3rd ed., pp. 134–148). Sudbury, MA: Jones & Bartlett.

Mager, R. F. (1962). *Preparing instructional objectives.* Belmont, CA: Fearon Publishers.

Mawn, B., & Reece, S. M. (2000). Reconfiguring a curriculum for the new Millennium: The process of change. *Journal of Nursing Education, 39(3),* 101–108.

McEwen, M., & Brown, S. C. (2002). Conceptual frameworks in undergraduate nursing curricula: Report of a national survey. *Journal of Nursing Education, 41(1),* 5–14.

Meleis, A. I. (2005). *Theoretical nursing: Development and progress* (3rd ed.). Philadelphia: Lippincott Williams & Wilkins.

Messecar, D. C., Van Son, C., & O'Meara, K. (2003). Reading statistics in nursing research: A self-study CD-ROM module. *Journal of Nursing Education, 42(5),* 220–226.

Metcalf, B. L., & Yankou, D. (2003). Using gaming to help nursing students understand ethics. *Journal of Nursing Education, 42(5),* 212–215.

National Council of State Boards of Nursing (NCSBN). (2005). Nursing Regulation; Boards of Nursing Contact Information. https://www.ncsbn.org/247.htm.

National League for Nursing (NLN). (1972). *Criteria for the appraisal of baccalaureate and higher degree programs in nursing.* New York: National League for Nursing Press.

National League for Nursing (NLN). (1977). *Criteria for evaluation of educational programs in nursing leading to an associate degree* (5th ed.). New York: National League for Nursing Press.

National League for Nursing Accrediting Committee (NLNAC). (2004). *Accreditation manual, 2004 for post secondary and higher degree programs in nursing.* New York: Author.

Papastrat, K., & Wallace, S. (2003). Teaching baccalaureate nursing students to prevent medication errors using a problem-based learning approach. *Journal of Nursing Education, 42(10),* 459–464.

Peterson, J. Z., Hennig, L. M., Dow, K. H., & Sole, M. L. (2001). Designing and facilitating class discussion in an internet class. *Nurse Educator, 26(1),* 28–32.

Quiring, J., & Gray, G. (1982). Organizing approaches used in curriculum design. *Journal of Nursing Education, 21(2),* 38–44.

Ramsey, R. W., & Clark, C. E. (2009). Teaching and learning at a distance. In D. M. Billings & J. A. Halstead (Eds.), *Teaching in nursing: A guide for faculty* (3rd ed., pp. 351–368). St. Louis: Elsevier.

Ramey, S. L., & Hay, M. L. (2003). Using electronic portfolios to measure student achievement and assess curricular integrity. *Nurse Educator, 28(1),* 31–36.

Rentschler, D. D., & Spegman, A. M. (1996). Curriculum revolution: Realities of change. *Journal of Nursing Education, 35(9),* 389–393.

Rhorer, J. H. (2000). Teaching strategies: Infuse fun into learning. *Nurse Educator, 25(1),* 13–15.

Richardson, K., & Trudeau, K. J. (2003). A case for problem-based collaborative learning in the nursing classroom. *Nurse Educator, 28(2),* 83–88.

Richardson, S. E. (2003). Complementary health and healing in nursing education. *Journal of Holistic Nursing, 21(1),* 20–35.

Rowles, C. J., & Russo, B. L. (2009). Strategies to promote critical thinking and active learning. In D. M. Billings & J. A. Halstead (Eds.), *Teaching in nursing: A guide for faculty* (3rd ed., pp. 238–261). St. Louis, Elsevier.

Salzer, J. S. (2004). Web-based instruction. In A. J. Lowenstein & M. J. Bradshaw (Eds.), *Fuszard's innovative teaching strategies in nursing* (3rd ed., pp. 210–225). Sudbury, MA: Jones & Bartlett.

Scales, F. S. (1985). *Nursing curriculum: Development, structure, function.* Norwalk, CT: Appleton-Century-Crofts.

Secrest, J. (2008). The role of tool development in an Orem-based curriculum. *Self-care, Dependent Care and Nursing, 16(2),* 25–33.

Seng, V. S., Mirenda, R., & Lowry, L. W. (1996). The Neuman systems model in nursing education. In P. H. Walker & B. Neuman (Eds.), *Blueprint for use of nursing models: Education, research, practice and administration* (publication no. 14-2696, pp. 91–140). New York: National League for Nursing Press.

Sok, S. R., Erlen, J. A., & Kim, K. B. (2004). Complementary and alternative therapies in nursing curricula: A new direction for nurse educators. *Journal of Nursing Education, 43(9),* 401–405.

Tanner, C. A. (1989). An analysis of the historical and political background of the revision of the NLN's criteria for the appraisal of baccalaureate and higher degree programs. In N. Diekelmann, D. Allen, & C. Tanner (Eds.), *The NLN criteria for appraisal of bac-calaureate programs: A critical hermeneutic analysis* (publication no. 15-2253, pp. 3–10). New York: National League for Nursing Press.

Watson, M. J. (1996). Watson's theory of transpersonal caring. In P. H. Walker & B. Neuman (Eds.), *Blueprint for use of nursing models: Education, research, practice and administration* (publication no. 14-2696, pp. 141–186). New York: National League for Nursing Press.

Watts, R. J., Cuellar, N. G., & O'Sullivan, A. L. (2008). Developing a blueprint for cultural competence education at Penn. *Journal of Professional Nursing, 24(3),* 136–142.

Webber, P. B. (2002). A curriculum framework for nursing. *Journal of Nursing Education, 41(1),* 15–23.

Wong, F. K. Y., Cheung, S., Chung, L., Chan, K., Chan, A., To, T., & Wong, M. (2008). Framework for adopting a problem-based learning approach in a simulated clinical setting. *Journal of Nursing Education, 47(11),* 508–514.

Wu, R. R. (1979). Designing a curriculum model. *Journal of Nursing Education, 18(3),* 13–21.

Youseffi, F., Caldwell, R., Hadnot, P., & Blake, B. J. (2000). Recall rummy: Learning can be fun . . . a card game to reinforce proper skill techniques. *Journal of Continuing Education in Nursing, 31(4),* 161–162.

Zwirn, E. E., & Muehlenkord, A. (2009). Using media, multimedia, and technology-rich learning environments. In D. M. Billings & J. A. Halstead (Eds.), *Teaching in nursing: A guide for faculty* (3rd ed., pp. 335–350). St. Louis: Elsevier.

# C H A P T E R

## 21

# Future Issues in Nursing Theory

## M e l a n i e   M c E w e n

*R*ebecca Jackson will graduate from a master's program in nursing in only a few weeks. She has learned a great deal about nursing practice, research, administration and management, and education from the various courses she has taken, and she is enthusiastic about the career opportunities she is considering. When she started the program she was confident that she wanted to become a nurse administrator, but midway through her studies she decided to focus on research. She ultimately wants to get her doctorate and become an educator and researcher.

Currently, Rebecca is working as a clinical supervisor at the public health department in a major metropolitan area. In the 10 years Rebecca has been with the health department, she has witnessed tremendous growth in the diversity of the population served. There are immigrant families from several Spanish-speaking countries, as well as from the Southeast Asian countries of Cambodia, Laos, Vietnam, and the Philippines. Recently, there has been an influx of refugees from Iraq, Croatia, Bosnia, and eastern Africa. Rebecca is intrigued by these groups' divergent perceptions of health and ways to promote health. Furthermore, she is concerned with communication issues and how to motivate health promotional practices. This is particularly important, she is determined, in working with children and in teaching parents ways to improve their health.

In her position, Rebecca has had several opportunities to be involved in funded research. At present, she is working with a sociologist, an anthropologist, a clinical psychologist, and an epidemiologist to write a grant for a research project that will examine and compare health beliefs, health practices, and health promotional behaviors among various cultural groups in the city. The study will be multilevel and multiphased and will incorporate both quantitative and qualitative data collection techniques and analysis.

Rebecca helped develop the conceptual framework for the study, which combines aspects of the Health Belief Model and Leininger's Culture Care Diversity Theory. The framework identifies cultural beliefs, practices, and values and incorporates them with knowledge of health threats and perceptions of illness severity, seriousness, and value for taking action. The researchers expect that the information provided by the study will allow the health *department to develop a series of health programs that are sensitive to the needs, beliefs, and practices of the many cultural groups in the department's catchment area.*

During the last two decades a number of shifts occurred in the demographic patterns of the United States. This has been coupled with major changes in the health care delivery system and changes in the causes of illness, disability, and death. Among other changes, there has been a growing emphasis on health care finance reform, community-based care, health promotion, and risk reduction. Additionally, significant cost reductions, restructuring of health care services, and growth in integrated health care systems using managed care are anticipated. Consequently, the increased severity of illness among persons in inpatient facilities and the increased incidence of chronic illnesses, particularly in the growing number of elderly, have taxed the health care system (Hinshaw, 2000; Johnston, Rogers, Cross, & Sochan, 2005; Long, 2004). These shifts are expected to continue and perhaps become even more pronounced well into the 21st century.

Despite system-wide changes, major problems still exist and must be addressed. For example, the health care system is not designed to provide convenient care to all who need it. The system is organized according to physicians' specialties and schedules, not according to the needs of their patients. Hospitals are used inappropriately, with access to care, supplemental insurance, and home care services still unevenly distributed.

There is also a growing need for health care providers, including nurses, who can meet the challenges of the changing system and evolving health and illness patterns. Nurses of the future must be capable of ensuring access to care and promoting high-quality outcomes. The American Association of Colleges of Nursing (AACN) (2008) has described the skills and practice capabilities currently expected for nurses (Box 21-1). In short, essential competencies include critical thinking and clinical judgment skills; ability to work in a variety of health care settings and with patients who have complex health problems; effective organizational and teamwork skills, understanding of evidence-based care; recognition of the influence of culture on health and ability to care for individuals from diverse backgrounds and across the lifespan; and a commitment to personal accountability and professional development.

Quinless and Elliot (2000) addressed the following three goals to be considered when planning for the health care system of the future:

1. Better health for all with an emphasis on reducing health disparities among racial and ethnic minority groups
2. Improved quality of life for an aging population
3. Cost-effective health care

---

**BOX 21-1** *Competencies and Skills Needed by Generalist Nurses*

| | |
|---|---|
| Practice from a holistic, caring framework | Practice in a variety of health care settings |
| Practice from an evidence base | Care for patients across the health–illness continuum |
| Promote safe, quality patient care | |
| Use clinical/critical reasoning to address simple to complex situations | Care for patients across the lifespan |
| | Care for diverse populations |
| Assume accountability for one's own and delegated nursing care | Engage in care of self in order to care for others |
| | Engage in continuous professional development |

Source: AACN (2008).

To meet these goals, the discipline of nursing should give increasing attention to certain theories, concepts, and models. Among these are primary health care (as opposed to "illness care"), health promotion, health protection, motivation, health as a resource for everyday life, health economics, patient safety, environmental concerns, and quality of life. Frameworks for practice will embrace community-based and community-focused care, changing identification of the client (aggregate versus individual), interprofessional collaboration, noninstitutional care settings, and multiple levels of decision-making authority (Manojlovich, Barnsteiner, Bolton, Disch, & Saint, 2008; Porter-O'Grady, 2001; Rutherford, 2008).

This chapter describes ongoing and anticipated changes that will affect the discipline of nursing during the next decade and examines how these changes will influence theory and knowledge development. Topics covered include future issues in nursing science and future issues in theory development. This is followed by an exploration of future theoretical issues related to nursing practice, research, administration and management, and education.

## Future Issues in Nursing Science

Nursing science is concerned with answering questions of interest to the profession and adding to the body of knowledge. Knowledge development is accomplished through the study of concepts, relationships, and theories relevant to the discipline, and generally occurs within the broad domain of one of the major worldviews of the discipline.

As discussed in Chapter 1, a paradigm is a pattern, model, or global concept accepted by most people in an intellectual community; it is a set of systematic beliefs or a worldview. Paradigms provide scientists with a general orientation to phenomena; a way of organizing perceptions; criteria for selecting problems; guidelines for investigations and methods; and limitations on possible solutions. The paradigm, or worldview, provides a guiding framework for resolving problems, conducting research, and deriving theories and laws in the discipline.

Nursing science has two predominant paradigms, broadly classified as empiricist and constructivist, which hold fundamentally opposing views of knowledge development and reality. Chapter 1 described the ongoing debate within the scientific nursing community about the appropriateness of the two philosophies and methodologies for directing and conducting research, as well as identifying questions of relevance to the discipline.

Many in the profession find the continuing philosophical debate inconclusive, frustrating, and not germane to nursing. A change of perspective is required for nursing science to reconcile the philosophical differences between the two extant paradigms. Many scholars believe that nursing should emphasize the benefits of inquiry per se, rather than the supremacy of one paradigm over the other, because neither method is more scientific than the other, and the process of inquiry is the same despite the methods used to acquire knowledge (Barrett, 2002; Chinn & Kramer, 2008; Kikuchi, 2003; Whall & Hicks, 2002).

In the 21st century, nursing science should work to eliminate obstacles to nursing research and promote acceptance of multiple methods of inquiry and use of research findings in practice. Because the problems of nursing are so diverse, use of differing viewpoints and paradigms are needed to help answer questions and provide solutions to questions of interest. Because multiple perspectives encourage appreciation of the uniqueness of individuals, use of various perspectives will encourage identifying answers to important problems. Also, applying different viewpoints provides new insights that can help nurses formulate new ideas for study.

Combining or triangulating methods can maximize the strengths and minimize the weaknesses of each method and should be encouraged. Integration of qualitative and quantitative methods has been suggested as one way to advance nursing science, because research traditions from both paradigms are complementary although the approaches are different. Qualitative methods can describe phenomena of interest in nursing and generate theories that propose relationships between identified concepts. Quantitative methods can test the relationships of qualitatively developed theories and suggest whether the theory should be accepted or revised (Foss & Ellefsen, 2002).

It is possible to unite the disparate views of nurse researchers, theorists, and practitioners by downplaying paradigmatic differences while enhancing the value of scholarly inquiry through multiple approaches. Quantitative approaches to research problems can be seen as compatible with qualitative methods; there should not be a commitment to mutually exclusive paradigms. Indeed, Chinn and Kramer (2008) observe that blending and using a variety of research processes and techniques in knowledge development indicates growing maturity in nursing scholarship. Nurses should be encouraged to be pragmatic regarding research methodology and use the right method for the task.

# Future Issues in Nursing Theory

According to the American Association of Colleges of Nursing (AACN, 1996) nurses in advanced practice should be prepared to critique, evaluate, and use theory. Nurses should be able to integrate and apply a wide range of theories from nursing and other sciences into a comprehensive and holistic approach to care. Thus, in addition to nursing theories, nurses prepared at the graduate level should be exposed to relevant theories from a wide range of fields, including natural sciences, social sciences, biologic sciences, and organizational and management concepts. Basic theoretical knowledge and skills proposed by the AACN are listed in Box 21-2.

As explained in Chapter 2, the discipline of nursing is currently in the "constructed knowledge stage" of theory development. In this stage, there is an increasing emphasis on philosophy and philosophy of science in nursing. Additionally, in

---

**BOX 21-2** *Theoretical Knowledge and Skills for Advanced Practice Nurses*

**MASTER'S-PREPARED NURSES SHOULD:**
1. Critique and evaluate a variety of theories from nursing and related fields
2. Apply and use appropriate theories from nursing and related fields to provide high-quality health care to clients
3. Understand the health care delivery system in which they practice through the application of appropriate theories

Source: AACN (1996, pp. 10–11).

this stage, there has been a shift in focus from grand theories to middle range and practice theories, and to the application of theory in research and practice. It is anticipated that the importance of middle range and practice theories will continue to be stressed, and there will be less attention given to grand theories and conceptual frameworks. See Chapters 10, 11, and 17 for detailed discussions of middle range and practice theories.

In a study of nursing theory instructors in master's programs, McEwen (2000) identified the issues that were perceived as "essential" for graduate nursing students. These were, in order: introduction to theory, the relationship of theory and research, middle range theories, grand nursing theories, nursing's metaparadigm, theory analysis, concept analysis, and theory evaluation. This study also identified content that instructors felt was overemphasized in graduate theory courses. The most commonly cited content areas were grand nursing theories and theory development/theory construction. On the other hand, content that nursing theory instructors believed needed increased emphasis were application of theory in practice, middle range theory, and the interdependent relationship of theory, research, and practice.

## IMPLICATIONS FOR THEORY DEVELOPMENT

The discipline of nursing has recognized several new trends for theory development. These include development of middle range theories, situation-specific (practice) theories, and evidence-based practice (EBP) protocols/procedures as the latest steps in knowledge development.

There has been broad acceptance of the need to develop middle range theories to support nursing practice (Chinn & Kramer, 2008; Fitzpatrick, 2008; Kim, 2006; Meleis, 2007; Smith & Liehr, 2008). This call for development of middle range theory is consistent with a desire to focus increased attention on substantive knowledge development. In the future, as additional middle range theories are developed, there will be a growing need to consider their analysis and evaluation (whether formal or informal). Indeed, nurses should direct considerable effort toward developing, testing, evaluating, and refining middle range theories to develop the discipline's substantive knowledge base.

In recent years, there has been enhanced attention to the application of theory in practice and the relationship of theory, practice, and research. Development of situation-specific (practice) theories and EBP models have consequently become increasingly emphasized (Chinn & Kramer, 2008; Im, 2005; Meleis, 2007). Furthermore, many nurse researchers use theories from other disciplines in their studies and, as a result, more emphasis and discussion should be given to borrowed theory, along with recognition that this practice does not negate the findings or make them less valuable to nursing.

It is important that nurses understand the interrelationship between theory, research, and practice and recognize the importance of this reciprocal relationship to the continuing development of nursing as a profession. In a practice discipline such as nursing, theory and practice are inseparable, and development and application of theory affiliated with research-based practice have been seen as fundamental to the development of professionalism and autonomous practice. Despite repeated calls to merge theory, practice, and research, there remains a confusing and fragmented mix. Progress has been made, however, because there has been increased emphasis on the interchange and interaction among research, clinical practice, and theory development. It is hoped that this trend will continue.

## Theoretical Perspectives on Future Issues in Nursing Practice, Research, Administration and Management, and Education

With accessibility, cost containment, and provision of quality care driving health care reform, the discipline of nursing must anticipate how these forces will affect nursing within the changing health care system. At the beginning of the 21st century, nurses are expected to assume a central role in helping to achieve cost-effective, quality health services. How these changes and related theoretical implications will affect nursing practice, nursing research, nursing administration and management, and nursing education are examined separately.

## FUTURE ISSUES AND NURSING PRACTICE

A transformation is occurring in nursing practice. This has been driven by socioeconomic factors as well as by developments in health care delivery. Many nursing leaders have identified relevant factors including changing demographics and increasing racial and ethnic diversity and related health disparities; the explosion of technology and information systems; globalization of the world's economy; more educated consumers; increasing acceptance and use of alternative therapies; genomic information; a shift to population-based care; and increasing complexity of care (Berry & Hern, 2004; Johnston et al., 2005; Long, 2004; Parker, 2005; Porter-O'Grady, 2001).

Increasingly, nurses are finding employment in home health and other ambulatory settings in which they provide care for well or chronically ill clients. Patients are getting older, and they are more likely to suffer from chronic illnesses. These trends will most likely continue throughout the near future and, in response, nursing interventions will focus more on comprehensive assessment and care planning, case management, and client teaching to achieve the goals of health promotion, health maintenance, and disease prevention. Further, in the future, nurses will routinely use diagnosis and intervention databases, as well as expert systems, to assist with decision making.

Nurses need to be prepared to function in some type of community-based health care system. They must be able to collaborate and cooperate within a multidisciplinary team and to demonstrate critical thinking and decision-making capabilities. They will be asked to resolve conflicts and affect health care at both the individual and aggregate level. Nurses must also have at least a basic knowledge of several disciplines including public health, biostatics, and behavioral sciences. In addition, they must possess management and administration skills. Specific nursing practice competencies needed for today's health care system were identified from a recent study of nurse administrators (Utley-Smith, 2004); these are shown in Table 21-1.

### Theoretical Implications for Nursing Practice

Based on current and anticipated changes, a number of models, concepts, and theories need to be developed and applied in nursing practice, and then studied and refined. New models should be based on community-based practice, population focus, case management, and interdisciplinary and interagency collaboration. Concepts and theories should be developed that focus on cultural competence, resource management, health promotion, risk reduction, motivation, management of chronic diseases, normal aging, maternal–child welfare, and social epidemics, among others.

The concept of EBP has grown dramatically and will help fill the gap among research, theory, and practice (Hudson, Duke, Haas, & Varnell, 2008; Simpson, 2004). This focus on EBP should assist in the integration of research findings into clinical

TABLE 21-1 *Nursing Practice Competencies for Today's Health Care System*

| Competency | Examples of Activities |
|---|---|
| Health promotion—Activities to enable clients to improve health, maximize health potential, and enhance well-being | Teach prevention and health promotion activities<br>Educate patients about lifestyle and its effect on health<br>Use community resources to enhance care<br>Advocate for policy change to promote health |
| Supervision—Ability to coordinate the implementation of the plan of nursing care by ancillary or subordinate members of the health care team | Supervise ancillary nursing staff<br>Delegate and monitor work tasks of ancillary staff<br>Assume responsibility for personnel under direct supervision |
| Interpersonal communication—Use relationship skills to work effectively on an interdisciplinary team | Organize daily routine in an efficient manner<br>Function as a participating member of the health care team<br>Function effectively in problem-solving situations<br>Apply effective communication skills<br>Collaborate with other members of the health care team |
| Direct care—Appropriately use psychomotor and/or technical skills in delivering patient care | Administer medications<br>Perform ADLs for assigned patients<br>Perform major care tasks (e.g., catheterization, Levine tube insertion) |
| Computer technology—Ability to use electronic and technological equipment to access, retrieve, and store information that assists in the delivery of effective care | Demonstrate computer literacy<br>Access and retrieve electronic data necessary for patient care<br>Use information technology to facilitate communication, manage data, and solve patient care problems |
| Caseload management—Ability to coordinate care of a number of clients | Organize care for a group of 2–10 patients (depending on the nurse's experience and responsibilities, patient needs, and patient acuity)—involves direct care, time management, and resource management |

Source: Utley-Smith (2004).

practice. As discussed in Chapter 17, EBP is relatively new in nursing, because many nursing practices are based on experience, tradition, intuition, common sense, and untested theories. Although the encouragement to move to EBP is growing, implementation has been stalled somewhat. This is attributed to the delay in implementation of nursing research findings in practice. More effort will be needed to identify and define "best practices" and to communicate them with both providers and consumers of health care. As the conceptualization of EBP becomes more established within nursing, however, the relationship between EBP and theory must become more explicit. Nursing theorists and scholars should focus attention on melding middle range theory and EBP, and turn attention to recognizing the association between EBP and situation-specific or prescriptive theories.

## FUTURE ISSUES AND NURSING RESEARCH

The new century challenges nursing research with many critical imperatives for improving health care. Health and illness challenges of the 21st century will necessitate reshaping health research as well as health care delivery. Likewise, the changes in the nation's population; its health needs and expectations; and changes in the health care system will have a dramatic impact on the direction of nursing research. Changes in technology and hospital systems; changes in staffing patterns; and scientific emphasis in areas such as genetics must also be addressed in nursing research. Furthermore, greater emphasis must be placed on reporting nursing research activities and findings to other researchers, clinicians, the media, and the public (National Institute of Nursing Research [NINR], 2009).

During the last three decades, there has been a significant increase in the amount and quality of nursing research. In the last 10 years, research priorities focused on topics such as end-of-life/palliative care, chronic illness experiences (i.e., managing symptoms, avoiding complications of disease and disability, supporting family caregivers, and promoting health behaviors), quality of life, and quality of care. Additional areas of interest related to these themes as well as additional ones have been identified by the NINR (2006) for more focused study in the future (Table 21-2).

### Theoretical Implications for Nursing Research

With the identification and promotion of these nursing research priorities, a number of concepts and theories should be studied and further developed over the next decade. These include such phenomena as transitions, quality of life, motivation, changing lifestyle habits, health promotion, symptom management, palliative care, economics of care, caregiver support, disparity, vulnerability, gender differences, informatics, telehealth, genetics, decision making and self-determination, and family interactions.

To improve health care and ultimately promote nursing science, nurses should continue developing and testing middle range and practice theories. They should test conceptual relationships and combine the study of concepts and relationships from various theories. Use of techniques such as meta-analysis and triangulation to synthesize findings will become increasingly important.

## FUTURE ISSUES AND NURSING LEADERSHIP AND ADMINISTRATION

A number of issues and developments will dramatically affect nursing administration and leadership in the future (Box 21-3). According to Roy (2000), concerns about health care costs affect nursing by determining how work is organized and treatment planned, and influencing clients' perception of, and participation in, care. Increasing calls for significant change in health care financing may serve to change reimbursement mechanisms. There will be an increase in state and federal regulation related to cost and managed care, and states will continue to define, measure, and assess quality and serve as contractors for corporate entities while enforcing accountability of managed care organizations. Case management will lead to greater levels of interdisciplinary and collaborative practice. Addressing problems related to the current nursing shortage and the essential need to promote integration of care through systems thinking and collaboration among

---

**BOX 21-3** *Issues Affecting Nursing Administration and Management in the Future*

- Cost of health care
- Challenge of managed care
- Impact of health policy and regulation
- Interdisciplinary education for collaborative practice
- Nursing shortage
- Opportunities for lifelong learning and workforce development
- Significant advances in nursing science and research

Source: Roy (2000).

TABLE 21-2 *Future Areas for Nursing Research Emphasis*

| Themes | Areas Targeted for Specific Study |
| --- | --- |
| Promoting health and preventing disease | Develop biomarkers to assess disease risk and response to treatment, identify susceptibility genes for at-risk individuals and design intervention to moderate risk.<br>Develop or improve biobehavioral methods, measures and intervention strategies to optimize health.<br>Identify factors that influence decision making that results in behavioural changes that promote health and prevent disease and disability.<br>Identify and develop individual and family interventions designed to sustain health-promoting behaviors over time (e.g., prevention of obesity, prevention of HIV/AIDS transmission).<br>Design intervention studies using community-based approaches to facilitate health promotion/risk reduction behaviors.<br>Investigate opportunities to identify and ameliorate the long-term consequences of prematurity, including near-term infants at risk for complications. |
| Improving quality of life: Self-management of chronic illnesses | Develop technologies to facilitate self-identification and self-reporting of symptoms.<br>Design self-management strategies to promote healthy lifestyle choices.<br>Define behaviors that support adherence to treatment for complex illnesses.<br>Evaluate factors that impact independence and self-care in long-term care settings.<br>Identify strategies for self-management and promotion of personal health among long-term survivors of disease and persons with chronic disabilities. |
| Improving quality of life: Symptom management | Delineate causative mechanisms underlying symptoms.<br>Improve recognition of symptoms by patients, their caregivers and health care providers.<br>Develop interventions that improve patient response and adaptation to symptoms and symptom clusters.<br>Design strategies to improve management of symptoms.<br>Develop strategies for assessment and intervention to improve health-related quality of life in persons with chronic or life-threatening illnesses. |
| Improving quality of life: Caregiving | Design interventions to improve physiological and cognitive function in residents of long-term care facilities.<br>Develop interventions to improve the quality of caregiving.<br>Evaluate factors that impact the health and quality of life of informal caregivers and recipients.<br>Identify factors that improve the transition from one setting to another.<br>Develop models for first responders in emergency situations. |
| Eliminating health disparities | Elucidate mechanisms underlying disparities (geography, minority status, underserved populations, and disability) and design interventions to eliminate them.<br>Design culturally appropriate interventions to communicate risks and susceptibility to at-risk populations.<br>Apply findings from biobehavioral, descriptive, and interventional studies to factors influencing health disparities among youth and adolescents.<br>Identify strategies that will reduce the long-term adverse consequences of poor maternal and reproductive health in minorities and underserved populations.<br>Evaluate and modify partnership and training programs to build capacity in minority-serving institutions and expand the pool of investigators from under-represented groups. |
| Setting directions for end-of-life research | Identify factors that influence, and develop strategies to improve decision-making and treatment strategies at the end of life.<br>Validate instruments and refine methodologies to address the complex issues of end-of-life research.<br>Develop interventions to improve palliative care and enhance quality of life for the dying patient and to support family and informal caregivers.<br>Explain factors related to the end-of-life among underserved groups.<br>Support the development of informatics tools that will facilitate the integration and analysis of data from end-of-life studies.<br>Increase efforts to expand end-of-life research. |

Source: NINR (2006).

health teams and changes in practice models to promote autonomy, empowerment and professional development are particularly important issues facing nursing administrators (Domino, 2005; Formella & Rovin, 2004; Rovin & Formella, 2004).

In nursing administration, collaboration and care coordination will be increasingly important with enhanced efforts to contain the costs associated with managing complex client needs. As a result, there should be some degree of interdisciplinary competence in all health professions. This will necessitate corresponding changes in leadership and management priorities that promote unity and collaboration (Rovin & Formella, 2004; Roy, 2000). As a result, nursing administrators have identified a number of competencies needed by future nurse managers. These include leadership skills, financial/budgeting knowledge, business acumen, communication skills, human resource and labor relations skills, as well as collaboration and team building skills (Scoble & Russell, 2003).

Nursing administrators must be able to identify institutional strengths and weaknesses and to assess human resources and environmental issues. Nursing administrators should also focus on maximizing human potential and accountability and work to encourage growth and development of employees. There is a need to use proven motivational techniques to encourage both staff and clients. The challenge is to integrate services in an efficient and effective way to improve care outcomes, while managing costs and meeting satisfaction needs (Domino, 2005; Scoble & Russell, 2003).

### Theoretical Implications for Nursing Administration and Management

For the future, models of care delivery must be developed that will achieve desired client outcomes and contribute to staff satisfaction, retention, and productivity. Furthermore, these models must contribute to the financial integrity of the organization for which they are developed, because there is a need to make the system efficient while ensuring quality care. Data management and processing of information are essential in every area, and administrators must be able to quantify changes in client acuity and to provide exact information about clients.

Models of care should provide greater integration of health services, more intense management of services, an increase in outcome-oriented management, and an increase in ambulatory and community-based health care. There will also be an increased emphasis on bioinformatics and communication skills, and health care financing will continue to be of paramount importance. Concepts to be developed and examined in nursing administration and management include cost, value, competency, utilization, quality measurement, productivity, innovation, integration, and outcomes (Porter-O'Grady & Malloch, 2003; Rutherford, 2008). Quinless and Elliot (2000) recommended that nursing students and administrators learn to apply basic economic theories and concepts and be aware of the costs involved in providing complex health care for the growing population. They also suggested that nurses understand how to balance care and cost and design cost-effective health care delivery. Finally, all nurses should constantly consider the ethical considerations that underlie health services.

## FUTURE ISSUES AND NURSING EDUCATION

In the past, nursing education supported passive learning, using structured, professional instruction and supervised practice. Nursing students have been socialized using mechanistic, rigid standards, where faculty demand that they meet the minimum standards of objective-based learning. To survive in the highly complex, challenging, and rapidly changing health care system, however, it will be increasingly important for nurses to use and apply creative and critical thinking skills. Nursing leaders have recognized that significant changes are needed in nursing education to promote these skills. Further, issues such as the shortage of nursing faculty, coupled with a serious shortage of nurses educated to teach nursing; the growing acceptance of virtual education and simulation; the increase in nontraditional students; and the explosion of accelerated programs have challenged previous nursing education models and traditions (Kelly, 2002; Speziale & Jacobson, 2005).

In recent years, there have been calls for nurse educators to review old assumptions and methods for educating nurses. Because nurses must be able to think critically and independently, content and learning experiences must be revamped to produce graduates with the competencies needed for current and future practice. A recent nationwide study for nursing education programs (Speziale & Jacobson, 2005) identified several content areas that will need enhanced emphasis now and in the future. These include diversity, informatics, and EBP. Furthermore, nursing educators expect to place greater emphasis in use of distance learning and Internet course simulations, case studies, active learning strategies, concept mapping, computer-assisted instruction, and virtual reality simulations in nursing programs in the future. Other teaching strategies or modalities that will be used increasingly in the future include listservs, problem-based learning, simulation, e-learning, mentoring, and video-conferencing.

To support these changes, nursing educators need to teach thinking skills as well as content. They should use active learning strategies to foster student responsibility for learning. They might restructure clinical experiences and change content to place less emphasis on hospital experiences and narrow medical specialty areas to de-emphasize illness care and emphasize wellness care. In addition, nursing students must learn to evaluate the effectiveness of nursing interventions.

Tanner (2007) outlined other curricular changes for the future that include increased emphasis on the process and procedure of learning. She encouraged the use of group work to promote communication and social skills, and increased use of projects that require months to complete to enhance understanding of the complexity of the real world. She also advocated incorporating alternative perspectives, such as providing greater diversity in clinical experiences, to broaden understanding. Box 21-4

---

**BOX 21-4** *Skill Categories for Future Nursing Curricula*

- *Effective, accurate communication skills:* Programs should focus on efficient, accurate, and useful oral and written communication skills.
- *Internal locus of control:* Programs should encourage students to recognize that behavior and abilities can influence outcomes and assist in decision making; this will enable professionals to cope with changing situations and resources.
- *Legislative policy awareness:* Nurses should be knowledgeable about public policy issues that affect client care delivery and the nurse's role; they must be advocates for their own and their clients' rights.
- *Leadership/influence skills:* Nurses must take a proactive leadership role in influencing how care is delivered and in improving client care goals.
- *Crisis management strategies:* Crisis management strategies must be learned and practiced; this will allow nurses to deal effectively with changing priorities and policies.
- *Effective organizational skills and time management strategies:* Increased workloads and shrinking resources make it critical for nurses to learn how to manage their time and resources well.

Source: Bowen, Lyons and Young (2000).

presents the types of skills that should be promoted through nursing curricula to meet current and future health care needs.

### Theoretical Implications for Nursing Education

Rather than teach traditional specialties (e.g., maternity nursing, pediatrics, psychiatric nursing), nursing educational programs in the future should stress essential concepts, theories, and models. These should include issues such as aging and care of elders, aspects of pharmacology, human growth and development, vulnerable populations, genetics, complementary and alternative therapies, environmental health issues, health policy, palliative care, and culture. Models should incorporate high-tech care, EBP, patient safety, and palliative care. Pathophysiology of chronic illnesses, health promotion, disease prevention and self-care, community health care, decision making, change processes, and management and leadership models should also be taught (AACN, 2008; Tanner, 2007).

Curricula should shift from being primarily content driven and controlled by the faculty to being outcome driven and focused on the needs of the learner, the profession, and the public. A diversity of theoretical and practice experiences should be encouraged, and experiences should include involvement in discharge planning, caring for clients in outpatient and ambulatory care settings, assisting families in well-baby clinic visits, and assisting individuals in gaining access to community resources. Further, interdisciplinary learning and collaborative practice experiences are essential.

Content for nursing education in the future should include leadership development, critical-thinking and problem-solving skills, EBP, clinical competency in a variety of settings, collaboration and communication, outcomes focus, cultural competence, and appreciation of research directed toward practice and educational evaluation. Other concepts to be stressed in nursing education programs are safety, teaching and learning, health promotion, illness prevention, lifelong learning, and professional development.

Experiential knowledge and active participation in learning can lead to the development of a knowledge base and a better ability to think critically and independently. Contemporary educational systems must provide opportunities for students to practice and use critical and creative processes within their basic nursing education. Programs should emphasize group and resource management, organizational and leadership skills, clinical management and coordination, technological capabilities, and professional judgment (Bellack & O'Neil, 2000).

## Summary

Increasingly, nurses will be coordinators of teams of care, where they will manage multiskilled workers and share accountability for clinical and financial outcomes. They will need to become adept at care coordination, delegation, interdisciplinary collaboration, setting of standards, and monitoring of outcomes across the continuum of care. For the future, it is important that the discipline continue to develop the broad knowledge base of nursing and work to understand the integration of theory, research, and practice. Additionally, the discipline should recognize how this reciprocal arrangement affects nursing practice, administration and management, and education.

Rebecca, the nurse in the opening case study, recognized some of the changes described in this chapter (e.g., increasing cultural diversity, the need to focus on health promotion, communication challenges) and wanted to address them in her practice and research. She also understood that to respond to these changes, she had much to learn about issues in nursing practice, research, administration and management, and education, particularly related to theory and development of nursing science.

Nurses are committed to a holistic view of the person, and as the health profession with the largest number of providers, nursing has the potential to have the greatest impact on health and health care delivery. But to prepare for the future, nurses must more clearly identify and communicate what they do. Ongoing development, application, analysis, and evaluation of concepts, principles, theories, and models are vital to this process; nurses must be encouraged to continue these activities to develop the discipline.

## LEARNING ACTIVITIES

1. Talk to a nurse administrator, a nurse educator, a nurse researcher, and an advanced practice nurse (nurse practitioner or clinical nurse specialist) about future issues in nursing and health care delivery. What changes do they anticipate in the next few years? How should currently practicing nurses prepare for future changes?

2. Select a nursing journal that deals primarily with education, research, or administration (e.g., *Journal of Nursing Education, Nursing Research, Journal of Nursing Administration*), and review issues from the past 3 years to analyze trends. What are the "hot topics"? Can any predictions be made for future issues?

3. Select a nursing journal that primarily discusses scholarly issues or topics related to nursing science (e.g., *Advances in Nursing Science, Image: Journal of Nursing Scholarship*) and review issues from the past 3 years to analyze trends. What are the "hot topics"? Can any predictions be made for future issues?

4. Select a nursing specialty journal (e.g., *MCN The American Journal of Maternal Child Nursing, Pediatric Nursing, Journal of Community Health Nursing*) that is primarily concerned with practice and review issues from the past 3 years to analyze trends. What are the "hot topics"? Can any predictions be made for future issues.

5. Join a listserv related to an advanced nursing role (e.g., education, administration, advanced practice) to examine current issues and to communicate with members about future issues.

## REFERENCES

American Association of Colleges of Nursing (AACN). (1996). *The essentials of master's education for advance practice nursing.* Washington, DC: Author.

American Association of Colleges of Nursing (AACN). (2008). *The essentials of baccalaureate education for professional nursing practice.* Washington, DC: Author.

Barrett, E. A. M. (2002). What is nursing science? *Nursing Science Quarterly, 15*(1), 51–60.

Bellack, J. P., & O'Neil, E. H. (2000). Recreating nursing practice for a new century: Recommendations and implications of the Pew Health Professions Commissions Final Report. *Nursing and Health Care Perspectives, 21*(1), 14–21.

Berry, T. A., & Hern, M. J. (2004). Genetic practice, education and research: An overview of advanced practice nurses. *Clinical Nurse Specialist, 18*(3), 126–136.

Bowen, M., Lyons, K. J., & Young, B. E. (2000). Nursing and health care reform: Implications for curriculum development. *Journal of Nursing Education, 39*(1), 27–33.

Chinn, P. L., & Kramer, M. K. (2008). *Theory and nursing: Integrated knowledge development* (7th ed.). St. Louis: Mosby.

Domino, E. (2005). Nurses are what nurses do—Are you where you want to be? *Association of periOperative Registered Nurses Journal, 81*(1), 187–201.

Fitzpatrick, J. J. (2008). Foreword. In M. J. Smith & P. R. Liehr (Eds.), *Middle range theory for nursing* (2nd ed., pp. xv–xvi). New York: Springer.

Formella, N., & Rovin, S. (2004). Creating a desirable future for nursing, Part 2: The issues. *Journal of Nursing Administration, 34*(6), 264–267.

Foss, C., & Ellefsen, B. (2002). The value of combining qualitative and quantitative approaches in nursing research by means of method triangulation. *Journal of Advanced Nursing, 40*(2), 242–248.

Hinshaw, A. S. (2000). Nursing knowledge for the 21st century: Opportunities and challenges. Image: *Journal of Nursing Scholarship, 32*(2), 117–123.

Hudson, K., Duke, G., Haas, B., & Varnell, G. (2008). Navigating the evidence-based practice maze. *Journal of Nursing Management, 16*(6), 409–416.

Im, E. O. (2005). Development of situation-specific theories: An integrative approach. *Advances in Nursing Science, 28*(2), 137–151.

Johnston, N., Rogers, M., Cross, N., & Sochan, A. (2005). Teaching as if the future matters. *Nursing Education Perspectives, 26*(3), 152–158.

Kelly, C. M. (2002). Investing in the future of nursing education: A cry for action. *Nursing Education Perspectives, 23*(1), 24–29.

Kikuchi, J. R. (2003). Nursing knowledge and the problem of worldviews. *Research and Theory for Nursing Practice: An International Journal, 17*(10), 7–17.

Kim, H. S. (2006). Introduction. In H. S. Kim & I. Kollak (Eds.), *Nursing theories: Conceptual and philosophical foundations* (2nd ed.). New York: Springer Publishing.

Long, K. A. (2004). Preparing nurses for the 21st century: Reenvisioning nursing education and practice. *Journal of Professional Nursing, 20*(2), 82–88.

Manojlovich, M., Barnsteiner, J., Bolton, L. B., Disch, J., & Saint, S. (2008). Nursing practice and work environment issues in the 21st century. *Nursing Research, 57*(1S), S11–S14.

McEwen, M. (2000). Teaching theory at the master's level: Report of a national survey of theory instructors. *Journal of Professional Nursing, 16*(6), 354–361.

Meleis, A. I. (2007). Theoretical nursing: *Development and progress* (4th ed.). Philadelphia: Lippincott Williams & Wilkins.

National Institute of Nursing Research (NINR). (2006). *NINR strategic plan: Changing practice, changing lives.* http://www.ninr.nih.gov/NR/rdonlyres/9021E5EB-B2BA-47EA-B5DB-1E4DB11B1289/

4894/NINR_StrategicPlanWebsite.pdf. Retrieved April 25, 2009.

National Institute of Nursing Research (NINR). (2009). 2008 *Areas of research opportunity.* http://www.ninr.nih.gov/NR/rdonlyres/5AC1595B-08BF-4A6C-A08B-3B2B2FF82829/4750/ExecutiveSummary.pdf. Retrieved April 2, 2009.

Parker, P. J. (2005). One nurse informatics specialties views the future: Technology in the crystal ball. *Nursing Administration Quarterly, 29*(2), 123–124.

Porter-O'Grady, T. (2001). Profound change: 21st century nursing. *Nursing Outlook, 49*(4), 182–186.

Porter-O'Grady, T., & Malloch, K. (2003). *Quantum leadership: A textbook of new leadership.* Sudbury, MA: Jones & Bartlett.

Quinless, F. W., & Elliot, N. L. (2000). The future in health care delivery: Lessons from history, demographics and economics. *Nursing and Health Care Perspectives, 21*(2), 84–89.

Rovin, S., & Formella, N. (2004). Creating a desirable future for nursing, Part 1: The nursing shortage is a lack of creative and systematic thinking. *Journal of Nursing Administration, 34*(4), 163–166.

Roy, C. (2000). A theorist envisions the future and speaks to nursing administrators. *Nursing Administration Quarterly, 24*(2), 1–12.

Rutherford, M. M. (2008). The how, what and why of valuation and nursing. *Nursing Economics, 26*(6), 347–352.

Scoble, K. B., & Russell, G. (2003). Vision 2020: Profile of the future nurse leader (part I). *Journal of Nursing Administration, 33*(6), 324–330.

Simpson, R. L. (2004). Evidence-based nursing offers certainty in the uncertain world of health care. *Nursing Management, 35*(10), 10–12.

Smith, M. C., & Liehr, P. R. (2008). Preface. In M. J. Smith & P. R. Liehr (Eds.), *Middle range theory for nursing* (2nd ed., pp. xvii–xx). New York: Springer.

Speziale, H. J. S., & Jacobson, L. (2005). Trends in registered nurse education programs 1998–2008. *Nursing Education Perspectives, 26*(4), 230–235.

Tanner, C. A. (2007). The curriculum revolution revisited. *Journal of Nursing Education, 46*(2), 51–52.

Utley-Smith, Q. (2004). Five competencies needed by new baccalaureate graduates. *Nursing Education Perspectives, 25*(4), 166–170.

Whall, A. L., & Hicks, F. D. (2002). The unrecognized paradigm shift in nursing: Implications, problems and possibilities. *Nursing Outlook, 50*(2), 72–76.

Page numbers followed by b indicate box; those followed by f indicate figure; those followed by t indicate table.